2nd EDITION

NETTER'S

SURGICAL ANATOMY
AND APPROACHES

Conor P. Delaney,
MD, MCh, PhD, FACS, FRCSI, FASCRS, FRCSI (Hon)

Chairman
Digestive Disease and Surgery Institute
Cleveland Clinic
Victor W. Fazio Endowed Professor of Colorectal Surgery
Cleveland Clinic Lerner College of Medicine
Cleveland, Ohio

Illustrations by
Frank H. Netter, MD

Contributing Illustrators
Carlos A. G. Machado, MD
Kristen Wienandt Marzejon, MS, MFA
James A. Perkins, MS, MFA
John A. Craig, MD
Paul Kim, MS
Sara M. Jarret, MFA

ELSEVIER

Elsevier
1600 John F. Kennedy Blvd.
Ste 1800
Philadelphia, PA 19103-2899

NETTER'S SURGICAL ANATOMY AND APPROACHES, SECOND EDITION   ISBN: 978-0-323-67346-4

Previous edition copyrighted 2014.

Library of Congress Control Number: 2020939762

Publisher: Elyse O'Grady
Senior Content Development Specialist: Marybeth Thiel
Publishing Services Manager: Catherine Jackson
Senior Project Manager: Daniel Fitzgerald
Designer: Patrick Ferguson

Printed in China.

Last digit is the print number: 9   8   7   6   5   4   3

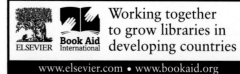

For my colleagues who have contributed to this book.

And their inspiring excellence, attention to detail, and care for optimizing

The standard of patient care

About the Artists

Frank H. Netter, MD

Frank H. Netter was born in 1906 in New York City. He studied art at the Art Students' League and the National Academy of Design before entering medical school at New York University, where he received his MD degree in 1931. During his student years, Dr. Netter's notebook sketches attracted the attention of the medical faculty and other physicians, allowing him to augment his income by illustrating articles and textbooks. He continued illustrating as a sideline after establishing a surgical practice in 1933, but he ultimately opted to give up his practice in favor of a full-time commitment to art. After service in the United States Army during World War II, Dr. Netter began his long collaboration with the CIBA Pharmaceutical Company (now Novartis Pharmaceuticals). This 45-year partnership resulted in the production of the extraordinary collection of medical art so familiar to medical professionals worldwide.

In 2005, Elsevier, Inc. purchased the Netter Collection and all publications from Icon Learning Systems. Over 50 publications featuring the art of Dr. Netter are available through Elsevier, Inc. (in the United States: https://www.us.elsevierhealth.com/ and outside the United States: www.elsevierhealth.com)

Dr. Netter's works are among the finest examples of the use of illustration in the teaching of medical concepts. The 13-book *Netter Collection of Medical Illustrations*, which includes the greater part of the more than 20,000 paintings created by Dr. Netter, became and remains one of the most famous medical works ever published. *The Netter Atlas of Human Anatomy*, first published in 1989, presents the anatomical paintings from the Netter Collection. Now translated into 16 languages, it is the anatomy atlas of choice among medical and health professions students the world over.

The Netter illustrations are appreciated not only for their aesthetic qualities, but, more important, for their intellectual content. As Dr. Netter wrote in 1949, "... clarification of a subject is the aim and goal of illustration. No matter how beautifully painted, how delicately and subtly rendered a subject may be, it is of little value as a *medical illustration* if it does not serve to make clear some medical point." Dr. Netter's planning, conception, point of view, and approach are what inform his paintings and make them so intellectually valuable.

Frank H. Netter, MD, physician and artist, died in 1991.

Learn more about the physician-artist whose work has inspired the Netter Reference collection: https://netterimages.com/artist-frank-h-netter.html.

Carlos Machado, MD

Carlos Machado was chosen by Novartis to be Dr. Netter's successor. He continues to be the main artist contributing to the Netter collection of medical illustrations.

Self-taught in medical illustration, cardiologist Carlos Machado has meticulously updated some of Dr. Netter's original plates and has created many original paintings of his own in the style of Netter as an extension of the Netter collection. Dr. Machado's photorealistic expertise and keen insight into the physician–patient relationship informs his vivid and unforgettable visual style. His dedication to researching each topic and subject he paints places him among the premier medical illustrators at work today.

Learn more about his background and see more of his art at: https://netterimages.com/artist-carlos-a-g-machado.html.

Preface

The *Atlas of Human Anatomy* by Frank H. Netter, MD, has been the pinnacle of demonstrating the anatomy of the human body for generations of students. To those who would wish to perform or understand surgical procedures, however, there has been no direct link between the beautiful images created by Dr. Netter and the surgical procedures being performed. In *Netter's Surgical Anatomy and Approaches*, we try to address a request by many *Netter* users to tie these anatomical diagrams to the procedures they perform, while advancing the book from the description and images used in the first edition.

This book portrays the curriculum of basic and common general surgical procedures in chapters that describe the relevant anatomy for each procedure. In his very first edition, Dr. Netter stated that "anatomy of course does not change, but our understanding of anatomy and its clinical significance does." Consequently, in some cases we have been able to pair the anatomy demonstrated in his illustrations with a modern intraoperative photograph or radiographic image, particularly focusing on the new approaches required for minimally invasive surgery. For many chapters, new *Netter*-style illustrations have been created to demonstrate key anatomical points for an operative procedure or to show a key surgical perspective or orientation that is not captured in the original *Netter* images. The result is a volume that covers the most important and common areas in surgery, as well as exploring complex areas such as transplantation and advanced cancer surgery.

A book like this would not be possible without the help of many people. Being fortunate to work at an institution like the Cleveland Clinic, I elected to enlist the support of my colleagues from many different surgical specialties. It is only with the guidance and assistance of the editorial team of Michael S. Benninger, MD, Tony R. Capizzani, MD, FACS, Tommaso Falcone, MD, FRCSC, FACOG, Stephen R. Grobmyer, MD, Jihad Kaouk, MD, Matthew Kroh, MD, Sean P. Lyden, MD, John H. Rodriguez, MD, FACS, Michael J. Rosen, MD, Christopher T. Siegel, MD, PhD, Allan Siperstein, MD, Scott R. Steele, MD, MBA, R. Matthew Walsh, MD, and the direction and guidance of the ever-patient Dan Fitzgerald and Marybeth Thiel at Elsevier that this project has been completed.

On behalf of my co-editors and myself, we hope you enjoy this second edition of *Netter's Surgical Anatomy and Approaches*.

Conor P. Delaney, MD, MCh, PhD, FACS, FRCSI, FASCRS, FRCSI (Hon)

Contributors

EDITOR

Conor P. Delaney, MD, MCh, PhD, FACS, FRCSI, FASCRS, FRCSI (Hon)
Chairman
Digestive Disease and Surgery Institute
Cleveland Clinic
Victor W. Fazio Endowed Professor of
Colorectal Surgery
Cleveland Clinic Lerner College of Medicine
Cleveland, Ohio

SECTION EDITORS

Michael S. Benninger, MD
Chairman
Head and Neck Institute
Cleveland Clinic
Professor of Surgery
Lerner College of Medicine of CWRU
Cleveland, Ohio
The Neck

Tony R. Capizzani, MD, FACS
Assistant Professor
General Surgery
Digestive Disease and Surgery Institute
Cleveland Clinic
Cleveland, Ohio
Vascular Access, Emergency and Trauma Procedures

Tommaso Falcone, MD, FRCSC, FACOG
Chief of Staff, Chief Academic Officer,
Medical Director
Cleveland Clinic London
Professor of Obstetrics, Gynecology and
Reproductive Biology
Cleveland Clinic Lerner College of Medicine
Cleveland, Ohio
Urology and Gynecology

Stephen R. Grobmyer, MD
Chairman
Oncology Institute
Cleveland Clinic Abu Dhabi
Abu Dhabi, United Arab Emirates
Breast and Oncology

Jihad Kaouk, MD
Director
Center for Robotics and Minimally Invasive
Surgery
Glickman Urological & Kidney Institute
Cleveland Clinic
Cleveland, Ohio
Urology and Gynecology

Matthew Kroh, MD
Chairman
Digestive Disease Institute
Cleveland Clinic Abu Dhabi
Abu Dhabi, United Arab Emirates
Upper Gastrointestinal

Sean P. Lyden, MD
Professor and Chairman
Vascular Surgery
Cleveland Clinic
Cleveland, Ohio
Vascular

John H. Rodriguez, MD, FACS
Director of Surgical Endoscopy
Advanced Laparoscopic and Bariatric Surgery
Digestive Disease and Surgery Institute
Cleveland Clinic
Cleveland, Ohio
Upper Gastrointestinal

Michael J. Rosen, MD
Professor of Surgery
Lerner College of Medicine
Cleveland Clinic
Cleveland, Ohio
Hernia

Christopher T. Siegel, MD, PhD
Associate Professor of Surgery
Digestive Disease and Surgery Institute
Cleveland Clinic Lerner College of Medicine
Cleveland Clinic
Cleveland, Ohio
Hepatobiliary
Organ Transplantation

Allan Siperstein, MD
Professor and Chair
Endocrine Surgery Department
Cleveland Clinic
Cleveland, Ohio
Endocrine

Scott R. Steele, MD, MBA
Chairman
Department of Colorectal Surgery
Rupert B. Turnbull, M.D. Endowed Chair in
Colorectal Surgery
Digestive Disease and Surgery Institute
Cleveland Clinic
Cleveland, Ohio
Lower Gastrointestinal

R. Matthew Walsh, MD
Professor and Chairman
General Surgery
Digestive Disease and Surgery Institute
Cleveland Clinic
Cleveland, Ohio
Hepatobiliary

CONTRIBUTORS

Robert Abouassaly, MD
Associate Professor
Glickman Urological & Kidney Institute
Cleveland Clinic
Louis Stokes Cleveland VA Medical Center
Cleveland, Ohio
Radical Prostatectomy

Kareem Abu-Elmagd, MD, PhD, FACS
Director
Center for Gut Rehabilitation &
Transplantation (CGRT)
Digestive Disease and Surgery Institute
Cleveland Clinic
Cleveland, Ohio
Intestinal and Multivisceral Transplantation

Usman Ahmad, MD, FACS
Assistant Professor of Surgery
Staff Surgeon
Thoracic Surgery
Cleveland Clinic
Cleveland, Ohio
Esophagectomy

Abdul Q. Alarhayem, MD
Clinical Fellow
Vascular Surgery
Cleveland Clinic
Cleveland, Ohio
*Radiocephalic, Brachiocephalic, and Brachiobasilic
Fistula*

Michael Antiporda, MD
Fellow
Advanced Gastrointestinal and Minimally
Invasive Surgery
Providence Portland Medical Center
Portland, Oregon
Gastrectomy

Sofya H. Asfaw, MD, FACS
Assistant Professor of Surgery
Department of General Surgery
Digestive Disease and Surgery Institute
Cleveland Clinic
Cleveland, Ohio
Chest Tube Placement

Federico Aucejo, MD
Associate Professor of Surgery
Transplantation Center
Digestive Disease and Surgery Institute
Cleveland Clinic
Cleveland, Ohio
Hepatectomy
Living Donor Liver Transplantation

Toms Augustin, MD, MPH, FACS
Assistant Professor
Department of General Surgery
Digestive Disease and Surgery Institute
Cleveland Clinic
Cleveland, Ohio
Distal Pancreatectomy

Jocelyn M. Beach, MD
Assistant Professor of Surgery
Section of Vascular Surgery
Dartmouth-Hitchcock Medical Center
Lebanon, New Hampshire
*Carotid Subclavian Bypass/Transposition and
Vertebral Transposition*

Cassandre Benay, MD
General Surgery
Hopital de LaSalle
Montreal, Quebec, Canada
Thyroidectomy and Parathyroidectomy

Eren Berber, MD
Staff Surgeon
Endocrine and General Surgery
Cleveland Clinic
Cleveland, Ohio
Hepatectomy

Riccardo Bertolo, MD
Urologist
Glickman Urological & Kidney Institute
Cleveland Clinic
Cleveland, Ohio
Laparoscopic Transperitoneal Radical Nephrectomy
Radical Prostatectomy
Radical Cystectomy

Vladimir Bolshinsky, MBBS, DipSurgAnat, FRACS
Clinical Associate
Colorectal Surgery
Digestive Disease and Surgery Institute
Cleveland Clinic
Cleveland, Ohio
Low Anterior Resection With Total Mesorectal Excision and Anastomosis

Paul C. Bryson, MD
Associate Professor of Otolaryngology—Head and Neck Surgery
Laryngology Section Head
Department of Otolaryngology
Cleveland Clinic Lerner College of Medicine
Cleveland, Ohio
Tracheostomy

Tony R. Capizzani, MD, FACS
Assistant Professor
General Surgery
Digestive Disease and Surgery Institute
Cleveland Clinic
Cleveland, Ohio
Tracheal Intubation and Endoscopic Anatomy
Central Line Anatomy

Francis J. Caputo, MD
Associate Professor and Program Director
Department of Vascular Surgery
Cleveland Clinic
Cleveland, Ohio
Aortic Aneurysm Repair and Thoracoabdominal Aneurysm Repair
Femoral Tibial Bypass

Walter S. Cha, MD
Staff Surgeon
Department of General Surgery
Digestive Disease and Surgery Institute
Cleveland Clinic
Cleveland, Ohio
Common Bile Duct Surgery and Choledochoduodenostomy

Bradley J. Champagne, MD
Professor of Surgery
Colorectal Surgery
Digestive Disease and Surgery Institute
Cleveland Clinic
Chair of Surgery
Fairview Hospital—Cleveland Clinic
Cleveland, Ohio
Right Colectomy

Julietta Chang, MD
Bariatric Surgeon
Department of Surgery
Marian Regional Medical Center
Santa Maria, California
Surgical Management of Achalasia

James M. Church, MB, ChB, MMedSci, FRACS
Staff Surgeon
Colorectal Surgery
Digestive Disease and Surgery Institute
Cleveland Clinic
Cleveland, Ohio
Perianal Abscess and Fistula in Ano

Giuseppe D'Amico, MD
Staff Surgeon
Hepato-Pancreato-Biliary/Liver and Intestinal Transplantation Surgery
General Surgery
Digestive Disease and Surgery Institute
Cleveland Clinic
Cleveland, Ohio
Liver Transplantation

Gerardo Davalos, MD
Research Scholar
Surgery
Duke University
Durham, North Carolina
Truncal and Selective Vagotomy

Robert DeBernardo, MD
Section Head Gynecologic Oncology
Laura J Fogarty Endowed Chair for Uterine Cancer Research
Director of the Peritoneal Surface Malignancy Program
Associate Professor of Surgery Lerner College of Medicine
Woman's Health Institute
Cleveland Clinic
Cleveland, Ohio
Oophorectomy for Benign and Malignant Conditions

Conor P. Delaney, MD, MCh, PhD, FACS, FRCSI, FASCRS, FRCSI (Hon)
Chairman
Digestive Disease and Surgery Institute
Cleveland Clinic
Victor W. Fazio Endowed Professor of
Colorectal Surgery
Cleveland Clinic Lerner College of Medicine
Cleveland, Ohio
*Low Anterior Resection With Total Mesorectal
Excision and Anastomosis*

Teresa Diago-Uso, MD
Assistant Professor of Surgery
Transplantation Center
Digestive Disease and Surgery Institute
Cleveland Clinic
Cleveland, Ohio
*Living Donor Liver Transplantation
Deceased Donor Organ Recovery*

Risal Djohan, MD
Vice Chairman
Plastic Surgery
Cleveland Clinic
Cleveland, Ohio
Breast Reconstruction

Nathan Droz, MD
Vascular Surgery Fellow
Vascular Surgery
Cleveland Clinic
Cleveland, Ohio
Visceral Bypass

Bijan Eghtesad, MD
Staff Surgeon
Hepato-Pancreato-Biliary/Liver
Transplantation Surgery
Digestive Disease and Surgery Institute
Cleveland Clinic
Cleveland, Ohio
*Liver Transplantation
Deceased Donor Organ Recovery*

Kevin El-Hayek, MD, FACS
Section Head
Endoscopic Surgery
Division of General Surgery
Section Head
Hepato-Pancreato-Biliary Surgery
Division of Surgical Oncology
Metro Health System
Assistant Professor of Surgery
Case Western Reserve University
Cleveland, Ohio
*Gastric Emptying Procedures
Pancreatoduodenectomy*

Aldo Fafaj, MD
General Surgery
Digestive Disease and Surgery
Cleveland Clinic
Cleveland, Ohio
Laparoscopic Inguinal Hernia Repair

Behzad S. Farivar, MD
Assistant Professor of Surgery
Department of Vascular Surgery
Cleveland Clinic
Cleveland, Ohio
*Carotid Subclavian Bypass/Transposition and
Vertebral Transposition*

Jeffrey M. Farma, MD
Professor
Surgical Oncology
Fox Chase Cancer Center
Philadelphia, Pennsylvania
Inguinal and Pelvic Lymphadenectomy

Alisan Fathalizadeh, MD, MPH
Associate Staff Surgeon
Department of General Surgery
Digestive Disease and Surgery Institute
Cleveland Clinic
Cleveland, Ohio
Gastric Emptying Procedures

Molly Flannagan, MD, FACS
Assistant Professor of Surgery
Digestive Disease and Surgery Institute
Cleveland Clinic
Cleveland, Ohio
Emergency Thoracotomy for Trauma

Masato Fujiki, MD
Assistant Professor of Surgery, Transplantation
Center
Digestive Disease and Surgery Institute
Cleveland Clinic
Cleveland, Ohio
*Living Donor Liver Transplantation
Intestinal and Multivisceral Transplantation*

Juan Garisto, MD
Urologist
Glickman Urological & Kidney Institute
Cleveland Clinic
Cleveland, Ohio
Radical Cystectomy

Keith Glover, MD
Resident
Vascular Surgery
Cleveland Clinic
Cleveland, Ohio
*Femoral Endarterectomy and Femoral Popliteal
Bypass*

David A. Goldfarb, MD
Professor of Surgery, CCLCM
Glickman Urological & Kidney Institute
Cleveland Clinic
Cleveland, Ohio
Kidney Transplantation

Emre Gorgun, MD
Director
Endoluminal Surgery Center
Department of Colorectal Surgery
Digestive Disease and Surgery Institute
Cleveland Clinic
Cleveland, Ohio
Ileal Pouch Anal Anastomosis

Stephen R. Grobmyer, MD
Chairman
Oncology Institute
Cleveland Clinic Abu Dhabi
Abu Dhabi, United Arab Emirates
Mastectomy: Partial and Total

Morgan Gruner, MD
OB-GYN Resident Physician
Department of Subspecialty Care for Women's
Health
Cleveland Clinic
Cleveland, Ohio
Oophorectomy for Benign and Malignant Conditions

Alfredo D. Guerron, MD
Assistant Professor of Surgery
General Surgery
Duke University Health System
Durham, North Carolina
Truncal and Selective Vagotomy

Georges-Pascal Haber, MD, PhD
Chairman
Department of Urology
Glickman Urological & Kidney Institute
Cleveland Clinic
Cleveland, Ohio
Retroperitoneal Lymph Node Dissection

David M. Hardy, MD, RPVI, FACS
Assistant Professor
Vascular Surgery
Cleveland Clinic
Cleveland, Ohio
Carotid Endarterectomy
Above-Knee and Below-Knee Amputation

Koji Hashimoto, MD, PhD
Director
Living Donor Liver Transplantation
Associate Professor of Surgery
Transplantation Center
Digestive Disease and Surgery Institute
Cleveland Clinic
Cleveland, Ohio
Living Donor Liver Transplantation

Barbara J. Hocevar, MSN, RN, CWOCN
Assistant Director, WOC Nursing Education
R. B. Turnbull, Jr. MD, School of WOC Nursing
Education
Digestive Disease and Surgery Institute
Cleveland Clinic
Cleveland, Ohio
Abdominal Wall Marking and Stoma Site Selection

Kristen Holler, DO
Critical Care Fellow
Anesthesiology Institute
Cleveland Clinic
Cleveland, Ohio
Tracheal Intubation and Endoscopic Anatomy

Stefan D. Holubar, MD, MS
Director of Research
Colorectal Surgery
Digestive Disease and Surgery Institute
Cleveland Clinic
Cleveland, Ohio
Abdominoperineal Resection

Farah A. Husain, MD
Division Chief
Bariatric Services
Associate Professor
Department of Surgery
Oregon Health & Science University
Portland, Oregon
Roux-en-Y Gastric Bypass and Sleeve Gastrectomy

Daniel J. Kagedan, MD, MSc, FRCSC
Surgical Oncology Fellow
Department of Surgical Oncology
Roswell Park Comprehensive Cancer Center
Buffalo, New York
Retroperitoneal Sarcoma

Matthew F. Kalady, MD
Professor of Surgery
Colorectal Surgery
Vice-Chairman
Colorectal Surgery
Cleveland Clinic
Director
Sanford R. Weiss, MD Center for Hereditary
Colorectal Neoplasia
Co-Director
Comprehensive Colorectal Cancer Program
Cleveland, Ohio
Left and Sigmoid Colectomy

Jihad Kaouk, MD
Director
Center for Robotics and Minimally Invasive
Surgery
Glickman Urological & Kidney Institute
Cleveland Clinic
Cleveland, Ohio
Radical Prostatectomy
Radical Cystectomy

Hermann Kessler, MD, PhD
Professor of Surgery
Section Head
Minimally Invasive Surgery
Colorectal Surgery
Digestive Disease and Surgery Institute
Cleveland Clinic
Cleveland, Ohio
Abdominoperineal Resection

Leena Khaitan, MD, MPH
Professor of Surgery
Department of Surgery
Director
Metabolic and Bariatric Surgery
Center Digestive Health Institute
Director
Esophageal and Swallowing Center
Digestive Health Institute
University Hospitals
Cleveland Medical Center
Cleveland, Ohio
Minimally Invasive Antireflux Surgery

Amit Khithani, MD, DABS
Faculty Surgeon
Surgical Oncology and Hepatopancreatobiliary
Surgery
Department of Surgery
Kendall Regional Medical Center
Miami, Florida
Pancreatoduodenectomy

Lee Kirksey, MD, MBA
Vice Chairman
Vascular Surgery
Cleveland Clinic
Cleveland, Ohio
Radiocephalic, Brachiocephalic, and Brachiobasilic Fistula

Eric A. Klein, MD
Chairman
Glickman Urological & Kidney Institute
Cleveland Clinic
Cleveland, Ohio
Retroperitoneal Lymph Node Dissection

Venkatesh Krishnamurthi, MD
Director
Kidney/Pancreas Transplant Program
Glickman Urological & Kidney Institute
Transplant Center
Cleveland Clinic
Associate Professor of Surgery
Cleveland Clinic Lerner College of Medicine
Cleveland, Ohio
Pancreas and Kidney Transplantation

Matthew Kroh, MD
Chairman
Digestive Disease Institute
Cleveland Clinic Abu Dhabi
Abu Dhabi, United Arab Emirates
Surgical Management of Achalasia

David M. Krpata, MD
Assistant Professor
Cleveland Clinic Lerner College of Medicine
Department of General Surgery
Digestive Disease and Surgery Institute
Cleveland Clinic
Cleveland, Ohio
Surgical Approach to Chronic Groin Pain Following Inguinal Hernia Repairs

Jamie A. Ku, MD
Staff
Head and Neck Institute
Cleveland Clinic
Cleveland, Ohio
Selective (Supraomohyoid) Neck Dissection, Levels I-III

Choon Hyuck David Kwon, MD, PhD
Professor of Surgery
Transplantation Center
Digestive Disease and Surgery Institute
Cleveland Clinic
Cleveland, Ohio
Hepatectomy
Living Donor Liver Transplantation

David J. Laczynski, MD
Vascular Surgery Resident
Vascular Surgery
Cleveland Clinic
Cleveland, Ohio
Above-Knee and Below-Knee Amputation

Judith Landis-Erdman, BSN, RN, CWOCN
Wound Ostomy Continence Nursing Team
Digestive Disease and Surgery Institute
Cleveland Clinic
Cleveland, Ohio
Abdominal Wall Marking and Stoma Site Selection

Kelsey E. Larson, MD
Assistant Professor of Surgery
General Surgery
University of Kansas
Kansas City, Kansas
Sentinel Lymph Node Biopsy

Pierre Lavertu, MD
Director of Head and Neck Surgery
Department of Otolaryngology—Head and
Neck Surgery
University Hospitals Case Medical Center
Professor
Case Western Reserve University School of
Medicine
Cleveland, Ohio
Selective (Supraomohyoid) Neck Dissection,
Levels I-III

Tripp Leavitt, MD
Resident Physician
Plastic Surgery
Cleveland Clinic
Cleveland, Ohio
Breast Reconstruction

Sungho Lim, MD
Fellow
Department of Vascular Surgery
Cleveland Clinic
Cleveland, Ohio
Aortic Aneurysm Repair and Thoracoabdominal
Aneurysm Repair

Jeremy M. Lipman, MD, MHPE
Program Director
General Surgery Residency
Colorectal Surgery
Digestive Disease and Surgery Institute
Cleveland Clinic
Cleveland, Ohio
Transverse Colectomy

Victoria Lyo, MD, MTM
Assistant Professor of Surgery
Foregut, Metabolic, and General Surgery
Division
University of California Davis
Sacramento, California
Roux-en-Y Gastric Bypass and Sleeve Gastrectomy

Gary N. Mann, MD
Associate Professor
Surgical Oncology
Roswell Park Comprehensive Cancer Center
Buffalo, New York
Retroperitoneal Sarcoma

Jeannine L. Marong, PA-C
Advanced Practice Coordinator of Trauma
Services
Hillcrest Hospital
Mayfield Heights, Ohio
Arterial Line Anatomy

Christopher Mascarenhas, MD, FACS
Assistant Professor
Division of Colon and Rectal Surgery
Columbia University Irving Medical Center
New York, New York
Left and Sigmoid Colectomy

Evan R. McBeath, MD
Otolaryngologist
Wood County Hospital
Bowling Green, Ohio
Selective (Supraomohyoid) Neck Dissection,
Levels I-III

Chad M. Michener, MD
Associate Professor of Surgery
Obstetrics, Gynecology and Women's Health
Institute
Cleveland Clinic Lerner College of Medicine
Vice Chair
Department of Obstetrics and Gynecology,
Main Campus
Obstetrics, Gynecology and Women's Health
Institute
Cleveland Clinic
Cleveland, Ohio
Hysterectomy for Benign and Malignant Conditions

Charles Miller, MD
Enterprise Director of Transplantation
Director
Transplantation Center
Professor of Surgery
Digestive Disease and Surgery Institute
Cleveland Clinic
Cleveland, Ohio
Hepatectomy
Living Donor Liver Transplantation

Eric T. Miller, MD
Transplantation and Urological Surgery
Glickman Urological & Kidney Institute
Cleveland Clinic
Cleveland, Ohio
Kidney Transplantation
Pancreas and Kidney Transplantation
Laparoscopic Donor Nephrectomy

Edwina C. Moore, BMedSci, MBBS, FRACS
Endocrine Surgeon
Cleveland Clinic
Cleveland, Ohio
Laparoscopic Adrenalectomy

Amit Nair, MS, MD, FRCS
Clinical Scholar
Transplantation Center
Digestive Disease and Surgery Institute
Cleveland Clinic
Cleveland, Ohio
Hepatectomy
Living Donor Liver Transplantation

Robert Naples, DO
General Surgery Resident
Department of General Surgery
Digestive Disease and Surgery Institute
Cleveland Clinic
Cleveland, Ohio
Splenectomy

Ahmed Nassar, MD
Transplant Surgery Fellow
Emory University
Atlanta, Georgia
*Common Bile Duct Surgery and
Choledochoduodenostomy*

Eileen A. O'Halloran, MD, MS
Complex General Surgical Oncology Fellow
Surgical Oncology
Fox Chase Cancer Center
Philadelphia, Pennsylvania
Inguinal and Pelvic Lymphadenectomy

Keita Okubo, MD, PhD
Clinical Research Fellow
Transplantation Center
Digestive Disease and Surgery Institute
Cleveland Clinic
Cleveland, Ohio
Hepatectomy
Living Donor Liver Transplantation

F. Ezequiel Parodi, MD
Associate Professor
Division of Vascular Surgery
University of North Carolina School of
Medicine
Durham, North Carolina
Visceral Bypass

Will Perry, MD, BS
Resident
Vascular Surgery
Cleveland Clinic
Cleveland, Ohio
Carotid Endarterectomy

Clayton C. Petro, MD
Assistant Professor of Surgery
Center for Abdominal Core Health
Digestive Disease and Surgery Institute
Cleveland Clinic
Cleveland, Ohio
Open Retromuscular Hernia Repair

Lee Ponsky, MD, FACS
Professor of Urology
Chief, Urologic Oncology
Leo and Charlotte Goldberg Chair of Advanced
Surgical Therapies
Master Clinician of Urologic Oncology Urology
Institute
University Hospitals Cleveland Medical Center
Case Western Reserve University School of
Medicine
Cleveland, Ohio
Laparoscopic Transperitoneal Radical Nephrectomy

Ajita Prabhu, MD
Assistant Professor of Surgery
Lerner College of Medicine
Center for Abdominal Core Health
Digestive Disease and Surgery Institute
Cleveland Clinic
Cleveland, Ohio
Open Flank and Lumbar Hernia Repair

Debra Pratt, MD
Medical Director
Fairview Breast Program
Cleveland Clinic Cancer Center Moll Pavilion
Cleveland, Ohio
Central Duct Excision and Nipple Discharge

Cristiano Quintini, MD
Director
Liver Transplantation
Professor of Surgery
Transplantation Center
Digestive Disease and Surgery Institute
Cleveland Clinic Lerner College of Medicine
Cleveland, Ohio
Hepatectomy
Liver Transplantation
Living Donor Liver Transplantation

Siva Raja, MD, PhD
Associate Professor of Surgery
Staff Surgeon
Thoracic Surgery
Cleveland Clinic
Cleveland, Ohio
Esophagectomy

Kevin M. Reavis, MD
Foregut and Bariatric Surgeon
Gastrointestinal and Minimally Invasive Surgery
The Oregon Clinic
Portland, Oregon
Gastrectomy

Saranya Reghunathan, MD
Department of Otolaryngology
Cleveland Clinic
Cleveland, Ohio
Tracheostomy

Beri M. Ridgeway, MD
Institute Chair
OB/GYN and Women's Health Institute
Cleveland Clinic
Cleveland, Ohio
Reconstructive Surgery for Pelvic Floor Disorders

John H. Rodriguez, MD, FACS
Director of Surgical Endoscopy
Advanced Laparoscopic and Bariatric Surgery
Digestive Disease and Surgery Institute
Cleveland Clinic
Cleveland, Ohio
Surgical Management of Achalasia

David R. Rosen, MD
Colorectal Surgery
Digestive Disease and Surgery Institute
Cleveland Clinic
Cleveland, Ohio
Transverse Colectomy

Steven Rosenblatt, MD
Associate Professor of Surgery
Department of General Surgery
Digestive Disease and Surgery Institute
Cleveland Clinic Lerner College of Medicine
Cleveland Clinic
Cleveland, Ohio
Splenectomy
Laparoscopic Inguinal Hernia Repair

Kazunari Sasaki, MD
Assistant Professor of Surgery
Transplantation Center
Digestive Disease and Surgery Institute
Cleveland Clinic
Cleveland, Ohio
Hepatectomy
Living Donor Liver Transplantation

Graham Schwarz, MD
Program Director
Microsurgery and Breast Reconstruction
Fellowship
Department of Plastic Surgery
Cleveland Clinic
Cleveland, Ohio
Axillary Lymphadenectomy and Lymphaticovenous Bypass

Sherief Shawki, MD, MSc, MBBCH
Staff Surgeon
Colon & Rectal Surgery
Digestive Disease and Surgery Institute
Cleveland Clinic
Assistant Professor of Surgery
Colon & Rectal Surgery
Lerner Medical School of Medicine
Cleveland, Ohio
Suture Rectopexy and Ventral Mesh Rectopexy

Christopher T. Siegel, MD, PhD
Associate Professor of Surgery
Digestive Disease and Surgery Institute
Cleveland Clinic Lerner College of Medicine
Cleveland Clinic
Cleveland, Ohio
Hepatectomy
Living Donor Liver Transplantation

Robert Simon, MD
Associate Staff
Division General and Hepatopancreaticobiliary
Surgery
Digestive Disease and Surgery Institute
Cleveland Clinic
Cleveland, Ohio
Cholecystectomy

Allan Siperstein, MD
Professor and Chair
Endocrine Surgery Department
Cleveland Clinic
Cleveland, Ohio
Thyroidectomy and Parathyroidectomy
Laparoscopic Adrenalectomy

Christopher J. Smolock, MD
Staff Vascular Surgeon
Department of Vascular Surgery
Cleveland Clinic
Cleveland, Ohio
Femoral Endarterectomy and Femoral Popliteal Bypass

Sean P. Steenberge, MD, MS
Resident
Vascular Surgery
Cleveland Clinic
Cleveland, Ohio
Femoral Tibial Bypass

Rachael C. Sullivan, MD, MS
Staff Physician
Digestive Disease and Surgery Institute
Cleveland Clinic
Cleveland, Ohio
Upper and Lower Extremity Fasciotomy

Andrew Tang, MD
Resident
Thoracic and Cardiovascular Surgery
Cleveland Clinic
Cleveland, Ohio
Esophagectomy

Patrick Tassone, MD
Fellow in Head & Neck Oncologic and
Reconstructive Surgery
Head and Neck Institute
Cleveland Clinic
Cleveland, Ohio
Selective (Supraomohyoid) Neck Dissection, Levels I-III

Luciano Tastaldi, MD
Clinical Research Fellow
Center for Abdominal Core Health
Digestive Disease and Surgery Institute
Cleveland Clinic
Cleveland, Ohio
Open Flank and Lumbar Hernia Repair

Lewis J. Thomas IV, MD
Urologic Oncology Fellow
Glickman Urological & Kidney Institute
Cleveland Clinic
Cleveland, Ohio
Retroperitoneal Lymph Node Dissection

Michael A. Valente, DO, FACS, FASCRS
Associate Professor
Residency Program Director
Colorectal Surgery
Digestive Disease and Surgery Institute
Cleveland Clinic
Cleveland, Ohio
Appendectomy

Stephanie A. Valente, DO, FACS
Breast Surgical Oncologist
Director
Breast Surgery Fellowship
General Surgery
Cleveland Clinic
Associate Professor of Surgery
Department of General Surgery
Cleveland Clinic Lerner College of Medicine
Case Western Reserve University
Cleveland, Ohio
Axillary Lymphadenectomy and Lymphaticovenous Bypass

Valery Vilchez, MD
Surgery Resident
Department of General Surgery
Digestive Disease and Surgery Institute
Cleveland Clinic
Cleveland, Ohio
Distal Pancreatectomy

Cynthia E. Weber, MD
Bariatric Surgery Fellow
Surgery
University Hospitals' of Cleveland
Cleveland, Ohio
Minimally Invasive Antireflux Surgery

Alvin C. Wee, MD, MBA
Surgical Director
Kidney Transplantation
Glickman Urological & Kidney Institute
Cleveland Clinic
Cleveland, Ohio
Kidney Transplantation
Laparoscopic Donor Nephrectomy

James S. Wu, MD, PhD
Staff Surgeon
Department of Colon and Rectal Surgery
Digestive Disease and Surgery Institute
Cleveland Clinic
Cleveland, Ohio
Abdominal Wall Marking and Stoma Site Selection

Chad A. Zender, MD, FACS
Assistant Professor
Department of Otolaryngology—Head and Neck Surgery
Case Western Reserve University School of Medicine
Cleveland, Ohio
Selective (Supraomohyoid) Neck Dissection, Levels I-III

Massarat Zutshi, MD
Staff Surgeon
Colorectal Surgery
Digestive Disease and Surgery Institute
Cleveland Clinic
Cleveland, Ohio
Hemorrhoids and Hemorrhoidectomy
Sphincter Repair and Sacral Neuromodulation

Contents

Video Contents

The Neck

Selective (Supraomohyoid) Neck Dissection, Levels I-III

Patrick Tassone, Chad A. Zender, Evan R. McBeath, Pierre Lavertu, and Jamie A. Ku

 VIDEO

1.1 Neck Dissection

INTRODUCTION

Neck dissection has been a standard method of removing at-risk or involved cancerous lymph nodes in the head and neck for more than 100 years. Crile first described the radical neck dissection in the early 1900s, but modifications by Bocca and others helped reduce the morbidity associated with lymph node removal, allowing for nerve and structure preservation when oncologically sound. This chapter discusses one of these modifications in detail, the *selective* or *supraomohyoid* neck dissection. A selective neck dissection, including levels I through III, is typically used for malignancies of the oral cavity in patients with N0 disease. When a larger nodal burden is present, an extended (levels I-IV) selective neck dissection or a modified radical neck dissection (levels I-V) is indicated. Lesions in the oral cavity that approach or cross the midline require treatment of both sides of the neck.

NECK ANATOMY FOR SURGICAL PLANNING

Understanding the regional lymphatic drainage pathways is critical when planning which type of neck dissection will be employed (Fig. 1.1). A supraomohyoid neck dissection is performed when treating patients who are at risk for micrometastasis in levels I, II, and III. The boundaries of levels I (submental and submandibular), II (upper jugular nodal chain), and III (midjugular nodal chain) are defined as follows:

Level Ia: Bounded laterally by the medial aspects of the anterior belly of the digastric muscles, and ending medially at a line drawn from the mandible to the hyoid bone at the anatomic midline.

Level Ib: Bounded by the lateral aspect of the anterior belly of the digastric muscle, the medial aspect of the posterior belly of the digastric and stylohyoid muscles, and the inferior border of the mandibular body superiorly.

Level IIa: Bounded anteriorly and superiorly by the posterior belly of the digastric and stylohyoid muscles, posteriorly by the vertical plane defined by the spinal accessory nerve and sternocleidomastoid muscle (SCM), and inferiorly by the horizontal plane defined by the inferior border of the hyoid bone.

Level IIb: Bounded anteriorly by the jugular vein and inferiorly by the vertical plane defined by the spinal accessory nerve, posteriorly by the posterior border of the SCM, and superiorly by the skull base.

Level III: Bounded superiorly by the horizontal plane defined by the inferior border of the hyoid bone, inferiorly by the horizontal plane defined by the inferior border of the cricoid cartilage and/or the omohyoid muscle as it crosses the internal jugular vein, anteriorly by the lateral border of the sternohyoid muscle, and posteriorly by the posterior border of the SCM.

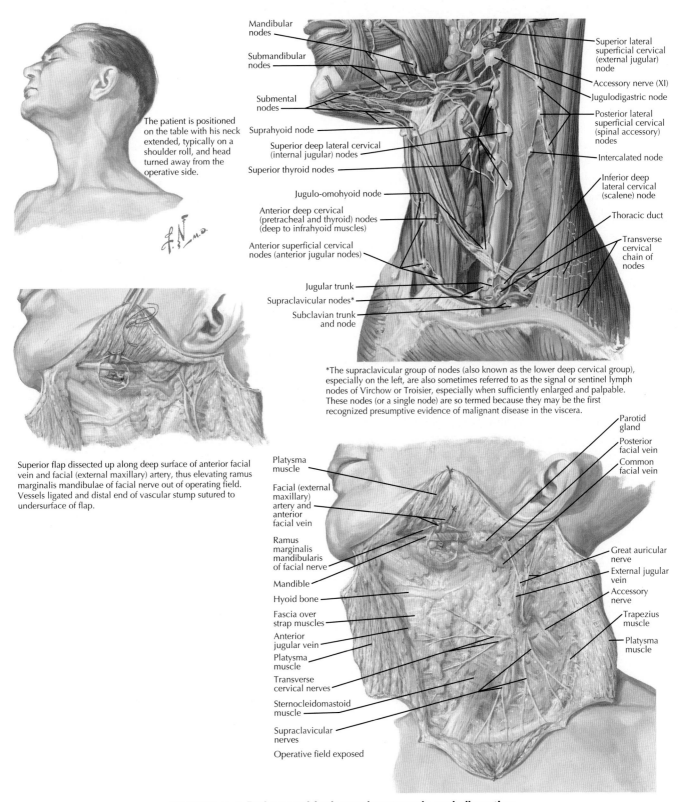

The patient is positioned on the table with his neck extended, typically on a shoulder roll, and head turned away from the operative side.

Superior flap dissected up along deep surface of anterior facial vein and facial (external maxillary) artery, thus elevating ramus marginalis mandibulae of facial nerve out of operating field. Vessels ligated and distal end of vascular stump sutured to undersurface of flap.

Mandibular nodes
Submandibular nodes
Submental nodes
Suprahyoid node
Superior deep lateral cervical (internal jugular) nodes
Superior thyroid nodes
Jugulo-omohyoid node
Anterior deep cervical (pretracheal and thyroid) nodes (deep to infrahyoid muscles)
Anterior superficial cervical nodes (anterior jugular nodes)
Jugular trunk
Supraclavicular nodes*
Subclavian trunk and node

Superior lateral superficial cervical (external jugular) node
Accessory nerve (XI)
Jugulodigastric node
Posterior lateral superficial cervical (spinal accessory) nodes
Intercalated node
Inferior deep lateral cervical (scalene) node
Thoracic duct
Transverse cervical chain of nodes

*The supraclavicular group of nodes (also known as the lower deep cervical group), especially on the left, are also sometimes referred to as the signal or sentinel lymph nodes of Virchow or Troisier, especially when sufficiently enlarged and palpable. These nodes (or a single node) are so termed because they may be the first recognized presumptive evidence of malignant disease in the viscera.

Platysma muscle
Facial (external maxillary) artery and anterior facial vein
Ramus marginalis mandibularis of facial nerve
Mandible
Hyoid bone
Fascia over strap muscles
Anterior jugular vein
Platysma muscle
Transverse cervical nerves
Sternocleidomastoid muscle
Supraclavicular nerves
Operative field exposed

Parotid gland
Posterior facial vein
Common facial vein
Great auricular nerve
External jugular vein
Accessory nerve
Trapezius muscle
Platysma muscle

FIGURE 1.1 Patient positioning and anatomy in neck dissection.

INCISION PLANNING AND PATIENT POSITIONING FOR NECK DISSECTION

Positioning for a neck dissection includes extending the neck and turning the patient's head away from the surgeon. This usually entails placing a shoulder roll under the patient to facilitate adequate extension.

Various types of incisions may be employed. A "hockey stick" incision that extends from the mastoid tip down the middle of the SCM and then across the neck in a crease, which is usually over the lowest level that will be surgically treated (Fig. 1.2), is typically used. The incision can be brought across the midline to the contralateral neck in the same manner, creating an "apron" incision, which will allow access to both sides of the neck when indicated to treat bilateral neck disease.

Raising the Subplatysmal Flap

Skin and subcutaneous incisions are continued down through the subcutaneous fat and platysma muscle but not through the superficial layer of the deep cervical fascia. A superior subplatysmal flap is then elevated up to the inferior border of the mandible. Care is taken to keep the plane of elevation immediately subplatysmal, to aid in identification and preservation of the marginal mandibular branch of the facial nerve. Laterally, the platysma muscle is not developed, and elevation must proceed over the external jugular vein and great auricular nerve. This allows for complete elevation of the flap (Fig. 1.3).

Inferior elevation is performed in a subplatysmal manner below where the omohyoid crosses the jugular vein. This allows for complete exposure of level III and for incorporation of level IV if needed. The flap elevation can be extended down to within 5 to 10 mm of the clavicle to aid visualization.

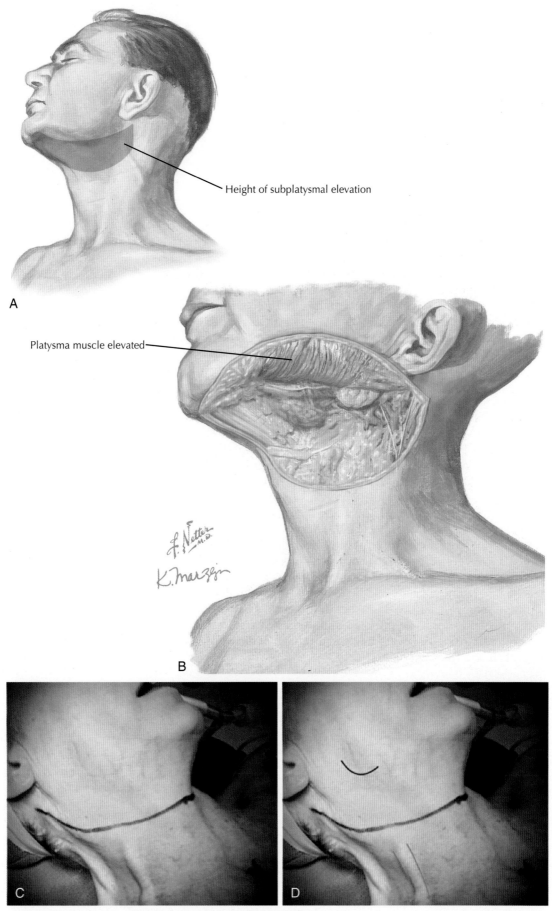

Height of subplatysmal elevation

A

Platysma muscle elevated

B

C

D

FIGURE 1.2 Incision design in selective neck dissection.
The incision is two fingerbreadths below the angle of the mandible (marked in *purple,* D) to protect the marginal mandibular nerve. The course of the external jugular vein (marked in *blue,* D) can also be seen through the skin.

LEVEL IA-IB NECK DISSECTION

After flap elevation, expose the anterior belly of the digastric muscle by making a midline incision from below the mentum to the hyoid bone. It is important to include all the fibrofatty contents from the contralateral medial edge of the digastric muscle. The elevation continues to the medial aspect of the submandibular gland to complete the level Ia dissection.

The marginal mandibular branch of the facial nerve can be located approximately 1 cm inferior to angle of the mandible. The nerve then travels superiorly to cross the mandible around the facial notch, where the nerve travels superficial to the facial artery and vein (Fig. 1.3). Incisions brought across the neck are always two fingerbreadths below the angle to prevent inadvertent injury to this nerve. The marginal mandibular branch of the facial nerve lies between the superficial layer of the deep cervical fascia and the adventitia investing the anterior facial vein. The superficial layer of the deep cervical fascia is incised at the inferior border of the submandibular gland. It must be elevated and may be tacked to the platysma muscle to aid in elevation.

Care must be taken to preserve the marginal mandibular branch of the facial nerve and reflect it superiorly, along with the superficial layer of the deep cervical fascia, and to remove any submandibular retrovascular (perifacial) lymph nodes in the area. This is accomplished by developing a plane between the vein and superficial layer of the deep cervical fascia, keeping the fat pad that contains the facial nodes down in the specimen, along with the submandibular gland, and elevating and protecting the nerve.

At this point the anterior belly of the digastric muscle is isolated, and the gland and fibrofatty contents of level Ia are brought posteriorly across the mylohyoid muscle.

Next, retract the mylohyoid muscle, identify and preserve the lingual and hypoglossal nerves, and identify, ligate, and divide the submandibular duct, submandibular ganglion, and corresponding vasculature. Branches of the facial artery into the submandibular gland can be numerous and must be controlled and divided to release the contents of Level 1B from its posterior attachments. Level I is released and left pedicled by the inferior fibrofatty attachments to levels II and III.

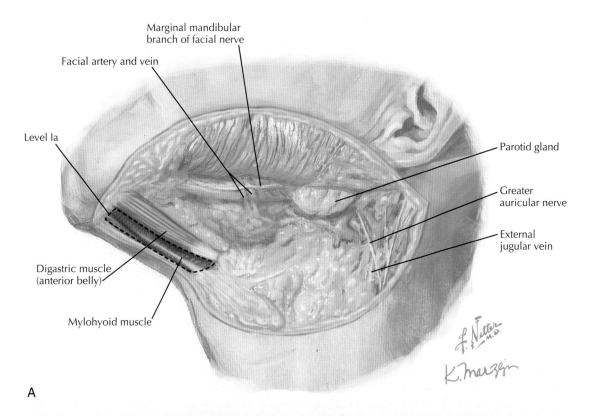

A

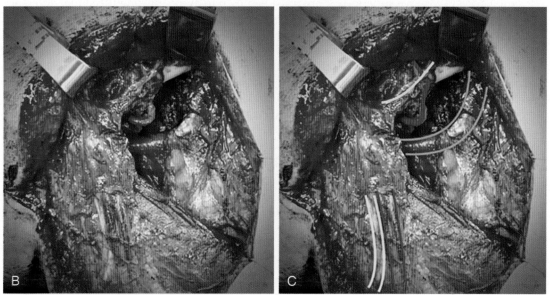

FIGURE 1.3 Subplatysmal flaps and level Ib dissection.
The greater auricular nerve (marked in *yellow,* C) and external jugular vein (marked in *blue,* C) can be seen coursing together over the superficial surface of the sternocleidomastoid muscle. The marginal mandibular nerve (marked in *yellow,* C) can be seen coursing over the facial artery (marked in *red,* C) at the facial notch of the mandible. The facial artery then travels deep and posterior into the neck, deep to the posterior belly of the digastric muscle (marked in *orange,* C), where it takes off from the external carotid artery.

LEVEL II-III NECK DISSECTION

Identify the posterior belly of the digastric muscle, creating the digastric tunnel back to the mastoid tip under the SCM.

Incise the investing fascial layer along the anterior border of the SCM, ligating and dividing the external jugular vein in the process. An attempt should be made to preserve the greater auricular nerve, if not involved with disease.

Unwrap the SCM from its investing fascia. This is accomplished along a broad, superior-to-inferior plane, from the digastric muscle superiorly to the omohyoid muscle inferiorly.

Identify the spinal accessory nerve at its entrance into the SCM, and trace it under the posterior belly of the digastric muscle. The spinal accessory nerve typically passes lateral to the internal jugular vein just before diving under the posterior belly of the digastric muscle (Fig. 1.4A, B, and C). The nerve will occasionally bisect or run deep to the jugular vein.

The spinal accessory nerve is released from the surrounding soft tissue, and then level IIb is released from the skull base, the back of the jugular vein, the SCM, and the deep cervical fascia. Level IIb is left attached to IIa and brought under the spinal accessory nerve.

Once the investing fascial layer is elevated off the SCM down to the level of the deep cervical rootlets, the dissection is taken medially across the rootlets from the omohyoid muscle to the spinal accessory nerve superiorly. Care must be taken to avoid injuring the spinal accessory nerve in this area as it exits the SCM posteriorly.

Dissect levels II and III medially in a plane lateral to the cervical rootlets and the carotid sheath, which invests the carotid artery, internal jugular vein, and vagus nerve (Fig. 1.4D and E).

Once the elevation reaches the jugular vein, the fascia from the internal jugular vein is unwrapped. Branches of the vein may be ligated and divided as the specimen is brought medially. The ansa cervicalis will be transected during the inferior dissection as the specimen is brought across the jugular vein to the lateral aspect of the strap muscles. Superiorly, the hypoglossal nerve, which runs lateral to the carotid artery and medial to the jugular vein, must be protected under the digastric muscle (Fig. 1.5). The ansa hypoglossi will likely have to be transected as the specimen is brought medially to the hyoid bone and strap musculature.

The specimen is then dissected away from the hypoglossal nerve and posterior belly of the digastric muscle until it can be easily removed. The anterior dissection will meet with the posterior dissection as the specimen is brought across the strap muscles, carotid artery, and jugular vein.

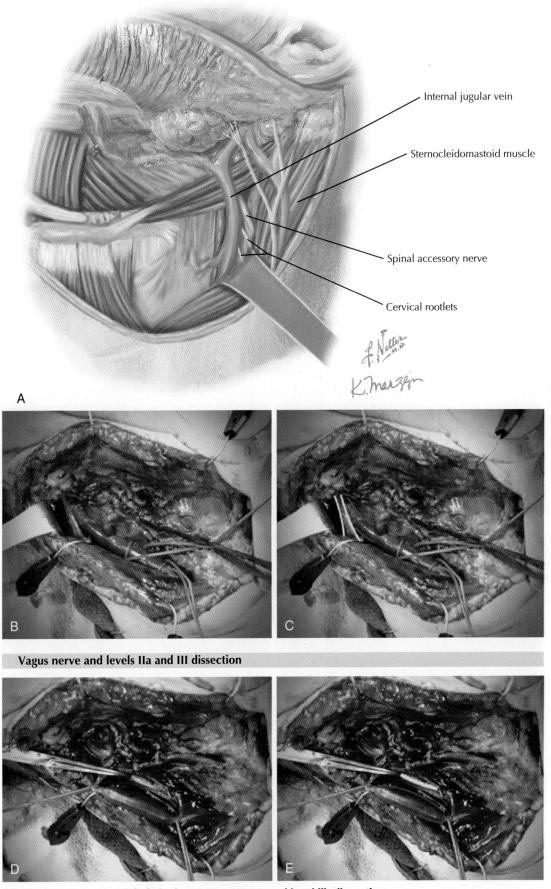

Spinal accessory nerve and level IIb dissection

Internal jugular vein

Sternocleidomastoid muscle

Spinal accessory nerve

Cervical rootlets

A

B

C

Vagus nerve and levels IIa and III dissection

D

E

FIGURE 1.4 A, B, and C, Spinal accessory nerve and level IIb dissection.
The spinal accessory nerve (marked in *yellow,* C) can be seen traveling from the jugular foramen through the sterno-cleidomastoid muscle. The spinal accessory nerve divides levels IIa and IIb and is seen in its typical relationship superficial to the internal jugular vein (marked in *blue,* C). D and E, Vagus nerve and levels IIa and III dissection. The vagus nerve (marked in *yellow,* E) can be seen traveling in the carotid sheath, medial to the internal jugular vein (marked in *blue,* E).

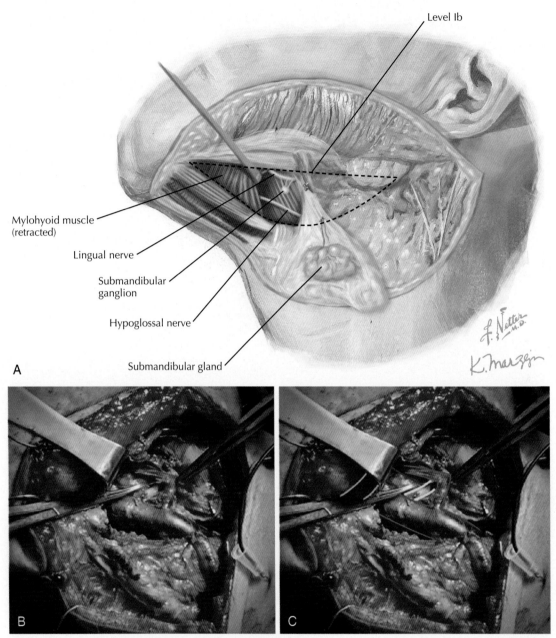

Level Ib

Mylohyoid muscle
(retracted)

Lingual nerve

Submandibular
ganglion

Hypoglossal nerve

A

Submandibular gland

FIGURE 1.5 Hypoglossal nerve and level IIa dissection.
The posterior belly of the digastric muscle (marked in *orange, right*) is retracted superiorly to reveal the hypoglossal nerve (marked in *yellow*, C). The hypoglossal nerve can be identified running deep to the internal jugular vein and its branches (marked in *blue*, C) but superficial to the external carotid artery (marked in *red*, C).

SUGGESTED READINGS

Janfaza P, editor. Cummings otolaryngology: head and neck surgery, 5th ed. Philadelphia: Saunders; 2010.

Myers EN, editor. Operative otolaryngology: head and neck surgery, 2nd ed. Philadelphia: Saunders; 2008.

Tracheostomy

Paul C. Bryson and Saranya Reghunathan

 VIDEO

2.1 Tracheostomy

INTRODUCTION

Tracheotomy (tracheostomy) is one of the oldest surgical procedures known, with the first reference in 3600 BCE. Chevalier Jackson is credited with standardizing the tracheotomy procedure in 1932, outlining the individual steps for establishing a direct airway through the anterior neck tissues and into the trachea. This technique was subsequently used during the polio epidemic. Throughout the years, this technique has evolved to include three primary techniques: percutaneous dilatational, open surgical, and other new percutaneous techniques. This chapter focuses primarily on the open technique and briefly reviews the classical percutaneous dilatation technique. At present, the tracheostomy is more commonly used for prolonged mechanical ventilation rather than for upper airway obstruction.

INDICATIONS AND PRINCIPLES OF TRACHEOTOMY

Indications for tracheotomy are multiple and include the need to bypass an airway obstruction caused by congenital anomaly, vocal cord paralysis, inflammatory disease, benign or malignant laryngeal pathology, laryngotracheal trauma, facial trauma, or severe sleep apnea refractory to other interventions. Currently, the most common indication for tracheostomy is acute respiratory failure with need for prolonged mechanical ventilation. The second most common indication is in patients with neurologic insult requiring a safe, comfortable airway with possible need for home mechanical ventilation. Upper airway obstruction is currently a less common indication for tracheostomy.

PREOPERATIVE CONSIDERATIONS

Once a tracheotomy is planned, certain factors influence whether patients should have an open tracheotomy or a *percutaneous dilatational* tracheotomy (PDT), as first described by Ciaglia in 1985.

If the consideration for PDT is present, the following ideally should also be present: (1) easily palpable tracheal landmarks, (2) a skilled bronchoscopist who helps guide the proceduralist and prevent extubation, and (3) knowledge of when conversion to open tracheostomy is necessary.

Regardless of the tracheotomy method chosen, a patient's overall medical condition must be optimized, body habitus assessed, and coagulation profile addressed, because these too help determine which tracheotomy method is most ideal. Other important considerations include the urgency of the procedure, which is often directly related to the current status of the airway.

In determining whether to perform the procedure open vs. percutaneously, surgeons must consider availability of proper equipment, patient portability, surgeon's experience (open vs. percutaneous technique), and capability of the institution to perform bedside procedures. This will determine which team performs the procedure and whether it will be done in the operating room or at the bedside in the intensive care unit.

PERIOPERATIVE CONSIDERATIONS

In anticipation of placement of the tracheostomy tube, it is prudent to consider the options for tracheostomy tube size and type. In choosing the size of the tube, both gender and age play the most important roles. Looking at the inner and outer diameter of tracheostomy tubes helps in choosing the most appropriately sized tube. In the absence of time for consideration, a Shiley 6 tracheostomy often fits the widest range of adult male and female patients.

SURGICAL ANATOMY AND OPEN TRACHEOTOMY PROCEDURE
External Anatomy

The patient is placed in the supine position, with the head facing toward the anesthesia team. It is to the surgeon's benefit to place the neck in extension, often with the aid of a shoulder roll, because it helps bring more of the trachea into the neck from the chest.

Next, it is critical to palpate and mark the following structures: the thyroid notch superiorly, cricoid cartilage, and suprasternal notch inferiorly (Fig. 2.1). Typically, the horizontal incision for the tracheostomy will be 2 cm above the sternal notch and be approximately 3 cm long. The area of proposed incision is injected with 1% lidocaine with 1:100,000 epinephrine solution for hemostasis and anesthesia. The local anesthesia is most critical in awake tracheostomy patients but remains beneficial from a hemostasis perspective in patients under general anesthesia.

Once the patient is appropriately prepped and draped according to surgeon preference, the horizontal incision is carried through the skin, soft tissue, platysma, until the midline strap muscles are identified (see Fig. 2.1).

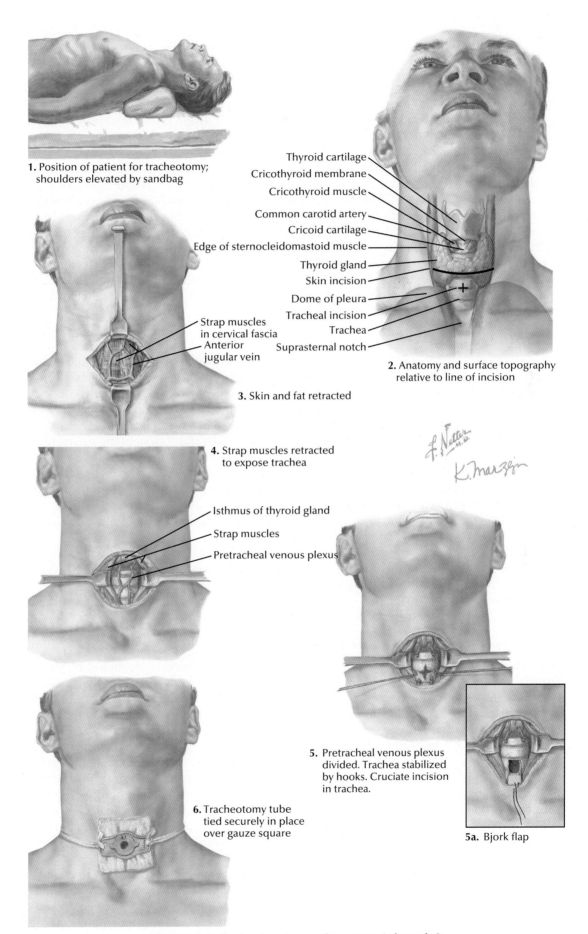

1. Position of patient for tracheotomy; shoulders elevated by sandbag

2. Anatomy and surface topography relative to line of incision

Thyroid cartilage
Cricothyroid membrane
Cricothyroid muscle
Common carotid artery
Cricoid cartilage
Edge of sternocleidomastoid muscle
Thyroid gland
Skin incision
Dome of pleura
Tracheal incision
Trachea
Suprasternal notch

3. Skin and fat retracted

Strap muscles in cervical fascia
Anterior jugular vein

4. Strap muscles retracted to expose trachea

Isthmus of thyroid gland
Strap muscles
Pretracheal venous plexus

5. Pretracheal venous plexus divided. Trachea stabilized by hooks. Cruciate incision in trachea.

5a. Bjork flap

6. Tracheotomy tube tied securely in place over gauze square

FIGURE 2.1 Tracheotomy procedure, steps 1 through 6.

Strap Muscles and Midline Raphe

The anterior jugular veins are deep to the platysma and typically located on the strap musculature and may require ligation if encountered in the midline (Fig. 2.2). In the lower neck, the surgeon must be conscious of the innominate artery.

The innominate (brachiocephalic) artery is the first branch of the aorta. It typically crosses the trachea at the level of the ninth cartilaginous ring and travels upward to divide behind the sternoclavicular joint into the right subclavian artery and right common carotid artery. Before dissection of the strap muscles, the surgeon should palpate for innominate pulsations in the suprasternal notch and should be cognizant of the pathway of the surgical dissection in the setting of a high-riding vessel.

Midline dissection is essential for hemostasis and avoidance of paratracheal structures, including the great vessels of the neck. The midline raphe between the paired sternohyoid and sternothyroid muscles can be easily identified. Lateral retraction of the strap muscles along the midline raphe will expose the underlying thyroid gland. In patients with suboptimal body habitus or difficult anatomy, palpation of the trachea, cricoid cartilage, and thyroid notch can help maintain a midline course of dissection (see Fig. 2.2).

Thyroid Isthmus

The strap muscles are separated in the midline through the avascular midline raphe and retracted to either side until the thyroid isthmus is visible. The isthmus of the thyroid gland generally lies across the first to fourth tracheal rings. It must be divided when overlying the tracheotomy site, because this will make reinsertion safer and easier in the setting of accidental dislodgement. Moreover, the isthmus is very vascular and is ideally managed in a controlled setting.

The isthmus can be addressed in one of several ways. First, the fascial attachments of the thyroid to the anterior trachea may be dissected free, thus allowing the gland to be retracted above or below the planned entry site into the trachea. If the thyroid is enlarged and cannot be retracted out of the way, it will have to be divided by further dissecting it from the anterior tracheal wall in the immediate pretracheal plane to establish a bloodless plane of dissection. By identifying the bright-white layer of the tracheal cartilage, the surgeon minimizes bleeding from trauma to the posterior aspect of the gland.

Once the thyroid isthmus is elevated from the trachea, the surgeon may use two clamps on either side, then cutting in the midline with a cautery device. Once divided, the two ends of isthmus are then suture-ligated using a running or figure-of-eight 2-0 silk stitch. If available, energy devices may be used, based on surgeon preference. Use of cautery alone to divide the thyroid may be appropriate in the case of a small isthmus.

Anatomy With Trachea Visualized

Once the bright white of the trachea is easily visualized, the cricoid hook should be used. It provides stability to the trachea and is especially useful in cases of difficult anatomy, where the trachea is deeper in the mediastinum. The cricoid hook can elevate the trachea out of the chest in the patient with kyphosis or a low-lying laryngotracheal complex. Once the anterior wall of the trachea is visualized, the space between the second and third tracheal rings is identified by palpation using a hemostat. At this juncture, it is important to notify the anesthesia team member that you are prepared to enter the airway. This allows them to free the endotracheal tube (ETT) by either deflating it before entering the airway or advancing it distally to prevent ETT cuff deflation. It is preferable to maintain the ETT inflated during the procedure. It allows ventilation and minimizes the spray of blood and secretions into the surgical field.

Surgeon preference and age of the patient may influence the type of tracheal incision used. In adults, a horizontal incision is made between the rings with a scalpel and can be extended laterally in each direction using scissors.

In children, a vertical incision may be used. In adults a common technique is to create an anterior tracheal window by removing a section of a single ring. Another common technique in either children or adults is to create an inferiorly based "trapdoor" flap (Björk flap) composed of an anterior portion of a single tracheal ring and interspace tissue below. After an intercartilaginous incision is made, scissors are used to cut downward on either side to create an inferiorly

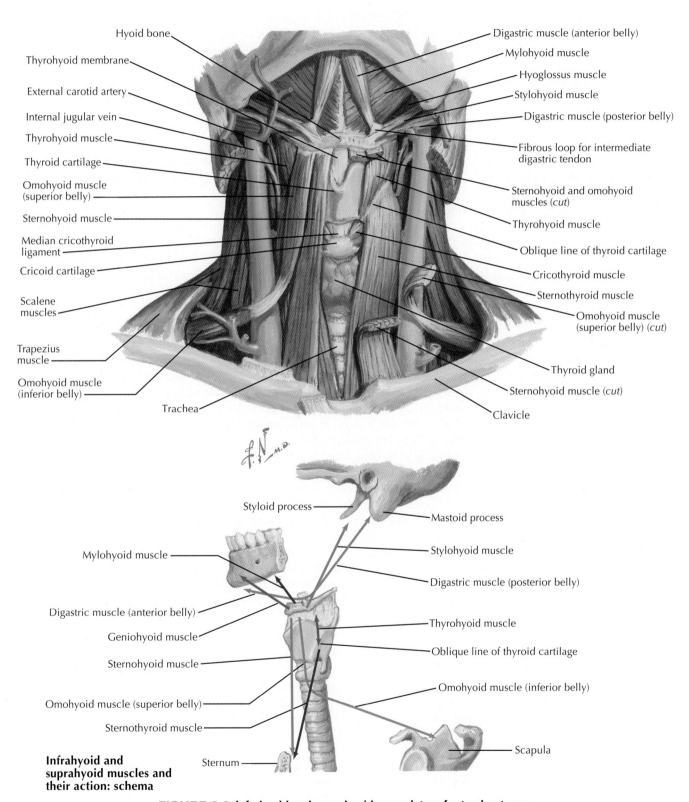

Hyoid bone

Thyrohyoid membrane

External carotid artery

Internal jugular vein

Thyrohyoid muscle

Thyroid cartilage

Omohyoid muscle (superior belly)

Sternohyoid muscle

Median cricothyroid ligament

Cricoid cartilage

Scalene muscles

Trapezius muscle

Omohyoid muscle (inferior belly)

Trachea

Digastric muscle (anterior belly)

Mylohyoid muscle

Hyoglossus muscle

Stylohyoid muscle

Digastric muscle (posterior belly)

Fibrous loop for intermediate digastric tendon

Sternohyoid and omohyoid muscles (cut)

Thyrohyoid muscle

Oblique line of thyroid cartilage

Cricothyroid muscle

Sternothyroid muscle

Omohyoid muscle (superior belly) (cut)

Thyroid gland

Sternohyoid muscle (cut)

Clavicle

Styloid process

Mastoid process

Stylohyoid muscle

Digastric muscle (posterior belly)

Mylohyoid muscle

Thyrohyoid muscle

Digastric muscle (anterior belly)

Oblique line of thyroid cartilage

Geniohyoid muscle

Sternohyoid muscle

Omohyoid muscle (inferior belly)

Omohyoid muscle (superior belly)

Sternothyroid muscle

Scapula

Sternum

Infrahyoid and suprahyoid muscles and their action: schema

FIGURE 2.2 Infrahyoid and suprahyoid musculature for tracheotomy.

Anatomy With Trachea Visualized (Continued)

based flap of tracheal tissue. The superior edge of this flap is then stitched to the skin edge to exteriorize and secure the trachea in an effort to reduce the distance from the skin to the airway and "dead space" that can create a false passage. Although some consider this to be the safest method because the airway is secured to the skin, this technique may lead to some scarring or tracheocutaneous fistula after decannulation, both of which can typically be managed with small procedures.

Anatomy With Tracheotomy Tube in Place

Once the airway is entered, the ETT is pulled out slowly by the anesthesiologist until it is just above the newly created tracheotomy. The purpose of this maneuver is to keep the endotracheal tube in the airway until adequate tube placement in the newly created airway is confirmed. Next, the tracheotomy tube or ETT is then placed through the opening into the trachea. After the airway is secured, as confirmed by CO_2 monitor or ventilator, the oral ETT is then removed. The tracheostomy tube is then sutured to the skin using 2-0 silk to minimize the risk of accidental dislodgement. In addition, a circumferential tie is placed and secured around the neck, allowing at least one finger to slide underneath to minimize constriction. In obese patients or those with fragile skin, a padded dressing may be indicated under the neck ties.

PERCUTANEOUS DILATATIONAL TRACHEOTOMY PROCEDURE

Traditionally, tracheostomy has been performed by surgeons or otolaryngologists in the operating room using standard surgical principles. Operational pressures and limited institutional resources have prompted a re-examination of the setting for tracheotomy and the exploration of transitioning patients from the ICU setting to longer-term ventilator facilities after tracheotomy tube placement. In addition, open tracheostomy has a number of possible complications, including the loss of the airway, injuries to nearby structures, bleeding, pneumothorax, tracheoinnominate fistula, infection, and tracheal stenosis. Thus other "less invasive" techniques that could be performed in the ICU at bedside have been introduced.

The most popular of these alternative surgical approaches is the PDT method proposed by Ciaglia in 1985. Similar to the open tracheostomy, general anesthesia is administered and the patient is prepped and draped. However, all steps are performed under bronchoscopic vision. In addition, unlike the open tracheostomy, there is no sharp dissection.

First, a skin incision is made. The pretracheal tissue is cleared with blunt dissection. The endotracheal tube is pulled back proximally. The bronchoscopist places the distal tip of the bronchoscope such that the light shines through the trachea into the surgical wound. The operator enters the tracheal lumen below the second tracheal ring with an introducer needle. This is then serially dilated over guidewire. The tracheostomy tube is then placed under direct visualization, which then also confirms its location.

SUMMARY

Tracheotomy is used to establish a surgical airway in patients requiring prolonged mechanical ventilation or those who require anatomic bypass because of either obstruction or lack of function. Surgeon mastery of anatomy and ability to use proper techniques in specific settings maximizes successful patient outcomes and minimizes potential complications.

SUGGESTED READINGS

Ciaglia P, Firsching R, Syniec C. Elective percutaneous dilatational tracheostomy: a new simple bedside procedure: preliminary report. Chest 1985;87:715–9.

Jackson C. Tracheotomy. Laryngoscope 1909;19:285–90.

Lassen HC. A preliminary report on the 1952 epidemic of poliomyelitis in Copenhagen with special reference to the treatment of acute respiratory insufficiency. Lancet 1953;1(6749):37–41.

Moore KL. The cardiovascular system. In: Moore KL, Persaud TVN, editors. The developing human: clinically oriented embryology, 8th ed. Philadelphia: Saunders; 2008. pp. 285–337.

Pierson DJ. Tracheostomy from A to Z: historical context and current challenges. Respir Care 2005;50(4):473–75.

SECTION 2

Endocrine

SECTION EDITOR: Allan Siperstein

Thyroidectomy and Parathyroidectomy

Allan Siperstein and Cassandre Benay

▶ **VIDEO**

3.1 Thyroidectomy and Parathyroidectomy

THYROIDECTOMY

Thyroidectomy is the most common endocrine surgical procedure. By definition, a total thyroidectomy requires the resection of both thyroid lobes and isthmus, whereas a thyroid lobectomy requires the resection of one lobe with the isthmus up to the contralateral lobe. Indications for thyroidectomy include benign causes such as mass effect of nodule(s) (on the aerodigestive tract, recurrent laryngeal nerve [RLN], major vessels), thyrotoxicosis (Graves disease refractory to medical therapy, Graves disease in the context of thyroid nodules, toxic nodular goiter), as well as malignancy or suspected malignancy on cytology from fine-needle aspirations.

Although thyroidectomy is a safe procedure in experienced hands of a high-volume endocrine surgeon, it carries inherent rare but serious risks: cervical hematoma, hypocalcemia, and RLN injury. Preoperative evaluation should include thyroid-stimulating hormone (TSH), comprehensive central and lateral neck ultrasonography to rule out metastatic disease, and, in selected patients, voice examination by laryngoscopy.

Surgical Anatomy for Thyroidectomy

The thyroid is a bilobed gland wrapped anteriorly to the trachea and joined by an isthmus. The pyramidal lobe, which represents the embryologic remnant of the thyroglossal duct, can be found on the left side of the isthmus in up to 60% of patients. The thyroid is attached posteriorly to the trachea by the suspensory ligament of Berry. Each thyroid lobe is supplied by the superior and inferior thyroid arteries arising from the carotid artery and thyrocervical trunk, respectively. Each hemithyroid is drained by the superior, middle, and inferior thyroid veins. The upper and middle veins empty in the internal jugular, whereas the inferior thyroid vein drains into the brachiocephalic vein (Fig. 3.1).

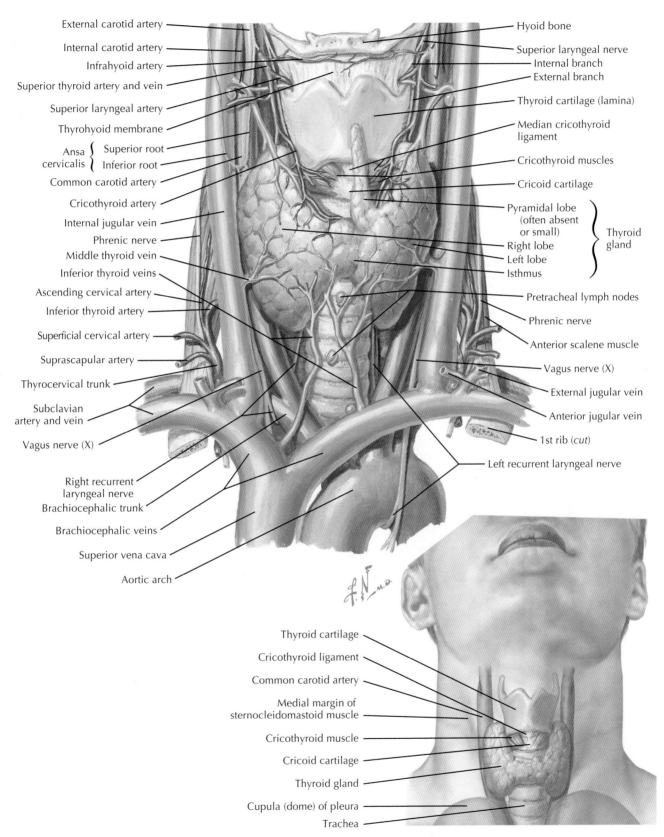

External carotid artery

Internal carotid artery

Infrahyoid artery

Superior thyroid artery and vein

Superior laryngeal artery

Thyrohyoid membrane

Ansa cervicalis { Superior root

Inferior root

Common carotid artery

Cricothyroid artery

Internal jugular vein

Phrenic nerve

Middle thyroid vein

Inferior thyroid veins

Ascending cervical artery

Inferior thyroid artery

Superficial cervical artery

Suprascapular artery

Thyrocervical trunk

Subclavian artery and vein

Vagus nerve (X)

Right recurrent laryngeal nerve

Brachiocephalic trunk

Brachiocephalic veins

Superior vena cava

Aortic arch

Hyoid bone

Superior laryngeal nerve

Internal branch

External branch

Thyroid cartilage (lamina)

Median cricothyroid ligament

Cricothyroid muscles

Cricoid cartilage

Pyramidal lobe (often absent or small)

Right lobe

Left lobe

Isthmus

} Thyroid gland

Pretracheal lymph nodes

Phrenic nerve

Anterior scalene muscle

Vagus nerve (X)

External jugular vein

Anterior jugular vein

1st rib (cut)

Left recurrent laryngeal nerve

Thyroid cartilage

Cricothyroid ligament

Common carotid artery

Medial margin of sternocleidomastoid muscle

Cricothyroid muscle

Cricoid cartilage

Thyroid gland

Cupula (dome) of pleura

Trachea

FIGURE 3.1 Thyroid gland, anterior view.

Surgical Anatomy of the Superior Recurrent Laryngeal Nerve

In the upper neck, the superior laryngeal nerve (SLN) branches off the vagus nerve. Two to three centimeters cephalad to the superior pole vessels, the SLN divides into an internal and external branch. The internal branch provides sensation to the supraglottic area of the larynx as well as the base of the tongue, whereas the external branch provides motor innervation to the cricothyroid muscle.

The external branch of the SLN (EBSLN) crosses the superior pole vessels 1 cm or more cephalad to the thyroid parenchyma, travels medially to the superior pole vessel, and provides motor innervation to the cricothyroid muscle. On rare occasion, the EBSLN crosses the superior pole vessels at the junction with the thyroid parenchyma junction, therefore increasing the likelihood of injury and emphasizing the importance of ligating individual vessels as close as possible to the thyroid capsule (see Fig. 3.2).

Surgical Anatomy of the Recurrent Laryngeal Nerve

The RLN is a branch of the vagus that wraps around the right subclavian artery and the aortic arch on the left. For this reason, the left RLN is more medial than the right RLN, which enters the neck more obliquely. The RLN travels cephalad and medial to the central neck through the thoracic inlet. As it enters the central neck, it crosses the inferior thyroid artery, then travels in the tracheoesophageal groove for approximately 1 cm before entering the larynx by diving posteriorly to the inferior edge of the pharyngeal constrictors. As the RLN travels cephalad, it passes posterior to the *tubercle of Zuckerkandl*, a posterolateral parenchyma protrusion of the thyroid gland. Finally, before entering the larynx, the RLN often bifurcates into an anterior motor branch and posterior sensory branch (Fig. 3.2).

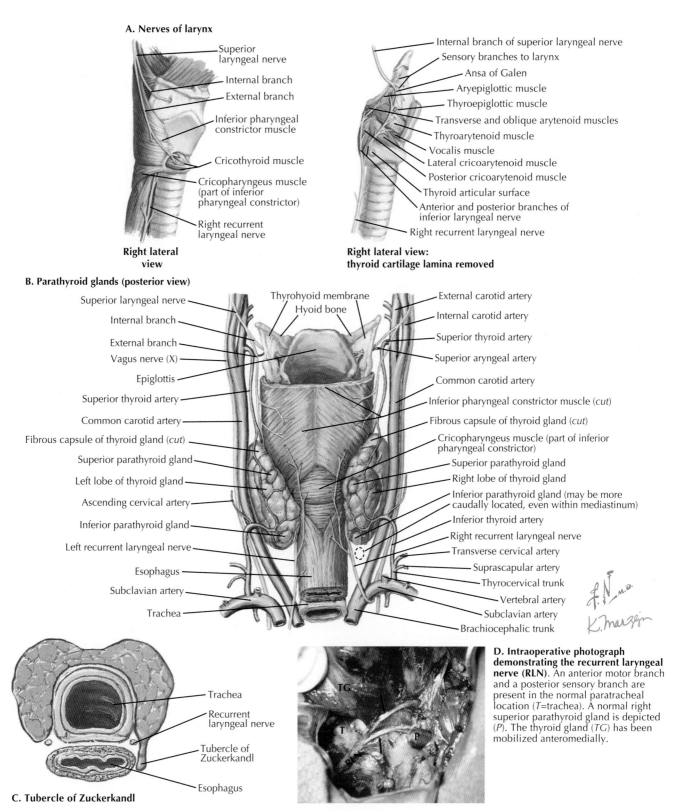

A. Nerves of larynx

- Superior laryngeal nerve
- Internal branch
- External branch
- Inferior pharyngeal constrictor muscle
- Cricothyroid muscle
- Cricopharyngeus muscle (part of inferior pharyngeal constrictor)
- Right recurrent laryngeal nerve

Right lateral view

- Internal branch of superior laryngeal nerve
- Sensory branches to larynx
- Ansa of Galen
- Aryepiglottic muscle
- Thyroepiglottic muscle
- Transverse and oblique arytenoid muscles
- Thyroarytenoid muscle
- Vocalis muscle
- Lateral cricoarytenoid muscle
- Posterior cricoarytenoid muscle
- Thyroid articular surface
- Anterior and posterior branches of inferior laryngeal nerve
- Right recurrent laryngeal nerve

Right lateral view: thyroid cartilage lamina removed

B. Parathyroid glands (posterior view)

- Superior laryngeal nerve
- Internal branch
- External branch
- Vagus nerve (X)
- Epiglottis
- Superior thyroid artery
- Common carotid artery
- Fibrous capsule of thyroid gland (cut)
- Superior parathyroid gland
- Left lobe of thyroid gland
- Ascending cervical artery
- Inferior parathyroid gland
- Left recurrent laryngeal nerve
- Esophagus
- Subclavian artery
- Trachea

- Thyrohyoid membrane
- Hyoid bone

- External carotid artery
- Internal carotid artery
- Superior thyroid artery
- Superior aryngeal artery
- Common carotid artery
- Inferior pharyngeal constrictor muscle (cut)
- Fibrous capsule of thyroid gland (cut)
- Cricopharyngeus muscle (part of inferior pharyngeal constrictor)
- Superior parathyroid gland
- Right lobe of thyroid gland
- Inferior parathyroid gland (may be more caudally located, even within mediastinum)
- Inferior thyroid artery
- Right recurrent laryngeal nerve
- Transverse cervical artery
- Suprascapular artery
- Thyrocervical trunk
- Vertebral artery
- Subclavian artery
- Brachiocephalic trunk

C. Tubercle of Zuckerkandl

- Trachea
- Recurrent laryngeal nerve
- Tubercle of Zuckerkandl
- Esophagus

D. Intraoperative photograph demonstrating the recurrent laryngeal nerve (RLN). An anterior motor branch and a posterior sensory branch are present in the normal paratracheal location (*T*=trachea). A normal right superior parathyroid gland is depicted (*P*). The thyroid gland (*TG*) has been mobilized anteromedially.

FIGURE 3.2 Anatomy of superior and recurrent laryngeal nerves.

Patient Positioning and Skin Incision

The patient is positioned supine, with arms tucked with a soft roll placed behind the shoulders with the head resting on a soft foam. Proper positioning is essential: neck hyperextension increases the surgical working space and places the trachea and thyroid more anteriorly.

Adequate knowledge of surface anatomy and patient-specific anatomy by means of intraoperative neck ultrasonography determines the location and the size of the incision. Ideally, a 3- to 5-cm incision in a natural skin crease should be made approximately at the isthmus and equidistant from each poles upper and lower poles of the thyroid (Fig. 3.3).

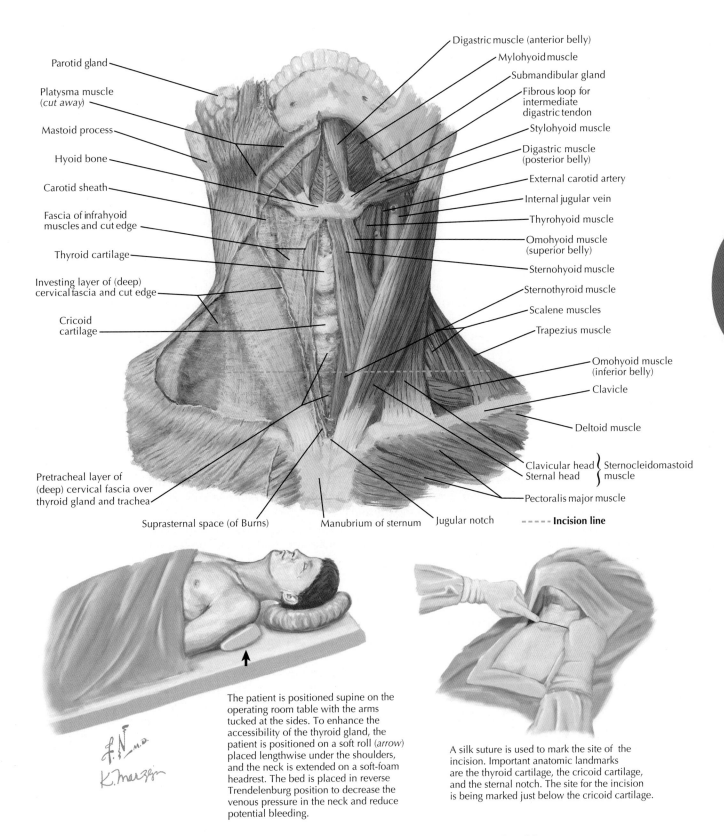

Digastric muscle (anterior belly)

Mylohyoid muscle

Submandibular gland

Fibrous loop for intermediate digastric tendon

Stylohyoid muscle

Digastric muscle (posterior belly)

External carotid artery

Internal jugular vein

Thyrohyoid muscle

Omohyoid muscle (superior belly)

Sternohyoid muscle

Sternothyroid muscle

Scalene muscles

Trapezius muscle

Omohyoid muscle (inferior belly)

Clavicle

Deltoid muscle

Clavicular head
Sternal head } Sternocleidomastoid muscle

Pectoralis major muscle

- - - - - **Incision line**

Parotid gland

Platysma muscle (*cut away*)

Mastoid process

Hyoid bone

Carotid sheath

Fascia of infrahyoid muscles and cut edge

Thyroid cartilage

Investing layer of (deep) cervical fascia and cut edge

Cricoid cartilage

Pretracheal layer of (deep) cervical fascia over thyroid gland and trachea

Suprasternal space (of Burns)

Manubrium of sternum

Jugular notch

The patient is positioned supine on the operating room table with the arms tucked at the sides. To enhance the accessibility of the thyroid gland, the patient is positioned on a soft roll (*arrow*) placed lengthwise under the shoulders, and the neck is extended on a soft-foam headrest. The bed is placed in reverse Trendelenburg position to decrease the venous pressure in the neck and reduce potential bleeding.

A silk suture is used to mark the site of the incision. Important anatomic landmarks are the thyroid cartilage, the cricoid cartilage, and the sternal notch. The site for the incision is being marked just below the cricoid cartilage.

FIGURE 3.3 Anatomical landmarks for thyroidectomy and parathyroidectomy.

Exposing the Thyroid Gland

After skin incision, dissection is carried down the subcutaneous fat and through the platysma muscle. Platysma flaps are created cephalad up to the prominence of the thyroid cartilage and caudal down to the sternal notch and lateral to the sternocleidomastoids. To avoid unnecessary bleeding from anterior jugular veins, dissection should be performed anterior to these veins and posterior to the platysma (Fig. 3.3).

The thyroid gland is exposed by dissecting the midline avascular plane between the bilateral sternothyroid and sternohyoid muscles. Note that with a large multinodular goiter, this avascular plane is occasionally distorted and therefore not always midline. It is not necessary to routinely divide the strap muscles, but this is a maneuver that can ease access to a very large goiter. The strap muscles are innervated by the ansa cervicalis caudally; therefore they should be divided cephalad to prevent denervation and muscle atrophy (Fig. 3.4).

The thyroid lobe is retracted anteromedially with a peanut dissector sponge. This increases the space between the thyroid and the important structures of the central neck. Then the areolar tissue in the central neck can be bluntly dissected with gentle sweeping motions using a peanut dissector sponge to expose the central neck and the carotid laterally. The middle thyroid vein should be ligated at this point.

Mobilizing the Thyroid Lobe

The superior pole of the thyroid is mobilized by applying gentle lateral and caudal traction, opening the avascular space of reeves. Superior pole vessels are then ligated one by one with an energy device as close as possible to the thyroid capsule to avoid injuring the EBSLN and the superior parathyroid, which is gently peeled down away from the thyroid's capsule. Ligation of pole vessels with an energy device has been shown to be safe, to decrease surgical time, and to reduce lymphatic leaks during modified radical neck dissections.

The inferior pole is approached in similar a fashion. The inferior thyroid pole is retracted cephalad and laterally, allowing ligation of individual inferior pole vessels and preservation of the inferior parathyroid and RLN.

If a parathyroid is inadvertently removed, it should be submitted to frozen section to confirm the presence of parathyroid tissue, then minced and autotransplanted into pockets in the sternocleidomastoid muscle.

The RLN should be identified before ligating any lateral structure. The thyroid is gently retracted anteriorly and medially to increase the central neck space. The RLN is identified using anatomic landmarks (tubercle of Zuckerkandl, tracheoesophageal groove, inferior thyroid pole vessels, anatomic relation with parathyroid glands), and only then can structures anterior to the RLN be ligated. Finally, the ligament of Berry is ligated.

A. Muscles of the neck (lateral view)

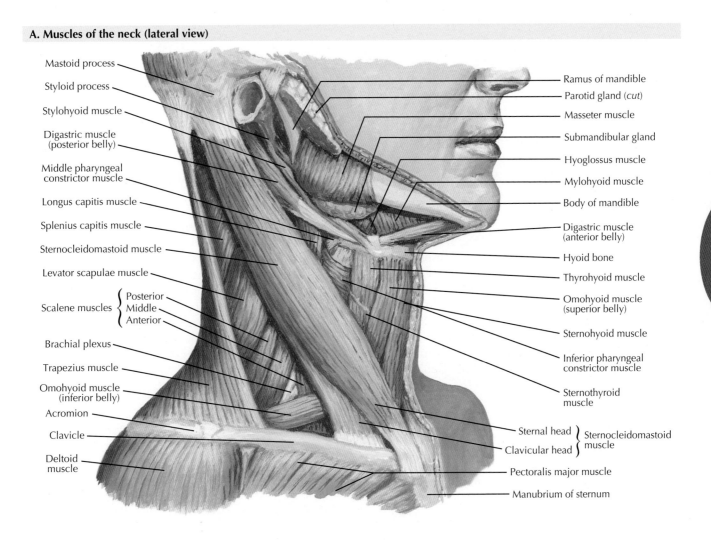

Mastoid process

Styloid process

Stylohyoid muscle

Digastric muscle
(posterior belly)

Middle pharyngeal
constrictor muscle

Longus capitis muscle

Splenius capitis muscle

Sternocleidomastoid muscle

Levator scapulae muscle

Scalene muscles { Posterior
Middle
Anterior

Brachial plexus

Trapezius muscle

Omohyoid muscle
(inferior belly)

Acromion

Clavicle

Deltoid
muscle

Ramus of mandible

Parotid gland (*cut*)

Masseter muscle

Submandibular gland

Hyoglossus muscle

Mylohyoid muscle

Body of mandible

Digastric muscle
(anterior belly)

Hyoid bone

Thyrohyoid muscle

Omohyoid muscle
(superior belly)

Sternohyoid muscle

Inferior pharyngeal
constrictor muscle

Sternothyroid
muscle

Sternal head } Sternocleidomastoid
Clavicular head } muscle

Pectoralis major muscle

Manubrium of sternum

B. Parathyroid glands (right lateral view)

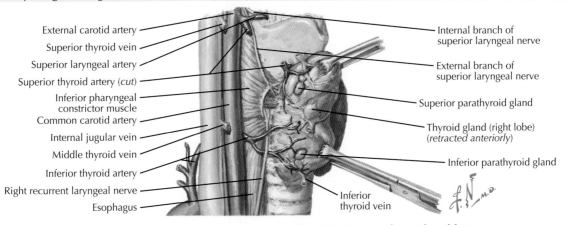

External carotid artery

Superior thyroid vein

Superior laryngeal artery

Superior thyroid artery (*cut*)

Inferior pharyngeal
constrictor muscle

Common carotid artery

Internal jugular vein

Middle thyroid vein

Inferior thyroid artery

Right recurrent laryngeal nerve

Esophagus

Internal branch of
superior laryngeal nerve

External branch of
superior laryngeal nerve

Superior parathyroid gland

Thyroid gland (right lobe)
(*retracted anteriorly*)

Inferior parathyroid gland

Inferior
thyroid vein

FIGURE 3.4 Surgical anatomy for thyroidectomy and parathyroidectomy.

PARATHYROIDECTOMY

Anatomy and Embryology of the Parathyroid Glands

A normal parathyroid gland is an oval, yellow or light-brown organ measuring a few millimeters (Fig. 3.5). Both superior and inferior parathyroids are supplied by the inferior thyroid artery.

Superior parathyroids develop from the fourth branchial pouch and are situated on the posteromedial surface of the superior thyroid pole. Because of embryologic migration, ectopic superior parathyroid glands can be found in the retropharyngeal, retroesophageal, posterior mediastinal, or intrathyroid location but are most commonly found in the tracheoesophageal groove. Superior parathyroids are more often subcapsular then the inferior parathyroids.

In contrast to the superior parathyroids, the inferior parathyroids undergo extensive migration; consequently their anatomic location is more variable. The most common ectopic location for the inferior parathyroid glands is within the thymus; however, it can be also found in the thyrothymic ligament, the anterosuperior mediastinum, undescended within the submandibular area, or within the thyroid gland (Fig. 3.6A).

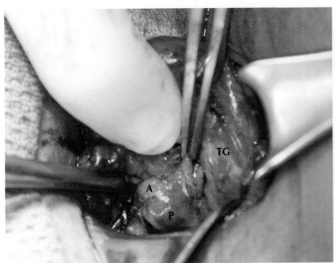
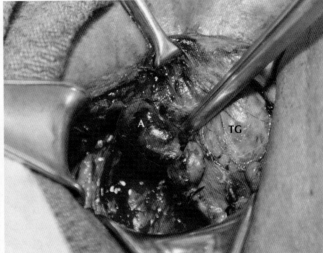

A. A normal superior parathyroid gland (*P*) surrounded by adipose tissue (*A*) is demonstrated with the thyroid gland (*TG*) retracted anteromedially.

B. A left inferior parathyroid adenoma (*A*) is depicted in its normal anatomic position with the thyroid gland (*TG*) mobilized anteromedially.

C. Development of the thyroid and parathyroid glands

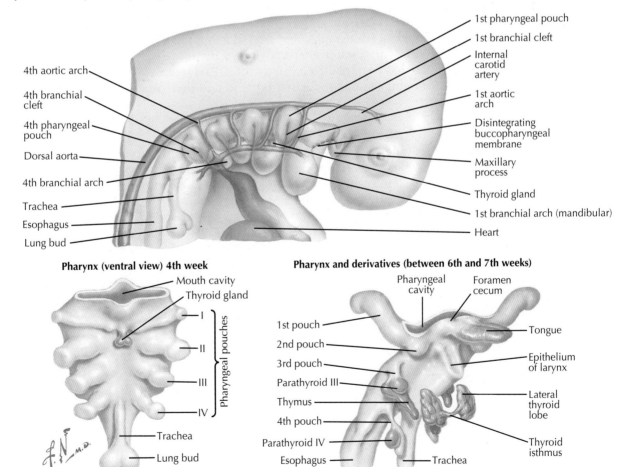

FIGURE 3.5 Anatomy and embryology of parathyroid glands.

Indication for Surgery

The only definitive treatment for primary, secondary, and tertiary hyperparathyroidism (HPT) is parathyroidectomy. For primary HPT, the extent of surgical exploration varies, even among high-volume centers. Some feel that focal parathyroid exploration guided by preoperative localizing tests and intra-operative PTH (IOPTH) measurement provides durable results. Others prefer routine four-gland exploration, regardless of localizing test results, because of the finding of multigland disease not suspected preoperatively. In opposition to primary HPT, in which single-gland adenoma is frequent, secondary and tertiary HPT patients have parathyroid hyperplasia, and therefore four-gland exploration is required.

Adjunct Tests

Preoperative imaging is routinely used to guide the surgical exploration. The procedures of choice are a surgeon-performed ultrasonography (that also identifies concomitant thyroid disease), technetium 99m sestamibi scintigraphy, and arterial enhanced CT (Fig. 3.6B).

A 50% decrease in IOPTH 10 minutes after excision of the diseased gland confirms that the hyperfunctioning tissue has been removed. Failure of IOPTH to drop 50% or greater indicates that the hyperfunctioning parathyroid is still present, and therefore further exploration is required.

Parathyroid Gland Exploration

The steps to expose the central neck are similar to a thyroidectomy but with a smaller incision. Ligating the middle thyroid vein is rarely necessary; however it can improve exposure of the central neck in certain cases. If the parathyroid glands are not found within their common positions, exploration should be continued in their ectopic location.

Management of parathyroid adenoma consists of resecting the diseased adenoma after visual confirmation that the other glands are normal and that the IOPTH decreases appropriately. Management of parathyroid hyperplasia consists of subtotal parathyroidectomy or total parathyroidectomy with autotransplant. During a subtotal parathyroidectomy, the parathyroid remnant should be created first, and its viability should be confirmed before resecting the other glands. Up to 15% of patients have a supernumerary gland; therefore, to avoid leaving one, the central neck should be thoroughly explored and a thymectomy should be routinely performed because this is the most common site of supernumerary glands.

A. Anatomic sites for ectopic parathyroid adenoma, with images of abnormal focus and a corresponding specimen

Sites for ectopic parathyroid glands.
Open circles depict the normal location for the superior and inferior parathyroid glands.

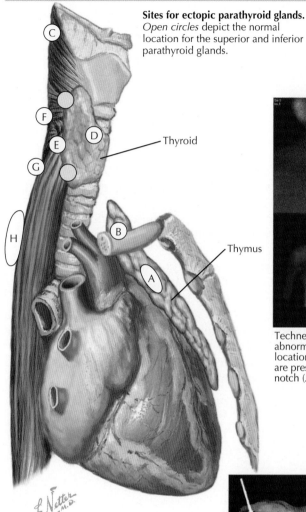

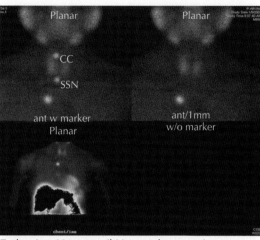

Technetium 99m sestamibi images demonstrating an abnormal focus of radiotracer accumulation in a retrosternal location on the right. In the first image, radiopaque markers are present on the cricoid cartilage (*CC*) and the suprasternal notch (*SSN*).

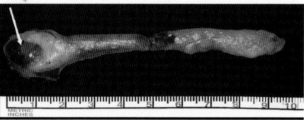

Intrathymic parathyroid adenoma (*arrow*) that corresponds to the abnormal focus of radiotracer accumulation seen on the technetium images.

B. Preoperative imaging of neck

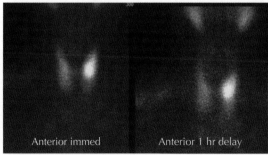

Technetium 99m sestamibi scan demonstrating an abnormal focus of radiotracer accumulation seen in the left side of the neck on immediate and 1-hour delayed images.

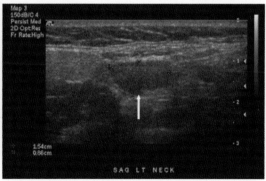

Static sonographic image in the sagittal plane demonstrating a homogeneous, hypoechoic mass inferior to the left lobe of the thyroid gland that corresponded to a left inferior parathyroid adenoma.

FIGURE 3.6 Anatomic sites for ectopic parathyroid adenoma and preoperative imaging of neck.

SUGGESTED READINGS

Irvin III GL, Dembrow VD, Prudhomme DL, et al. Operative monitoring of parathyroid gland hyperfunction. Am J Surg 1991;162.

Monteiro R, Han A, Etiwy M, et al. Importance of surgeon-performed ultrasound in the preoperative nodal assessment of patients with potential thyroid malignancy. Surgery 2018;163(1):112–7.

Pusztaszeri M, Rossi ED, Auger M, et al. The Bethesda system for reporting thyroid cytopathology: proposed modifications and updates for the second edition from an international panel. Acta Cytol 2016;60(5):399–405.

Siperstein S, Berber E, Barbosa GF, et al. Predicting the success of limited exploration for primary hyperparathyroidism using ultrasound, sestamibi, and intraoperative parathyroid hormone. Ann Surg 2008(3);248.

Wallace LB, Parikh RT, Ross LV, et al. The phenotype of primary hyperparathyroidism with normal parathyroid hormone levels: how low can parathyroid hormone go? Surgery 2011;150(6):1102–12.

Laparoscopic Adrenalectomy

Allan Siperstein and Edwina C. Moore

INTRODUCTION

The adrenals are paired retroperitoneal glands that lie partially anterior, superior, and medial to the upper pole of the kidneys, bounded by retroperitoneal fat and Gerota's fascia. The right adrenal gland is posteromedial to the right lobe of the liver and posterior to the inferior vena cava (IVC). The left adrenal gland is lateral to the aorta and posterior to the splenic artery and pancreatic tail (Figs. 4.1 and 4.2). The most common morphologic configuration is an inverted V or Y-shape, with an anteromedial body and two posterolateral limbs. A normal adrenal gland is 2 to 6 mm thick and 2 to 4 cm in length (Fig. 4.2, *inset*). Rarely small rests of adrenal tissue can be found near the adrenal bed or in the pelvis, which may be important in refractory cases.

The arterial supply is via the superior, middle, and inferior adrenal arteries, which branch from the inferior phrenic, abdominal aorta, and renal arteries, respectively. From a clinical perspective, the surgeon also encounters multiple, small, and unnamed branches. The venous drainage consists of one dominant vein that must be formally ligated and divided. The left adrenal vein often joins the medially located left inferior phrenic vein to form a common channel before entering the left renal vein. The right adrenal vein is short and drains directly into the posterolateral aspect of the IVC.

The adrenal gland is composed of a capsule, an outer cortex with three distinct functional layers (zona glomerulosa, zona fasciculata, zona reticularis), and an inner medulla (Fig. 4.3). Each cortical sublayer and the medulla secrete specific hormones with individual functions.

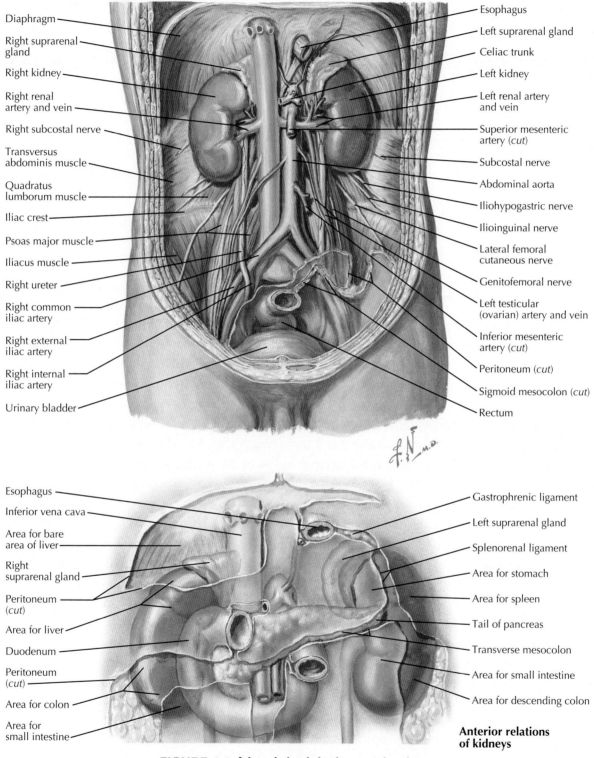

Diaphragm

Right suprarenal gland

Right kidney

Right renal artery and vein

Right subcostal nerve

Transversus abdominis muscle

Quadratus lumborum muscle

Iliac crest

Psoas major muscle

Iliacus muscle

Right ureter

Right common iliac artery

Right external iliac artery

Right internal iliac artery

Urinary bladder

Esophagus

Left suprarenal gland

Celiac trunk

Left kidney

Left renal artery and vein

Superior mesenteric artery (cut)

Subcostal nerve

Abdominal aorta

Iliohypogastric nerve

Ilioinguinal nerve

Lateral femoral cutaneous nerve

Genitofemoral nerve

Left testicular (ovarian) artery and vein

Inferior mesenteric artery (cut)

Peritoneum (cut)

Sigmoid mesocolon (cut)

Rectum

Esophagus

Inferior vena cava

Area for bare area of liver

Right suprarenal gland

Peritoneum (cut)

Area for liver

Duodenum

Peritoneum (cut)

Area for colon

Area for small intestine

Gastrophrenic ligament

Left suprarenal gland

Splenorenal ligament

Area for stomach

Area for spleen

Tail of pancreas

Transverse mesocolon

Area for small intestine

Area for descending colon

Anterior relations of kidneys

FIGURE 4.1 Adrenal glands in situ, anterior views.

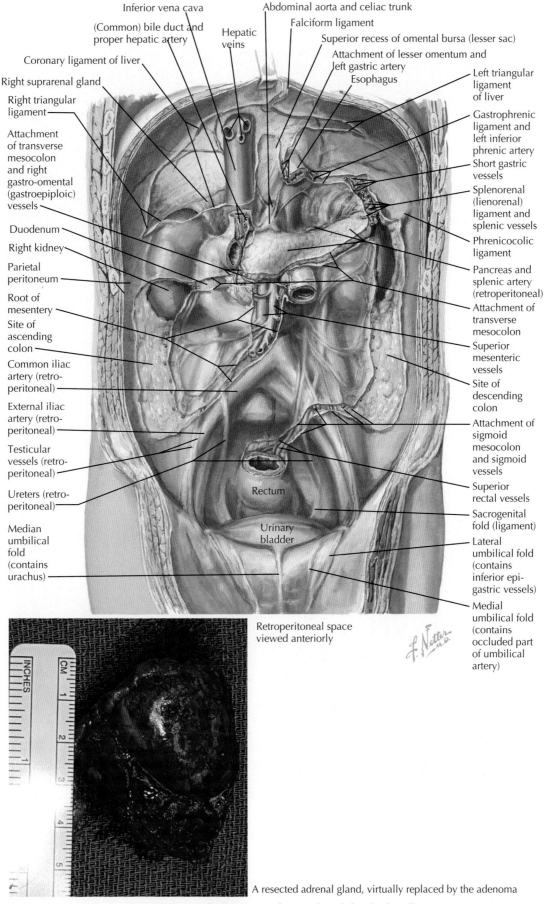

Inferior vena cava

(Common) bile duct and proper hepatic artery

Coronary ligament of liver

Right suprarenal gland

Right triangular ligament

Attachment of transverse mesocolon and right gastro-omental (gastroepiploic) vessels

Duodenum

Right kidney

Parietal peritoneum

Root of mesentery

Site of ascending colon

Common iliac artery (retro-peritoneal)

External iliac artery (retro-peritoneal)

Testicular vessels (retro-peritoneal)

Ureters (retro-peritoneal)

Median umbilical fold (contains urachus)

Hepatic veins

Abdominal aorta and celiac trunk

Falciform ligament

Superior recess of omental bursa (lesser sac)

Attachment of lesser omentum and left gastric artery

Esophagus

Left triangular ligament of liver

Gastrophrenic ligament and left inferior phrenic artery

Short gastric vessels

Splenorenal (lienorenal) ligament and splenic vessels

Phrenicocolic ligament

Pancreas and splenic artery (retroperitoneal)

Attachment of transverse mesocolon

Superior mesenteric vessels

Site of descending colon

Attachment of sigmoid mesocolon and sigmoid vessels

Superior rectal vessels

Sacrogenital fold (ligament)

Lateral umbilical fold (contains inferior epigastric vessels)

Medial umbilical fold (contains occluded part of umbilical artery)

Rectum

Urinary bladder

Retroperitoneal space viewed anteriorly

A resected adrenal gland, virtually replaced by the adenoma

FIGURE 4.2 Peritoneum of posterior abdominal wall.

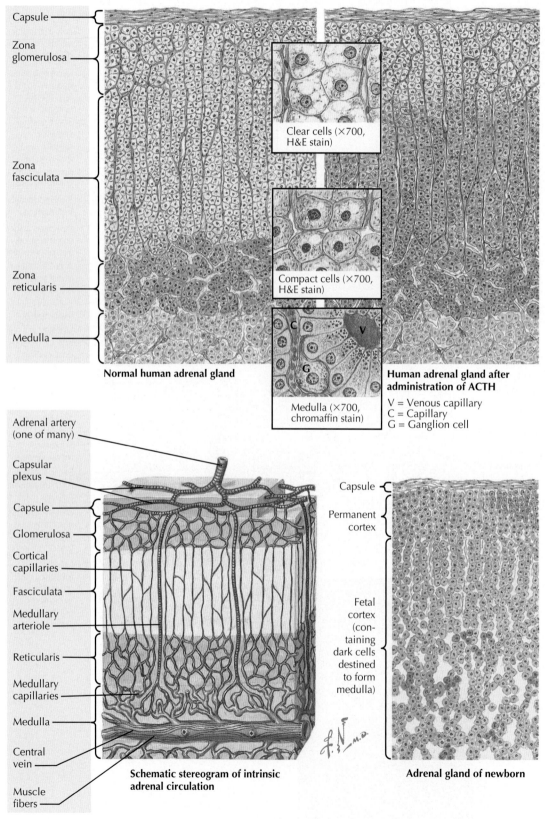

Normal human adrenal gland

Clear cells (×700, H&E stain)

Compact cells (×700, H&E stain)

Medulla (×700, chromaffin stain)

Human adrenal gland after administration of ACTH

V = Venous capillary
C = Capillary
G = Ganglion cell

Capsule
Zona glomerulosa
Zona fasciculata
Zona reticularis
Medulla

Adrenal artery (one of many)
Capsular plexus
Capsule
Glomerulosa
Cortical capillaries
Fasciculata
Medullary arteriole
Reticularis
Medullary capillaries
Medulla
Central vein
Muscle fibers

Schematic stereogram of intrinsic adrenal circulation

Capsule
Permanent cortex
Fetal cortex (containing dark cells destined to form medulla)

Adrenal gland of newborn

FIGURE 4.3 **Histology of the adrenal glands.** *ACTH,* Adrenocorticotropic hormone; *H&E,* hematoxylin and eosin.

SURGICAL PRINCIPLES

Cross-sectional imaging via a noncontrast computed tomography (CT) or magnetic resonance imaging (MRI) is integral in the workup of adrenal nodules (Fig. 4.4A and B). A CT with adrenal protocol is a three-phase scan that includes a nonenhanced phase, a postcontrast portal venous phase (70 seconds after intravenous injection of iodinated contrast), and a delayed phase (15 minutes after injection). It is important to calculate the contrast washout characteristics of an adrenal lesion, especially for lipid-poor adenomas. The Hounsfield scale is a quantitative measure of radiodensity and is best determined on a noncontrast image. The radiodensity of distilled water at standard pressure and temperature is defined as zero Hounsfield units (HU). Adrenal masses with low (<10U) HU are considered benign.

MRI evaluation of adrenal lesions may also be useful, although typically less sensitive than CT. A normal adrenal gland appears hypointense (dark) on T1- and T2-weighted images, relative to surrounding soft tissue. MRI enables excellent morphologic delineation of adrenal masses but, similar to CT, cannot distinguish the cortex from the medulla and therefore cannot differentiate cortical tumors from medullary tumors, adenomas from phaechromocytomas. The role of positron emission tomography-computed tomography (PET-CT) imaging for adrenal disease is limited to patients with a prior history of cancer. False negatives may be seen with necrotic or hemorrhagic metastases and non-fluorodeoxyglucose (FDG) avid cancers (e.g., neuroendocrine tumors [NETs]). Adrenal venous sampling has become the gold-standard practice for lateralization in primary aldosteronism (Fig. 4.4C and D).

Not all adrenal lesions warrant removal. Adrenalectomy should be considered in three independent scenarios:

1. Functional tumors with hypersecretion of adrenal hormones
2. Potentially malignant (indeterminate) tumors: unequivocal growth on serial imaging 6 months apart or HU >10 on noncontrast CT scan
3. Malignant tumors

Biopsy may be considered in very rare situations to obtain a tissue diagnosis in patients with adrenal metastases before initiating systemic treatment.

Subtotal or cortical-sparing adrenalectomy may be considered in patients with bilateral adrenal tumors or a heredity associated with high risk of recurrence (e.g., Von Hippel Lindau [VHL]), obviating the incidence of iatrogenic adrenal insufficiency and its numerous sequelae. Where possible, it is preferable to perform subtotal resection on the left as it is often harder to re-operate on the right.

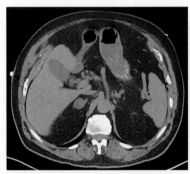

A. Noncontrast (axial cut) abdominal CT showing indeterminate right adrenal lesion (HU 20).

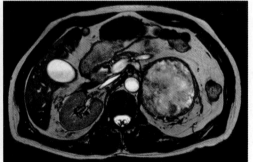

B. Abdominal MRI (axial cut) showing left adrenal phaeochromocytoma.

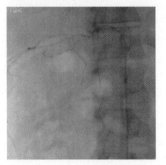

C. Right adrenal angiogram during adrenal venous sampling for a patient with primary hyperaldosteronism.

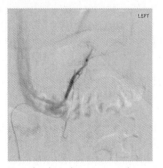

D. Left adrenal angiogram for patient in part C.

FIGURE 4.4 Adrenal gland in computed tomography (CT), magnetic resonance imaging (MRI), and positron emission tomography (PET).

SURGICAL TECHNIQUE

A minimally invasive approach has become the gold standard of care for adrenal surgery despite a paucity of RCTs comparing it with open surgery.

The location of the adrenals in the upper retroperitoneal space has led to the development of several surgical approaches: anterior transperitoneal, lateral transperitoneal, and posterior retroperitoneal. Each approach is associated with unique but important patient positioning to maximize exposure. When deciding the best approach for a patient, surgeons should consider body habitus, history of prior abdominal surgery, and tumor size and locality. Typically, lateral transabdominal adrenalectomy provides the widest operative field, and anatomic landmarks are most familiar. It is also easier to convert to an open approach in rare emergency settings and uses gravity for natural retraction of the liver/spleen. By contrast, the posterior retroperitoneal is advantageous for bilateral resections because it avoids the need to reposition and re-prep the patient. Relative contraindications to a retroperitoneal resection are tumors larger than 7 cm (difficult to create adequate working space), body mass index (BMI) exceeding 45 (difficult to create room on the operating table for the pannus), increased intraocular pressure (IOP; prone positioning increases IOP and, if prolonged, may cause optic nerve injury and blindness), and the need to explore the peritoneal cavity (e.g., to examine for metastatic disease).

Lateral Transperitoneal Approach

The patient is positioned in a lateral decubitus position with the side of the adrenal pathology facing upward (Fig. 4.5A). Three laparoscopic ports are usually adequate on the left; however, in obese patients, a fourth port may be required. On the right side, an extra port is always necessary for liver retraction. The ports are evenly placed between the midaxillary and midabdominal lines, approximately 2 cm below the costal margin. Once pneumoperitoneum is established, pressure is maintained at 16 to 18 mm Hg.

Right Lateral Transperitoneal Approach

The peritoneal cavity is visually inspected. The triangular ligament is divided, enabling medial rotation of the liver, to expose the right adrenal gland and IVC. The dissection is continued upwards toward the diaphragm. The peritoneum overlying the lateral border of the IVC is incised and the adrenal gland is gently retracted laterally. The areolar tissue posterior and lateral to the gland is divided with an energy device until the retroperitoneal muscles are seen. The superior pole is then mobilized off the diaphragm, being mindful of inferior phrenic venous tributaries. Once the adrenal vein is readily exposed, it is ligated and divided (Fig. 4.5B–E). By gently retracting the caudal aspect of the gland away from the renal hilum, the surgeon can avoid inadvertent injury to superior pole renal vessels (which may subsequently manifest as renovascular hypertension). The dissection is completed by dividing the superolateral and posterior attachments, which are done last to preserve access for the remainder of the operation.

Left Lateral Transperitoneal Approach

To access the retroperitoneal space, the splenic flexure is mobilized and gently retracted inferiorly. The spleen and tail of pancreas are medially rotated to expose Gerota's fascia. It is important not to dissect too far laterally and enter a plane behind the kidney. Mobilization of the adrenal gland is commenced in a top-down technique, starting superomedially and continuing circumferentially until the left adrenal vein is identified medially, often directly opposite the valley from the splenic vein. It is prudent to formally dissect the left adrenal vein, inferior phrenic, and common channel to avoid inadvertent injury. Once exposed, the adrenal vein is ligated and divided.

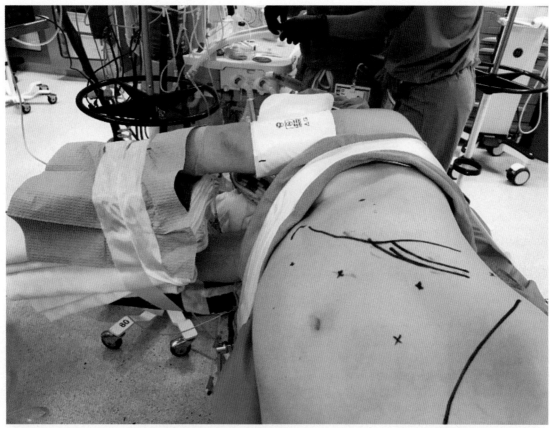

A. Patient placed in lateral decubitus position prior to a left laparoscopic transabdominal adrenalectomy

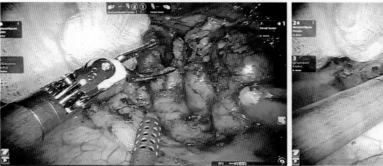

B. The right adrenal gland is mobilized circumferentially

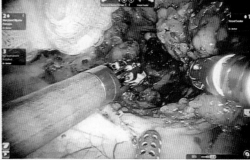

C. The right kidney is identified as the adrenal gland is retracted

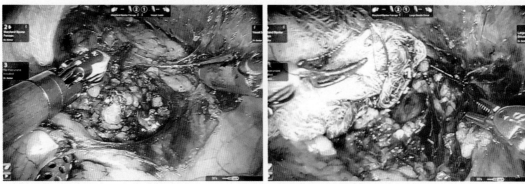

D. The adrenal vein as it inserts into the IVC

E. Ligation of the adrenal vein

FIGURE 4.5 Lateral transperitoneal approach.

Posterior Retroperitoneal Approach

The patient is positioned in a prone jackknife position (Fig. 4.6A). The chest and hips are placed on noncompressible bolsters. This creates a space for the abdomen and pannus to lie elevated off the table, which is important to maximize expansion of the retroperitoneal space. The hip bolster is placed at the joint in the bed where the torso meets the lower extremity. The bed is flexed 30 degrees at the junction of the upper and lower torso and 45 degrees at the junction of the lower torso and legs. In this position, the boundaries of the retroperitoneal space are paraspinal muscles medially, kidney/adrenals/peritoneum anteriorly (closer to the operating table), and thorax/ribs posteriorly (closer to the surgeon).

Three ports are standard in the posterior approach on the right and left sides. A 10-mm incision is made 2 cm inferior to the costal margin, halfway between the paraspinal muscles and the proposed lateral port. The subcutaneous space is bluntly dissected medially and laterally to allow for controlled insertion of the remaining ports. The lateral port is placed just inferior to the costal margin, ideally as far lateral as possible, and the medial port is placed just lateral to the paraspinal muscles. Pneumoperitoneum in the retroperitoneum is maintained at 18 to 22 mm Hg, which is slightly higher than for transperitoneal laparoscopy.

Intraoperative ultrasound can be used at this point to confirm the location of the adrenal gland and is especially useful in patients with copious fat or small tumors (e.g., primary aldosteronism). Using mostly blunt dissection, the surgeon divides flimsy posterior attachments of the perinephric and periadrenal fat from the peritoneum (laterally) and paraspinal muscles (medially). The adrenal gland is carefully mobilized circumferentially with blunt and sharp dissection, starting from the superolateral aspect and continuing caudally. A plane between the adrenal and paraspinal muscles is dissected to expose the inferior phrenic veins (on the left side) and IVC (on the right side). Inferior and medial retraction of the kidney helps to identify the adrenal vein (Fig. 4.6B–D). On the right, the adrenal vein can be traced to the midpoint of the adrenal gland on its anterior surface (closer to the table). On the left there is often a tongue of tissue extending along the left adrenal vein, which is important to fully dissect and remove.

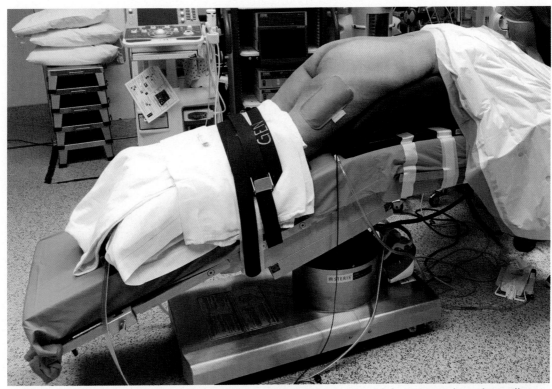

A. Patient placed in prone jackknife position prior to a retroperitoneal dissection with face supported on a foam pillow

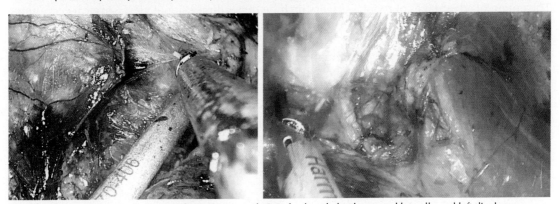

B. Loose areolar retroperitoneal tissue, first encountered after port placement in a posterior approach adrenalectomy

C. Left adrenal gland retracted laterally and left diaphragm

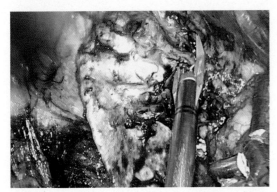

D. Left adrenal gland and left adrenal vein prior to clipping and division

FIGURE 4.6 **Posterior retroperitoneal approach.**

Robotic

The potential advantages of robotic surgery include three-dimensional view, surgical economics (wristed instruments), and a stable camera platform; however, the cost is higher for currently unproven patient gain.

Patient positioning and port placement are the same as for the laparoscopic approach. Once the trocars are inserted, the robot is docked at 11 o'clock from the patient's head for right adrenalectomy and one o'clock for left side. The robotic instruments are then attached to the robotic patient trolley. The primary surgeon moves to the console, while the assistant remains scrubbed at bedside (Fig. 4.7). Robotic dissection mirrors the laparoscopic approach. The appropriate plane of dissection corresponds to the anterior margin of the iliopsoas muscle in the periadrenal tissue, with a small margin away from the edge of the gland to avoid capsular effraction. The main adrenal vein is exposed, dissected, and divided between two clips.

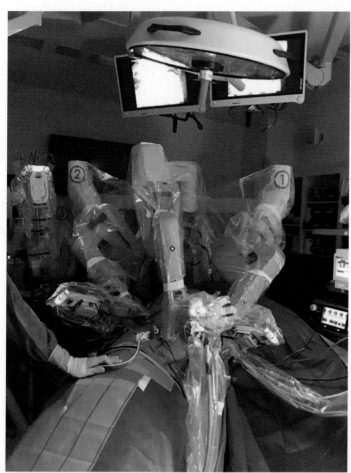

Robot docked during a transabdominal adrenalectomy. Four ports are used on the right: camera (10 mm), suction (5 mm), Maryland forceps (5 mm), and vessel sealer (5 mm)

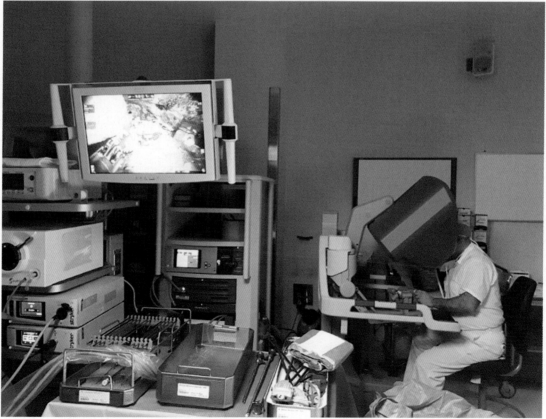

Surgeon at robotic console

FIGURE 4.7 **Robotic approach to adrenalectomy.**

TIPS AND TRICKS

- To avoid venous engorgement and a bloody operative field, it is prudent to control the fine arterial vessels supplying the adrenal gland before ligation of the adrenal vein.
- If bleeding occurs, it is usually low-pressure bleeding. Pack the area with hemostatic agents and gauze and wait. In most cases, the bleeding will stop spontaneously. The insufflation pressure can also be temporarily increased (up to 30 mm Hg) to assist with control but requires careful communication with the anesthetic team and being mindful of systemic CO_2 levels.
- Pneumoperitoneum via CO_2 insufflation can obscure low-pressure venous bleeding. At the conclusion of the case, lower the cavity pressure and inspect for occult bleeding.
- An indwelling catheter may be required during a posterior approach surgery, because the elevated local pressure can impair urine output.

SUGGESTED READINGS

Goenka AH, Shah SN, Remer EM, Berber E. Adrenal imaging: a primer for oncosurgeons. J Sur Oncol 2012;106:543–8.

Kebebew E, Siperstein AE, Clark OH, Duh QY. Results of laparoscopic adrenalectomy for suspected and unsuspected malignant adrenal neoplasms. Arch Surg 2002;137:948–51.

Mazzaglia PA, Vezeridis MP. Laparoscopic adrenalectomy: balancing the operative indications with technical advances. J Sur Oncol 2010;101:739–44.

Okoh AK, Berber E. Laparoscopic and robotic adrenal surgery: transperitoneal approach. Gland Surgery 2015;4(5):435–41.

Taskin HE, Siperstein AE, Mercan S, Berber E. Laparoscopic posterior retroperitoneal adrenalectomy. J Sur Oncol 2012;106:619–21.

SECTION 3

Upper Gastrointestinal

SECTION EDITORS: **Matthew Kroh and
John H. Rodriguez**

Esophagectomy

Andrew Tang, Usman Ahmad, and Siva Raja

INTRODUCTION

Franz Torek performed the first successful esophagectomy in 1913, after 30 years of dismal results without any survivors. Improvements in technique and patient care have reduced morbidity and mortality; however, esophagectomy remains a high-risk procedure because of the challenging anatomic position of the esophagus, involvement of multiple body cavities in the resection (Fig. 5.1), tenuous blood supply of all reconstruction options, and the patient's often malnourished status.

SURGICAL APPROACHES

Active controversy surrounds the necessity for surgery in esophageal cancer, with minimalists stressing the poor cancer survival despite morbidity of radical surgery. However, it has been well validated that esophagectomy can be performed with low morbidity (33%) and mortality (3%).

The three most commonly employed approaches to esophagectomy are transhiatal, Ivor Lewis, and/or modified McKeown approach. In select patients a left thoracoabdominal esophagectomy can also be effective. Increasingly, many of these approaches are being performed minimally invasively and are broadly labeled as minimally invasive esophagectomy (MIE). The approach used depends on the surgical indication (e.g., transhiatal approach for benign conditions and small cancers), cancer stage, tumor location (e.g., modified McKeown for upper and middle esophageal cancers), and, above all, surgeon preference. There is no overwhelming evidence demonstrating the superiority of any one specific technique. The tumor location should be well established and generous proximal and distal margins ensured, because esophageal cancers spread not only to the regional lymph nodes but also along the submucosal lymphatic channels of the esophagus.

Reconstruction most often uses the stomach, with varying degrees of tubularization. Alternatives include colonic interposition or jejunal interposition, which requires microvascular augmentation or free flap, depending on the segment of esophagus that will be replaced, and rarely other soft tissue flaps for short segment reconstruction. Because any of these conduits have tenuous vascularity, the surgeon needs to be familiar with all esophageal reconstruction options.

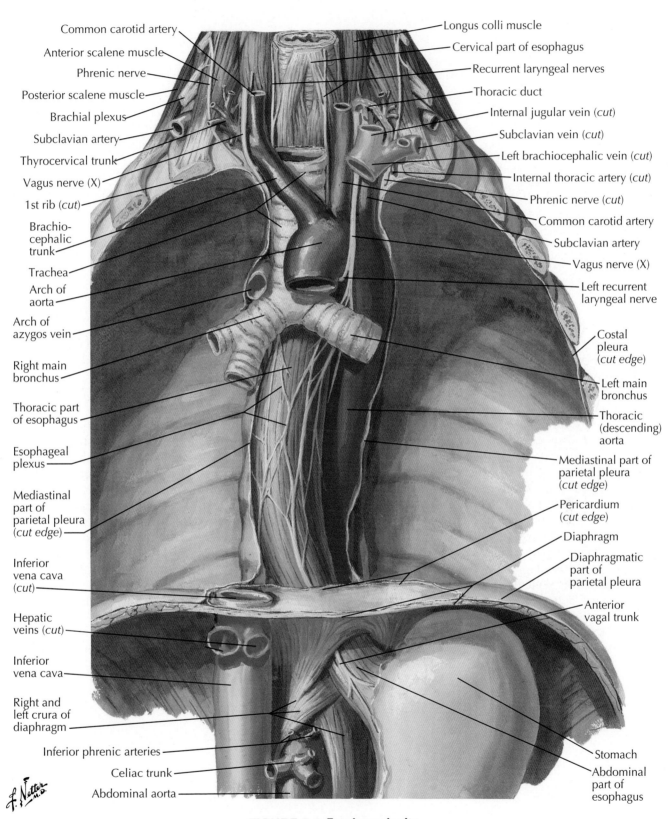

Common carotid artery

Anterior scalene muscle

Phrenic nerve

Posterior scalene muscle

Brachial plexus

Subclavian artery

Thyrocervical trunk

Vagus nerve (X)

1st rib (*cut*)

Brachio-
cephalic
trunk

Trachea

Arch of
aorta

Arch of
azygos vein

Right main
bronchus

Thoracic part
of esophagus

Esophageal
plexus

Mediastinal
part of
parietal pleura
(*cut edge*)

Inferior
vena cava
(*cut*)

Hepatic
veins (*cut*)

Inferior
vena cava

Right and
left crura of
diaphragm

Inferior phrenic arteries

Celiac trunk

Abdominal aorta

Longus colli muscle

Cervical part of esophagus

Recurrent laryngeal nerves

Thoracic duct

Internal jugular vein (*cut*)

Subclavian vein (*cut*)

Left brachiocephalic vein (*cut*)

Internal thoracic artery (*cut*)

Phrenic nerve (*cut*)

Common carotid artery

Subclavian artery

Vagus nerve (X)

Left recurrent
laryngeal nerve

Costal
pleura
(*cut edge*)

Left main
bronchus

Thoracic
(descending)
aorta

Mediastinal part of
parietal pleura
(*cut edge*)

Pericardium
(*cut edge*)

Diaphragm

Diaphragmatic
part of
parietal pleura

Anterior
vagal trunk

Stomach

Abdominal
part of
esophagus

FIGURE 5.1 Esophagus in situ.

Transhiatal Esophagectomy

The transhiatal esophagectomy is performed with the patient supine and the left side of the neck exposed. This approach begins in the abdomen, then traverses the hiatus to bluntly dissect the thoracic esophagus free, and reaches the neck to conclude the operation.

Abdominal exposure is achieved through either an upper midline incision (Fig. 5.2) or appropriate laparoscopic access.

Exploration is performed to rule out disseminated tumor, which would obviate resection. The dissection starts at the short gastric vessels and moves toward the left crus. Key steps include mobilizing the greater curvature while preserving the right gastroepiploic artery, then dividing the retrogastric adhesions to the pancreas. Many surgeons use a Kocher maneuver to mobilize the duodenum to provide additional conduit length, but this is not always necessary. Gastroesophageal (GE) junction dissection involves dividing the gastrohepatic ligament and phrenoesophageal attachments to the GE junction, and exposing the aorta at the diaphragmatic hiatus. The right gastric artery and its perforators are also preserved to maintain additional blood supply to the gastric conduit.

For distal esophageal cancers and gastroesophageal junction cancers, lymph node dissection includes skeletonizing the left gastric pedicle and proximal common hepatic artery as needed (Fig. 5.2C and D). The extensive lymphadenectomy of gastric cancer surgery is not routinely performed unless there is lymphadenopathy on imaging. Nodal tissue is left en bloc with the specimen.

The hiatus is opened, excising a rim of the hiatal musculature and entering the mediastinum in the plane of the mediastinal pleura, pericardium, and preaortic/prespinal planes.

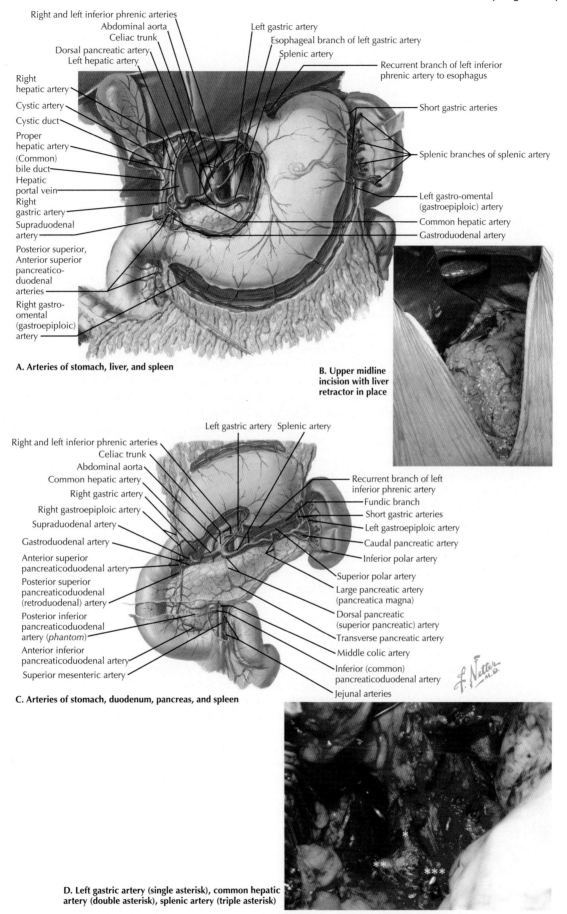

A. Arteries of stomach, liver, and spleen

Right and left inferior phrenic arteries
Abdominal aorta
Celiac trunk
Dorsal pancreatic artery
Left hepatic artery
Right hepatic artery
Cystic artery
Cystic duct
Proper hepatic artery
(Common) bile duct
Hepatic portal vein
Right gastric artery
Supraduodenal artery
Posterior superior, Anterior superior pancreatico-duodenal arteries
Right gastro-omental (gastroepiploic) artery

Left gastric artery
Esophageal branch of left gastric artery
Splenic artery
Recurrent branch of left inferior phrenic artery to esophagus
Short gastric arteries
Splenic branches of splenic artery
Left gastro-omental (gastroepiploic) artery
Common hepatic artery
Gastroduodenal artery

B. Upper midline incision with liver retractor in place

C. Arteries of stomach, duodenum, pancreas, and spleen

Right and left inferior phrenic arteries
Celiac trunk
Abdominal aorta
Common hepatic artery
Right gastric artery
Right gastroepiploic artery
Supraduodenal artery
Gastroduodenal artery
Anterior superior pancreaticoduodenal artery
Posterior superior pancreaticoduodenal (retroduodenal) artery
Posterior inferior pancreaticoduodenal artery (phantom)
Anterior inferior pancreaticoduodenal artery
Superior mesenteric artery

Left gastric artery Splenic artery
Recurrent branch of left inferior phrenic artery
Fundic branch
Short gastric arteries
Left gastroepiploic artery
Caudal pancreatic artery
Inferior polar artery
Superior polar artery
Large pancreatic artery (pancreatica magna)
Dorsal pancreatic (superior pancreatic) artery
Transverse pancreatic artery
Middle colic artery
Inferior (common) pancreaticoduodenal artery
Jejunal arteries

D. Left gastric artery (single asterisk), common hepatic artery (double asterisk), splenic artery (triple asterisk)

FIGURE 5.2 Anatomy of the lesser curve, second portion of the duodenum, and gastrohepatic ligament (stomach is rotated cephalad).

Transhiatal Esophagectomy (Continued)

Open transhiatal surgery is performed by cupping the esophagus in the extended fingers, bluntly stripping the esophagus up to the proximal mediastinum to the thoracic inlet. This maneuver may cause temporary hypotension resulting from cardiac compression; therefore it is important to communicate with the anesthesia team when this is being performed. Similar dissection can be performed laparoscopically.

At the same time, a 5- to 7-cm incision is made in the left neck from the sternal notch along the anterior sternocleidomastoid muscle border. The platysma muscle is divided and the sternocleidomastoid is retracted laterally. After the omohyoid muscle is divided, dissection is carried out in the tracheoesophageal groove. The fat pad, containing the left recurrent laryngeal nerve, is mobilized toward the airway, and circumferential control of the esophagus is obtained by encircling the esophagus with a soft drain (Fig. 5.3). Placing a nasogastric tube helps define the esophageal anatomy to facilitate blunt dissection. The upper mediastinal dissection is then performed bluntly inferiorly to meet the dissection from below. The esophagus is pulled into the neck and transected with a tissue stapler cutter, after pulling back the nasogastric tube (see Fig. 5.3). The distal staple line is sewn to a Penrose drain and reduced back into the abdomen along with the drain to maintain the track.

The gastric conduit is prepared by stretching the gastric cardia into the left upper quadrant (see Fig. 5.3E). Starting at the right gastric perforator just below the left gastric pedicle, the stomach is divided along the lesser curvature using a linear stapler, parallel to the greater curvature, to create a gastric conduit about 5 cm in width.

Some have advocated using narrow conduits to improve conduit emptying. The staple line can be started lower on the lesser curve if necessary to maintain a negative distal margin, making sure not to injure the right gastric artery (see Fig. 5.3F).

During laparoscopic tubularization, the conduit tip is either left attached to the specimen or sewn to the specimen before being pulled up into the neck. A hand-sewn or hybrid stapled anastomosis (modified collard anastomosis) is created to restore continuity (see Fig. 5.3G). The nasogastric tube is advanced into the conduit for decompression. Although some surgeons perform an intraoperative endoscopy to examine the anastomosis, we, and most others, do not routinely perform this.

A feeding jejunostomy tube is then placed 30 cm from the ligament of Treitz (see Fig. 5.3H).

Pyloric drainage, which includes pyloromyotomy, pyloroplasty, or injection of botulinum toxin A to the pylorus, is also typically performed. Some surgeons who use narrow gastric conduits no longer perform drainage procedures.

The excess conduit is reduced into the abdomen and secured to the hiatus to prevent herniation of abdominal viscera into the mediastinum (see Fig. 5.3I).

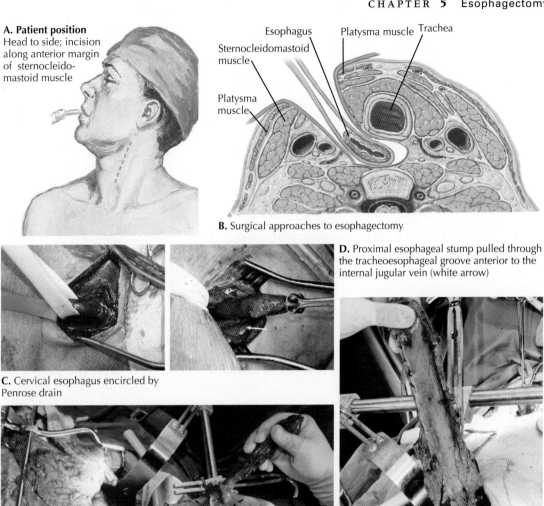

A. Patient position
Head to side; incision along anterior margin of sternocleido-mastoid muscle

Esophagus

Platysma muscle   Trachea

Sternocleidomastoid muscle

Platysma muscle

B. Surgical approaches to esophagectomy

C. Cervical esophagus encircled by Penrose drain

D. Proximal esophageal stump pulled through the tracheoesophageal groove anterior to the internal jugular vein (white arrow)

E. Gastric mobilization with preservation of right gastroepiploic artery arcade (black arrow), black dotted lines show the planned staple line for creation of the conduit

F. Gastric conduit prior to being pulled into the neck

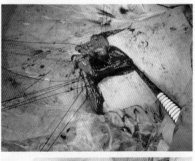

G. Modified Collard anastomosis

H. Stamm jejunostomy with 12 Fr T-tube

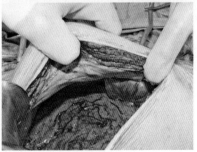

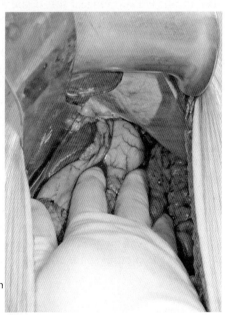

I. Reduction of excess conduit into the abdomen and pexy to the hiatus

FIGURE 5.3 Transhiatal esophagectomy.

Ivor Lewis and McKeown Approaches

The McKeown and Ivor Lewis approaches require transthoracic access, through right postero-lateral thoracotomy in the fifth intercostal space or thoracoscopy. The Ivor Lewis approach is defined by an intrathoracic anastomosis, whereas the McKeown approach is characterized by cervical anastomosis. The order in which the dissection is performed also differs between techniques.

The Ivor Lewis approach starts with gastric mobilization, then proceeds with thoracic (or thoracoscopic) dissection and intrathoracic anastomosis. The modified McKeown procedure starts with right thoracoscopy or thoracotomy to dissect the mediastinal esophagus from a left lateral decubitus position. The patient is then placed supine for the abdominal dissection and gastric conduit creation. The gastric conduit is created along the greater curve of the esophagus and then brought through the left neck to perform the anastomosis.

Ivor Lewis Esophagectomy

The patient is initially positioned supine and the abdomen is accessed through an upper abdominal incision or by five-port upper abdomen laparoscopy. Robotically assisted abdominal dissection ports are often placed slightly lower than their laparoscopic counterparts to avoid instrument collision.

After careful staging examination, the stomach is mobilized as described for the transhiatal approach. To wrap the intrathoracic anastomosis, an omental flap is created by maintaining the vascular pedicle from the distal one or two gastroepiploic arcade perforators (Fig. 5.4A).

The patient is then repositioned in a left lateral decubitus position for access to the right chest (5th intercostal posterolateral thoracotomy or thoracoscopy). The mediastinal pleura is widely excised in continuity with the esophagus. The esophagus is encircled and retracted using a Penrose drain. Periesophageal soft tissue and lymphatic tissue are resected en bloc. An advantage of this approach is the ability to skeletonize the pericardium and descending aorta under direct visualization. This allows for en bloc resection of periesophageal tissue, which is important oncologically for locally advanced esophageal tumors. The esophagus is divided above the azygos vein, which may require transecting the azygous vein. Identification and preservation of the membranous airway is vital, because thermal injury can result in delayed airway perforation, increasing the risk of conduit-airway fistulae. The specimen attached to the gastric conduit is delivered into the chest. Care should be taken to maintain the anatomic orientation of the conduit as it is delivered into the chest. A staple or hand-sewn esophago-gastric anastomosis can be performed (Fig. 5.4B).

This is typically an end-to-side functional end-to-end anastomosis performed between the esophagus and the greater curve of the stomach; as close as possible to the end of the right gastroepiploic artery to maximize conduit viability. The excess conduit is then resected with a tissue stapler cutter. The preserved omental pedicle is then placed between the gastric conduit and membranous airway and secured to the conduit. Sometimes the mediastinal pleura and the azygous vein can be preserved to act as a tissue barrier between the airway and anastomosis. Drains in the pleural space and can also control potential anastomotic leak.

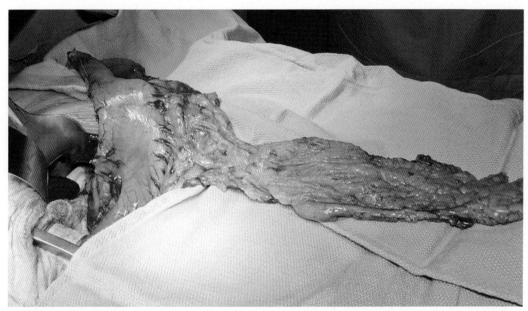

A. Gastric conduit preparation for Ivor-Lewis esophagectomy preserving the greater omentum to buttress the intrathoracic anastomosis

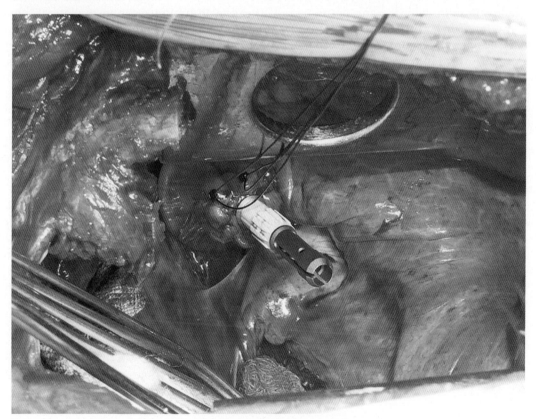

B. Double purse string around the EEA anvil for an intrathoracic anastomosis

FIGURE 5.4 Ivor Lewis esophagectomy.

Modified McKeown (Three-Hole) Esophagectomy

This is the best choice for middle and upper cancers or when thoracic staging is important to determine resectability. The three-hole procedure begins with the patient in the left lateral decubitus position with the arm positioned overhead. A fifth intercostal posterolateral thoracotomy (or four-port thoracoscopic access) is used for wide resection of the right mediastinal pleura, leaving the pleura over the esophagus, particularly over the tumor. Again, the dissection is performed in the subvagal plane when adjacent to the membranous airway to prevent immediate or delayed injury. The azygos vein may be divided, but preserving it allows for mediastinal anastomotic coverage and helps prevent thoracic leak (Fig. 5.5A, B, and C). The esophagus is retracted using an encircled Penrose drain. The esophagus and its surrounding lymph node tissues are mobilized, using cautery or ultrasonic shears.

The proximal dissection should be taken as superiorly as possible into the thoracic outlet and the distal dissection inferiorly to the crura. Similar to the thoracic dissection of an Ivor Lewis esophagectomy, care must be taken around the carina, where the membranous mainstem bronchi are at risk of sharp or thermal injury (Fig. 5.5D).

Once the thoracic dissection is complete, a chest drain is placed and the chest is closed. The patient is repositioned supine and the abdominal portion is performed as described for transhiatal esophagectomy. Small tumors can be brought through the neck incision, pulling the conduit up at the same time. Larger cancers should be pulled into the abdomen, placed in an impermeable specimen bag, and withdrawn through a small abdominal incision. The anastomosis is performed with staples (circular or double linear firing) or is hand-sewn. Drains are placed and the incisions are closed.

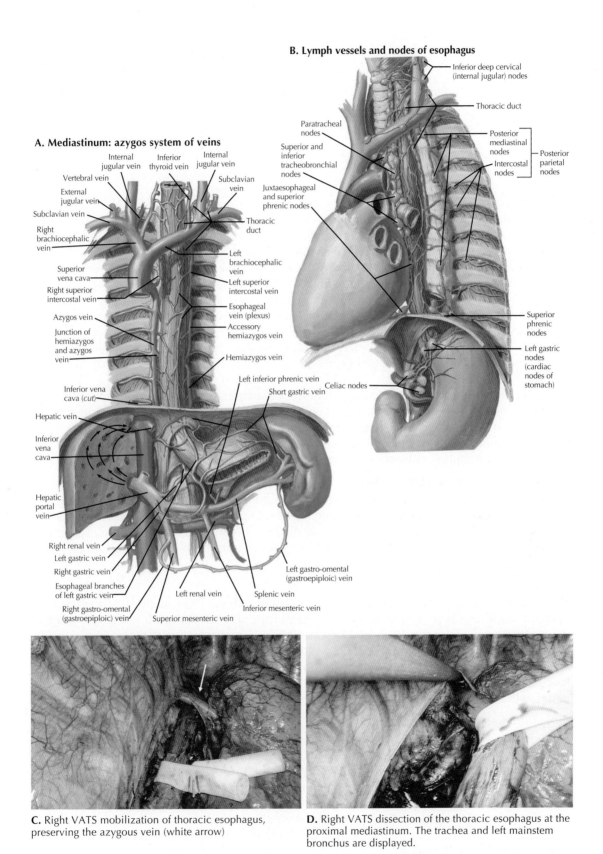

B. Lymph vessels and nodes of esophagus

Inferior deep cervical (internal jugular) nodes

Thoracic duct

Paratracheal nodes

Posterior mediastinal nodes

Posterior parietal nodes

Superior and inferior tracheobronchial nodes

Intercostal nodes

Juxtaesophageal and superior phrenic nodes

Superior phrenic nodes

Left gastric nodes (cardiac nodes of stomach)

Celiac nodes

A. Mediastinum: azygos system of veins

Internal jugular vein

Inferior thyroid vein

Internal jugular vein

Vertebral vein

Subclavian vein

External jugular vein

Subclavian vein

Right brachiocephalic vein

Thoracic duct

Superior vena cava

Left brachiocephalic vein

Right superior intercostal vein

Left superior intercostal vein

Azygos vein

Esophageal vein (plexus)

Junction of hemiazygos and azygos vein

Accessory hemiazygos vein

Hemiazygos vein

Inferior vena cava (cut)

Left inferior phrenic vein

Short gastric vein

Hepatic vein

Inferior vena cava

Left gastro-omental (gastroepiploic) vein

Hepatic portal vein

Right renal vein

Left gastric vein

Right gastric vein

Splenic vein

Esophageal branches of left gastric vein

Left renal vein

Inferior mesenteric vein

Right gastro-omental (gastroepiploic) vein

Superior mesenteric vein

Celiac nodes

C. Right VATS mobilization of thoracic esophagus, preserving the azygous vein (white arrow)

D. Right VATS dissection of the thoracic esophagus at the proximal mediastinum. The trachea and left mainstem bronchus are displayed.

FIGURE 5.5 Modified McKeown (three-hole) esophagectomy.

Left Thoracoabdominal Esophagectomy

A less common approach is the left thoracoabdominal esophagectomy, which has value in morbidly obese patients, prior upper midline abdominal surgery, or when the extent of disease is unclear. The incision is made in the left chest in the seventh interspace, crossing the costal arch, and is predominantly in the chest with limited abdominal extension (Fig. 5.6A). The diaphragm is divided close to the chest wall until the inferior tip of the spleen is visualized.

After the retractors are placed, the short gastric vessels are divided to gain access to the lesser sac, allowing for gastric conduit creation as previously described. The thoracic dissection is performed en bloc from the hiatus to the level of the inferior pulmonary vein and into the mediastinum in a subvagal plane similar to a transhiatal approach. The neck dissection allows for circumferential control of the esophagus, facilitating the standard gastric pull-up and anastomosis (Fig. 5.6B).

Closing the thoracoabdominal incision requires the diaphragm to be closed with interrupted horizontal mattress sutures. The pericostal sutures and the sutures used to close the arch are placed without excess tension to avoid arch subluxation (Fig. 5.6C).

The abdominal fascia is closed separately. This approach, when used regularly, can be performed in a short time, because the entire surgery can be done without repositioning the patient.

Minimally Invasive Esophagectomy

The three main approaches to the esophagectomy can employ a hybrid of open and minimally invasive approaches. However, to be deemed a true minimally invasive esophagectomy (MIE), the entire procedure is performed laparoscopically and thoracoscopically, including the critical steps of creating the gastric conduit and esophagogastric anastomosis (intrathoracically for Ivor-Lewis, at the base of the neck in McKeown).

Intrathoracic

The patient is placed in the left lateral decubitus position with slight flexion at the hips. Four ports are used (Fig. 5.7). A 10-mm port is placed in the seventh or eighth intercostal space in the midaxillary line for the 30-degree laparoscope. A 5-mm port is placed anteriorly for the ultrasonic shears or bipolar vessel sealer. Two additional ports are placed for retraction as shown later (see Fig. 5.7). The esophageal mobilization extends more superiorly in McKeown versus Ivor-Lewis. The inferior portion of the dissection should not extend too far into the peritoneum, which can cause loss of CO_2 insufflation into the abdomen.

Intraabdominal

The patient is placed supine in reverse Trendelenburg on a split-leg table for the abdominal portion. During dissection five ports are used: three 5-mm and two 12-mm ports (Fig. 5.7C). A 30-degree 10-mm laparoscope is used in the midline through a 12-mm port, and a laparoscopic linear stapler is used in the right upper quadrant through a 12-mm port. A liver retractor is placed through the right lateralmost 5-mm port. The left two 5-mm ports are used by the assistant to provide retraction. The steps of the dissection are similar to what was stated earlier; however, the phrenoesophageal ligament is divided last to prevent escape of the pneumoperitoneum into the mediastinum.

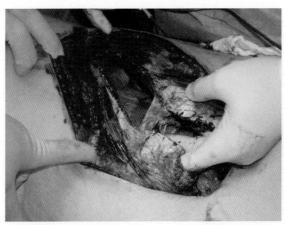

A. Left thoracoabdominal incision through the 7th intercostal space, dividing the diaphragm

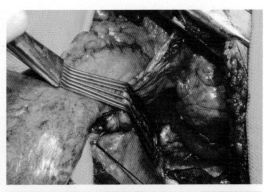

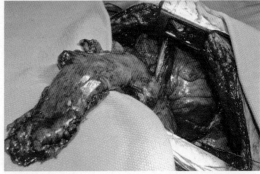

B. Creation of gastric conduit in preparation for pull-up into the chest

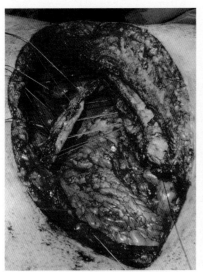

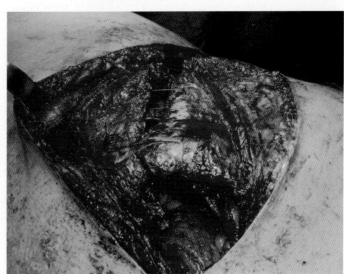

C. Closure of the subcostal arch

FIGURE 5.6 Left thoracoabdominal esophagectomy.

Anastomosis

During the Ivor-Lewis approach, the intrathoracic anastomosis is created thoracoscopically. The anvil is attached to the remnant esophagus either by suturing it in intracorporeally or by using an Orvil device. The EEA stapler is placed through the anterior axillary port into the gastric conduit and connected to the Orvil in a fashion in which staple lines do not overlap.

During the modified McKeown, the anastomosis is created in the neck in the same manner as during the open procedure.

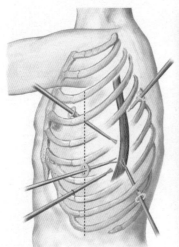

A. Ivor Lewis esophagectomy: five-port laparascopic placement

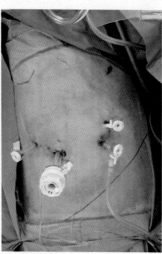

B. Right VATS ports

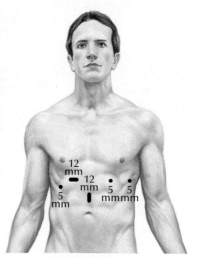

C. Intraabdominal: five-port placement

FIGURE 5.7 **Intrathoracic.**

SUGGESTED READINGS

Ercan S, Rice TW, Murthy SC, Rybicki LA, Blackstone EH. Does esophagogastric anastomotic technique influence the outcome of patients with esophageal cancer? J Thorac Cardiovasc Surg 2005;129(3):623–31. https://doi.org/10.1016/j.jtcvs.2004.08.024.

Gaur P, Blackmon SH. Jejunal graft conduits after esophagectomy. J Thorac Dis 2014;6(SUPPL. 3):333–40. https://doi.org/10.3978/j.issn.2072-1439.2014.05.07.

Lewis I. The surgical treatment of carcinoma of the oesophagus with special reference to a new operation for growths of the middle third. Br J Surg 1946;34(133):18–31.

Low DE, Alderson D, Cecconello I, et al. International consensus on standardization of data collection for complications associated with esophagectomy: Esophagectomy Complications Consensus Group (ECCG). Ann Surg 2015;262(2):286–94. https://doi.org/10.1097/SLA .0000000000001098.

Luketich JD, Pennathur A, Awais O, et al. Outcomes after minimally invasive esophagectomy. Ann Surg 2012;256(1):95–103. https://doi.org/10.1097/SLA.0b013e3182590603.

McKeown KC. Total three-stage oesophagectomy for cancer of the oesophagus. Br J Surg 1976;63(4):259–62. https://doi.org/10.1002/bjs.1800630403.

Orringer MB. Transhiatal esophagectomy: how I teach it. Ann Thorac Surg 2016;102(5): 1432–7. https://doi.org/10.1016/j.athoracsur.2016.09.044.

Rice TW, Rusch VW, Apperson-Hansen C, et al. Worldwide esophageal cancer collaboration. Dis Esophagus 2009;22(1):1–8. https://doi.org/10.1111/j.1442-2050.2008.00901.x.

Seder CW, Raymond D, Wright CD, et al. The Society of Thoracic Surgeons General Thoracic Surgery database 2018 update on outcomes and quality. Ann Thorac Surg 2018;105(5): 1304–7. https://doi.org/10.1016/j.athoracsur.2018.02.006.

Minimally Invasive Antireflux Surgery

Cynthia E. Weber and Leena Khaitan

▶ VIDEO

6.1 Laparoscopic Nissen Fundoplication

INTRODUCTION

Gastroesophageal reflux disease (GERD) remains one of the most common diseases for which patients seek medical treatment. Surgical intervention is offered after failure of maximal medical therapy and/or when an anatomic defect, such as a hiatal hernia, is detected, or if the patient is suffering a complication of reflux such as a stricture. Minimally invasive antireflux surgery serves to reestablish the original anatomic barriers to reflux and reinforce the closing function of the lower esophageal sphincter (LES) by wrapping the gastric fundus around the gastroesophageal junction (GEJ).

SURGICAL PRINCIPLES

Successful antireflux surgery results in recreation of a functional LES complex. This begins with circumferential dissection of the diaphragmatic crura and identification of a possible hiatal defect. If herniated, the GEJ is reduced below the diaphragm with the goal of at least 4 cm of intraabdominal esophageal length. The crura are reapproximated with sutures to allow only the esophagus to fit through the hiatal opening. After closure of the crura, a "floppy" 360-degree Nissen fundoplication is formed around the distal esophagus as the most commonly performed procedure to augment the lower esophageal sphincter (Figs. 6.1 to 6.3).

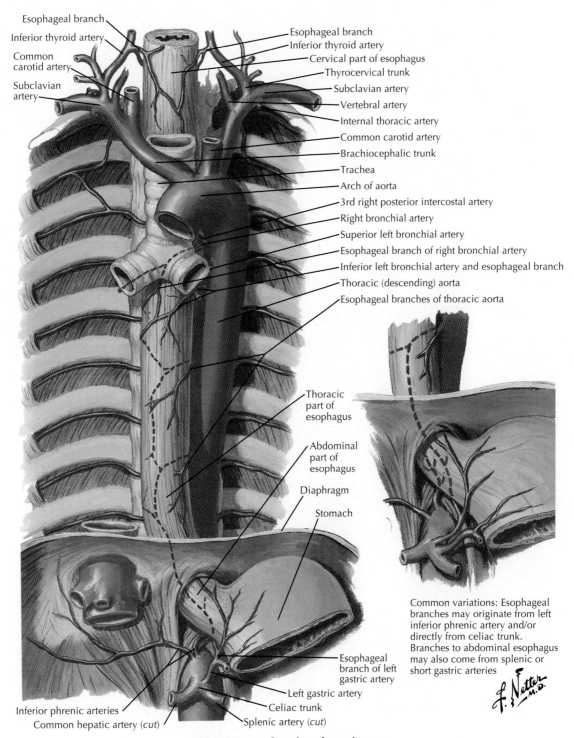

Esophageal branch
Inferior thyroid artery
Common carotid artery
Subclavian artery

Esophageal branch
Inferior thyroid artery
Cervical part of esophagus
Thyrocervical trunk
Subclavian artery
Vertebral artery
Internal thoracic artery
Common carotid artery
Brachiocephalic trunk
Trachea
Arch of aorta
3rd right posterior intercostal artery
Right bronchial artery
Superior left bronchial artery
Esophageal branch of right bronchial artery
Inferior left bronchial artery and esophageal branch
Thoracic (descending) aorta
Esophageal branches of thoracic aorta

Thoracic part of esophagus

Abdominal part of esophagus

Diaphragm

Stomach

Esophageal branch of left gastric artery

Left gastric artery
Celiac trunk
Splenic artery (cut)

Inferior phrenic arteries
Common hepatic artery (cut)

Common variations: Esophageal branches may originate from left inferior phrenic artery and/or directly from celiac trunk. Branches to abdominal esophagus may also come from splenic or short gastric arteries.

f. Netter M.D.

FIGURE 6.1 **Arteries of esophagus.**

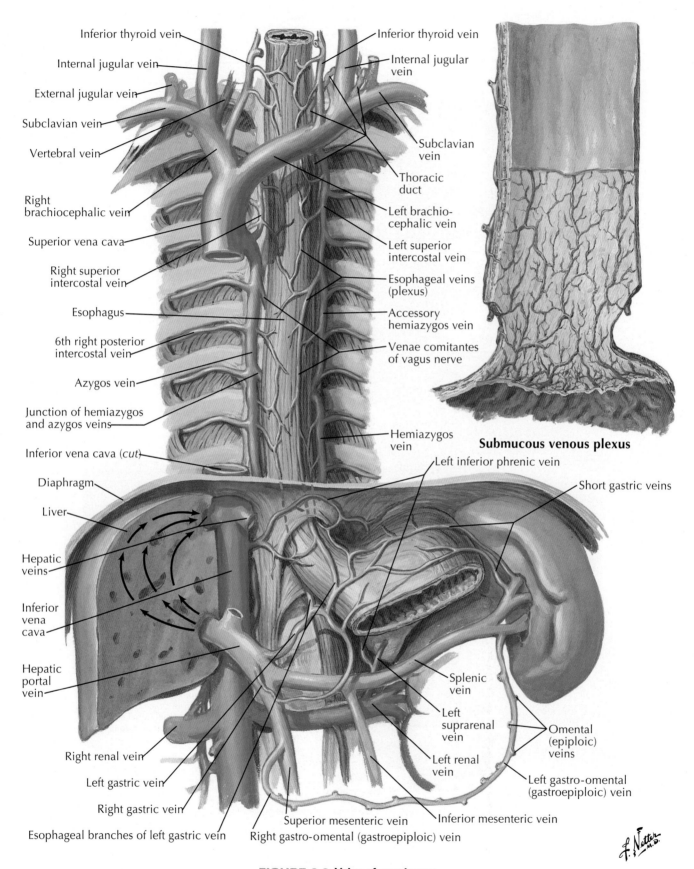

Inferior thyroid vein

Internal jugular vein

External jugular vein

Subclavian vein

Vertebral vein

Right brachiocephalic vein

Superior vena cava

Right superior intercostal vein

Esophagus

6th right posterior intercostal vein

Azygos vein

Junction of hemiazygos and azygos veins

Inferior vena cava (*cut*)

Diaphragm

Liver

Hepatic veins

Inferior vena cava

Hepatic portal vein

Right renal vein

Left gastric vein

Right gastric vein

Esophageal branches of left gastric vein

Inferior thyroid vein

Internal jugular vein

Subclavian vein

Thoracic duct

Left brachio-cephalic vein

Left superior intercostal vein

Esophageal veins (plexus)

Accessory hemiazygos vein

Venae comitantes of vagus nerve

Hemiazygos vein

Submucous venous plexus

Left inferior phrenic vein

Short gastric veins

Splenic vein

Left suprarenal vein

Left renal vein

Omental (epiploic) veins

Left gastro-omental (gastroepiploic) vein

Inferior mesenteric vein

Superior mesenteric vein

Right gastro-omental (gastroepiploic) vein

FIGURE 6.2 Veins of esophagus.

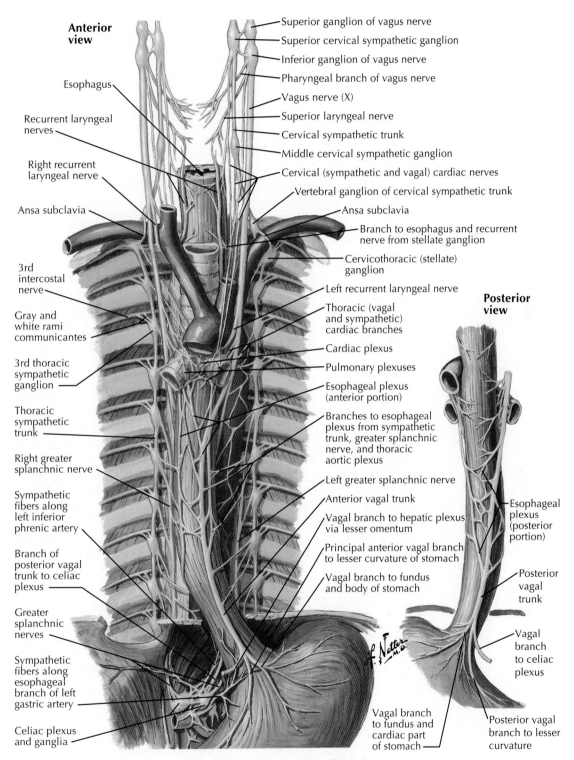

Anterior view

Esophagus

Recurrent laryngeal nerves

Right recurrent laryngeal nerve

Ansa subclavia

3rd intercostal nerve

Gray and white rami communicantes

3rd thoracic sympathetic ganglion

Thoracic sympathetic trunk

Right greater splanchnic nerve

Sympathetic fibers along left inferior phrenic artery

Branch of posterior vagal trunk to celiac plexus

Greater splanchnic nerves

Sympathetic fibers along esophageal branch of left gastric artery

Celiac plexus and ganglia

Superior ganglion of vagus nerve

Superior cervical sympathetic ganglion

Inferior ganglion of vagus nerve

Pharyngeal branch of vagus nerve

Vagus nerve (X)

Superior laryngeal nerve

Cervical sympathetic trunk

Middle cervical sympathetic ganglion

Cervical (sympathetic and vagal) cardiac nerves

Vertebral ganglion of cervical sympathetic trunk

Ansa subclavia

Branch to esophagus and recurrent nerve from stellate ganglion

Cervicothoracic (stellate) ganglion

Left recurrent laryngeal nerve

Thoracic (vagal and sympathetic) cardiac branches

Cardiac plexus

Pulmonary plexuses

Esophageal plexus (anterior portion)

Branches to esophageal plexus from sympathetic trunk, greater splanchnic nerve, and thoracic aortic plexus

Left greater splanchnic nerve

Anterior vagal trunk

Vagal branch to hepatic plexus via lesser omentum

Principal anterior vagal branch to lesser curvature of stomach

Vagal branch to fundus and body of stomach

Vagal branch to fundus and cardiac part of stomach

Posterior view

Esophageal plexus (posterior portion)

Posterior vagal trunk

Vagal branch to celiac plexus

Posterior vagal branch to lesser curvature

FIGURE 6.3 Innervation of esophagus.

PREOPERATIVE WORKUP

Preoperative studies are essential to aid in appropriate surgical decision making and define any anatomic abnormalities that are contributing to symptomology. These include upper endoscopy, upper gastrointestinal series (UGI), esophageal manometry (with or without impedance), and gastroesophageal reflux (GER) testing with or without impedance. Upper endoscopy can reveal intraluminal pathology, esophagitis, gastritis, peptic ulcer disease, hiatal hernia (Fig. 6.4), and characterize the gastroesophageal valve by Hill-Grade classification. UGI further defines anatomy and relation of GEJ to the diaphragm as well as the presence or absence of a hiatal hernia. GER testing allows quantification of reflux and symptom correlation with the presence of reflux. Traditional GER testing is pH based and greater than 4% acid exposure is considered pathologic. The addition of impedance allows detection of non-acid reflux. These tests can be performed with a nasogastric probe or an endoscopically deployed wireless capsule.

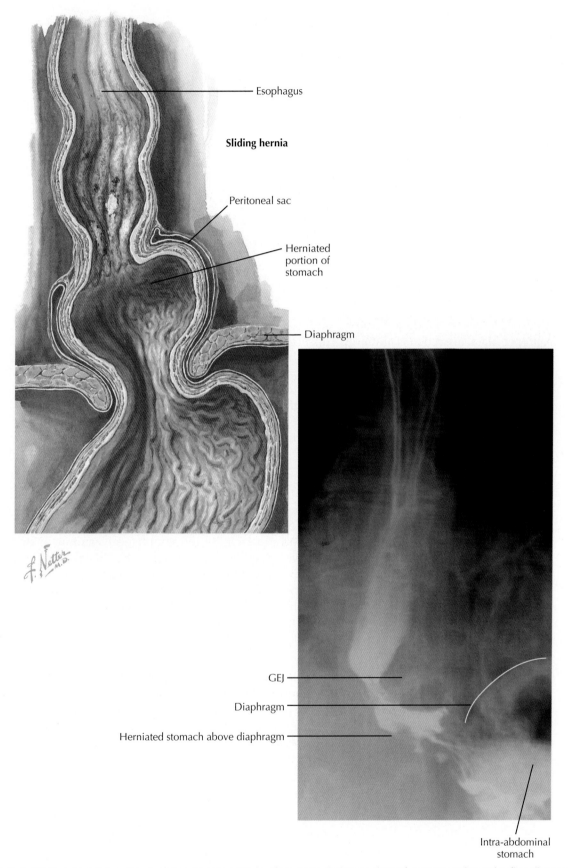

FIGURE 6.4 Sliding hiatal hernia. A sliding hiatal hernia is often seen during workup of gastroesophageal reflux disease (GERD). Other types of hiatal hernias, types II to IV, are less common. *GEJ,* Gastroesophageal junction.

DIAPHRAGMATIC CRURA

A proper hiatal dissection is primarily a dissection of the diaphragmatic crura (Fig. 6.5). In most people, the right and left pillars of the right diaphragmatic crus form the esophageal hiatus. Abdominal exposure of this region requires retraction of the left lobe of the liver anteriorly with a self-retaining retractor. The filmy part of the gastrohepatic ligament, known as the pars flaccida, is incised to reveal the base of the right crus. In this region of the lesser omentum, the hepatic branch of the anterior vagus traverses horizontally and a replaced left hepatic artery may be encountered. Medial to the crus, the inferior vena cava (IVC) and the caudate lobe are identified to prevent injury.

RIGHT CRURAL PILLAR

The right pillar is bluntly dissected from the esophagus and the mediastinum is entered in the anatomic avascular plane. This dissection is carried along the medial edge of the pillar anteriorly to the apex of the hiatus and posteriorly to create a retroesophageal window, taking care to preserve the endoabdominal fascia overlying the muscular pillar. If a hiatal hernia sac is encountered, the avascular plane exists circumferentially between the hernia sac and the mediastinum. The posterior vagus nerve is identified at the 6 to 7 o'clock position relative to the esophagus and is preserved against the esophagus. Concentrating the dissection on the crura and not the esophagus helps to avoid vagal injury.

LEFT CRURAL PILLAR

The left pillar is approached laterally once the esophagus is encircled with the Penrose. The angle of His is identified and the pillar is bluntly dissected from the esophagus in the same avascular plane entered on the right side. The anterior vagus nerve is identified between the 11 and 2 o'clock position relative to the esophagus and is preserved. Once again, if a hernia sac is encountered, the dissection is performed between the sac and mediastinum.

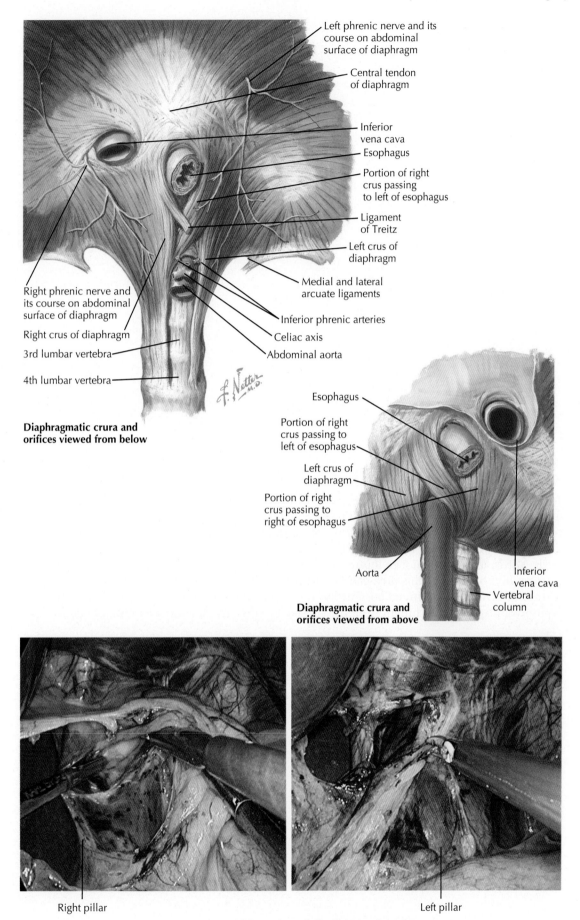

Diaphragmatic crura and orifices viewed from below

Left phrenic nerve and its course on abdominal surface of diaphragm

Central tendon of diaphragm

Inferior vena cava

Esophagus

Portion of right crus passing to left of esophagus

Ligament of Treitz

Left crus of diaphragm

Medial and lateral arcuate ligaments

Inferior phrenic arteries

Celiac axis

Abdominal aorta

Right phrenic nerve and its course on abdominal surface of diaphragm

Right crus of diaphragm

3rd lumbar vertebra

4th lumbar vertebra

Esophagus

Portion of right crus passing to left of esophagus

Left crus of diaphragm

Portion of right crus passing to right of esophagus

Aorta

Inferior vena cava

Vertebral column

Diaphragmatic crura and orifices viewed from above

Right pillar

Left pillar

FIGURE 6.5 Dissection of diaphragmatic crura.

SHORT GASTRIC VESSELS

To reach the base of the left pillar, the gastric fundus is grasped and the short gastric vessels arising from the splenic artery are divided using an energy device (ultrasonic shears or bipolar electrocautery). This dissection begins at the base of the fundus with entry into the lesser sac along the greater curvature of the stomach. The short gastric vessels are divided cephalad toward the angle of His, taking care not to injure the stomach or spleen. Meticulous hemostasis is critical because hemorrhage in this area can be difficult to control. After takedown of these vessels, further dissection is continued posteriorly to mobilize the posterior fundus (Fig. 6.6). There is typically a posterior attachment from the stomach to the anterior surface of the pancreas.

View with stomach reflected cephalad

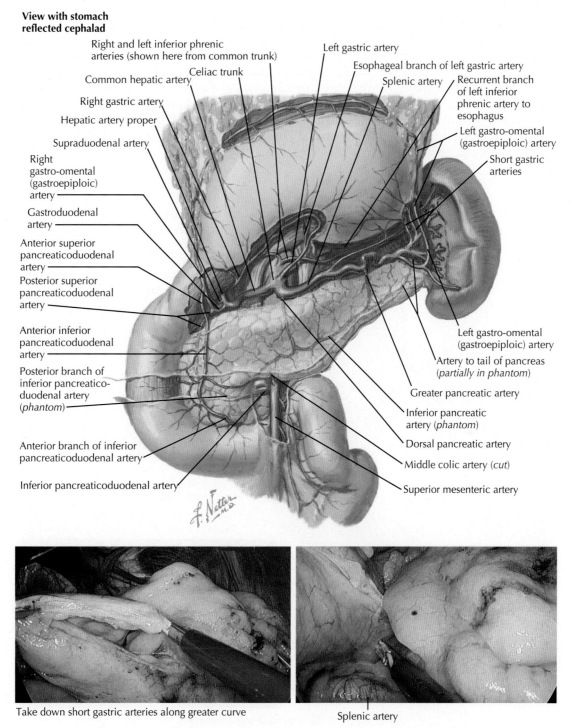

Right and left inferior phrenic arteries (shown here from common trunk)

Celiac trunk

Common hepatic artery

Right gastric artery

Hepatic artery proper

Supraduodenal artery

Right gastro-omental (gastroepiploic) artery

Gastroduodenal artery

Anterior superior pancreaticoduodenal artery

Posterior superior pancreaticoduodenal artery

Anterior inferior pancreaticoduodenal artery

Posterior branch of inferior pancreatico-duodenal artery (*phantom*)

Anterior branch of inferior pancreaticoduodenal artery

Inferior pancreaticoduodenal artery

Left gastric artery

Esophageal branch of left gastric artery

Splenic artery

Recurrent branch of left inferior phrenic artery to esophagus

Left gastro-omental (gastroepiploic) artery

Short gastric arteries

Left gastro-omental (gastroepiploic) artery

Artery to tail of pancreas (*partially in phantom*)

Greater pancreatic artery

Inferior pancreatic artery (*phantom*)

Dorsal pancreatic artery

Middle colic artery (*cut*)

Superior mesenteric artery

Take down short gastric arteries along greater curve

Splenic artery

FIGURE 6.6 Anatomy of posterior stomach and short gastric arteries.

PHRENOESOPHAGEAL LIGAMENT

The phrenoesophageal ligament is a tough, fibrous projection of transversalis fascia from the under surface of the diaphragm that attaches to the intraabdominal esophagus about 2 cm proximal to the GEJ. It is an important part of the LES complex because it prevents superior displacement of the esophagus into the thoracic cavity by elastic recoil. Complete esophageal mobilization requires division of the phrenoesophageal ligament at the confluence of the right and left pillars (Fig. 6.7). At this point, a Penrose drain is passed through the retroesophageal window and used to encircle the esophagus to aid with retraction. The left lateral portion of the phrenoesophageal ligament along the medial border of the left pillar is generally the thickest portion of the ligament.

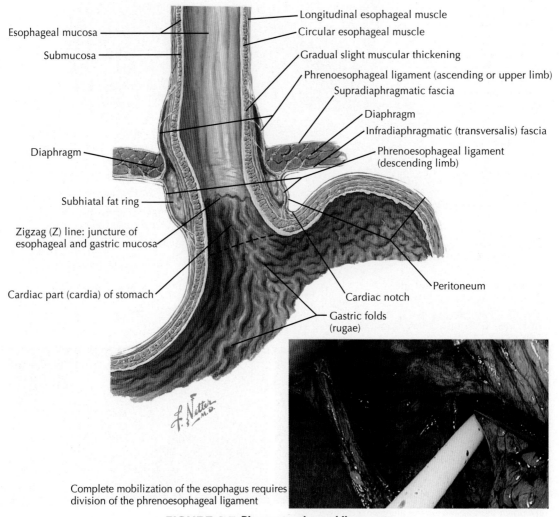

Complete mobilization of the esophagus requires division of the phrenoesophageal ligament

FIGURE 6.7 Phrenoesophageal ligament.

CRURAL CLOSURE

After passage of a 56- to 60-Fr bougie, thick bites of crura are taken with nonabsorbable suture, ensuring healthy bites of endoabdominal fascia as well as underlying muscle. Pledgets are used to buttress the repair, especially when the tissue is under tension. During suturing it is important to be cognizant of the aorta posteriorly in the mediastinum and the IVC located medial to the right pillar to prevent injury (Fig. 6.8). This closure can be reinforced with a mesh in some cases that is placed posteriorly.

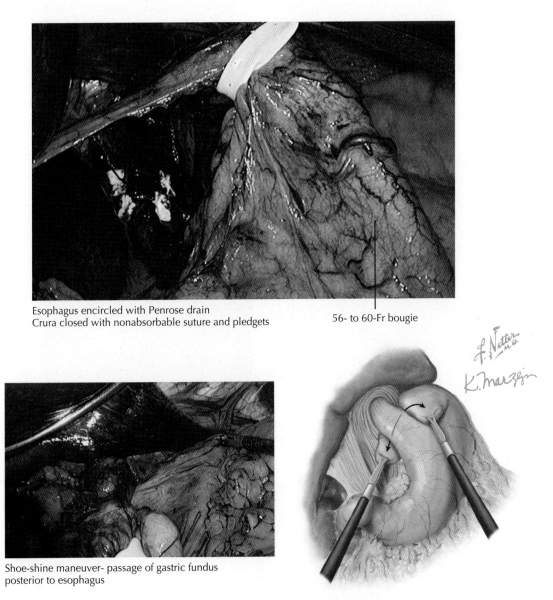

Esophagus encircled with Penrose drain
Crura closed with nonabsorbable suture and pledgets

56- to 60-Fr bougie

Shoe-shine maneuver- passage of gastric fundus
posterior to esophagus

FIGURE 6.8 Crural closure and shoe-shine maneuver.

FUNDOPLICATION CREATION AROUND ESOPHAGUS

After the right and left pillar are reapproximated around the esophagus, the gastric fundus is passed posterior to the esophagus in the retroesophageal window from left to right. The "shoe-shine" maneuver is used, which involves applying gentle retraction as the fundus is pulled back and forth behind the esophagus to prevent twisting, appropriately orient and size the wrap, and ensure that the wrap is "floppy" (see Fig. 6.8). The fundoplication is created using nonabsorbable sutures starting 2 cm proximal to the GEJ to ensure the entire wrap sits on the esophagus and not the stomach. A sizing device such as a bougie is kept within the esophagus during creation of the plication to avoid making it too tight. The first two sutures involve both sides of the fundus and a mural bite of the esophagus, whereas the third suture is a fundus-to-fundus bite. Injury to the anterior vagus should be avoided. A Nissen fundoplication is a 360-degree wrap. In certain situations, especially in the setting of dysphagia, a partial wrap may be considered: either a Toupet (270-degree posterior) or Dor (180-degree anterior) fundoplication. At the completion of the wrap, upper endoscopy is performed to confirm appropriate orientation and location of the fundoplication. The plication should be 2 cm in length, sitting at the base of the esophagus, and allow passage of an instrument beneath it with the bougie in place (Fig. 6.9).

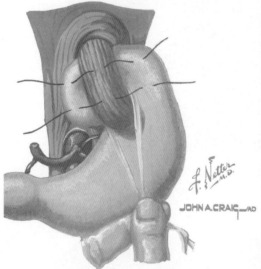

Heavy interrupted silk sutures passed through seromuscular layers of fundus, lightly incorporating anterior esophageal wall

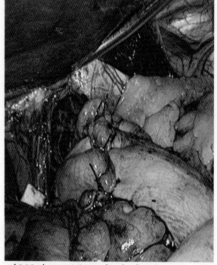

Creation of 360-degree Nissen fundoplication
First two sutures incorporate fundus and anterior esophageal wall
Third suture is fundus to fundus

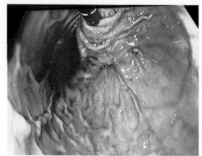

Endoscopic view of completed fundoplication

FIGURE 6.9 **Laparoscopic Nissen (360-degree) fundoplication and endoscopy.**

SUGGESTED READINGS

Nissen R. Hiatus hernia and it's surgical indication. Dtsch Med Wochenschr 1995;80(14):467–9.
Singhal V, Khaitan L. Preoperative evaluation of gastroesophageal reflux disease. Surg Clin North Am 2015;95(3):615–27.

Truncal and Selective Vagotomy

Gerardo Davalos and Alfredo D. Guerron

 VIDEO

7.1 Laparoscopic Truncal Vagotomy

INTRODUCTION

Gastric acid production contributes to duodenal and gastric ulcer formation. Intraluminal gastric acid is released by parietal cells, which in turn are stimulated via three mechanisms: gastrin, histamine, and acetylcholine. All three mechanisms activate the hydrogen-potassium ATPase-releasing hydrogen ions into the stomach lumen. Specifically, acetylcholine is released in response to parasympathetic stimulation, which travels in the fibers of the vagus nerves (Fig. 7.1). When pharmacologic therapy is not enough to decrease acid production, surgical vagotomy intervention can be applied to interrupt this neural pathway anatomically. There are three different techniques options described: truncal vagotomy (TV), selective vagotomy (SV), and highly selective vagotomy (HSV). Furthermore, technological advances have allowed for these operations to be performed with minimally invasive techniques, which have translated into fewer procedure-related complications.

Although acid-reducing surgery has become an operation with few indications, it is still an essential tool in the surgeon armamentarium. Vagotomy is currently indicated for intractability or complication of peptic ulcer disease in a stable patient who has failed maximum medical therapy and more recently, owing to the rapid increase of bariatric surgeries worldwide, as a surgical treatment alternative for marginal ulcers post-Roux-en-Y gastric bypass (RYGB). When performing acid-reducing surgeries, surgeons must understand the anatomy, physiopathology, and clinical implications of different techniques and approaches as well as their potential postoperative complications.

ANATOMY: INNERVATION OF THE STOMACH

Sympathetic innervation follows that of the arterial supply of the stomach (Figs. 7.2 through 7.4). Parasympathetic innervation, on the other hand, is controlled by the right and left vagus nerves, which enter the thoracic cavity along with the esophagus. As the two trunks enter the abdomen, they rotate so that the left trunk becomes anterior and the right trunk posterior to the esophagus. Both trunks innervate the stomach along the lesser curvature and induce the parietal cells to secrete hydrochloric acid as well as control the motor activity of the stomach. The left vagus nerve gives off branches that innervate the liver, biliary tract, and gallbladder. The right vagus nerve innervates the colon, small intestine, and pancreas. Importantly, the right branch also creates a small branch behind the esophagus named the "criminal nerve of Grassi," which, if missed and not divided, can lead to recurrent disease.

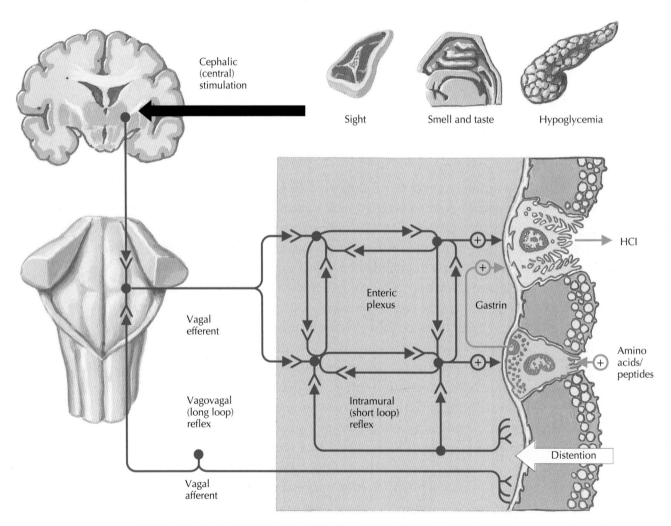

Gastric acid secretion initiated and modulated by nervous system via central stimulation through vagal efferents and enteric plexus and by intramural (short) feedback loop and a second (long, or vagovagal) feedback loop, both stimulated by gastric antral distention

JOHN A.CRAIG—AD

FIGURE 7.1 Vagal stimulation and acid secretion.

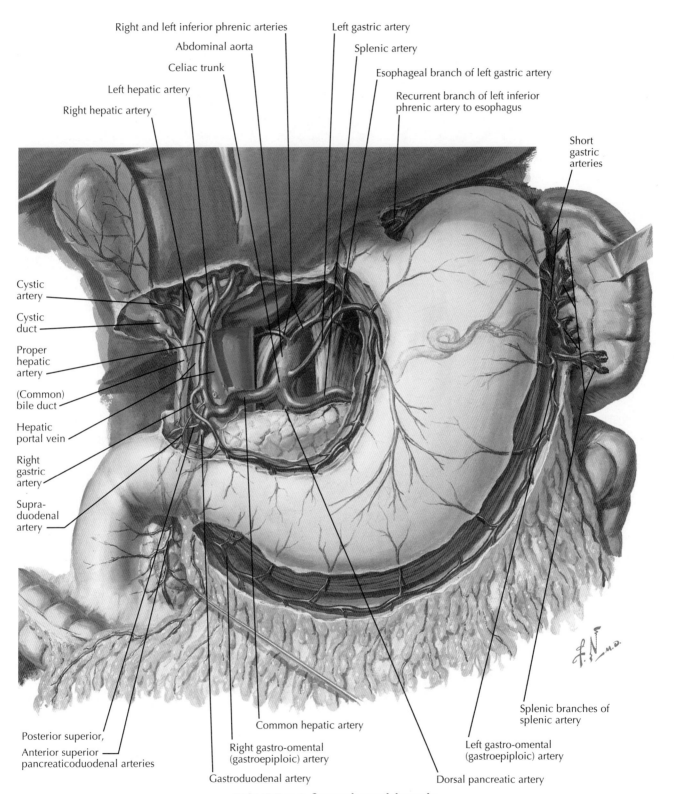

Right and left inferior phrenic arteries

Abdominal aorta

Celiac trunk

Left hepatic artery

Right hepatic artery

Left gastric artery

Splenic artery

Esophageal branch of left gastric artery

Recurrent branch of left inferior phrenic artery to esophagus

Short gastric arteries

Cystic artery

Cystic duct

Proper hepatic artery

(Common) bile duct

Hepatic portal vein

Right gastric artery

Supra-duodenal artery

Posterior superior, Anterior superior pancreaticoduodenal arteries

Gastroduodenal artery

Right gastro-omental (gastroepiploic) artery

Common hepatic artery

Dorsal pancreatic artery

Left gastro-omental (gastroepiploic) artery

Splenic branches of splenic artery

FIGURE 7.2 Stomach arterial supply.

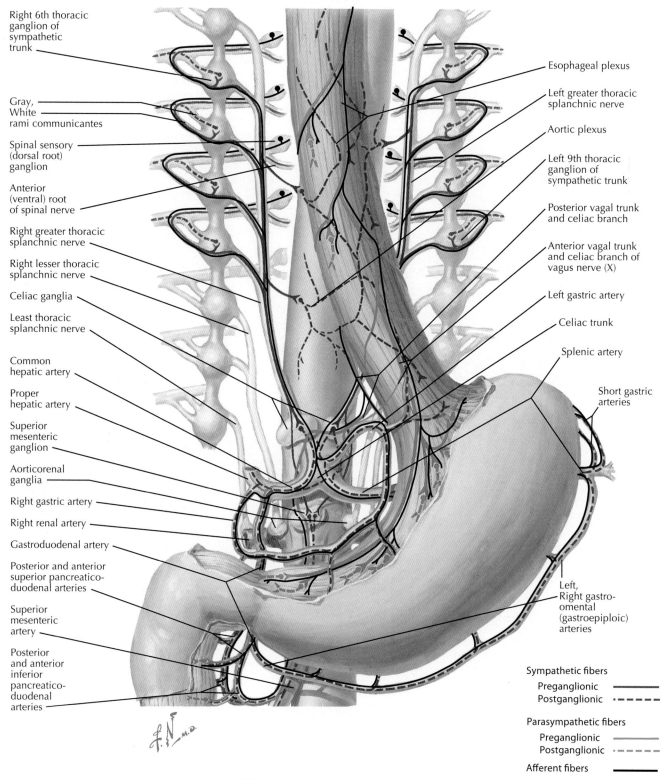

Right 6th thoracic ganglion of sympathetic trunk

Gray, White rami communicantes

Spinal sensory (dorsal root) ganglion

Anterior (ventral) root of spinal nerve

Right greater thoracic splanchnic nerve

Right lesser thoracic splanchnic nerve

Celiac ganglia

Least thoracic splanchnic nerve

Common hepatic artery

Proper hepatic artery

Superior mesenteric ganglion

Aorticorenal ganglia

Right gastric artery

Right renal artery

Gastroduodenal artery

Posterior and anterior superior pancreatico-duodenal arteries

Superior mesenteric artery

Posterior and anterior inferior pancreatico-duodenal arteries

Esophageal plexus

Left greater thoracic splanchnic nerve

Aortic plexus

Left 9th thoracic ganglion of sympathetic trunk

Posterior vagal trunk and celiac branch

Anterior vagal trunk and celiac branch of vagus nerve (X)

Left gastric artery

Celiac trunk

Splenic artery

Short gastric arteries

Left, Right gastro-omental (gastroepiploic) arteries

Sympathetic fibers

Preganglionic
Postganglionic

Parasympathetic fibers

Preganglionic
Postganglionic

Afferent fibers

FIGURE 7.3 Stomach innervation.

A. Association of innervation and arterial supply – anterior view

Anterior and posterior layers of lesser omentum

Right greater thoracic splanchnic nerve

Right and left inferior phrenic arteries and plexuses

Hepatic branch of anterior vagal trunk

Anterior vagal trunk

Celiac branch of posterior vagal trunk

Celiac branch of anterior vagal trunk

Left gastric artery and plexus

Vagal branch from hepatic plexus to pyloric part of stomach

Hepatic plexus

Right gastric artery and plexus

Anterior gastric branch of anterior vagal trunk

Left greater thoracic splanchnic nerve

Left lesser thoracic splanchnic nerve

Splenic artery and plexus

Celiac ganglia and plexus

Plexus on gastro-omental (gastroepiploic) arteries

Superior mesenteric artery and plexus

Plexus on anterior superior and anterior inferior pancreaticoduodenal arteries (posterior pancreaticoduodenal arteries and plexuses not visible in this view)

B. Innervation of the stomach – posterior view

Plexus on gastro-omental (gastroepiploic) arteries

Posterior gastric branch of posterior vagal trunk

Hepatic plexus

Right gastric artery and plexus

View with stomach reflected cephalad

Greater,
Lesser,
Least
thoracic splanchnic nerves

Plexus on gastroduodenal artery

Plexus on anterior superior and anterior inferior pancreaticoduodenal arteries

Plexus on posterior superior and posterior inferior pancreaticoduodenal arteries

Hepatic branch of anterior vagal trunk via lesser omentum

Branch from hepatic plexus to cardia via lesser omentum

Right inferior phrenic artery and plexus

Posterior vagal trunk

Celiac branch of posterior vagal trunk

Celiac branch of anterior vagal trunk

Left gastric artery and plexus

Left inferior phrenic artery and plexus

Celiac ganglia and plexus

Greater, lesser, and least thoracic splanchnic nerves

Splenic artery and plexus

Aorticorenal ganglia

Superior mesenteric ganglion and plexus

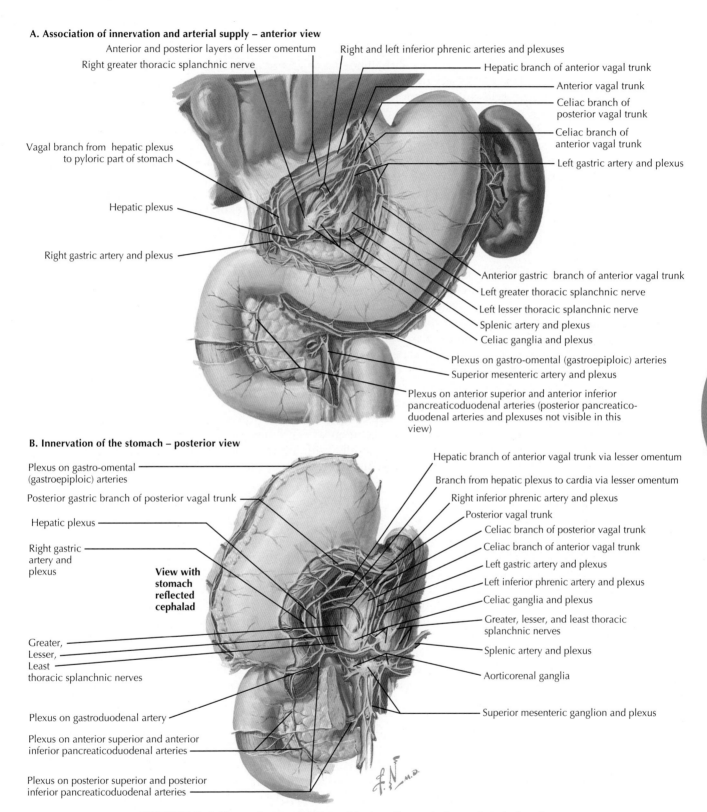

FIGURE 7.4 Stomach vasculature and innervation anterior and posterior views.

CLINICAL INDICATIONS

Refractory Peptic Ulcer Disease

Historically, management of patients with duodenal or gastric ulcers was initially confined to surgical intervention, specifically by way of vagotomy procedures. However, with the introduction of effective acid suppression medication and the crucial discovery and treatment of *Helicobacter pylori* as one of the primary causes of the pathology, the role of such procedures has fundamentally decreased. The current use of vagotomy for peptic ulcer disease (PUD) is reserved for carefully selected patients who have failed maximum medical therapy or are allergic to proton pump inhibitors, have undergone treatment and eradication of *H. pylori,* and have recalcitrant complications of the disease such as bleeding, obstruction, or intractable pain. Additionally, vagotomies in a PUD scenario are rarely performed by themselves and are generally implemented in conjunction with a primary resection, drainage, or a diversion procedure. For PUD these primary procedures are chosen to treat the complications, whereas vagotomy is usually added to decrease the risk of ulcer recurrence.

Recalcitrant Marginal Ulcers After Roux-en-Y-Gastric Bypass

Roux-en-Y gastric bypass is the second most common bariatric procedure, with more than 40,000 cases performed annually in the United States. Marginal ulcers are a common complication after Roux-en-Y gastric bypass, with an incidence rate of up to 16%. It is defined as an ulcer at or near the gastrojejunal anastomosis. Although the majority of marginal ulcers resolve with medical management and lifestyle changes, in the rare case of a nonhealing marginal ulcer, acid suppression surgery can be considered. Current surgical management for this type of ulcer typically consists of resection and subsequent revision of the gastrojejunal anastomosis, which entails considerable morbidity and complications. For this reason, some have proposed the use of truncal vagotomy as a less-invasive procedure with potentially better outcomes. Moreover, advances in minimally invasive techniques have allowed this type of procedure to be approached thoracoscopically and laparoscopically, with initial studies reporting feasibility and favorable results when compared with a traditional revision of the gastrojejunal anastomosis.

PROCEDURES

Truncal Vagotomy

Truncal vagotomy involves a complete transection of the vagus nerve and can be accomplished through either an abdominal or thoracic approach. Open, laparoscopic, or thoracoscopic methods have been described; however, the type of procedure performed depends on multiple factors, which include patient age, the risk for ulcer recurrence, the severity of symptoms, clinical status, body mass index, and, more important, the surgeon's expertise. Because the vagus nerve also supplies motor function innervation to the circular muscle fibers of the antrum and pylorus, a complete transection of the fibers does not allow the pylorus to relax effectively, which in turn increases intragastric pressure and delays gastric emptying; this is the reason why most surgeons will perform concomitant drainage procedures. Additionally, complete vagal transection at this level can also lead to postvagotomy syndrome symptoms, which include diarrhea, hypergastrinemia, and dumping syndrome.

Abdominal Approach

The surgery can be performed open or laparoscopically and initiates by accomplishing entrance to the abdominal cavity. Depending on the surgical approach, the patient can be placed in a supine or lithotomy position. If the patient is in a supine position, the operating surgeon stands on the right side of the patient while the assistant is on the contralateral side. If the lithotomy position is used, the surgeon stands between the legs. After induction of anesthesia and intubation, the patient's abdomen is then prepped and draped in sterile fashion. In an open approach, an upper midline incision from the xiphoid to the umbilicus is made. In laparoscopic approaches, pneumoperitoneum is achieved via Veress needle. A 5-mm optical port and a 0-degree laparoscope are then used to enter the abdominal cavity in a left subcostal position. Additional 5-mm ports are placed in the left supraumbilical region and right upper quadrant. A 12-mm port is also placed in the right supraumbilical position.

After the peritoneal cavity is inspected, a self-retaining liver retractor is placed to facilitate access to the lesser curve and the diaphragmatic hiatus. The right and left crus are identified. The hiatus is entered via the right crus, and a circumferential esophageal dissection is performed to achieve distal esophageal mobilization. Dissection is performed for a distance of 4 to 5 cm above the gastroesophageal junction (GEJ). The left or anterior vagal trunk can typically be found 2 to 4 cm superior to the GEJ on the anterior surface of the intra-abdominal esophagus as it indents the anterior wall of the esophagus (Fig. 7.5A). Once identified, the trunk is clipped proximally and distally with medium clips and divided for a minimum specimen of 2 cm. Notably, careful inspection for multiple smaller additional anterior vagus nerves on the anterior surface of the esophagus should be done using a nerve hook; if found, these should also be divided to complete the vagotomy. The posterior or right trunk can be found along the right edge of the esophagus. Exposure can be facilitated by retracting the esophagus to the left. Additional care must be taken to identify the criminal nerve of Grassi (Fig. 7.5B), a branch of the right/posterior vagus nerve. Lack of division of this branch can lead to continued parietal cell stimulation and resultant recurrent peptic ulcer disease. Once recognized, a segment is resected in a similar fashion. Both resected specimens should later be sent to pathology for verification.

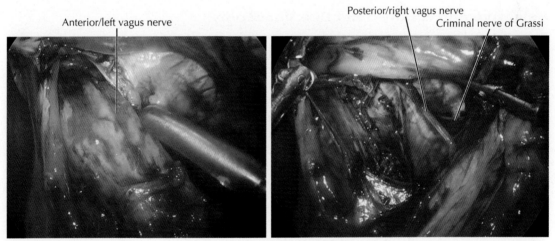

A. Anterior/left vagus nerve   B. Posterior/right vagus nerve and criminal nerve of Grassi

FIGURE 7.5 **Right and left vagus nerves.**

Thoracic Approach

The thoracic approach to vagotomy can be either open or thoracoscopic and only applies for TV; SV and HSV cannot be performed through the thoracic approach. After general anesthesia has been induced using a double-lumen endotracheal tube, the patient is placed in a right lateral position. The transthoracic approach can be performed through a left eighth or ninth intercostal space anterolateral incision. The thoracoscopic approach involves an incision over the ninth intercostal space where a 10-mm trocar is placed. A second 5-mm trocar is placed anterior to the first, and a third 5-mm trocar is placed at the seventh interspace. If downward retraction of the diaphragm is required for exposure, a fourth 5-mm trocar is added. The inferior pulmonary ligament is then incised, and the lung is retracted cephalad. The posterior mediastinum is entered by incising the parietal pleura longitudinally anterior to the aorta just above the hiatus. The esophagus is identified, and the anterior and posterior vagus nerves are clipped proximally, distally divided, and sent for specimen verification, as described earlier.

Selective and Highly Selective Vagotomy

Because complete truncal vagotomy halts parasympathetic innervation to most of the gastrointestinal tract and can lead to a postvagotomy syndrome, less radical and more focused options have been described. SV transects only the anterior and posterior gastric nerves of Latarjet. It spares the celiac and hepatic branches but results in denervation of the pylorus, thus requiring additional gastric drainage procedures. In contrast, HSV consists of denervation of the parietal cell mass by dividing the nerve branches of the anterior and posterior vagus as they enter the stomach (Fig. 7.6). Because the terminal and most distal divisions of the vagus nerve (crow's foot) are preserved, pyloric sphincter mechanisms are spared, thus eliminating the need for gastric emptying procedures. Both selective and highly selective vagotomies, however, are rarely performed these days. Some of the drawbacks of both procedures include narrowing indications, a steep surgeon's learning curve, and high recurrence rates, which have ultimately limited their use.

The surgical approach can be achieved either in an open or laparoscopic fashion. In both cases, the main trunks are first recognized as described in truncal vagotomy. In SV, although the celiac and hepatic branches are carefully preserved, the anterior and posterior Latarjet nerves (which lie approximately 1 to 2 cm from the lesser curve) are identified and divided. In HSV the procedure starts by examining the lesser curve of the stomach and identifying the left gastric vessels and the gastric branch of the anterior vagus nerve. Distal branches that go in the direction of the stomach wall are individually ligated and divided proximal to the cardia and toward the incisura angularis, leaving the crow's foot intact for gastric emptying. Dissection starts approximately 7 cm proximal to the pylorus and should be continued toward the GEJ, taking care to stay close to the stomach to not compromise the main trunk of the vagus. It is recommended that at least three terminal branches of the anterior gastric nerve of Latarjet, which supply the antrum and the pylorus, be identified and preserved. Next, the greater omentum is divided, and the stomach is turned upward and to the right to expose the posterior surface. Similarly, branches proceeding toward the stomach are identified and divided as close to the wall as possible. The distal esophagus should be denervated for 6 cm in length to ensure adequate parietal cell signal disruption.

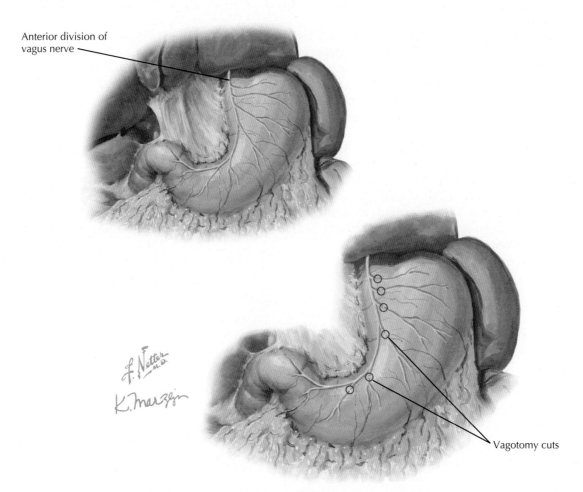

FIGURE 7.6 Selective and highly selective vagotomy.

SUGGESTED READINGS

Bonanno A, Tieu B, Dewey E, Husain F. Thoracoscopic truncal vagotomy versus surgical revision of the gastrojejunal anastomosis for recalcitrant marginal ulcers. Surg Endosc 2018 Aug 21. https://doi.org/10.1007/s00464-018-6386-7. [Epub ahead of print] PubMed PMID: 30132208.

Chang PC, Huang CK, Tai CM, Huang IY, Hsin MC, Hung CM. Revision using totally hand-sewn gastrojejunostomy and truncal vagotomy for refractory marginal ulcer after laparoscopic Roux-en-y gastric bypass: a case series. Surg Obes Relat Dis 2017;13(4):588–93. https://doi.org/10.1016/j.soard.2016.09.035. Epub 2016 Oct 4. PubMed PMID: 28215394.

Chau E, Youn H, Ren-Fielding CJ, Fielding GA, Schwack BF, Kurian MS. Surgical management and outcomes of patients with marginal ulcer after Roux-en-Y gastric bypass. Surg Obes Relat Dis 2015;11(5):1071–5.

Hunter J, Stahl RD, Kakade M, Breitman I, Grams J, Clements RH. Effectiveness of thoracoscopic truncal vagotomy in the treatment of marginal ulcers after laparoscopic Roux-en-Y gastric bypass. Am Surg 2012;78(6):663–8. PubMed PMID: 22643261.

Lagoo J, Pappas TN, Perez A. A relic or still relevant: the narrowing role for vagotomy in the treatment of peptic ulcer disease. Am J Surg 2014;207(1):120–6. https://doi.org/10.1016/j.amjsurg.2013.02.012. Epub 2013 Oct 16. Review. PubMed PMID: 24139666.

CHAPTER

8

Gastrectomy

Michael Antiporda and Kevin M. Reavis

 VIDEO

8.1 Laparoscopic Total Gastrectomy With D2 Lymphadenectomy

INTRODUCTION

The indications and approaches for gastrectomy have evolved in recent years. Before the introduction of effective diagnostic modalities and medical therapies for peptic ulcer disease (PUD) and *Helicobacter pylori* infection, most gastric operations were performed for complications of those diseases. Now, malignancy is the most common indication for gastric resection, with more than 26,000 new cases of gastric cancer occurring in the United States per year. Although it is one of the least commonly diagnosed cancers in the United States, it remains the third most common cause of cancer-related mortality worldwide. Underlying histologies include adenocarcinoma, lymphoma, carcinoid, gastrointestinal stromal tumor (GIST), and leiomyosarcoma. Indications for resection in the context of PUD include failure of healing despite appropriate medical management, hemorrhage, perforation, and obstruction. Other benign indications for resection include intractable hemorrhagic gastritis and end-stage gastroparesis refractory to medical management, pyloromyotomy, or gastric neurostimulator placement.

PREOPERATIVE WORKUP

Surgery is the cornerstone of treatment for gastric cancer. Integral to this treatment is appropriate staging. Endoscopy is used for biopsy and localization. Endoscopic ultrasound facilitates assessment of locoregional extent, and concomitant fine-needle aspiration improves accuracy of nodal staging. Combined PET-CT is used to rule out distant metastatic disease. Staging laparoscopy with peritoneal washings for cytology is important to assess for occult peritoneal disease and may reveal unresectable disease in 31% of cases.

When gastrectomy for benign causes is considered, endoscopy remains important for localization and assessment of landmarks for limited resection. In the setting of gastroparesis, gastric emptying study with nuclear scintigraphy is diagnostic when greater than 10% retention is noted at 4 hours. The presence of a bezoar on endoscopy may also be used as a diagnostic equivalent.

ANATOMY

The regions of the stomach are noted in Fig. 8.1. The blood supply of the stomach is from branches of the celiac axis. The important named branches are shown in Fig. 8.2. Variables not demonstrated include a posterior gastric artery seen in 62% of patients and aberrant left hepatic artery originating from the left gastric artery in 20% of cases. Lymph node stations are diagrammed along with venous drainage in Fig. 8.3.

SURGICAL APPROACH FOR GASTRECTOMY

Approaches to gastric resection increasingly use minimally invasive approaches. Early gastric cancer may even be treatable entirely endoscopically via endoscopic mucosal resection or endoscopic submucosal dissection techniques when the following criteria are met: stage Tis or T1a, less than 2 cm in diameter, well to moderate differentiation, absence of lymphovascular invasion, absence of lymph node metastases, and absence of ulceration. This approach is more common in Asia, where screening programs that detect early disease are broadly implemented because of the relatively high regional prevalence of gastric malignancy. Many references suggest that minimally invasive approaches offer various benefits, including decreased length of stay and estimated blood loss, and equivalence in oncologic outcomes with regard to lymph node yield and disease-free survival and overall survival. Whether resection is performed using an open, laparoscopic, or robotic approach, National Comprehensive Cancer Network (NCCN) guidelines recommend margins at least 4 cm, and lymphadenectomy to include harvest of 15 or more lymph nodes. The classifications of lymphadenectomy are according to the Japanese nomenclature, which includes D1, all lymph-bearing tissue within 3 cm of the lesion including perigastric lymph node stations along the lesser curvature (stations 1, 3, and 5) and greater curvature (stations 2, 4, and 6); D2, including celiac (station 9), CHA (station 8), LGA (station 7), and splenic artery and hilar lymph nodes (stations 10 and 11); and D3, including portahepatic (station 12) and para-aortic regions (station 16).

When performed via open means, laparoscopy is typically performed first to rule out carcinomatosis. Access is gained via an upper midline or bilateral chevron incision. When performed via laparoscopic or robot-assisted means, trocars are placed per surgeon preference, with objective of triangulation on the body of the stomach. The liver is retracted anterolaterally to expose the stomach. The greater omentum is mobilized off the transverse colon and kept with the stomach. The lesser sac is entered and assessed for spread of disease or posterior invasion of retroperitoneal structures, which may preclude resection. The greater curvature of the stomach is mobilized outside the gastroepiploic arcade. Short and posterior gastric arteries are mobilized. The junction of the right gastroepiploic artery with the gastroduodenal artery is exposed close to the head of the pancreas.

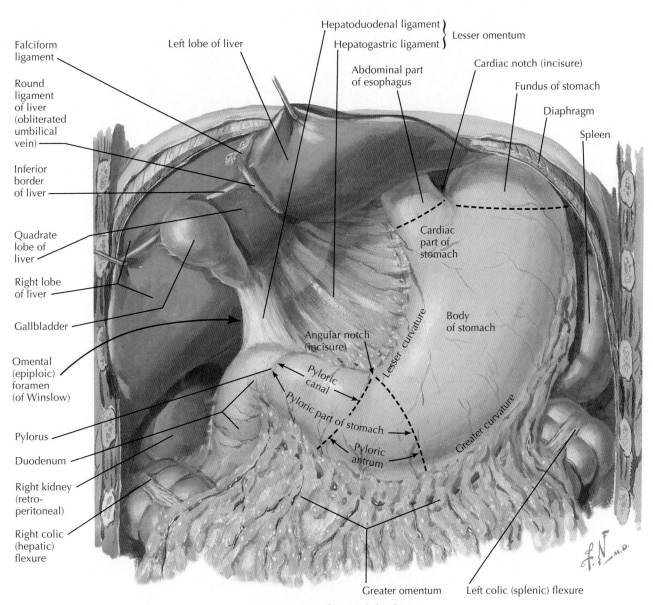

Falciform
ligament

Round
ligament
of liver
(obliterated
umbilical
vein)

Inferior
border
of liver

Quadrate
lobe of
liver

Right lobe
of liver

Gallbladder

Omental
(epiploic)
foramen
(of Winslow)

Pylorus

Duodenum

Right kidney
(retro-
peritoneal)

Right colic
(hepatic)
flexure

Left lobe of liver

Hepatoduodenal ligament ⎫
Hepatogastric ligament ⎭ Lesser omentum

Abdominal part
of esophagus

Cardiac notch (incisure)

Fundus of stomach

Diaphragm

Spleen

Cardiac
part of
stomach

Body
of stomach

Lesser curvature

Greater curvature

Angular notch
(incisure)

Pyloric
canal

Pyloric part of stomach

Pyloric
antrum

Greater omentum

Left colic (splenic) flexure

FIGURE 8.1 **Stomach in situ.**

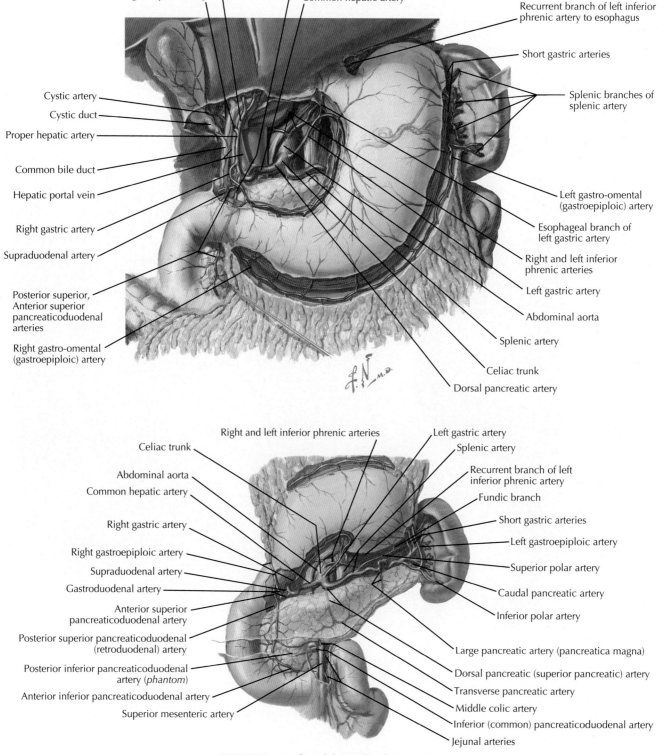

Left hepatic artery

Right hepatic artery

Gastroduodenal artery

Common hepatic artery

Recurrent branch of left inferior phrenic artery to esophagus

Short gastric arteries

Cystic artery

Cystic duct

Proper hepatic artery

Common bile duct

Hepatic portal vein

Right gastric artery

Supraduodenal artery

Posterior superior, Anterior superior pancreaticoduodenal arteries

Right gastro-omental (gastroepiploic) artery

Splenic branches of splenic artery

Left gastro-omental (gastroepiploic) artery

Esophageal branch of left gastric artery

Right and left inferior phrenic arteries

Left gastric artery

Abdominal aorta

Splenic artery

Celiac trunk

Dorsal pancreatic artery

Right and left inferior phrenic arteries

Celiac trunk

Abdominal aorta

Common hepatic artery

Right gastric artery

Right gastroepiploic artery

Supraduodenal artery

Gastroduodenal artery

Anterior superior pancreaticoduodenal artery

Posterior superior pancreaticoduodenal (retroduodenal) artery

Posterior inferior pancreaticoduodenal artery (*phantom*)

Anterior inferior pancreaticoduodenal artery

Superior mesenteric artery

Left gastric artery

Splenic artery

Recurrent branch of left inferior phrenic artery

Fundic branch

Short gastric arteries

Left gastroepiploic artery

Superior polar artery

Caudal pancreatic artery

Inferior polar artery

Large pancreatic artery (pancreatica magna)

Dorsal pancreatic (superior pancreatic) artery

Transverse pancreatic artery

Middle colic artery

Inferior (common) pancreaticoduodenal artery

Jejunal arteries

FIGURE 8.2 Arterial supply of stomach.

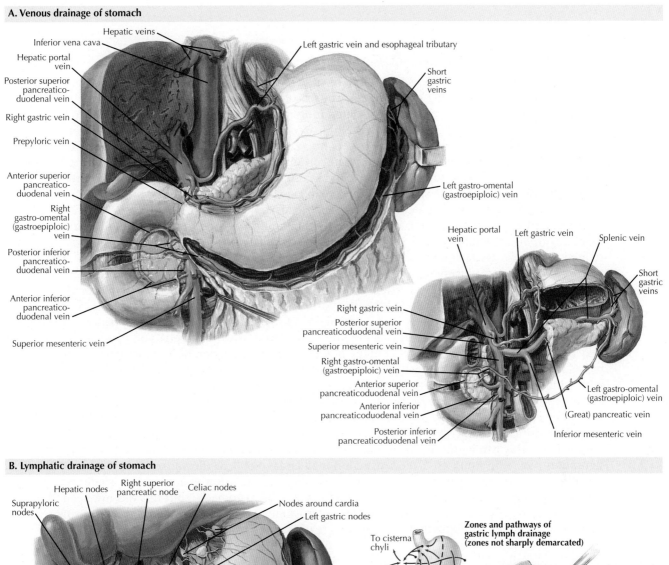

A. Venous drainage of stomach

Hepatic veins

Inferior vena cava

Left gastric vein and esophageal tributary

Hepatic portal vein

Short gastric veins

Posterior superior pancreatico-duodenal vein

Right gastric vein

Prepyloric vein

Anterior superior pancreatico-duodenal vein

Right gastro-omental (gastroepiploic) vein

Left gastro-omental (gastroepiploic) vein

Posterior inferior pancreatico-duodenal vein

Anterior inferior pancreatico-duodenal vein

Superior mesenteric vein

Hepatic portal vein

Left gastric vein

Splenic vein

Short gastric veins

Right gastric vein

Posterior superior pancreaticoduodenal vein

Superior mesenteric vein

Right gastro-omental (gastroepiploic) vein

Anterior superior pancreaticoduodenal vein

Anterior inferior pancreaticoduodenal vein

Posterior inferior pancreaticoduodenal vein

Left gastro-omental (gastroepiploic) vein

(Great) pancreatic vein

Inferior mesenteric vein

B. Lymphatic drainage of stomach

Hepatic nodes

Right superior pancreatic node

Celiac nodes

Suprapyloric nodes

Nodes around cardia

Left gastric nodes

Sub-pyloric nodes

To cisterna chyli

Zones and pathways of gastric lymph drainage (zones not sharply demarcated)

Left gastric nodes

Left gastro-omental (gastroepiploic) node

Nodes around cardia

Splenic nodes

Left gastro-omental (gastroepiploic) node

Right gastro-omental (gastroepiploic) nodes

Suprapyloric, retropyloric, and subpyloric nodes

Right gastro-omental (gastroepiploic) nodes

Right superior pancreatic node

Splenic nodes

Left superior pancreatic nodes

Celiac nodes

Superior mesenteric nodes

FIGURE 8.3 Venous and lymphatic drainage of stomach.

SURGICAL APPROACH FOR GASTRECTOMY (Continued)

D2 template lymphadenectomy is the standard of care in Asian centers. In Western centers, this template is recommended but not yet standard of care because of conflicting reports in the Western literature with regard to associated morbidity and long-term rates of overall survival. The pancreas and spleen are also typically spared in Western centers. Lymphadenectomy is performed starting at medial to the left hepatic artery, carried across the common hepatic artery, to the base of the left gastric artery, then continued across to the splenic artery with all lymph-bearing tissue including that between the inferior vena cava (IVC) and right crus of the diaphragm dissected with the specimen. The celiac axis is thus skeletonized as shown in Fig. 8.4. The left gastric artery is divided with a vascular load stapler.

The extent of gastric resection is determined by the location of the tumor. Distal tumors are treated with distal or subtotal gastrectomy. Proximal tumors or diffusely infiltrative tumors are treated with total gastrectomy. Hiatal dissection is completed with circumferential division of the phrenoesophageal ligament, and the distal esophagus is dissected several centimeters up into the mediastinum to release tension for anastomosis. Next, a gentle Kocher maneuver is performed to mobilize the pylorus and the first portion of the duodenum, and the duodenum is transected just distal to the pylorus with a vascular load stapler. Excess periduodenal dissection is avoided to minimize ischemia. The staple line is imbricated with Lembert-type sutures and may be additionally reinforced with a tongue of omentum. Mobilization of the stomach is completed by dividing remaining attachments within the lesser sac. The esophagus is then divided with a linear stapler several centimeters above the gastroesophageal junction.

The optimal postgastrectomy reconstruction is subject to some debate, and choice may be limited by extent of resection. Billroth I gastroduodenostomy is an option when distal gastrectomy is performed and permits preservation of duodenal passage. Otherwise reconstruction is performed with gastrojejunostomy or esophagojejunostomy via Billroth II or Roux-en-Y configuration (Fig. 8.5). Roux-en-Y reconstruction may be favorable as the various complications of Billroth I or II reconstruction are typically treatable with revision to Roux-en-Y anatomy. Further variations include creation of jejunal pouch as a "neo-stomach," but this has not been shown to be clearly superior. A Braun enteroenterostomy can be performed after Billroth II esophago-/gastrojejunostomy to divert biliopancreatic secretions away from the esophagus.

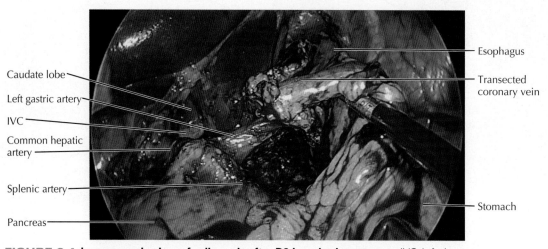

Caudate lobe

Left gastric artery

IVC

Common hepatic artery

Splenic artery

Pancreas

Esophagus

Transected coronary vein

Stomach

FIGURE 8.4 **Laparoscopic view of celiac axis after D2 lymphadenectomy.** *IVC,* Inferior vena cava.

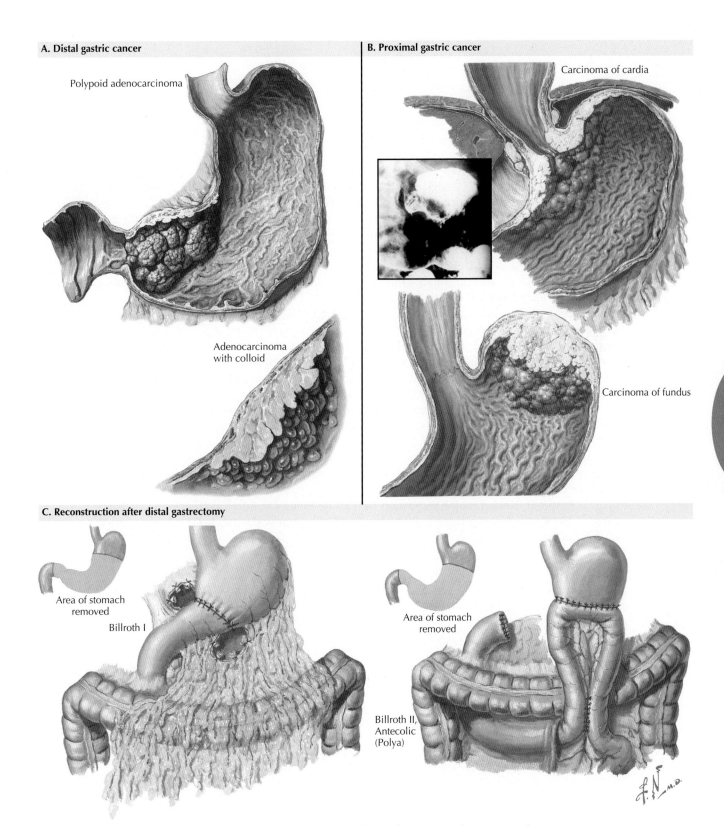

A. Distal gastric cancer

Polypoid adenocarcinoma

Adenocarcinoma
with colloid

B. Proximal gastric cancer

Carcinoma of cardia

Carcinoma of fundus

C. Reconstruction after distal gastrectomy

Area of stomach
removed

Billroth I

Area of stomach
removed

Billroth II,
Antecolic
(Polya)

FIGURE 8.5 Distal and proximal gastric cancer and reconstruction.

SUGGESTED READINGS

Al-Batran SE, Hofheinz RD, Pauligk C, et al. Histopathological regression after neoadjuvant docetaxel, oxaliplatin, fluorouracil, and leucovorin versus epirubicin, cisplatin, and fluorouracil orcapecitabine in patients with resectable gastric or gastro-oesophageal junction adenocarcinoma (FLOT4-AIO): results from the phase 2 part of a multicentre, open-label, randomised phase 2/3 trial. Lancet Oncol 2016;17(12):1697–708.

Bhayani NH, Sharata AM, Dunst CM, Kurian AA, Reavis KM, Swanstrom LL. End of the road for a dysfunctional end organ: laparoscopic gastrectomy for refractory gastroparesis. J Gastrointest Surg 2015;19(3):411–7.

Bonenkamp JJ, Hermans J, Sasako M, van de Velde CJ. Extended lymph node dissection for gastric cancer. N Engl J Med 1999;340:908.

Cunningham D, Allum WH, Stenning SP, et al. Perioperative chemotherapy versus surgery alone for resectable gastroesophageal cancer. N Engl J Med 2006;355:11.

Cuschieri A, Weeden S, Fielding J, et al. Patient survival after D1 and D2 resections for gastric cancer: long-term results of the MRC randomized surgical trial. Br J Cancer 1999;79:1522.

Hartgrink HH, van de Velde CJ, Putter H, et al. Extended lymph node dissection for gastric cancer: who may benefit? Final results of the randomized Dutch Gastric Cancer Group trial. J Clin Oncol 2004;22:2069.

MacDonald JS, Smalley SR, Benedetti J, et al. Chemoradiotherapy after surgery compared with surgery alone for adenocarcinoma of the stomach or gastroesophageal junction. N Engl J Med 2001;345:725.

Songun I, Putter H, Kranenbarg EM, Sasako M, van de Velde CJ. Surgical treatment of gastric cancer: 15-year follow-up results of the randomised nationwide Dutch D1D2 trial. Lancet Oncol 2010;11(5):439–49.

Gastric Emptying Procedures

Kevin El-Hayek and Alisan Fathalizadeh

▶ VIDEO

9.1 Per-Oral Pyloromyotomy (POP) and Laparoscopic Pyloromyotomy

INTRODUCTION

Gastric emptying procedures may play a role in the management of various disease processes, including benign or malignant gastric outlet obstruction, gastroparesis, and pyloric stenosis. Depending on the diagnosis, treatment options may include medical management, enteral or decompressive access tubes, surgical endoscopy, and surgical resection. A thorough understanding of gastric and duodenal anatomy is important when considering endoscopic and surgical gastric emptying procedures (Fig. 9.1A through C).

PRINCIPLES OF TREATMENT

Generally, the treatment for gastric outlet obstruction (GOO) should be managed in the least invasive manner that is appropriate in the context of the disease process. Benign GOO may result from ulcer disease, which may necessitate surgery in medically refractory situations. Malignant GOO may be managed by surgical or endoscopic treatment options based on the individual patient's needs. Gastroparesis treatment should begin with medical management followed by endoscopic per-oral pyloromyotomy (POP), gastric electric stimulator, laparoscopic pyloroplasty, and, ultimately, gastrectomy if necessary. Pyloric stenosis may also be managed endoscopically or surgically.

NONSURGICAL OPTIONS

Nonsurgical options may be implemented for some forms of gastric outlet obstruction. Although results have been disappointing, botulinum toxin, endoscopic dilation, and stenting have been implemented in the treatment of gastroparesis. Stenting remains a valid treatment option in the management of inoperable gastric outlet obstruction.

ENTERAL ACCESS

Patients with gastric outlet obstruction usually have intractable nausea and bloating. Palliative venting gastrostomy tubes (G-tubes) have been used and validated in patients with malignant obstructions. Its use has also been more widely applied to patients with severe medically refractory gastroparesis. The American College of Gastroenterology guidelines also conditionally recommend jejunostomy tubes for delivery of nutrition in patients with gastroparesis or GOO. A combination of a gastrostomy and jejunostomy tube may provide palliative venting in addition to nutritional access.

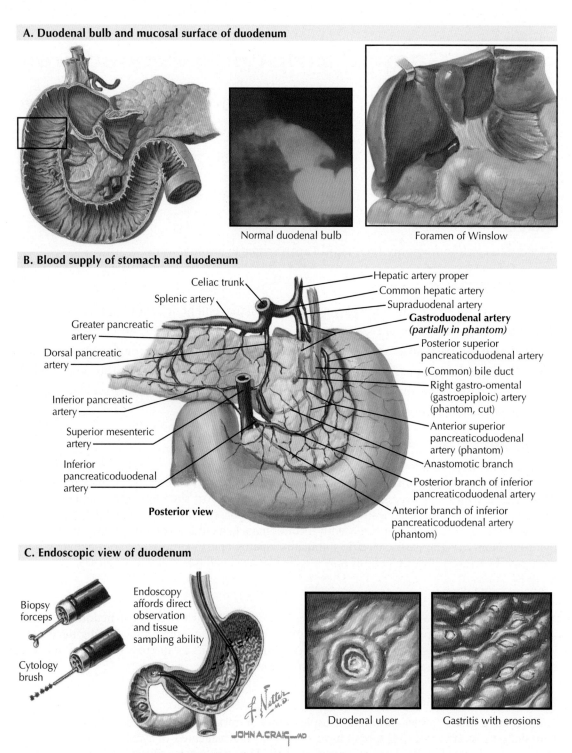

A. Duodenal bulb and mucosal surface of duodenum

Normal duodenal bulb

Foramen of Winslow

B. Blood supply of stomach and duodenum

Celiac trunk

Splenic artery

Greater pancreatic artery

Dorsal pancreatic artery

Inferior pancreatic artery

Superior mesenteric artery

Inferior pancreaticoduodenal artery

Posterior view

Hepatic artery proper

Common hepatic artery

Supraduodenal artery

Gastroduodenal artery (partially in phantom)

Posterior superior pancreaticoduodenal artery

(Common) bile duct

Right gastro-omental (gastroepiploic) artery (phantom, cut)

Anterior superior pancreaticoduodenal artery (phantom)

Anastomotic branch

Posterior branch of inferior pancreaticoduodenal artery

Anterior branch of inferior pancreaticoduodenal artery (phantom)

C. Endoscopic view of duodenum

Biopsy forceps

Cytology brush

Endoscopy affords direct observation and tissue sampling ability

Duodenal ulcer

Gastritis with erosions

FIGURE 9.1 Duodenal bulb, blood supply, and endoscopic view.

SURGICAL ENDOSCOPIC APPROACHES

First performed in 2012 on a porcine model, the POP, also called the gastric per-oral endoscopic myotomy (G-POEM), was modeled after per-oral endoscopic myotomy (POEM) for the treatment of achalasia. POP provides an endoscopic option for patients with gastroparesis while maintaining comparable outcomes with less associated morbidity, operative time, estimated blood loss, and hospital length of stay when compared with a traditional surgical pyloroplasty.

In brief, the procedure involves the concepts and equipment used in endoscopic submucosal dissection (ESD). Using a standard flexible endoscope fitted with a beveled cap, dye is injected into the submucosal plane 2 to 4 cm proximal to the pylorus (Fig. 9.2A). An electrocautery knife is used to create a 1.5- to 2-cm transverse mucosal incision (Fig. 9.2B). A submucosal tunnel is extended to the pyloric muscle fibers, which are then divided (Fig. 9.2C and D). The mucosotomy is then closed with sequential endoscopic clips. (Fig. 9.2E).

An endoscopic pyloromyotomy for infants with congenital hypertrophic pyloric stenosis has also been described. The technique in pediatric patients does not involve a submucosal tunnel but comprises two incisions from the mucosal surface into the anterior and posterior walls of the pylorus.

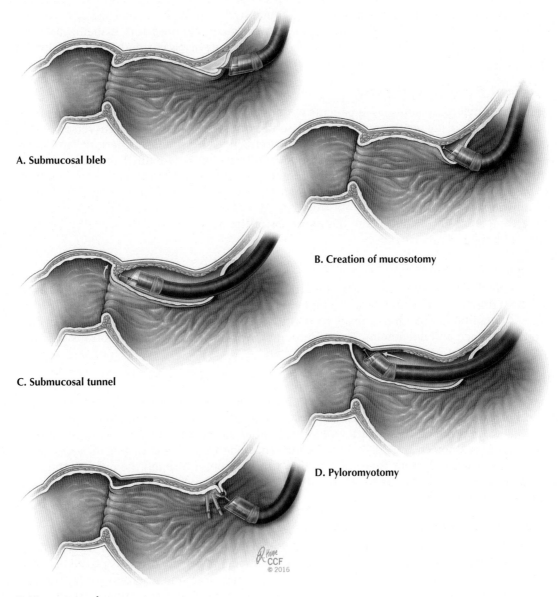

A. Submucosal bleb

B. Creation of mucosotomy

C. Submucosal tunnel

D. Pyloromyotomy

E. Mucosotomy closure

FIGURE 9.2 Per-oral pyloromyotomy.
(Reprinted with permission, Cleveland Clinic Center for Medical Art & Photography © 2016–2019. All Rights Reserved.)

SURGICAL APPROACHES

Surgical gastric emptying procedures can be performed in an open manner via an upper midline or right subcostal incision or minimally invasively using laparoscopic or robotic techniques. An increasing emphasis is being placed on performing minimally invasive interventions as a means of improving overall patient outcomes while also reducing length of stay and hospital cost.

Gastric Electric Stimulator

Gastric electric stimulators (GES) may be offered for the treatment of patients with medically refractory diabetic or idiopathic gastroparesis. Both open and minimally invasive approaches have been described involving the placement of 2 leads roughly 10 cm proximal to the pylorus within the "antral pump" of the stomach. These leads are then connected to an externally adjustable generator that is secured to the abdominal wall. Although the mechanism of action is not clearly understood, it appears that patients with medically refractory diabetic gastroparesis respond better than those with idiopathic causes. The device is currently approved by the FDA as a humanitarian use exemption at select centers.

Surgical Pyloromyotomy

To perform a pyloromyotomy, as in patients with hypertrophied pyloric stenosis, the omentum is first mobilized using gentle traction to expose the transverse colon. The transverse colon is drawn caudally to visualize the gastric antrum. Retracting the stomach inferiorly and laterally helps visualize the pylorus. The gastroduodenal junction is identified by the prepyloric vein (Fig. 9.3). An incision is made along the anterior surface of the pylorus extending from the prepyloric vein to the antrum of the stomach. The incision is taken through the serosal and muscle layers until the submucosa is visualized bulging into the cleft (Figs. 9.3, and 9.4). At the completion of the dissection, the two sides of the hypertrophied pylorus should move independently.

Heineke-Mikulicz Pyloroplasty

With a Heineke-Mikulicz pyloroplasty, initially, a Kocher maneuver is performed by releasing the lateral duodenal attachments and completely freeing the duodenum from the retroperitoneum. A longitudinal incision is made over the pylorus, extending several centimeters onto both the stomach and duodenum. The longitudinal incision is then closed in a transverse orientation to prevent narrowing the outlet (Fig. 9.5).

Finney U-Shaped Pyloroplasty

After an extensive Kocher maneuver is performed, a traction suture is placed in the superior margin of the midpylorus. A second traction suture is placed 5 cm proximal to the pylorus on the greater curvature of the stomach and 5 cm distal to the pyloric ring on the duodenal wall. The walls of the stomach and duodenum are then sutured together. A U-shaped incision is then made into the stomach from above the traction suture, around through the pylorus and onto the duodenum a similar distance. A side-to-side sutured gastroduodenal anastomosis is then performed in two layers.

Jaboulay Gastroduodenostomy

An initial extensive Kocher maneuver is performed. The gastric wall is then mobilized for about 6 to 8 cm proximally and brought toward the duodenal wall. A suture is placed between the gastric wall and duodenum as near the pylorus as practical, and a second suture is taken between the stomach and duodenum to allow about 6 to 8 cm of approximation. A two-layered side-to-side gastroduodenal anastomosis is made with preservation of the pylorus.

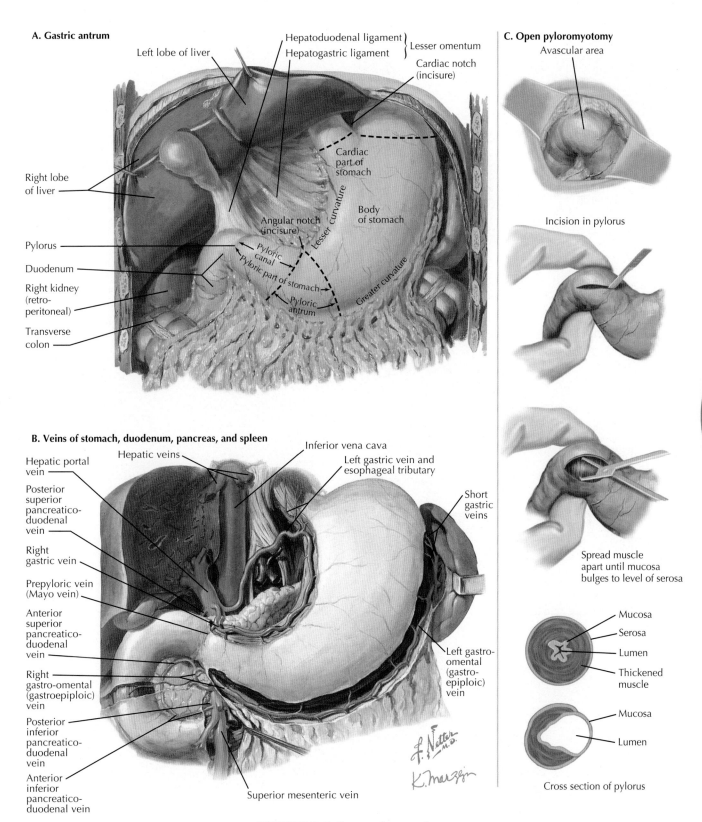

A. Gastric antrum

Left lobe of liver

Hepatoduodenal ligament ⎱
Hepatogastric ligament ⎰ Lesser omentum

Cardiac notch (incisure)

Right lobe of liver

Cardiac part of stomach

Body of stomach

Pylorus

Duodenum

Angular notch (incisure)

Lesser curvature

Right kidney (retro-peritoneal)

Pyloric canal
Pyloric part of stomach

Pyloric antrum

Greater curvature

Transverse colon

B. Veins of stomach, duodenum, pancreas, and spleen

Hepatic veins

Inferior vena cava

Hepatic portal vein

Left gastric vein and esophageal tributary

Posterior superior pancreatico-duodenal vein

Short gastric veins

Right gastric vein

Prepyloric vein (Mayo vein)

Anterior superior pancreatico-duodenal vein

Right gastro-omental (gastroepiploic) vein

Left gastro-omental (gastro-epiploic) vein

Posterior inferior pancreatico-duodenal vein

Anterior inferior pancreatico-duodenal vein

Superior mesenteric vein

C. Open pyloromyotomy

Avascular area

Incision in pylorus

Spread muscle apart until mucosa bulges to level of serosa

Mucosa
Serosa
Lumen
Thickened muscle

Mucosa
Lumen

Cross section of pylorus

FIGURE 9.3 Open pyloromyotomy.

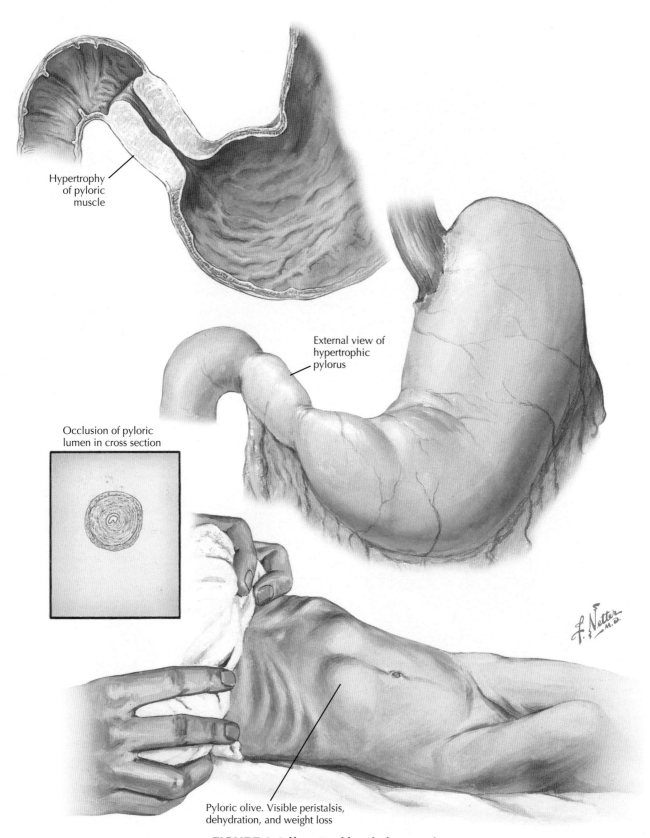

Hypertrophy
of pyloric
muscle

External view of
hypertrophic
pylorus

Occlusion of pyloric
lumen in cross section

Pyloric olive. Visible peristalsis,
dehydration, and weight loss

FIGURE 9.4 Hypertrophic pyloric stenosis.

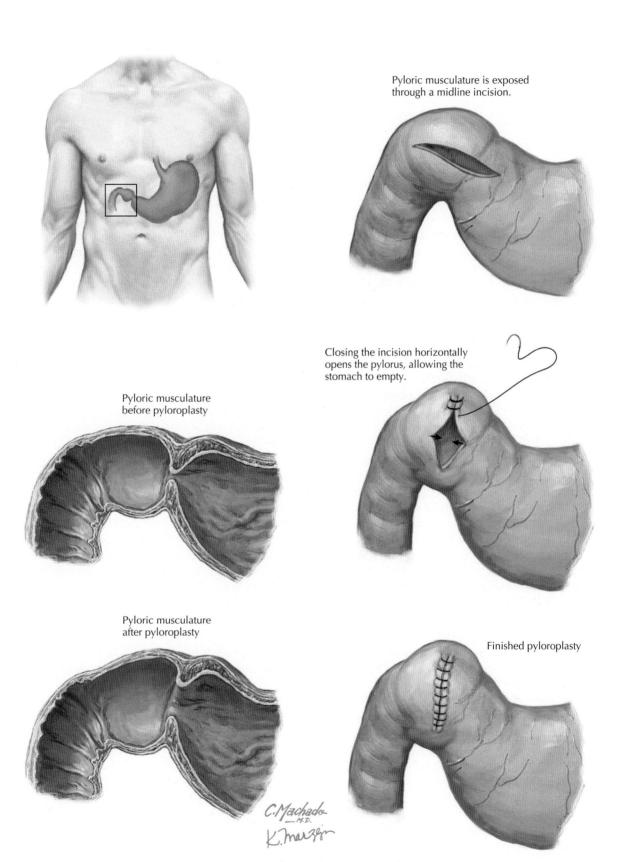

Pyloric musculature is exposed through a midline incision.

Pyloric musculature before pyloroplasty

Closing the incision horizontally opens the pylorus, allowing the stomach to empty.

Pyloric musculature after pyloroplasty

Finished pyloroplasty

FIGURE 9.5 **Pyloroplasty constructions.**

Distal Gastrectomy and Billroth I, Billroth II, or Roux-en-Y Reconstruction

After intra-abdominal inspection, a Kocher maneuver is performed to mobilize the duodenum. The greater omentum is detached from the transverse colon. The gastroesophageal junction and gastric fundus are mobilized. The halfway point of the stomach is selected where the gastroepiploic artery most closely approximates the greater curvature of the stomach. On the lesser curvature, the stomach is divided just distal to the third prominent vein. The hepatic flexure of the colon is mobilized away from the duodenum. The avascular duodenal attachments are released. A truncal vagotomy may be performed in cases of refractory ulcer disease. The stomach is mobilized and any posterior attachments are released creating a retrogastric plane between the lesser and greater curvature. Once the point of resection is identified and a window is created, the stomach and duodenum are divided between staplers. For a Billroth I (gastroduodenal) anastomosis, an end-to-end or end-to-side handsewn or stapled EEA anastomosis is created between the proximal stomach and the duodenum (Fig. 9.6).

To create a Billroth II (gastrojejunal) anastomosis after antrectomy, the stomach is mobilized and resected as previously described. A portion of jejunum that reaches without tension to the stomach is selected beyond the ligament of Treitz. The jejunal loop may be brought up either retrocolic (Fig. 9.7A) or antecolic (Fig. 9.7B), and the anastomosis performed in either a retrogastric or antegastric position. A hand-sewn or stapled anastomosis is created between the jejunum and the posterior portion of the stomach (see Fig. 9.6).

To perform a Roux-en-Y gastrojejunostomy, a portion of jejunum is selected roughly 40 cm distal to the ligament of Treitz. The jejunum is divided and the Roux limb is brought to the stomach in an antecolic or retrocolic fashion. To prevent bile reflux, a jejunojejunal anastomosis is created at least 40 cm from the gastrojejunal anastomosis. If an antecolic Roux limb is used, it is advisable to close pseudo-Peterson's defect, which is created between the Roux limb and the transverse colon. If a retrocolic limb is chosen, the mesenteric defect and Peterson's defect should also be closed.

Total Gastrectomy

A total gastrectomy is the most definitive gastric emptying procedure and is reserved for gastric malignancies or benign disorders not amenable to the above procedures. After laparoscopic ports are placed or midline laparotomy is made, the gastrohepatic ligament is divided close to the liver. The gastroesophageal junction and esophagus are mobilized into the abdomen. The omentum and lesser sac are removed en bloc from the transverse colon. The short gastric vessels are divided, and the celiac, splenic, and common hepatic arteries are skeletonized with a lymph node harvest in cases of malignancy. The left and right gastric and gastroepiploic arteries are ligated at their bases. The esophagus, stomach, and jejunum are then divided to complete specimen resection. Typical reconstruction is then with a Roux-en-Y esophagojejunostomy and jejunojejunostomy using the principles previously described (Fig. 9.8).

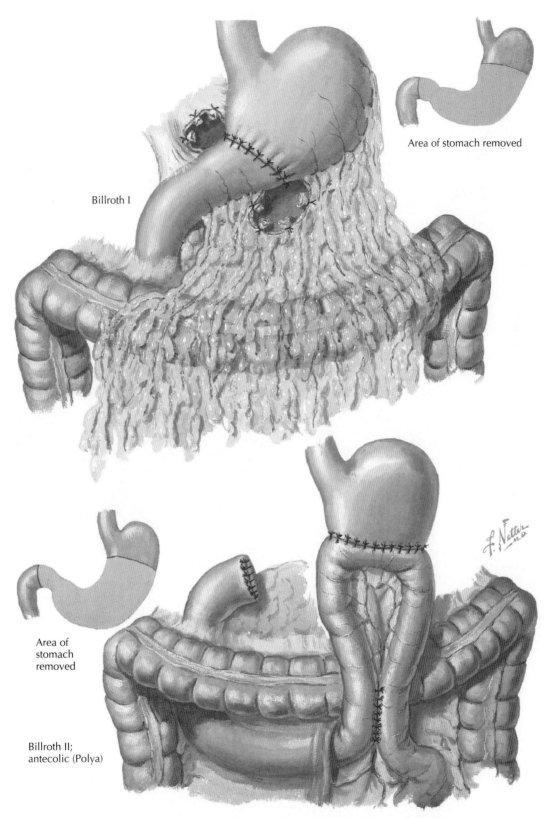

Billroth I

Area of stomach removed

Area of stomach removed

Billroth II; antecolic (Polya)

FIGURE 9.6 Principles of operative procedures: partial gastrectomy and Billroth anastomoses.

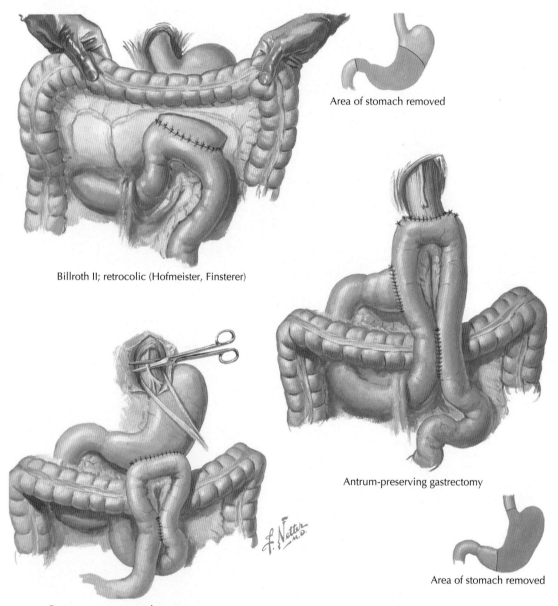

Area of stomach removed

Billroth II; retrocolic (Hofmeister, Finsterer)

Antrum-preserving gastrectomy

Area of stomach removed

Gastro-enterostomy and vagotomy

FIGURE 9.7 **Principles of operative procedure.**

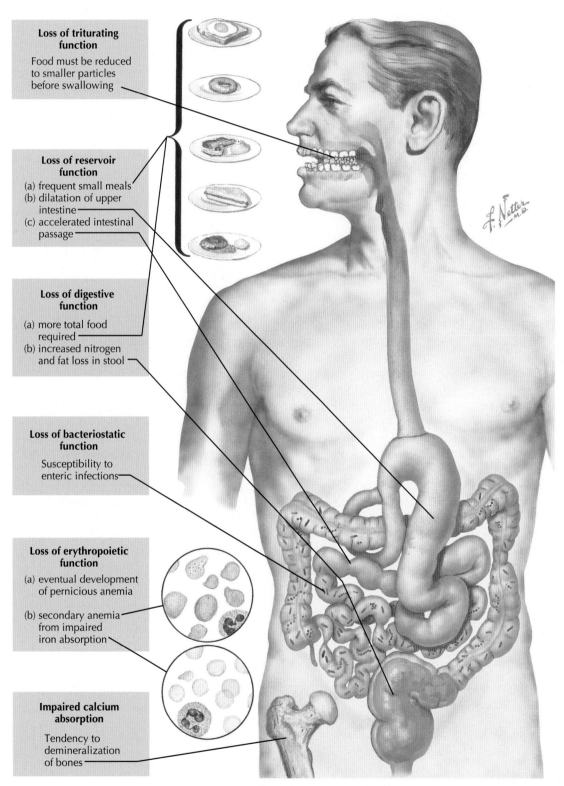

Loss of triturating function

Food must be reduced to smaller particles before swallowing

Loss of reservoir function

(a) frequent small meals
(b) dilatation of upper intestine
(c) accelerated intestinal passage

Loss of digestive function

(a) more total food required
(b) increased nitrogen and fat loss in stool

Loss of bacteriostatic function

Susceptibility to enteric infections

Loss of erythropoietic function

(a) eventual development of pernicious anemia

(b) secondary anemia from impaired iron absorption

Impaired calcium absorption

Tendency to demineralization of bones

FIGURE 9.8 Effects of total gastrectomy.

SUGGESTED READINGS

Allemang MT, Strong AT, Haskins IN, et al. How I do it: per-oral pyloromyotomy (POP). J Gastrointest Surg 2017;21(11):1963–8.

Choi YB. Laparoscopic gatrojejunostomy for palliation of gastric outlet obstruction in unresectable gastric cancer. Surg Endosc 2002;16(11):1620–6.

Clarke JO, Snape Jr WJ. Pyloric sphincter therapy: botulinum toxin, stents, and pyloromyotomy. Gastroenterol Clin North Am 2015;44:127–36.

Khashab MA, Stein E, Clarke JO, et al. Gastric peroral endoscopic myotomy for refractory gastroparesis: first human endoscopic pyloromyotomy (with video). Gastrointest Endosc 2013;78(5):764–8.

Landreneau J, Strong AT, El-Hayek K, et al. Laparoscopic pyloroplasty versus endoscopic per-oral pyloromyotomy for the treatment of gastroparesis. Surg Endosc 2019;33:773–81.

St Peter SD, Holcomb 3rd GW, Calkins CM, et al. Open versus laparoscopic pyloromyotomy for pyloric stenosis: a prospective, randomized trial. Ann Surg 2006;244(3):363–70.

Storm AC, Ryou M. Advances in the endoscopic management of gastric outflow disorders. Curr Opin Gastroenterol 2017;33:455–60.

Roux-en-Y Gastric Bypass and Sleeve Gastrectomy

Victoria Lyo and Farah A. Husain

▶ VIDEOS

10.1 Linear Stapled Gastric Bypass (Antecolic, Antegastric)
10.2 EEA Stapled Gastrojejunal Anastomosis (Antecolic, Antegastric)
10.3 Sleeve Gastrectomy

INTRODUCTION

Obesity is a major health problem worldwide and has reached an epidemic proportion in both developed and developing regions, with one-third of the world's population overweight or obese. A major risk factor for many diseases, obesity is associated with significant morbidity and mortality.

Bariatric surgery is currently the only modality that provides significant, long-term weight loss for the patient who is morbidly obese, with resultant improvement in obesity-related comorbidities. Gastric bypass is the "gold standard" for surgical management of morbid obesity in the United States, whereas sleeve gastrectomy is now the most commonly performed operation.

SURGICAL CRITERIA

Surgery for obesity should be considered after dieting, exercise, psychotherapy, and drug treatments have failed. National Institutes of Health (NIH) criteria for surgical treatment include a body mass index (BMI) of greater than 40 kg/m^2 or a BMI of greater than 35 kg/m^2 in combination with high-risk comorbid conditions. Sleeve gastrectomy provides durable weight loss and improved medical comorbidities similar to gastric bypass. However, sleeve gastrectomy should not be performed in patients with pre-existing gastroesophageal reflux disease because symptoms persist postoperatively, whereas gastric bypass is an anti-reflux procedure.

SURGICAL ANATOMY FOR GASTRIC BYPASS

Gastric bypass provides two components to aid in weight loss: restriction and malabsorption, which are both demonstrated in the depiction of a Roux-en-Y gastric bypass (Fig. 10.1A). Excessive intra-abdominal fat can make identification of the anatomy difficult, but with laparoscopic approaches, it is possible to perform the operation safely and achieve critical views of the anatomy.

Creation of a constricted, vertically oriented 20- to 30-mL gastric pouch based on the lesser curvature of the stomach provides the restrictive component of gastric bypass. The lesser curvature musculature is thick and less likely to distend than the fundus of the stomach (Fig. 10.1B).

Identification and dissection of the *angle of His* (the angle between the fundus and abdominal esophagus) is a crucial step during construction of the gastric pouch. The angle of His is just to the left of the midline and the gastroesophageal fat pad of Belsey. Transection of the stomach at the angle of His will separate the gastric fundus from the gastric pouch, because the gastric fundus can otherwise distend, with resultant weight gain (Fig. 10.1C). This approach also avoids stapling of the esophagus.

The anterior and posterior nerves of Latarjet descend along the lesser curvature of the stomach and usually lie 0.5 to 1 cm from the gastric wall. On opening the gastrohepatic ligament, the surgeon must perform dissection perigastrically to avoid injury of the anterior or posterior nerve of Latarjet. Injury of these nerves may result in delayed emptying of the distal stomach. A retrogastric window is created on the lesser curvature of the stomach 4 cm from the gastroesophageal junction, and retrogastric adhesions are taken down to allow complete mobilization of the stomach (Fig. 10.1D). This eliminates any redundant posterior wall of the pouch and exclude the fundus from the gastric pouch.

The three options to bring the Roux limb up to the gastric pouch are antecolic antegastric, retrocolic retrogastric, and retrocolic antegastric. Retrocolic retrogastric is the shortest path to the gastric pouch (tension free), whereas antecolic antegastric is the simplest of the three approaches.

The greater omentum is divided vertically in the midline, starting from the inferior edge of the omentum to the transverse colon. This approach will decrease the distance that the antecolic antegastric Roux limb must reach, while decreasing tension on the limb.

The ligament of Treitz is identified to the left of midline, with the inferior mesenteric vein to its left (Fig. 10.2). On creating a retrocolic path for the Roux limb, a defect in the transverse mesocolon must be anterior and to the left of ligament of Treitz to avoid injury to the middle colic vessels and to the pancreas.

The left gastric artery is the main arterial supply to the gastric pouch, which arises from the celiac artery. Initially, it runs superiorly and to the left to approach the gastroesophageal junction, where it gives rise to esophageal branches, turns inferiorly to follow the lesser curvature of the stomach, and terminates by anastomosing with the much smaller right gastric artery. In 25% of cases, the left gastric artery also gives rise to the left hepatic artery (or accessory left hepatic arteries), which runs through the superior part of the gastrohepatic ligament (Fig. 10.3A).

During Roux-en-Y gastric bypass, several internal defects must be closed with running non-absorbable suture to avoid internal hernia. These defects include Peterson's defect (between the Roux limb mesentery and the transverse mesocolon), the intermesenteric defect, and the defect in the transverse mesocolon (in retrocolic technique) (Fig. 10.3B). Bleeding and leakage may also occur but are minimized with good surgical technique without tension. Marginal ulcers, late fistulization to the remnant stomach, and stenosis of the gastrojejunal anastomosis are potential complications after surgery.

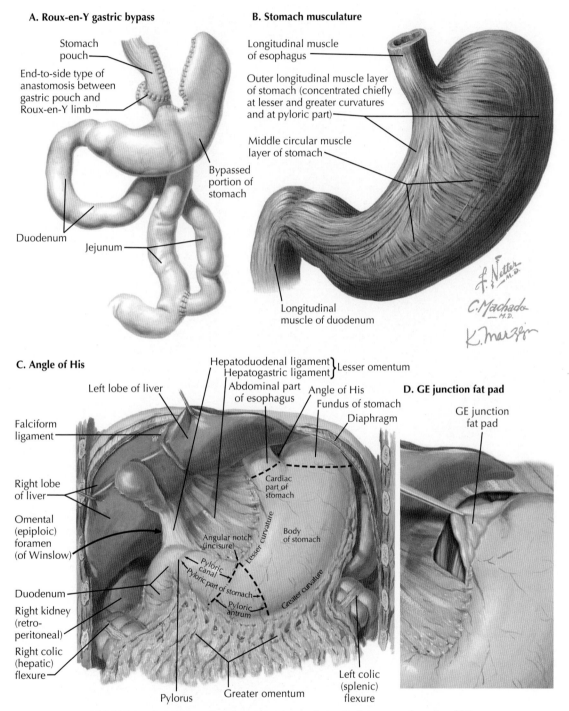

A. Roux-en-Y gastric bypass

Stomach pouch

End-to-side type of anastomosis between gastric pouch and Roux-en-Y limb

Duodenum

Jejunum

Bypassed portion of stomach

B. Stomach musculature

Longitudinal muscle of esophagus

Outer longitudinal muscle layer of stomach (concentrated chiefly at lesser and greater curvatures and at pyloric part)

Middle circular muscle layer of stomach

Longitudinal muscle of duodenum

C. Angle of His

Left lobe of liver

Falciform ligament

Right lobe of liver

Omental (epiploic) foramen (of Winslow)

Duodenum

Right kidney (retro-peritoneal)

Right colic (hepatic) flexure

Pylorus

Greater omentum

Hepatoduodenal ligament
Hepatogastric ligament } Lesser omentum

Abdominal part of esophagus

Angle of His
Fundus of stomach
Diaphragm

Cardiac part of stomach

Lesser curvature

Body of stomach

Angular notch (incisure)

Pyloric canal
Pyloric part of stomach
Pyloric antrum

Greater curvature

Left colic (splenic) flexure

D. GE junction fat pad

GE junction fat pad

FIGURE 10.1 Roux-en-Y bypass, stomach musculature, and angle of His.

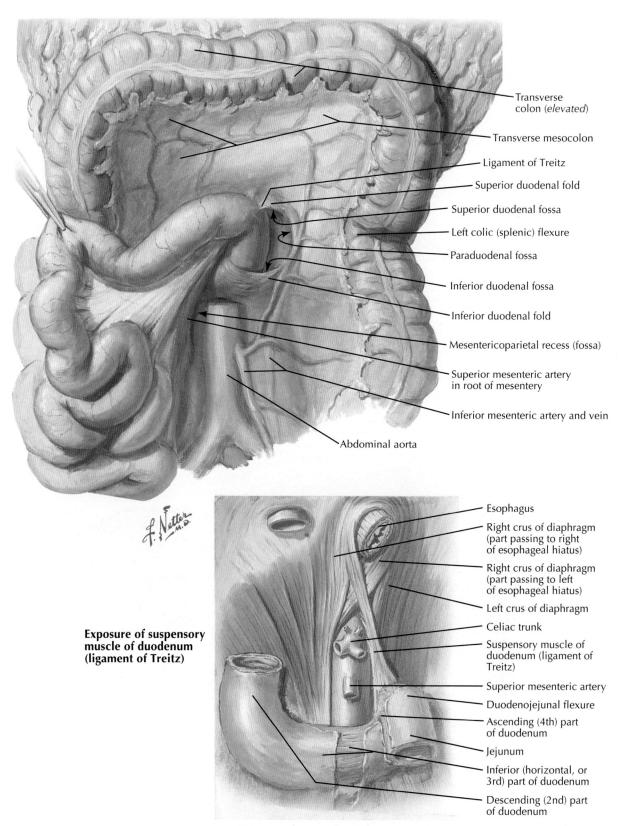

Transverse colon (*elevated*)

Transverse mesocolon

Ligament of Treitz

Superior duodenal fold

Superior duodenal fossa

Left colic (splenic) flexure

Paraduodenal fossa

Inferior duodenal fossa

Inferior duodenal fold

Mesentericoparietal recess (fossa)

Superior mesenteric artery in root of mesentery

Inferior mesenteric artery and vein

Abdominal aorta

Exposure of suspensory muscle of duodenum (ligament of Treitz)

Esophagus

Right crus of diaphragm (part passing to right of esophageal hiatus)

Right crus of diaphragm (part passing to left of esophageal hiatus)

Left crus of diaphragm

Celiac trunk

Suspensory muscle of duodenum (ligament of Treitz)

Superior mesenteric artery

Duodenojejunal flexure

Ascending (4th) part of duodenum

Jejunum

Inferior (horizontal, or 3rd) part of duodenum

Descending (2nd) part of duodenum

FIGURE 10.2 Roux-en-Y approach and ligament of Treitz.

A. Cross section of abdominal vasculature (coronal view)

Common hepatic artery

Left hepatic artery

Proper hepatic artery

Right hepatic artery

Gastroduodenal artery

Splenic artery

Left gastric artery

Celiac artery

Superior mesenteric artery

B. Potential herniation sites

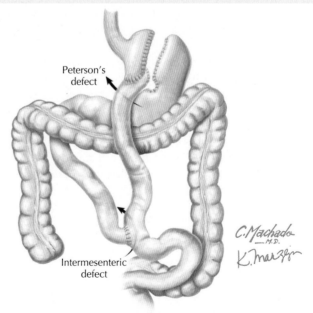

Peterson's defect

Intermesenteric defect

Transverse mesocolon defect (not shown)

FIGURE 10.3 Gastric arterial supply and closing of internal defects.

SURGICAL ANATOMY FOR SLEEVE GASTRECTOMY

Sleeve gastrectomy is considered a predominantly restrictive procedure with less malabsorption than a bypass or duodenal switch. The goal of the sleeve gastrectomy operation is to create a tubularized stomach along the lesser curvature of the stomach. This smaller stomach should hold approximately 60 to 100 mL of liquid.

The lesser curvature musculature is thick and less likely to distend than the fundus of the stomach. Starting at the distal body of the stomach along the greater curvature, the gastrocolic ligament is divided just caudal to the stomach using a bipolar or ultrasonic energy device, thus entering the lesser sac. The gastroepiploic artery is preserved and left in the greater omentum (Fig. 10.4).

Dissection is continued cephalad along the greater curvature and continued up to divide all the short gastric vessels. As the stomach is retracted to the right and anteriorly, the posterior stomach is identified and any posterior gastric adhesions to the retroperitoneum should be divided. The fundus is rotated medially and then completely separated from the spleen and diaphragm by dividing the lienogastric and gastrophrenic ligaments until the left crus is visible.

The gastroesophageal fat pad of Belsey at the angle of His should be dissected off of the stomach along the left lateral aspect so that the fundus and gastroesophageal junction is easily visible.

The gastrocolic ligament is then divided distally from the greater curve until 4 cm from the pylorus (Fig. 10.5). A 30- to 40-Fr bougie or endoscope is then placed to size the sleeve, and the stomach is transected using multiple fires of staplers. At the proximal stomach, care is taken to divide the stomach just to the left of the gastroesophageal junction at the angle of His to maximally remove fundus of the stomach but not to impinge upon the gastroesophageal junction (see Fig. 10.5). The remnant stomach is then removed.

An anatomically successful sleeve must not narrow the incisura, and the sleeve should lay flat without twisting or torsion of the staple line so as to avoid obstruction and stricture resulting in oral intolerance.

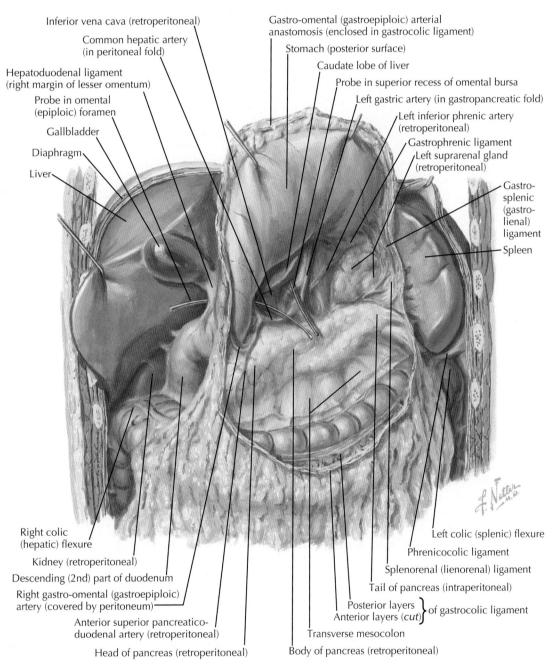

Inferior vena cava (retroperitoneal)

Common hepatic artery (in peritoneal fold)

Hepatoduodenal ligament (right margin of lesser omentum)

Probe in omental (epiploic) foramen

Gallbladder

Diaphragm

Liver

Gastro-omental (gastroepiploic) arterial anastomosis (enclosed in gastrocolic ligament)

Stomach (posterior surface)

Caudate lobe of liver

Probe in superior recess of omental bursa

Left gastric artery (in gastropancreatic fold)

Left inferior phrenic artery (retroperitoneal)

Gastrophrenic ligament

Left suprarenal gland (retroperitoneal)

Gastro-splenic (gastro-lienal) ligament

Spleen

Right colic (hepatic) flexure

Kidney (retroperitoneal)

Descending (2nd) part of duodenum

Right gastro-omental (gastroepiploic) artery (covered by peritoneum)

Anterior superior pancreatico-duodenal artery (retroperitoneal)

Head of pancreas (retroperitoneal)

Left colic (splenic) flexure

Phrenicocolic ligament

Splenorenal (lienorenal) ligament

Tail of pancreas (intraperitoneal)

Posterior layers
Anterior layers (cut) } of gastrocolic ligament

Transverse mesocolon

Body of pancreas (retroperitoneal)

FIGURE 10.4 Division of stomach from gastrocolic ligament.

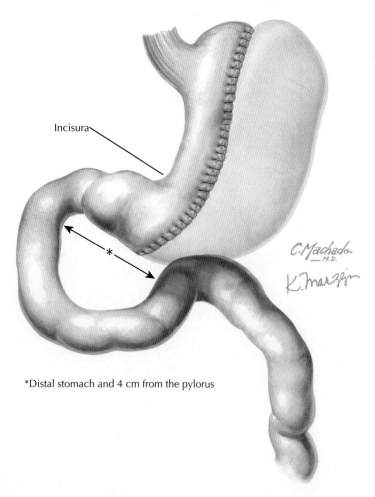

Incisura

*Distal stomach and 4 cm from the pylorus

FIGURE 10.5 Sleeve gastrectomy.

SUGGESTED READINGS

Berbiglia L, Zografakis JG, Dan AG. Laparoscopic roux-en-Y gastric bypass: surgical technique and perioperative care. Surg Clin North Am 2016;96(4):773–94.

Courcoulas AP, King WC, Belle SH, et al. Seven-year weight trajectories and health outcomes in the Longitudinal Assessment of Bariatric Surgery (LABS) Study. JAMA Surg 2018;153(5):427–34.

Hayes K, Eid G. Laparoscopic sleeve gastrectomy: surgical technique and perioperative care. Surg Clin North Am 2016;96(4):763–71.

Higa KD, Ho T, Tercero F, Yunus T, Boone KB. Laparoscopic Roux-en-Y gastric bypass: 10-year follow-up. Surg Obes Relat Dis 2011;7:516–25.

Nguyen NT, Blackstone RP, Morton JM, Ponce J, Rosenthal RJ. The ASMBS textbook of bariatric surgery. New York: Springer; 2015.

Rondelli F, Bugiantella W, Desio M, et al. Antecolic or retrocolic alimentary limb in laparoscopic roux-en-Y gastric bypass? A meta-analysis. Obes Surg 2016;26(1):182–95.

Rosenthal RJ. International sleeve gastrectomy expert panel consensus statement: best practice guidelines based on >12,000 cases. Surg Obes Relat Dis 2012;8:8–19.

Salminen P, Melmiö M, Ovaska J, et al. Effect of laparoscopic sleeve gastrectomy vs laparoscopic roux-en-Y gastric bypass on weight loss at 5 years among patients with morbid obesity; the SLEEVEPASS randomized clinical trial. JAMA 2018;319(3):241–54.

Schauer PR, Bhatt DL, Kirwan JP, et al. Bariatric surgery versus intensive medical therapy for diabetes—5-year outcomes. N Engl J Med 2017;376(7):641–51.

Shoar S, Saber AA. Long-term and midterm outcomes of laparoscopic sleeve gastrectomy versus Roux-en-Y gastric bypass: a systematic review and meta-analysis of comparative studies. Surg Obes Relat Dis 2017;13(2):170–80.

Surgical Management of Achalasia

Matthew Kroh, John H. Rodriguez, and Julietta Chang

INTRODUCTION

Achalasia is a rare disorder of the esophagus. From the Greek *khalasis* (to loosen, and Latin *a-*, without), the disease is characterized by dysphagia and reflux symptoms secondary to inability of the lower esophageal sphincter (LES) to relax, with varying degrees of esophageal dysmotility. Idiopathic achalasia secondary to immune-mediated chronic ganglionitis of the myenteric plexus is the most common variant; rarer causes of achalasia include pseudo-achalasia resulting from obstruction after foregut surgery, malignant infiltration of the gastroesophageal (GE) junction, or as a sequelae of paraneoplastic disease, or after destruction of the myenteric neurons by *Trypanosoma cruzi* in Chagas disease. Still, idiopathic achalasia remains rare, with an incidence of 1.6 cases per 100,000 patients.

PREOPERATIVE WORKUP

A barium esophagram in an achalasia may show a classic "bird's beak" appearance with delayed emptying of timed contrast (Fig. 11.1). However, up to one-third of patients with achalasia may not have abnormal esophagram findings. However, this gives the surgeon information about the esophageal anatomy, for example, if the patient has a hiatal hernia or a tortuous esophagus. Patients should undergo an endoscopy to rule out pseudoachalasia or an obstructing mass as cause of their obstruction. However, as with the esophagram, up to one-third will have a nondiagnostic esophagogastroduodenoscopy (EGD), so this is not the diagnostic test of choice for achalasia.

The gold standard for diagnosis remains high-resolution esophageal manometry, which will reveal high-resting pressure of the LES (>45 mm Hg); failure of LES relaxation with swallow (residual pressure > 10 mm Hg); as well as aperistalsis of the esophageal body ("classic" achalasia, or type I), pan-esophageal pressurization (type II), or spastic contractions (type III).

THERAPEUTIC CONSIDERATIONS

Unfortunately, no treatment currently exists that addresses the underlying pathophysiology of achalasia, and therapy is palliative and aims to relieve the symptoms of achalasia. Medical and endoscopic therapies available that are discussed elsewhere aim to relieve obstruction at the LES through pharmacotherapy or mechanical disruption of the muscle fibers. There are currently two surgical options that are offered to patients with achalasia: Heller myotomy with partial fundoplication, which has been offered laparoscopically since the 1990s; and the newer per-oral endoscopic myotomy (POEM) procedure, which was described in 2010.

Both therapies aim to disrupt the hypertrophic muscle fibers of the LES but do not address the poor motility of the esophagus, relying on gravity to allow the esophagus to drain once the downstream obstruction is relieved. In a patient with end-stage achalasia and a patulous, sigmoid esophagus (Fig. 11.2), a myotomy alone will not allow the esophagus to properly drain; these patients may require a palliative esophagectomy, which is not within the scope of this chapter.

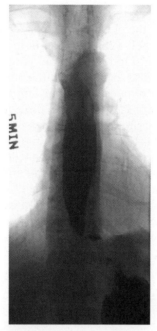

FIGURE 11.1 Barium swallow demonstrating classic bird's-beak appearance with a dilated esophagus and tapering at the gastroesophageal junction.

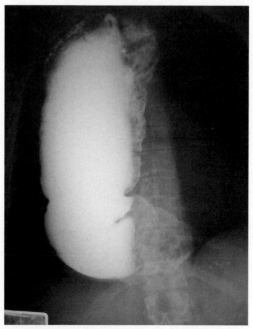

FIGURE 11.2 Barium swallow demonstrating end-stage achalasia with massive dilation and tortuous curving of the distal esophagus—the so-called *sigmoid esophagus*.

SURGICAL ANATOMY

The esophagus travels through the hiatus into the abdomen; the intra-abdominal portion is approximately 2 cm long and is covered by the phrenoesophageal ligament, which arises as a continuation of the subdiaphragmatic fascia, itself a continuation of the transversalis fascia (Fig. 11.3). The intra-abdominal esophagus is subject to intra-abdominal positive pressure and contributes to the LES. The musculature of the esophagus is composed of the outer longitudinal fibers and the inner circular layer. The upper esophagus is composed of striated muscle and subject to voluntary control, whereas the lower third is composed of smooth muscle fibers and the middle third is a mixture of both. Surgical myotomy should target the smooth muscle of the distal third of the esophagus. The sling muscle of the proximal stomach also contributes to the LES and extends onto the proximal 2 to 3 cm of the stomach, and it is imperative that these be divided to provide a complete myotomy.

The paired vagus nerves run along the esophagus and enter the abdomen through the hiatus to provide parasympathetic and sympathetic innervation to the viscera (Fig. 11.4). Proximally, they run in the tracheoesophageal groove but then course anterior and posterior to the esophagus as they enter the abdomen. The anterior vagus nerve enters from the mediastinum from the left, whereas the posterior vagus enters from the right. These should be identified and preserved during surgery.

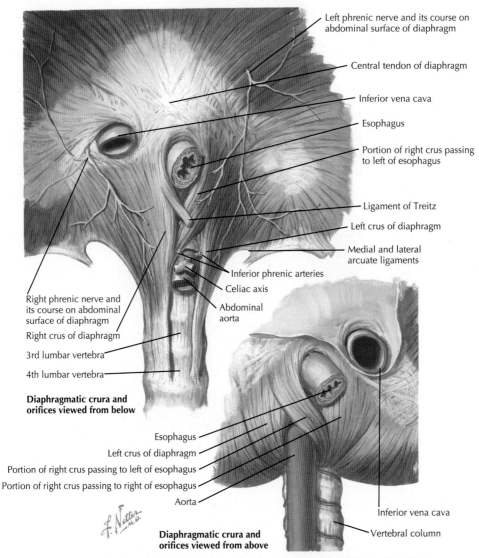

FIGURE 11.3 **View of the esophagus coursing through the diaphragmatic crura.**

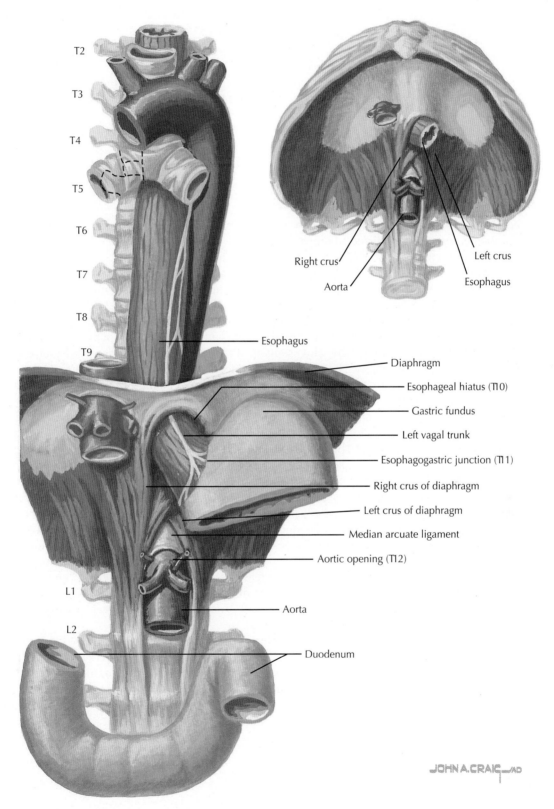

FIGURE 11.4 Relationship of the anterior vagus to the esophagus as it courses through the diaphragmatic hiatus.

LAPAROSCOPIC HELLER MYOTOMY

The beginning of the operation is similar to a laparoscopic anti-reflux procedure (Chapter 6). The esophagus must be mobilized to allow for a generous myotomy. The left lateral segment of the liver is retracted with a flexible retractor to allow for adequate visualization. The gastro-hepatic ligament is divided (Fig. 11.5) and phrenoesophageal ligament is incised over the right crus. The peritoneum over the anterior crura is incised, and the esophagus is mobilized circumferentially (Fig. 11.6). A Penrose drain can be passed around the esophagus at this step to aid in mediastinal dissection of the esophagus. If a hiatal hernia is present, this should be reduced to allow adequate intraesophageal length. The goal is to visualize at least 5 cm of anterior esophagus to perform an adequate myotomy. The esophageal fat pad is excised to clearly visualize the anterior surface of the esophagus. The anterior vagus nerve is identified and preserved.

The short gastric vessels are next divided starting at the lower pole of the spleen using an energy device in preparation for fundoplication after myotomy (Fig. 11.7).

If the anterior vagus nerve crosses the anterior surface of the esophagus, a tunnel may be created under the nerve to create the myotomy. If it lies relatively straight, the myotomy can be created to the left of the nerve. The esophageal muscle fibers are grasped by the surgeon and assistant to give adequate traction, and electrocautery is used to create a dotted line along the esophagus to mark the path of the myotomy and to aid in hemostasis. The muscular fibers are then sharply divided using laparoscopic shears (Fig. 11.8). Bulging from the esophageal mucosa indicates that the surgeon is in the correct plane, and that the circular muscle has been completely divided. Bleeding from the muscle edges can be controlled with an epinephrine-soaked sponge and pressure; electrocautery should be used judiciously in this area to avoid mucosal injury. The myotomy is continued proximally onto the esophagus for at least 5 to 6 cm and then distally onto the sling fibers of the stomach for at least 2 to 3 cm. An endoscopy at the completion of the myotomy helps confirm that all circular fibers of the LES have been divided, and a saline-leak test can be performed at this time as well. Inadvertent esophageal mucosotomies can be repaired with interrupted 4-0 Vicryl suture.

A partial fundoplication is performed in addition to the myotomy. The addition of a fundoplication does not affect postoperative dysphagia, but it does significantly decrease postoperative reflux symptoms from 31.5% vs. 8.8%. A posterior Toupet fundoplication helps to pull the circular fibers of the LES of the myotomy apart and, we believe, may decrease postoperative dysphagia (Fig. 11.9). However, if an inadvertent mucosotomy was repaired, an anterior Dor fundoplication helps buttress the repair.

A. Relationships of the right and left crura of the diaphragm. Note that the right and left pillars of the right crus form the esophageal hiatus.

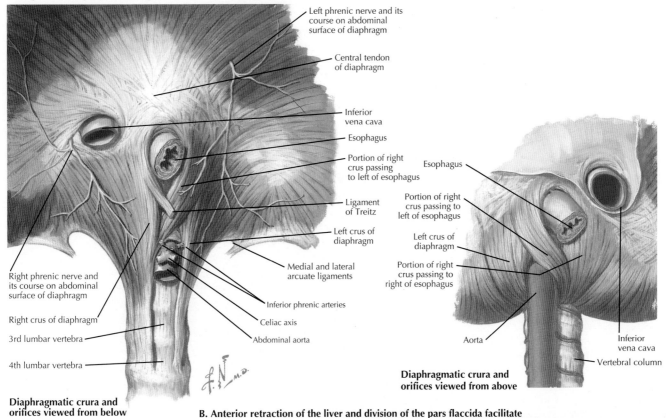

Left phrenic nerve and its course on abdominal surface of diaphragm

Central tendon of diaphragm

Inferior vena cava

Esophagus

Portion of right crus passing to left of esophagus

Ligament of Treitz

Left crus of diaphragm

Medial and lateral arcuate ligaments

Inferior phrenic arteries

Celiac axis

Abdominal aorta

Right phrenic nerve and its course on abdominal surface of diaphragm

Right crus of diaphragm

3rd lumbar vertebra

4th lumbar vertebra

Diaphragmatic crura and orifices viewed from below

Esophagus

Portion of right crus passing to left of esophagus

Left crus of diaphragm

Portion of right crus passing to right of esophagus

Aorta

Inferior vena cava

Vertebral column

Diaphragmatic crura and orifices viewed from above

B. Anterior retraction of the liver and division of the pars flaccida facilitate exposure of the right pillar of the right diaphragmatic crus.

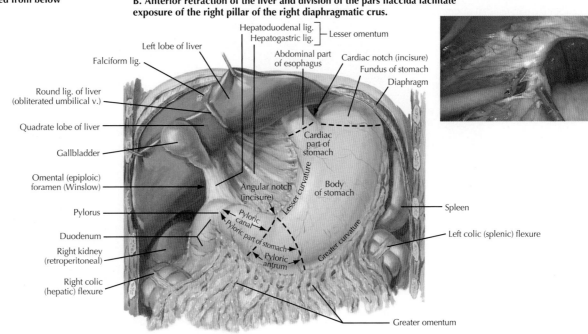

Hepatoduodenal lig.
Hepatogastric lig. — Lesser omentum

Left lobe of liver

Falciform lig.

Abdominal part of esophagus

Cardiac notch (incisure)

Fundus of stomach

Diaphragm

Round lig. of liver (obliterated umbilical v.)

Quadrate lobe of liver

Gallbladder

Omental (epiploic) foramen (Winslow)

Pylorus

Duodenum

Right kidney (retroperitoneal)

Right colic (hepatic) flexure

Cardiac part of stomach

Angular notch (incisure)

Lesser curvature

Body of stomach

Pyloric canal

Pyloric part of stomach

Pyloric antrum

Greater curvature

Spleen

Left colic (splenic) flexure

Greater omentum

FIGURE 11.5 Intraoperative diagram demonstrating incision of the pars flaccida to begin dissection toward the right crus of the diaphragm.

Phrenoesophageal ligament and relation to the esophageal hiatus. Complete mobilization of the esophagus requires division of the phrenoesophageal ligament.

Longitudinal esophageal muscle

Circular esophageal muscle

Gradual slight muscular thickening

Phrenoesophageal ligament (ascending or upper limb)

Supradiaphragmatic fascia

Diaphragm

Infradiaphragmatic (transversalis) fascia

Phrenoesophageal ligament (descending limb)

Peritoneum

Cardiac notch

Gastric folds (rugae)

Esophageal mucosa

Submucosa

Diaphragm

Subhiatal fat ring

Zigzag (Z) line: juncture of esophageal and gastric mucosa

Cardiac part (cardia) of stomach

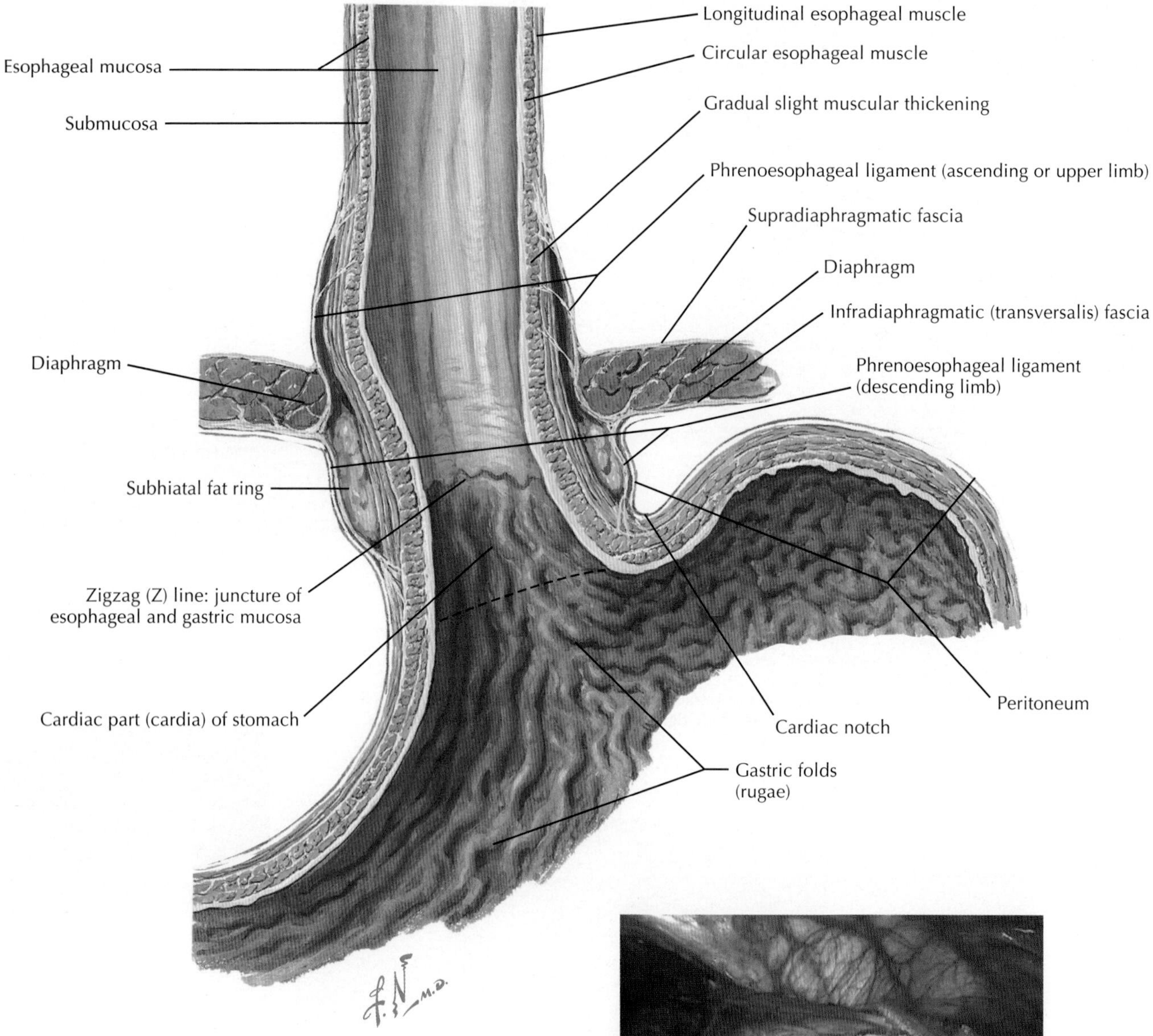

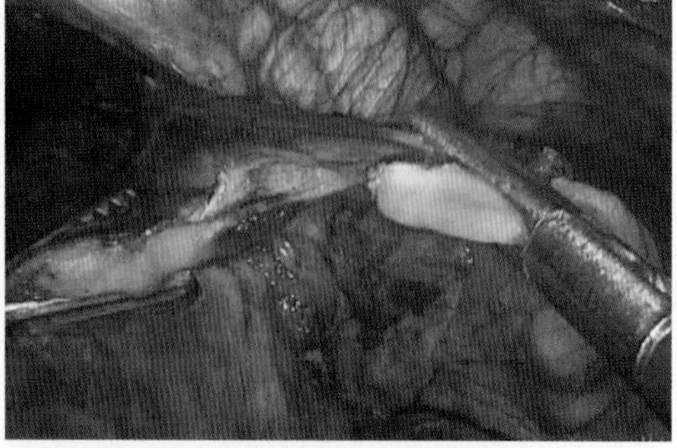

The sac is completely mobilized from the mediastinum and separated from the crural pillars, leaving endoabdominal fascia on the pillars.

FIGURE 11.6 Intraoperative diagram illustrating dissection of the left crus for circumferential mobilization of the esophagus.

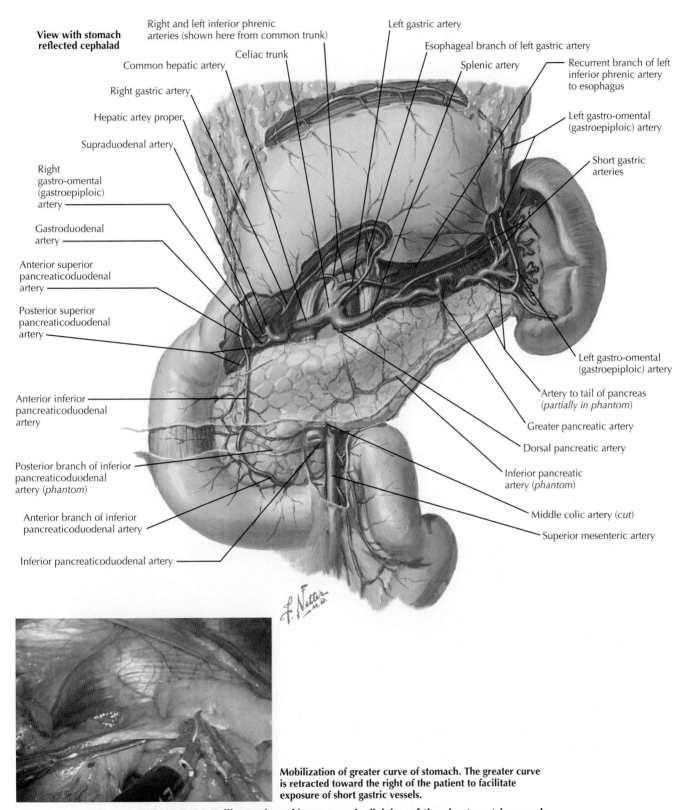

View with stomach reflected cephalad

Right and left inferior phrenic arteries (shown here from common trunk)

Celiac trunk

Common hepatic artery

Right gastric artery

Hepatic artey proper

Supraduodenal artery

Right gastro-omental (gastroepiploic) artery

Gastroduodenal artery

Anterior superior pancreaticoduodenal artery

Posterior superior pancreaticoduodenal artery

Anterior inferior pancreaticoduodenal artery

Posterior branch of inferior pancreaticoduodenal artery (*phantom*)

Anterior branch of inferior pancreaticoduodenal artery

Inferior pancreaticoduodenal artery

Left gastric artery

Esophageal branch of left gastric artery

Splenic artery

Recurrent branch of left inferior phrenic artery to esophagus

Left gastro-omental (gastroepiploic) artery

Short gastric arteries

Left gastro-omental (gastroepiploic) artery

Artery to tail of pancreas (*partially in phantom*)

Greater pancreatic artery

Dorsal pancreatic artery

Inferior pancreatic artery (*phantom*)

Middle colic artery (*cut*)

Superior mesenteric artery

Mobilization of greater curve of stomach. The greater curve is retracted toward the right of the patient to facilitate exposure of short gastric vessels.

FIGURE 11.7 Illustration of laparoscopic division of the short gastric vessels.

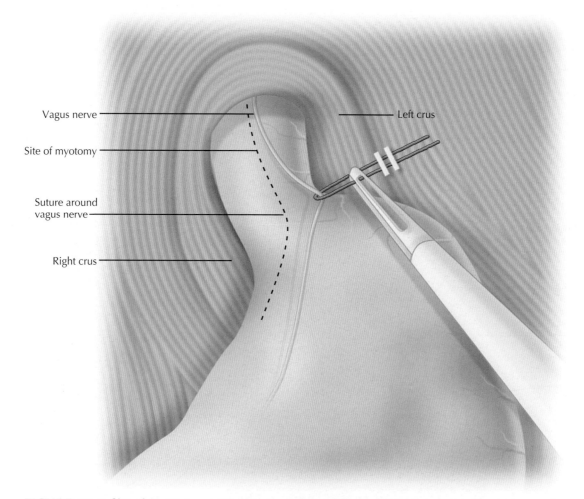

Vagus nerve

Left crus

Site of myotomy

Suture around
vagus nerve

Right crus

FIGURE 11.8 **Site of myotomy on the anterior surface of the esophagus, crossing the gastroesopha-geal junction.**
(Reused with permission from Rosen MJ. Heller myotomy. In: Ponsky JR, Rosen MJ, ed. Atlas of Surgical Techniques for the Upper GI Tract and Small Bowel. *Philadelphia: Elsevier; 2010:65–71, Fig. 8-1.)*

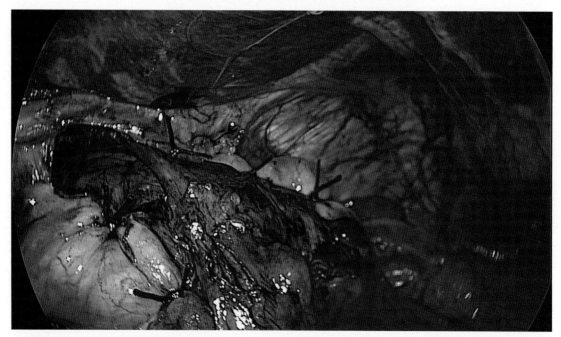

FIGURE 11.9 **Intraoperative picture of a completed Toupet fundoplication after Heller myotomy.**

PER-ORAL ENDOSCOPIC MYOTOMY (POEM)

POEM is a newer procedure in which the circular muscle of the esophagus is divided endo-scopically. The principles of surgical myotomy remain: to perform a complete myotomy that involves at least 5 cm of the distal esophagus, extending onto the sling muscles of the stomach. Because the procedure is performed endoscopically, there is no concomitant fundoplication; however, as the phrenoesophageal ligament is not disturbed and the ligament of His is pre-served, some postoperative reflux may be mitigated. However, studies comparing pH studies in patients undergoing POEM versus laparoscopic Heller myotomy with antireflux procedures have found that those who undergo POEM are more likely to have abnormal DeMeester scores.

Under general anesthesia, a diagnostic endoscopy is first performed to identify the GE junc-tion and assess how difficult it is to pass the endoscope through the LES. Any retained liquid in the esophagus is thoroughly suctioned. An overtube is placed per-orally at this time to facilitate the procedure. The endoscope is removed and a cap is placed over the tip of the endoscope. A triangle-tip (TT) knife is used through the working channel; 10 cm proximal to the GE junction, a submucosal weal is created using methylene-blue–tinged epinephrine solution. The TT knife is used to create a 2-cm mucosotomy and, with the aid of the cap, the endoscope is advanced into the tunnel. The TT knife is used to create a submucosal tunnel distally toward the GE junc-tion, staying the 4 o'clock to 6 o'clock position on the screen corresponding to patient right, the rationale being to avoid the short gastric vessels when performing the gastric portion of the myotomy. The mucosal tunnel will become tighter at the GE junction; palisading vessels in the submucosal area are another indication that the surgeon has reached the GE junction. Continued injection of the methylene blue solution with the needle withdrawn into the sub-mucosal plane can aid in dissecting this plane as well. Withdrawal of the scope from the tunnel and visualization of the true lumen into the stomach with retroflexion will confirm adequate creation of the submucosal tunnel once staining of the blue dye is visible onto the cardia of the stomach (Fig. 11.10).

Measuring at least 5 cm proximal to the GE junction, the myotomy is created using the TT knife. The longitudinal muscle fibers of the esophagus should be visible beyond this. The myotomy is continued distally onto the stomach, as far as the tunnel was created. At the con-clusion of the myotomy, a completion endoscopy should be performed to ensure easy passage of the endoscopy through the LES compared with prior. The stomach is desufflated, and the mucosotomy is closed with clips.

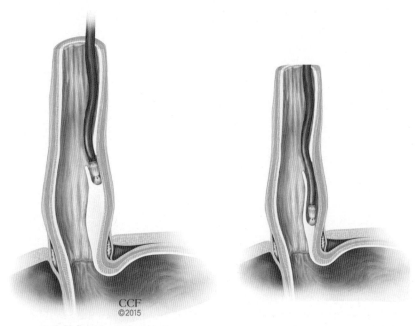

A–B. Creation of submucosal tunnel

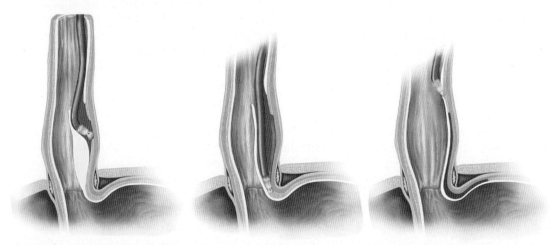

C–D. Endoscopic myotomy with division of
the circular muscle fibers of the esophagus

E. Closure of the mucosotomy with
endoscopic clips

FIGURE 11.10 Steps of a peroral endoscopic myotomy (POEM) procedure.
*(Reprinted with permission, Cleveland Clinic Center for Medical Art & Photography © 2015–2019. All Rights
Reserved.)*

SUGGESTED READINGS

Boeckxstaens GE, Zaninotto G, Richter JE. Achalasia. Lancet 2014;383:83–93. https://doi.org/
   10.1016/S0140-6736(13)60651-0.

Inoue H, Minami H, Kobayashi Y, Sato Y, Kaga M, Suzuki M, et al. Peroral endoscopic myotomy
   (POEM) for esophageal achalasia. Endoscopy 2010;42:265–71. https://doi.org/10.1055/
   s-0029-1244080.

Pandolfino JE, Gawron AJ. Achalasia. JAMA 2015;313:1841. https://doi.org/10.1001/
   jama.2015.2996.

Sanaka MR, Thota PN, Parikh MP, Hayat U, Gupta NM, Gabbard S, et al. Peroral endoscopic
   myotomy leads to higher rates of abnormal esophageal acid exposure than laparoscopic Heller
   myotomy in achalasia. Surg Endosc 2018. https://doi.org/10.1007/s00464-018-6522-4.

Stefanidis D, Richardson W, Farrell TM, Kohn GP, Augenstein V, Fanelli RD, et al. SAGES
   guidelines for the surgical treatment of esophageal achalasia. Surg Endosc 2012;26:296–311.
   https://doi.org/10.1007/s00464-011-2017-2.

Hepatobiliary

SECTION EDITORS: **Christopher T. Siegel and R. Matthew Walsh**

Cholecystectomy

Robert Simon

▶ **VIDEO**

12.1 Laparoscopic Cholecystectomy

INTRODUCTION

Cholecystectomy is one of the most common abdominal surgeries performed. There are many potential complications, and understanding the correct indications is imperative so that the benefits outweigh the risks. Knowing the proper and safe techniques is critical to help minimize those risks, and this begins with an understanding of anatomy and physiology.

ANATOMY

The gallbladder is located between segments IVb and V of the liver. It is one of the landmarks of the Cantlie line that divides the left and right lobes of the liver. The regions of the gallbladder include the fundus, body, infundibulum, neck, and the cystic duct (Fig. 12.1). The cystic duct drains into the common hepatic duct to form the common bile duct. There are many variants of cystic duct anatomy, and being familiar with these variations helps to avoid bile duct injuries during a cholecystectomy (Fig. 12.2). Bile fills the gallbladder via the cystic duct. The valves of Heister, located in the cystic duct, prevent passive reflux of bile from the gallbladder. The venous and lymphatic drainage of the gallbladder is via small tributaries into the gallbladder fossa. There are no named veins draining the gallbladder. The arterial supply is from the cystic artery. The most common origin of the cystic artery is from the right hepatic artery, but this is also subject to variation (Fig. 12.3).

PHYSIOLOGY

Bile is made in the liver and drains via the right and left hepatic ducts through the common hepatic duct and common bile duct into the second portion of the duodenum. The function of bile is to aid digestion of lipids by creating micelles. The function of the gallbladder is to concentrate bile by absorbing water and sodium. After an individual eats a fatty meal, cells in the duodenum release cholecystokinin, stimulating gallbladder contraction and relaxation of the sphincter of Oddi, releasing the concentrated bile into the duodenum. Bile is made up of bile salts, phospholipids, and cholesterol. When the concentrations of these are imbalanced, stones can precipitate in the gallbladder. The most common type of stones in the West are nonpigmented cholesterol stones. The other category of stones is pigmented stones, further divided into black stones from hemolytic disorders, and brown stones, from bile stasis and bacterial infection.

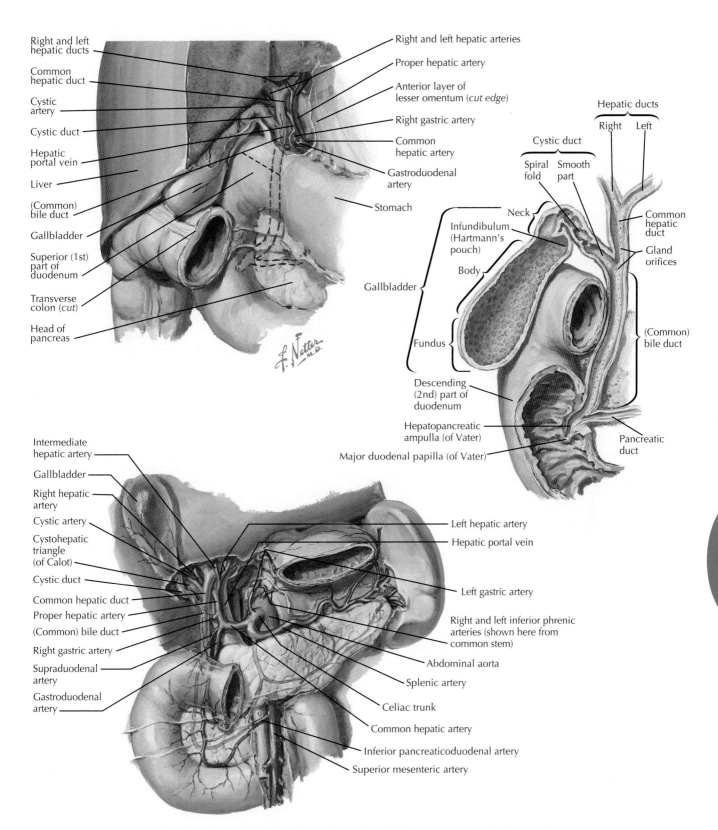

FIGURE 12.1 Gallbladder and extrahepatic bile ducts and arterial supply.

Variations in cystic duct

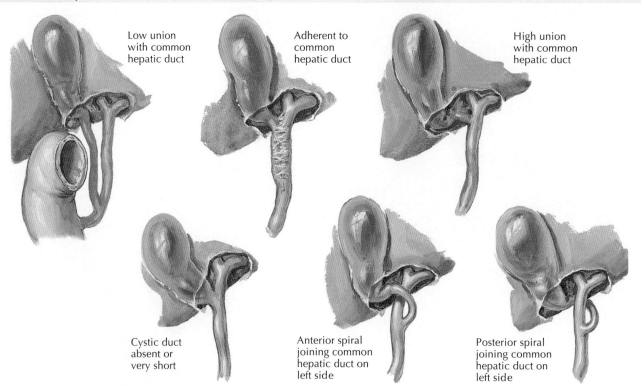

Low union with common hepatic duct

Adherent to common hepatic duct

High union with common hepatic duct

Cystic duct absent or very short

Anterior spiral joining common hepatic duct on left side

Posterior spiral joining common hepatic duct on left side

Accessory (aberrant) hepatic ducts

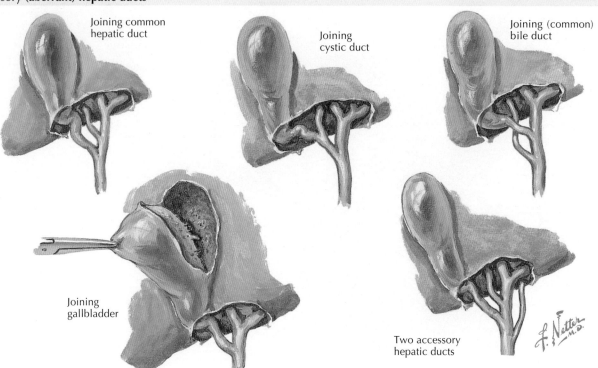

Joining common hepatic duct

Joining cystic duct

Joining (common) bile duct

Joining gallbladder

Two accessory hepatic ducts

FIGURE 12.2 Variations in cystic and hepatic ducts.

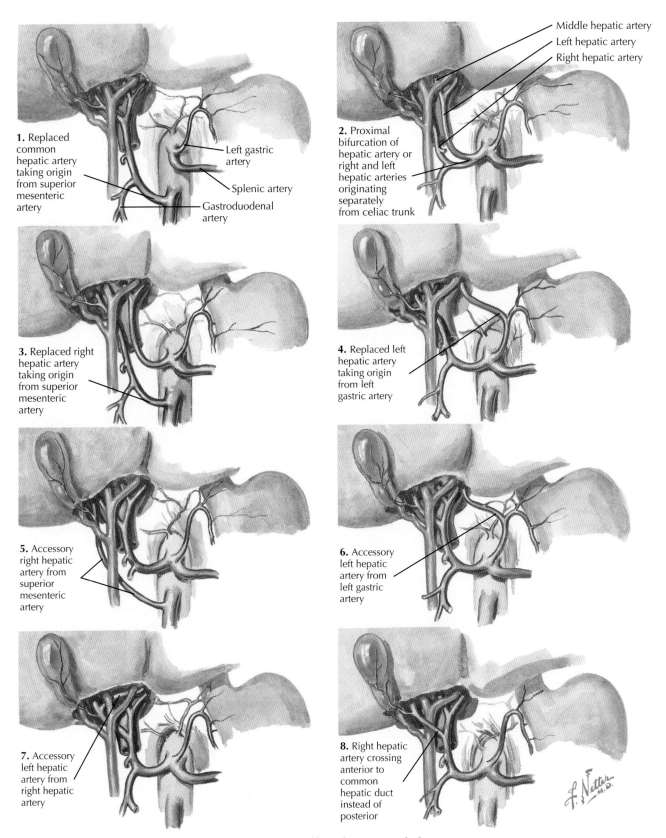

1. Replaced common hepatic artery taking origin from superior mesenteric artery

Left gastric artery

Splenic artery

Gastroduodenal artery

Middle hepatic artery
Left hepatic artery
Right hepatic artery

2. Proximal bifurcation of hepatic artery or right and left hepatic arteries originating separately from celiac trunk

3. Replaced right hepatic artery taking origin from superior mesenteric artery

4. Replaced left hepatic artery taking origin from left gastric artery

5. Accessory right hepatic artery from superior mesenteric artery

6. Accessory left hepatic artery from left gastric artery

7. Accessory left hepatic artery from right hepatic artery

8. Right hepatic artery crossing anterior to common hepatic duct instead of posterior

FIGURE 12.3 Hepatic artery variations.

INDICATIONS

Benign

- Acute calculous cholecystitis: Clinical biliary pain (biliary colic), imaging showing gallstones and signs of infection: Murphy sign, leukocytosis, fever
- Chronic calculous cholecystitis: Biliary colic and gallstones but not signs of inflammation
- Acute acalculous cholecystitis: Same as acute calculous disease, but no gallstones on imaging
- Chronic acalculous cholecystitis (biliary dyskinesia): Biliary colic but no gallstones

Symptomatic cholelithiasis is the most common benign indication for a cholecystectomy. Biliary colic is typically located in the epigastrium and/or right upper quadrant and resolves within a couple of hours. It can also radiate to the right back and right shoulder. Cholecystitis occurs when the cystic duct is obstructed. The gallbladder mucosa continues to make mucus and fill the gallbladder, causing distention and increased wall tension. This typically impairs venous drainage of the gallbladder, which causes inflammation and can ultimately lead to gangrene and potentially perforation. Cholecystitis can be divided radiologically into calculous and acalculous. Clinically they can also be divided into acute and chronic.

Acute calculous cholecystitis occurs when a stone obstructs the cystic duct and is accompanied by prolonged right upper quadrant and/or epigastric pain. The pain typically lasts longer than 24 hours. A classic physical exam finding is Murphy sign, in which inspiration is involuntarily halted with deep palpation of the right upper quadrant (Fig. 12.4). Patients tend to have a leukocytosis signifying inflammation. If fevers are present, this can imply an associated infection. Chronic calculous cholecystitis occurs when a stone may be stuck in the neck of the gallbladder and presents with biliary colic. Acute acalculous cholecystitis is a disease process typically found in patients with significant comorbidities, particularly cardiac disease, when bile stasis can occur. Chronic acalculous cholecystitis is termed *biliary dyskinesia* when the gallbladder is not contracting appropriately. This is diagnosed by classic symptoms and occasionally a hepatobiliary iminodiacetic acid (HIDA) scan with cholecystokinin administration. A gallbladder ejection fraction can be calculated, and if less than 35% with reproduction of symptoms after cholecystokinin administration, this is typically classified as biliary dyskinesia.

When stones escape the gallbladder and travel into the common bile duct, this is termed *choledocholithiasis*. When the stones obstruct the common bile duct, the bile can become infected, which is called *cholangitis*. This is a clinical diagnosis defined by Charcot's triad of jaundice, fever, and right upper quadrant abdominal pain. The treatment of this involves antibiotics, relief of the obstruction, and cholecystectomy to remove the source of the stones. Stones traveling through the common bile duct can also cause pancreatitis, again requiring timely removal of the gallbladder once the acute episode of pancreatitis resolves.

Sudden obstruction (biliary colic)

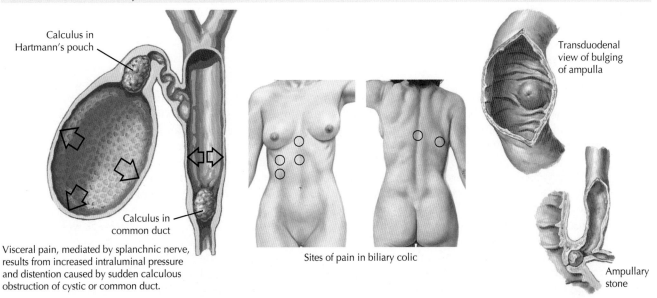

Calculus in
Hartmann's pouch

Calculus in
common duct

Transduodenal
view of bulging
of ampulla

Ampullary
stone

Visceral pain, mediated by splanchnic nerve,
results from increased intraluminal pressure
and distention caused by sudden calculous
obstruction of cystic or common duct.

Sites of pain in biliary colic

Persistent obstruction (acute cholecystitis)

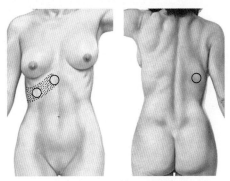

Sites of pain and hyperesthesia in
acute cholecystitis

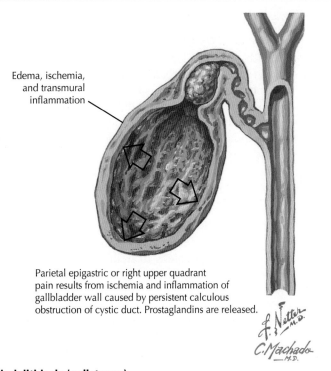

Edema, ischemia,
and transmural
inflammation

Parietal epigastric or right upper quadrant
pain results from ischemia and inflammation of
gallbladder wall caused by persistent calculous
obstruction of cystic duct. Prostaglandins are released.

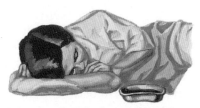

Patient lies motionless because jarring or
respiration increases pain. Nausea is common.

FIGURE 12.4 **Cholelithiasis (gallstones).**

Malignant

Cancer of the gallbladder is rare, with a poor prognosis. The incidence has been reported as about 1 in 100,000 with advanced disease having an estimated 5-year survival of up to 25%. The poor prognosis is largely related to the difficulty in early diagnosis because it usually does not lead to symptoms. It is difficult to diagnose preoperatively and often found incidentally on the final pathology report after a routine cholecystectomy. Further treatment is dictated by the T staging on final pathology. If it is T1a disease, meaning it is localized to the lamina propria, then a cholecystectomy alone is sufficient with an overall survival of over 95%. It is recommended that a patient undergo a radical cholecystectomy for T1b and T2 cancers because of the increased risk of lymph node metastasis. A radical cholecystectomy involves a portal lymphadenectomy, extending medially to the station 8 lymph node and skeletonizing the portal structures, as well as a partial hepatectomy of segments IVb and V. If the cystic duct margin at the common bile duct is involved by the cancer, then an extrahepatic bile duct resection is also warranted.

Of note, in patients found to have large gallbladder polyps, defined as greater than 1 cm, or large gallstones, defined as greater than 3 cm, it is recommended they undergo a cholecystectomy because of the increased risk of cancer.

TECHNIQUES

Laparoscopic

As with all other laparoscopic operations, proper port placement is imperative. For a cholecystectomy, four ports are usually used. A periumbilical port, which also typically doubles as the specimen extraction site, is usually a 10- to 12-mm port. Three additional 5-mm ports are placed: one in the subxiphoid region that is used for dissecting, and two in the right upper quadrant that are used for retracting the gallbladder and aiding with visualization. Visualization is also aided by placing the patient in steep reverse Trendelenburg position. The most lateral port is used to grasp the fundus of the gallbladder and retract it superolaterally. The remaining 5-mm port is used to grasp the infundibulum and retract it to help dissect the hepatocystic triangle. It is key to retract the infundibulum inferolaterally because this helps separate the cystic duct from the common bile duct and prevent bile duct injuries (Fig. 12.5).

Safe Cholecystectomy Program

The safe cholecystectomy program was developed by SAGES. A task force was initiated in 2014, which created six steps to help guide surgeons during laparoscopic cholecystectomy to help prevent injuries to the biliary tree. The first component of the program is obtaining a critical view of safety. This has been described since the mid-1990s and urges the surgeon to identify two and only two structures entering the gallbladder with liver seen in between. The proximal third of the hilar plate should also be dissected to ensure no tubular structures are going back into the liver. The remaining components of the program are understanding aberrant anatomy, liberal use of intraoperative cholangiography (or equivalent assessment: intraoperative ultrasound or indocyanine green), using an intraoperative time-out to ensure everyone agrees with the structures visualized before ligating anything; recognizing when the dissection is getting dangerous and knowing alternative options, such as subtotal cholecystectomy, conversion to open, or cholecystostomy tube placement; and last, calling in a second surgeon for help.

Cholecystectomy

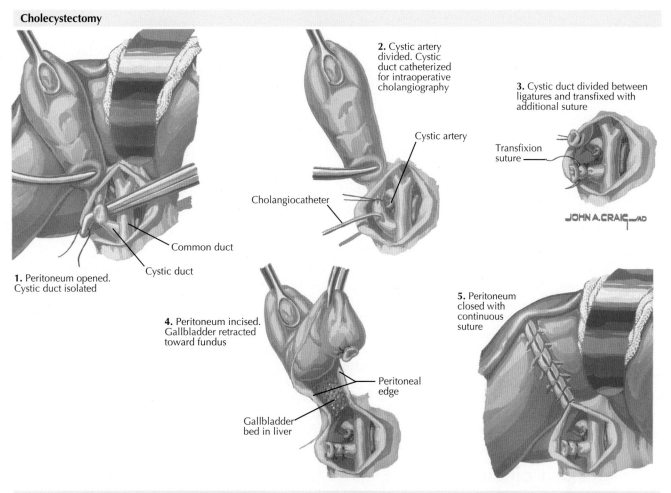

1. Peritoneum opened. Cystic duct isolated

Common duct

Cystic duct

2. Cystic artery divided. Cystic duct catheterized for intraoperative cholangiography

Cystic artery

Cholangiocatheter

3. Cystic duct divided between ligatures and transfixed with additional suture

Transfixion suture

JOHN A.CRAIG—AD

4. Peritoneum incised. Gallbladder retracted toward fundus

Peritoneal edge

Gallbladder bed in liver

5. Peritoneum closed with continuous suture

Critical view in open and laparoscopic cholecystectomy

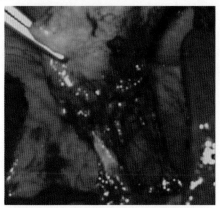

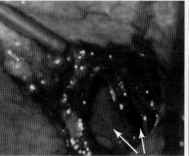

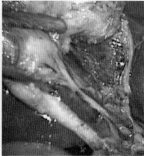

The critical view in open cholecystectomy. Note the GB is retracted in a cephalad fashion by its fundus while the infundibulum is retracted in a lateral way, opening the critical view with demonstration of the cystic duct, artery, and no other structure in between.

The critical view in laparoscopic cholecystectomy. Although similar retraction is exercised as in an open cholecystectomy (GB is retracted in a cephalad fashion by its fundus while the infundibulum is retracted in a lateral way, opening the critical view), not enough dissection is initially seen between the cystic duct and cystic artery (*first arrow*) and between the cystic artery and the cystic plate on the liver (*second arrow*). Further dissection was performed with a clear demonstration of the critical view.

FIGURE 12.5 Cholecystectomy and the critical view. *GB,* Gallbladder.

Rouviere's Sulcus

Rouviere's sulcus is a landmark that can be used to help avoid injuring the common bile duct. Rouviere's sulcus is present in the vast majority of individuals and in about ¾ of those cases, the right posterior branches of the hepatic artery and duct travel within it. The cystic duct and artery typically lay anterior and superior to this, whereas the common bile duct typically sits inferiorly. Therefore keeping the dissection superior to Rouviere's sulcus can theoretically help reduce the risk of a common bile duct injury.

Open

An open cholecystectomy is typically performed via a right subcostal incision. A self-retaining retractor helps to elevate the costal margin for sustained and adequate retraction. The gallbladder is typically dissected off of the liver bed via a "top-down" approach beginning at the fundus to isolate the cystic artery and duct last.

Intraoperative Cholangiogram

Intraoperative cholangiography is an important skill to have, not only to help prevent bile duct injuries but also to help identify and treat choledocholithiasis intraoperatively. Whether done using a laparoscopic or open approach, there are multiple ways it can be performed. There are multiple different catheters available to help cannulate the cystic duct. Dilute (50%) contrast should be used, because if the contrast is too concentrated, it can obscure stones. If a cholangiogram cannot be performed via the cystic duct, another option is to place a small-bore needle into the common bile duct. The puncture site can then be repaired with a 5-0 absorbable monofilament suture. Another alternative is to perform an intraoperative ultrasound to trace the cystic duct and common bile duct looking for shadowing stones. If stones are found, then a common bile duct exploration can be performed. This procedure will be discussed further in another chapter. Recently indocyanine green immunofluorescence can be used for biliary imaging if given preoperatively and equipment is available.

SPECIAL CIRCUMSTANCES

To help clinicians determine the appropriate treatment pathway for patients coming in with suspected acute cholecystitis, the Tokyo Guidelines flowchart was developed. It is a tool that grades acute cholecystitis into mild, moderate, and severe, taking into account the patient's comorbidities. A meta-analysis of available literature was used to answer a series of questions and develop the flowcharts. The article is available for free, and there are available online calculators for quick reference.

Cholecystitis or severe symptomatic cholelithiasis in pregnant patients can be treated with a cholecystectomy. Surgery should be avoided in the first or third trimester because of the risk of fetal loss or premature labor, respectively.

SUGGESTED READINGS

Dahmane, et al. Anatomy and surgical relevance of rouviere's sulcus. The Scientific World Journal 2013;2013:254287.

Okamoto, et al. Tokyo guidelines 2018: flowchart for the management of acute cholecystitis. J Hepatobiliary Pancreat Sci 2018;25:55–72.

Pucher, et al. SAGES expert delphi concensus: critical factors for safe surgical practice in laparoscopic cholecystectomy. Surg Endosc 2015;29(11):3074–85.

Rahman, et al. Trend analysis and survival of primary gallbladder cancer in the United States: a 1973-2009 population based study. Cancer Med 2017;6(4):874–80.

Soreide, et al. Systemic review of management of incidental gallbladder cancer after cholecystectomy. Br J Surg 2019;106(1):32–45.

Strasburg, et al. An analysis of the problem of biliary injury during laparoscopic cholecystectomy. J Am Coll Surg 1995;180(1):101–25.

You, et al. What is an adequate extent of resection for T1 gallbladder cancers? Ann Surg 2008;247(5):835–8.

Common Bile Duct Surgery and Choledochoduodenostomy

Walter S. Cha and Ahmed Nassar

 VIDEO

13.1 Laparoscopic Transcystic Common Bile Duct Exploration

INTRODUCTION

Approximately 15% of patients with gallbladder stones will also have stones within the common bile duct (CBD). Options for managing CBD stones include endoscopic treatment, including endoscopic retrograde cholangiopancreatography (ERCP) with biliary sphincterotomy, percutaneous interventions, and laparoscopic and open surgical procedures. Individual patient factors, available expertise, and desire for one- versus two-stage treatment will guide management strategy. Currently, the majority of patients with CBD stones are managed by using endoscopic techniques. However, endoscopic management of CBD stones may be problematic in patients with multiple large stones, stones above a stricture, and in patients with difficult access to the ampulla of Vater (stenosis, diverticulum, or altered anatomy, i.e., gastric bypass). Patients who are not candidates for endoscopic or percutaneous procedures may require surgical intervention. Surgical approaches to the CBD include laparoscopic CBD exploration through a transcystic approach or a choledochotomy, open CBD exploration, and biliary-enteric anastomosis.

CYSTIC DUCT ANATOMY AND VARIANTS

In most individuals (64% to 75%) the cystic duct joins the hepatic duct at approximately a 40-degree angle (Fig. 13.1). Less frequently (17% to 23%) the cystic duct runs parallel to the hepatic duct for a distance and may even enter the duodenum separately. In 8% to 13% of individuals the cystic duct may enter the hepatic duct on the left side after passing in front of or behind the common hepatic duct. Infrequently, the gallbladder may be sessile, with little to no cystic duct.

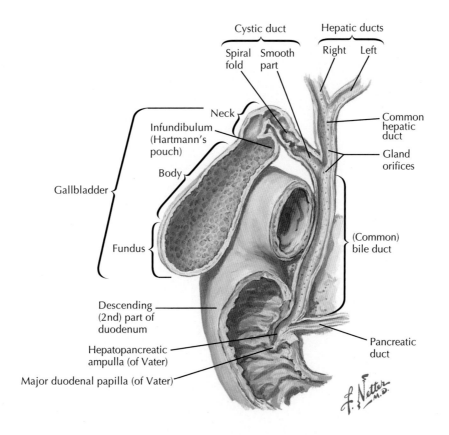

Variations in cystic duct

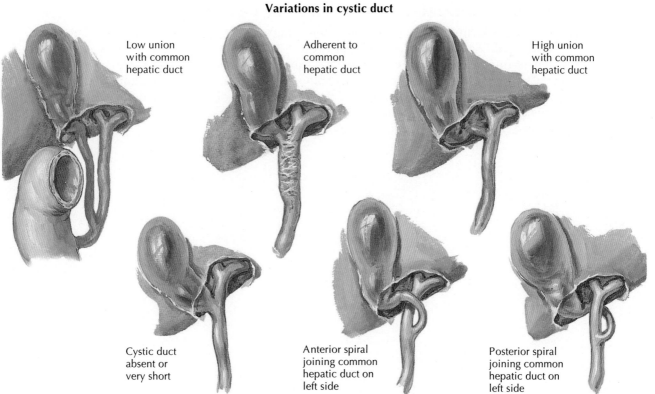

Low union
with common
hepatic duct

Adherent to
common
hepatic duct

High union
with common
hepatic duct

Cystic duct
absent or
very short

Anterior spiral
joining common
hepatic duct on
left side

Posterior spiral
joining common
hepatic duct on
left side

FIGURE 13.1 Cystic duct anatomy and variants.

LAPAROSCOPIC COMMON BILE DUCT EXPLORATION

If CBD stones are identified at laparoscopic cholecystectomy, laparoscopic CBD exploration may be warranted (Fig. 13.2). Successful laparoscopic CBD exploration avoids the risks associated with deferring treatment of a CBD stone or a subsequent endoscopic procedure.

Trocar placement for laparoscopic CBD exploration is similar to the port configuration used during laparoscopic cholecystectomy. An additional port in the right upper abdomen may be used for the choledochoscope or catheters. Robot-assisted common bile duct explorations have been described that mimic the laparoscopic approaches.

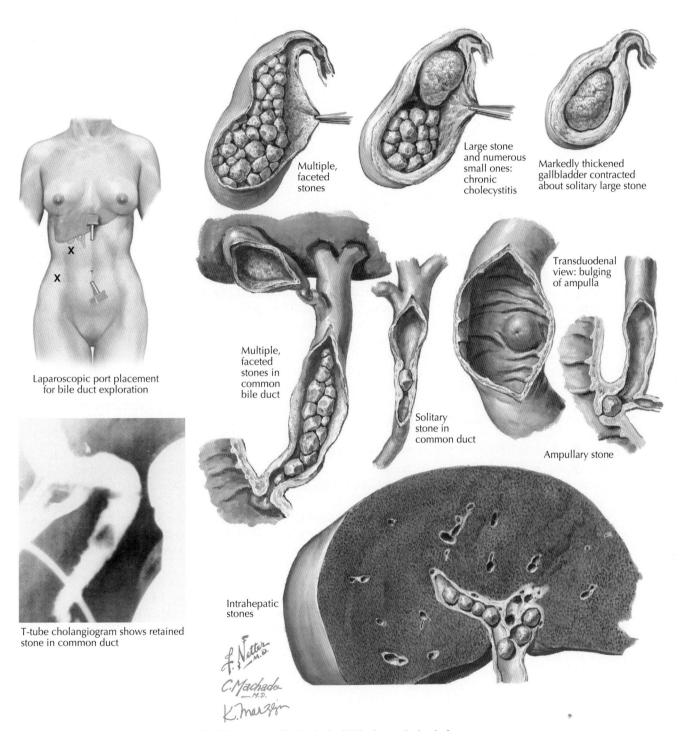

Laparoscopic port placement
for bile duct exploration

T-tube cholangiogram shows retained
stone in common duct

Multiple,
faceted
stones

Large stone
and numerous
small ones:
chronic
cholecystitis

Markedly thickened
gallbladder contracted
about solitary large stone

Multiple,
faceted
stones in
common
bile duct

Solitary
stone in
common duct

Transduodenal
view: bulging
of ampulla

Ampullary stone

Intrahepatic
stones

FIGURE 13.2 **Choledocholithiasis: pathologic features.**

Transcystic Approach

The transcystic approach to CBD exploration avoids a choledochotomy and eliminates the subsequent need for a T tube. After the cystic duct is controlled on the gallbladder side, a cystic ductotomy is created and a cholangiocatheter placed. The cystic duct may have to be dilated with a balloon before subsequent interventions to extract calculi (Fig. 13.3A).

The CBD is irrigated with saline to flush the stone. If unsuccessful, balloon catheters or wire baskets can be passed into the CBD under fluoroscopic guidance to capture and retrieve the stones. An additional option is antegrade balloon dilation of the sphincter under fluoroscopic guidance, followed by flushing to clear the duct of stones (Fig. 13.3B to D). This technique is not preferred because of the risk of pancreatitis occurring after dilation of the ampulla. After clearance of the CBD, the cystic duct is ligated with clips or an endoloop.

Transductal/Choledochotomy Approach

Transcystic extraction may not be feasible with large stones, small cystic ducts, or stone locations in the proximal bile ducts. Laparoscopic choledochotomy may provide access to these stones for subsequent removal.

With the gallbladder retracted cephalad, a longitudinal incision is made on the anterior aspect of the distal CBD because blood supply to the duct is lateral. The length of the incision is typically limited to 1 cm or the size of the largest stone. The stones are cleared by flushing, followed by basket or balloon retrieval.

Choledochoscopy may be a useful adjunct. The choledochotomy is typically closed using laparoscopic suturing techniques with monofilament absorbable sutures (Fig. 13.3E). The choledochotomy can be closed over a T tube to enable future access but T tubes are rarely indicated in current practices. Alternately, an antegrade stent can also be placed through the sphincter before closing the choledochotomy.

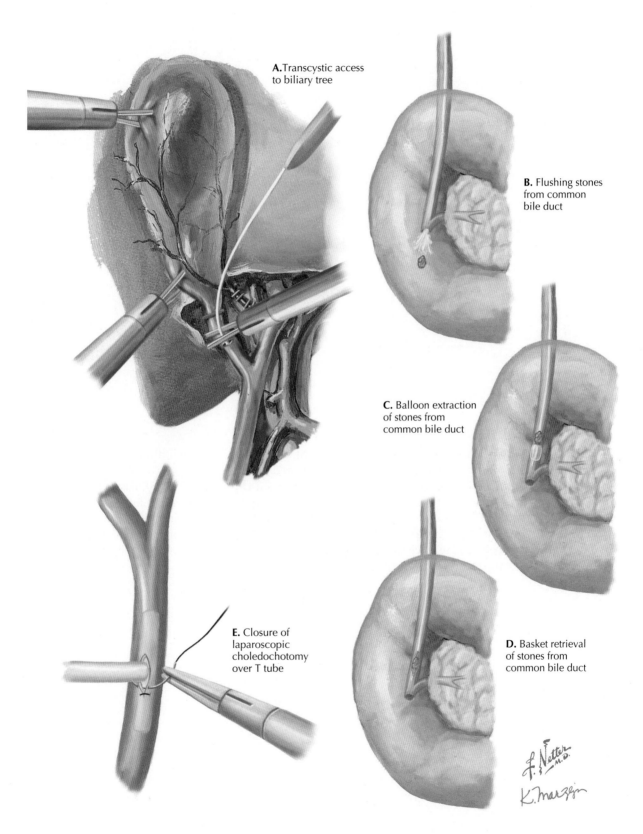

A. Transcystic access to biliary tree

B. Flushing stones from common bile duct

C. Balloon extraction of stones from common bile duct

D. Basket retrieval of stones from common bile duct

E. Closure of laparoscopic choledochotomy over T tube

FIGURE 13.3 Transcystic and transductal/choledochotomy approaches.

OPEN COMMON DUCT EXPLORATION

When minimally invasive options are not feasible or fail, open CBD exploration may be warranted. In addition, open exploration may be performed at open cholecystectomy when CBD stones are identified. The procedure is generally performed through a right subcostal incision (Fig. 13.4A). An upper midline incision may be used as an alternative. After a wide Kocher maneuver, a choledochotomy is created (Fig. 13.4B). A variety of instruments can be used to extract the stones: irrigation catheters, balloon catheters, biliary scoops, stone forceps, and flexible choledochoscopes. After clearance of the CBD, the choledochotomy may rarely be closed over a T tube using absorbable sutures (Fig. 13.4 C to E).

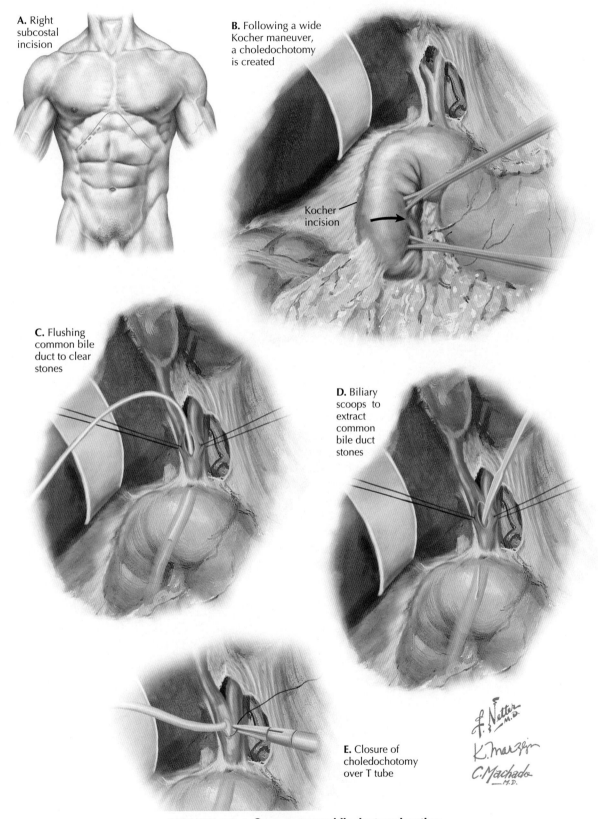

A. Right subcostal incision

B. Following a wide Kocher maneuver, a choledochotomy is created

Kocher incision

C. Flushing common bile duct to clear stones

D. Biliary scoops to extract common bile duct stones

E. Closure of choledochotomy over T tube

FIGURE 13.4 Open common bile duct exploration.

CHOLEDOCHODUODENOSTOMY

Choledochoduodenostomy may be useful after common duct exploration if there is concern about retained stones, as well as in patients with primary or recurrent biliary stones or a distal biliary stricture with a dilated common bile duct (>2.0 cm).

A wide Kocher maneuver is performed and the distal CBD is exposed. A choledochotomy of 2-cm length is made as close to the duodenum as possible. The biliary tree is cleared of calculi. A longitudinal duodenotomy is created, also 2 cm in length and adjacent to the choledochotomy (Fig. 13.5). An anastomosis is created between the CBD and the duodenum using interrupted synthetic absorbable sutures in a fish-mouth fashion.

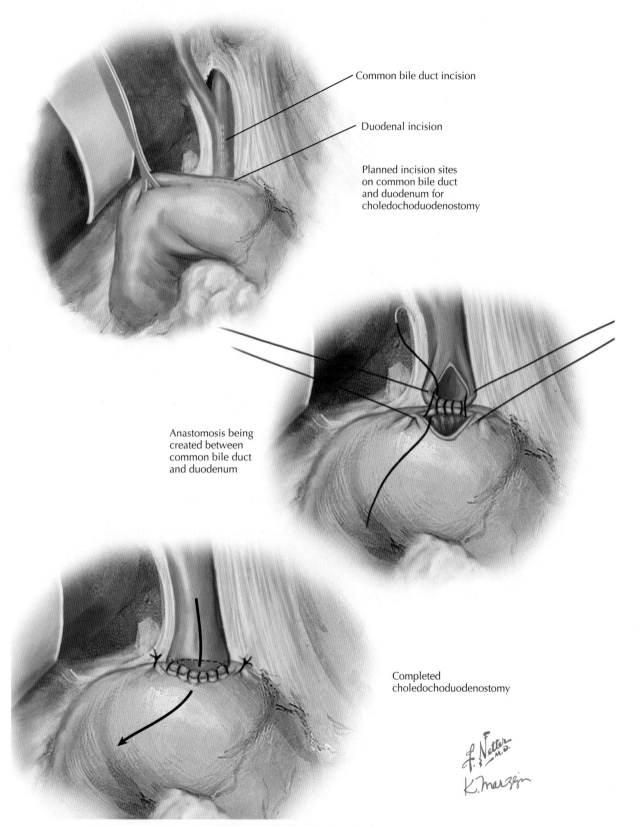

Common bile duct incision

Duodenal incision

Planned incision sites
on common bile duct
and duodenum for
choledochoduodenostomy

Anastomosis being
created between
common bile duct
and duodenum

Completed
choledochoduodenostomy

FIGURE 13.5 **Choledochoduodenostomy.**

SUGGESTED READINGS

Alkhamesi NA. Robot-assisted common bile duct exploration as an option for complex choledocholithiasis. Surg Endosc 2013;(1):263–6.

Cameron J, Sandone C, editors. Atlas of gastrointestinal surgery. 2nd ed. Hamilton: BC Decker; 2007.

DeAretxabala X, Bahamondes J. Choledochoduodenostomy for common bile duct stones. World J Surg 1998;22:1171–4.

Extrahepatic biliary tract and gallbladder. In: Skandalakis J, Colborn G, Weidman T, et al., editors. Skandalakis' surgical anatomy. Athens: BMP; 2004.

Okamoto H. Current assessment of choledochoduodenostomy: 130 consecutive series. Ann R Coll Surg Engl 2017;99(7):545–9.

Petelin JB. Laparoscopic common bile duct exploration. Surg Endosc 2003;17(11):1705–14.

Shojaiefard A, et al. Various techniques for the surgical treatment of common bile duct stones: a meta review. Gastroenterol Res Pract 2009;2009:840208.

Hepatectomy

Federico Aucejo, Kazunari Sasaki, Charles Miller, Eren Berber, Keita Okubo, Cristiano Quintini, Choon Hyuck David Kwon, Christopher T. Siegel, and Amit Nair

▶ VIDEOS

14.1 Laparoscopic Right Hepatectomy
14.2 Laparoscopic Left Hepatectomy
14.3 Robotic Left Hepatectomy

INTRODUCTION

Multiple factors have contributed to a significant increase in the current number of liver surgeries performed annually. Improvements in surgical and anesthetic techniques as well as patient selection have reduced the mortality associated with liver resection to between 1% and 5% at experienced centers, with acceptable associated morbidity. The improved surgical outcomes associated with the increased incidence of newly diagnosed cancers of the liver and biliary tree, along with substantial improvement in the adjuvant treatment of metastatic colon cancer to the liver, has helped to establish liver resection as the primary treatment modality for many patients with hepatocellular carcinoma, cholangiocarcinoma, and metastatic colon cancer to the liver. Of note, minimally invasive liver surgery via laparoscopy and robotic technology has developed substantially during the last decade.

SURGICAL PRINCIPLES

A major advance in the ability to perform liver resections is the understanding of the segmental anatomy of the liver, as described by Couinaud in 1957. In addition to the portal vein, the arterial supply, biliary drainage, and hepatic outflow must also be considered in planning the resection. Because of the significant variations in liver mass, vascular and biliary anatomy, tumor location, and extent of resection margin, adequate preoperative imaging is critical. For primary liver tumors, a margin of 1 to 2 cm is preferred. The resection margin for metastatic lesions is somewhat more controversial, but recent studies on resection of colorectal liver metastasis demonstrated a survival advantage with a resection margin of at least 1 cm. When a liver resection is planned, the remnant liver must have adequate mass for the patient as well as adequate arterial, portal, and hepatic vein flow. The remnant must also have adequate biliary drainage.

The liver is composed of eight segments based on the portal inflow into the organ (Fig. 14.1). Segments I to IV constitute the left lobe (colored purple, blue, and green on illustration) and segments V to VIII, the right lobe. Preoperative understanding of the patient's underlying liver anatomy is critical when planning a liver resection. Because of the wide variability in all the hepatic vascular and biliary structures, as well as a considerable amount of variability in the relative sizes of the right and left lobes, imaging is performed to delineate the key structures that may be encountered during the resection (Fig. 14.2). The most useful studies are triple-phase computed tomography or a high-resolution magnetic resonance imaging with contrast (Fig. 14.3).

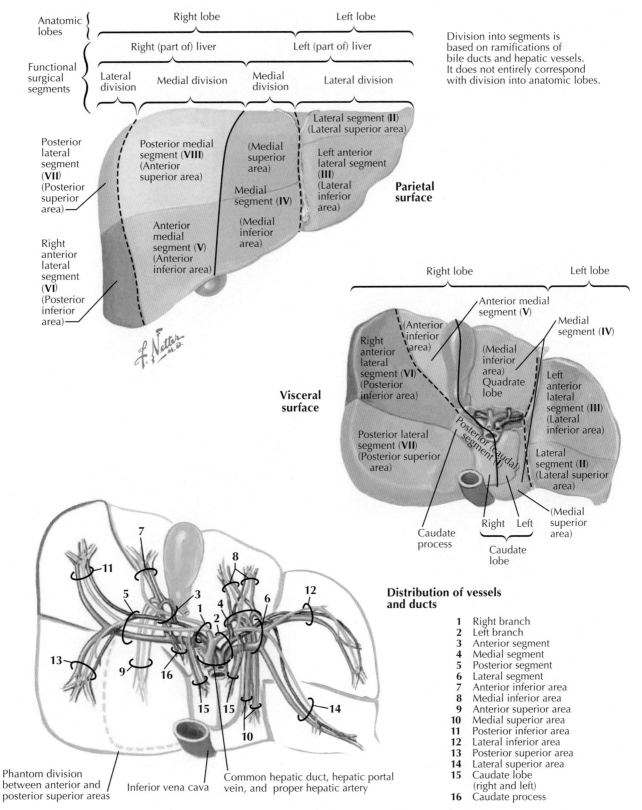

Anatomic lobes

Right lobe

Left lobe

Functional surgical segments

Right (part of) liver

Left (part of) liver

Lateral division

Medial division

Medial division

Lateral division

Division into segments is based on ramifications of bile ducts and hepatic vessels. It does not entirely correspond with division into anatomic lobes.

Posterior lateral segment (**VII**) (Posterior superior area)

Right anterior lateral segment (**VI**) (Posterior inferior area)

Posterior medial segment (**VIII**) (Anterior superior area)

Anterior medial segment (**V**) (Anterior inferior area)

(Medial superior area)

Medial segment (**IV**)

(Medial inferior area)

Lateral segment (**II**) (Lateral superior area)

Left anterior lateral segment (**III**) (Lateral inferior area)

Parietal surface

F. Netter
M.D.

Visceral surface

Right lobe

Left lobe

Right anterior lateral segment (**VI**) (Posterior inferior area)

(Anterior inferior area)

Anterior medial segment (**V**)

(Medial inferior area) Quadrate lobe

Medial segment (**IV**)

Left anterior lateral segment (**III**) (Lateral inferior area)

Posterior lateral segment (**VII**) (Posterior superior area)

Posterior (caudal) segment (I)

Lateral segment (**II**) (Lateral superior area)

(Medial superior area)

Caudate process

Right   Left

Caudate lobe

Distribution of vessels and ducts

Phantom division between anterior and posterior superior areas

Inferior vena cava

Common hepatic duct, hepatic portal vein, and proper hepatic artery

1	Right branch
2	Left branch
3	Anterior segment
4	Medial segment
5	Posterior segment
6	Lateral segment
7	Anterior inferior area
8	Medial inferior area
9	Anterior superior area
10	Medial superior area
11	Posterior inferior area
12	Lateral inferior area
13	Posterior superior area
14	Lateral superior area
15	Caudate lobe (right and left)
16	Caudate process

FIGURE 14.1 **Liver segments and lobes: vessels and duct distribution.**

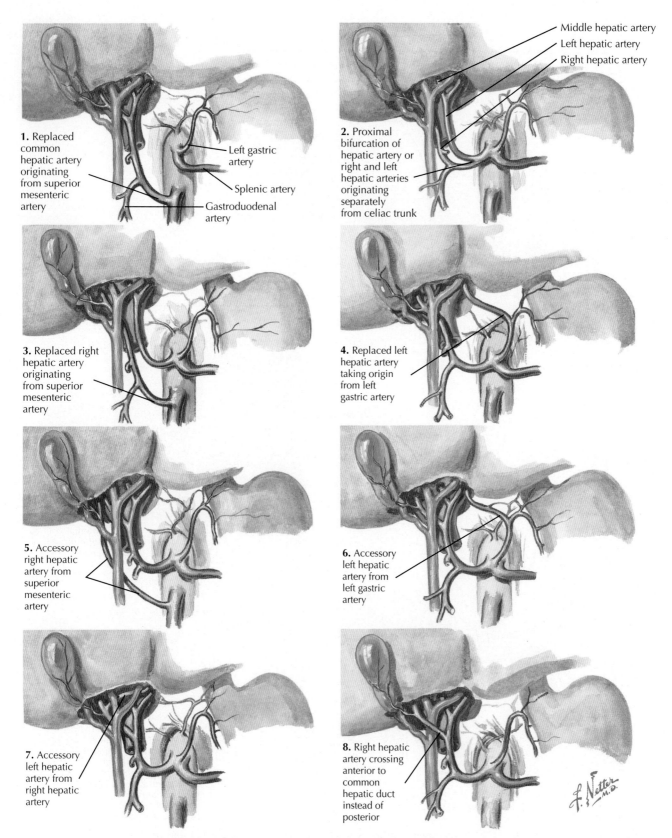

1. Replaced common hepatic artery originating from superior mesenteric artery

Left gastric artery

Splenic artery

Gastroduodenal artery

Middle hepatic artery
Left hepatic artery
Right hepatic artery

2. Proximal bifurcation of hepatic artery or right and left hepatic arteries originating separately from celiac trunk

3. Replaced right hepatic artery originating from superior mesenteric artery

4. Replaced left hepatic artery taking origin from left gastric artery

5. Accessory right hepatic artery from superior mesenteric artery

6. Accessory left hepatic artery from left gastric artery

7. Accessory left hepatic artery from right hepatic artery

8. Right hepatic artery crossing anterior to common hepatic duct instead of posterior

FIGURE 14.2 Variations in origin and course of hepatic artery and branches.

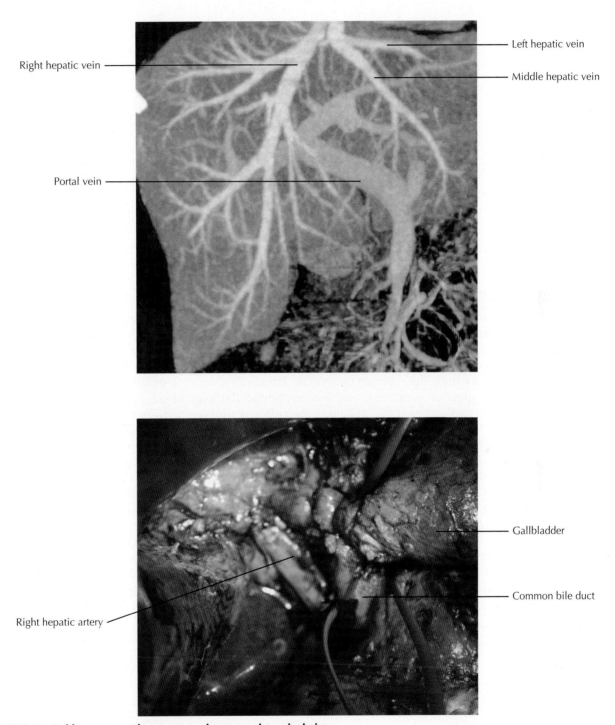

Right hepatic vein

Portal vein

Left hepatic vein

Middle hepatic vein

Gallbladder

Common bile duct

Right hepatic artery

FIGURE 14.3 Liver: magnetic resonance image and surgical view.
(CT image from Kamel IR, Liapi E, Fishman E. Liver and biliary system: evaluation by multidetector CT. Radiol Clin North Am 2005;43[6]:977–97.)

SURGICAL PRINCIPLES (Continued)

Arterial supply to the liver is through the hepatic artery, which supplies branches to the right and left lobes. Variations in the arterial supply to the liver include accessory or replaced right or left hepatic artery and an aberrant origin of the common hepatic artery (Fig. 14.2). The most common variants of the arterial blood supply to the liver include an accessory or replaced right hepatic artery from the superior mesenteric artery. This vessel is usually one of the first branches off the superior mesenteric and courses behind the head of the pancreas, posterior to the portal vein and common bile duct, traveling directly into the right lobe of the liver. The biliary tree also has significant variations (Fig. 14.4), which can add to the risk of biliary leaks from the cut edge of the liver. Bile leaks are one of the more common and problematic complications of liver resection. Maintaining adequate drainage of the remaining segments is critical in preventing biliary complications. Comparison of preoperative imaging with intraoperative cholangiography can often help clarify areas of confusion. After parenchymal transection has been performed, measures such as air insufflation or propofol injection (via the cystic duct stump) may aid in the detection of cut-surface biliary leakage.

Considerable variations exist in the relative size of the right and left lobes of the liver (Fig. 14.5). In addition to the size of each lobe, the underlying health of the liver parenchyma must also be factored into the decision regarding the minimum amount of liver that must remain for the patient to avoid liver insufficiency. Patients with cirrhosis or hepatic steatosis may need larger residual volumes after resection to maintain adequate function (Fig. 14.6).

Variations in cystic ducts

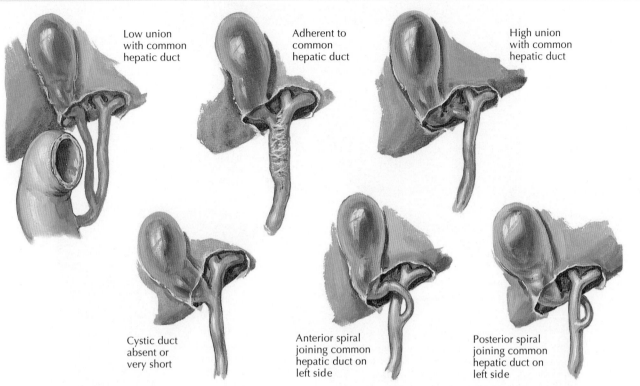

Low union with common hepatic duct

Adherent to common hepatic duct

High union with common hepatic duct

Cystic duct absent or very short

Anterior spiral joining common hepatic duct on left side

Posterior spiral joining common hepatic duct on left side

Accessory (aberrant) hepatic ducts

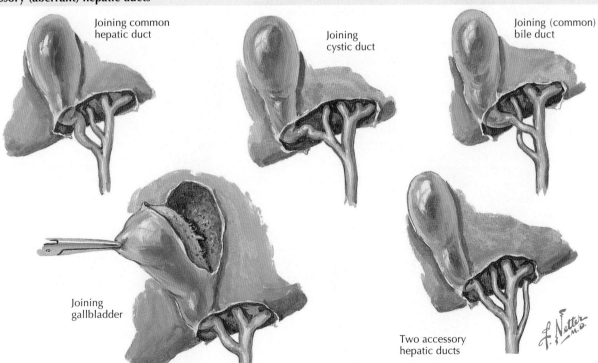

Joining common hepatic duct

Joining cystic duct

Joining (common) bile duct

Joining gallbladder

Two accessory hepatic ducts

FIGURE 14.4 Variations in cystic and hepatic ducts.

Anterior view of the liver. Hepatic lobes and perihepatic ligaments.

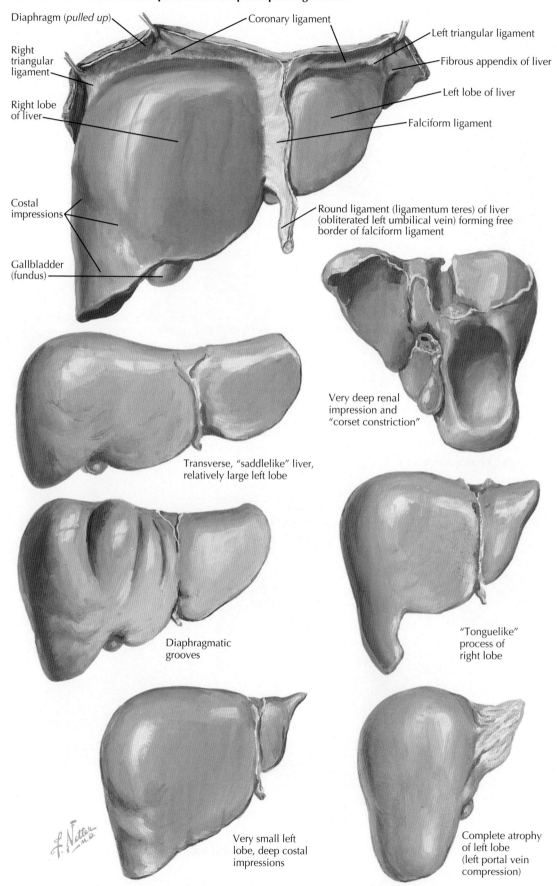

Diaphragm (*pulled up*)

Coronary ligament

Left triangular ligament

Right triangular ligament

Fibrous appendix of liver

Right lobe of liver

Left lobe of liver

Falciform ligament

Costal impressions

Round ligament (ligamentum teres) of liver (obliterated left umbilical vein) forming free border of falciform ligament

Gallbladder (fundus)

Transverse, "saddlelike" liver, relatively large left lobe

Very deep renal impression and "corset constriction"

Diaphragmatic grooves

"Tonguelike" process of right lobe

Very small left lobe, deep costal impressions

Complete atrophy of left lobe (left portal vein compression)

FIGURE 14.5 **Variations in form of liver.**

Fatty septal cirrhosis

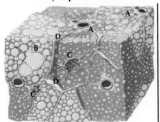

Micromembranes develop, radiating from portal tracts (*A*), around fatty cysts (*B*), in necrotic areas (*C*), and in "stress fissures" between areas of irregularly distributed fat (*D*). Simultaneously regeneration (purple) starts diffusely around lobular periphery.

Nonfatty septal cirrhosis

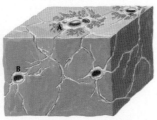

Micromembranes radiate diffusely through parenchyma, often originating at portal triads (*A*), as result of irritation (granulomatous disease, hemachromatosis, viral hepatitis?); or from central fields (*B*) (passive congestion, intoxications). Regeneration starts (*purple*).

Biliary cirrhosis

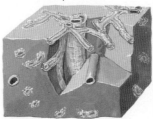

In infected or prolonged extra-hepatic biliary obstruction or in primary ductal disease, fibers form around diseased bile ducts and may also extend around intralobular ductules. Strands, not sheets, traverse the lobules as a network (pseudocirrhosis).

Postnecrotic cirrhosis

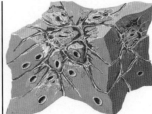

Circumscribed collapse after massive or submassive necrosis causes stress in surrounding tissue, and fissures appear. Septa develop in these as well, as a result of less severe involvement of surrounding parenchyma. Regeneration starts (*purple*).

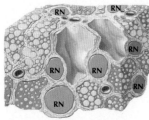

Micromembranes aggregate into thicker two-dimensional irregularly radiating sheets or septa, which dissect the lobules. Regenerative nodules (*RN*) further alter the architecture.

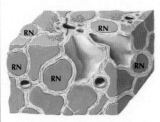

As in fatty type, membranes aggregate into dissecting septa and regenerative nodules (*RN*) develop. Note septa connecting portal triads and central veins.

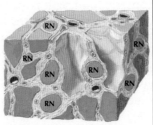

In later stages, as result of inflammation or other irritation, septa form, partly between strands, in part independently, dissecting lobules and compromising the circulation. Regenerative nodules (*RN*) appear.

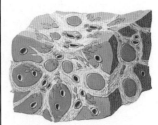

Broad bands of connective tissue result from massive collapse, whereas surrounding tissue is subdivided into small and multi-lobular nodules because of developing membranes, while regeneration takes place in nodules and in lobules.

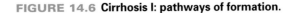

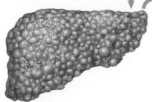

Regular formation of small nodules and thin septa, characteristic of "Laennec's" cirrhosis

Massive or relentless piecemeal necrosis and extensive regeneration

Irregular distribution of variable-sized nodules, many multilobular, and of septa, many of which are broad bands; postnecrotic cirrhosis

FIGURE 14.6 Cirrhosis I: pathways of formation.

RIGHT HEPATIC LOBECTOMY

This is a case of right hepatectomy performed for hepatocellular carcinoma (HCC) located between the right anterior and right posterior portal veins as shown in Fig. 14.7A. In this particular instance, the left portal vein and the bifurcation of the right portal vein occur at the same level, giving rise to a trifurcation of the main portal vein.

Various types of incisions can provide adequate exposure for a right lobe liver resection. One of the most common is the upper abdominal Mercedes incision, a bilateral subcostal incision with midline extension. Other variations include midline, bilateral subcostal, or a right subcostal incision with upper midline extension. Adequate exposure with a self-retaining retractor is essential (Fig. 14.7B).

In case of laparoscopic hepatectomy, total 5 to 7 trocars are inserted (Fig. 14.7C).

The liver is initially mobilized by dividing the perihepatic ligaments. The liver dissection is begun in the hilum by mobilizing the gallbladder off the liver bed. The lateral border between segments IV and V approximates the dissection plane between the right and left lobes of the liver. The retroperitoneum and Gerota's fascia, attached to the posterior right lobe of the liver, are incised to prevent liver lacerations of segments VI and VII, as the mobilization of the right lobe is begun (Fig. 14.7D). Once the inferior right lobe is free, the triangular ligament is divided along the liver to mobilize the right lobe out of the retroperitoneum. This dissection is continued superiorly to the entrance of the right hepatic vein into the vena cava. This maneuver separates the right lobe from the diaphragm. The dissection is continued posteriorly until the vena cava and short hepatic veins are fully exposed (Fig. 14.7E).

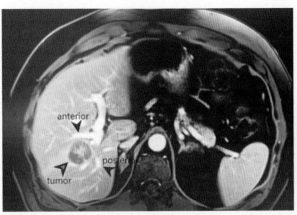

A. Hepatocellular carcinoma (HCC) located in the right lobe, between the right anterior and right posterior portal veins (arrows).

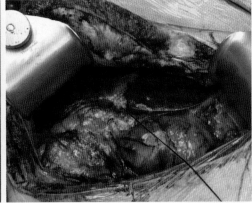

B. Hockey stick incision.

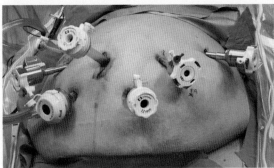

C. Positions of trocars in case of laparoscopic hepatectomy.

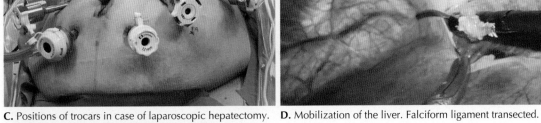

D. Mobilization of the liver. Falciform ligament transected.

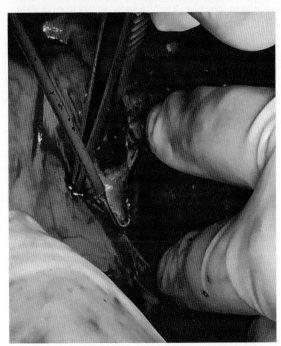

E. Mobilization of right lobe. Right triangular ligament transected.

FIGURE 14.7 Right hepatic lobectomy.

RIGHT HEPATIC LOBECTOMY (Continued)

Once all the short hepatic veins are divided, the right hepatic vein can be dissected in preparation for transection as the last step of the right hepatectomy. At this time, attention returns to the hilum. Dissection of the right liver hilum structures is performed (Fig. 14.7F). Intraoperative cholangiogram can be performed to display the biliary anatomy (Fig. 14.7G).

At this time, a demarcation plane should be evident on the surface of the liver. Although inflow vessels have been taken, better homeostasis can be obtained if inflow occlusion (i.e., Pringle maneuver) is performed. After a 10-minute course of pre-ischemic conditioning with an adequate recovery, the porta hepatis is clamped, the right hepatic vein is taken, and the liver parenchyma is divided (Fig. 14.7H). Intraoperative ultrasound is useful at this point to mark a plane of dissection lateral to the middle hepatic vein and to mark branches from the right lobe that drain through the middle vein, if present. Liver parenchymal dissection can be done with a crush technique, an ultrasonic device, or high-pressure water dissection (Fig. 14.7I, J, and K). Other techniques include using a stapler to divide the tissue or a bipolar cautery device.

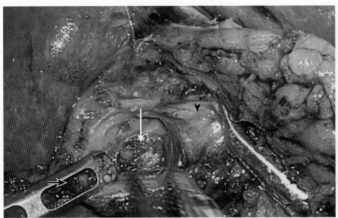

F. Right hepatic artery (black arrow), portal vein (white arrow), bile duct (black arrowhead).

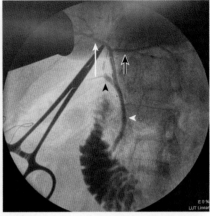

G. Intraoperative cholangiogram displaying biliary anatomy. Common hepatic duct (white arrowhead), cystic duct stump (black arrowhead), right hepatic duct (white arrow), left hepatic duct (black arrow). Scheme of liver hilum anatomy.

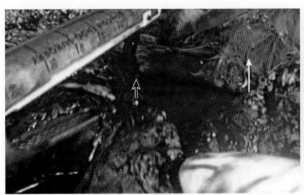

H. Right hepatic vein (black arrow). Vena cava (white arrow). Variations of right hepatic vein.

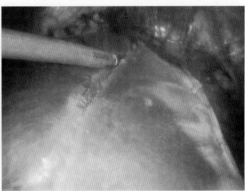

I. Marking parenchymal transection line following the Cantlie line (middle hepatic vein trajectory).

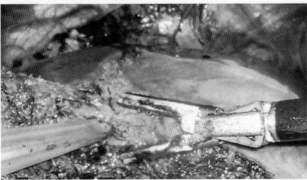

J. Parenchymal transection.

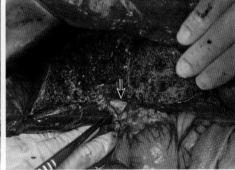

K. Liver parenchyma transected. Right hepatic artery (pointed by forceps) and right portal vein (arrow).

FIGURE 14.7 Right hepatic lobectomy (continued).

LEFT HEPATECTOMY

The left lobe of the liver comprises segments I to IV. The segments are defined by the portal branches. The left lobe lends itself better to segmental resection than the right lobe because of the easy access to the segmental branches of the left portal system. Segmental resection of the left lateral segment (segment II-III) or segment II-III-IV requires dissection further out into the porta hepatis to preserve the branches to the remaining segments. The hilar structures enter the lobe between segments III and IVb. Often, a bridge of liver tissue overlying the structures will have to be divided if segmental resections are planned. This allows access to the segmental portal and bile duct branches. Anomalous arterial and biliary anatomy is common for the left lobe.

Accessory or replaced left hepatic arteries will arise from the left gastric artery and travel in the gastrohepatic ligament to the liver. For planning a segmental resection of the left lateral segment, knowledge of the anatomy of the bile duct to segment IV is important to avoid inadvertent ligation or injury to the draining duct.

Exposure for surgery can be performed with a bilateral subcostal incision, a bilateral subcostal with a midline extension, or a midline incision.

Here a laparoscopic left lobe hepatectomy performed for colorectal cancer liver metastasis (CRLM) is shown (Fig. 14.8A). The left lateral segment of the liver is mobilized by dividing the left triangular ligament (Fig. 14.8B and C). The left segment is then retracted laterally and the gastrohepatic ligament opened. If present, an accessory or replaced left hepatic artery will travel in the gastrohepatic ligament to the liver. It can be ligated at this point in the dissection; otherwise, the peritoneum over the proximal hepatic artery lymph node is incised and the hepatic artery exposed. The hepatic artery is dissected proximally into the hilum to expose the left hepatic artery. If a formal left hepatectomy is being performed, the left hepatic artery can be ligated after it leaves the main hepatic artery. If segment I is to be left, the artery should be taken after it gives off the branch to segment I. Often, segment IV will have a separate branch off the main hepatic artery. If a formal left hepatic lobectomy is to be performed, the main hepatic artery can be followed to the common bile duct to see if segmental arteries to segment IV are present (Fig. 14.8D).

Once the left hepatic artery is taken, the gallbladder can be dissected off the liver bed and the cystic artery and duct ligated and divided. The common bile duct is then followed to the bifurcation, and the main left duct is encircled with a vessel loop. If segment I is to be left, the duct must be taken distal to the segment I bile duct takeoff. The duct can be taken early if performing a formal left lobectomy. If segmental resections are planned, it is often better to leave the duct until the parenchymal dissection, to facilitate identification of small ducts that travel into segments to be left.

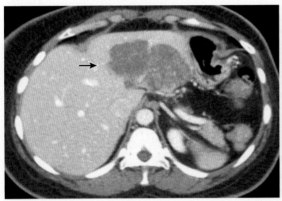

A. Left lobe mass (arrow).

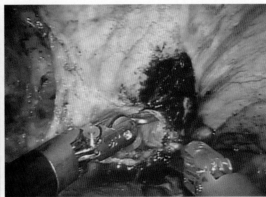

B. Left lobe mobilization. Left triangular ligament division.

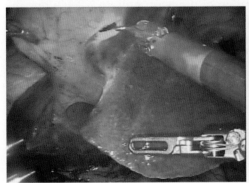

C. Left lobe mobilization. Falciform ligament division.

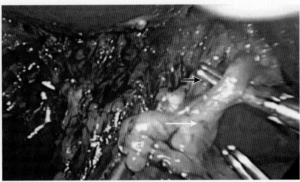

D. Middle hepatic artery (black arrow) and left hepatic artery (white arrow).

FIGURE 14.8 Left hepatectomy.

LEFT HEPATECTOMY (Continued)

At this time, the main left portal vein can be identified and encircled with a vessel loop (Fig. 14.8E). The portal vein can be taken with a stapler or can be controlled with clamps, divided, and then oversewn. If the caudate lobe is to be left, the portal branch to the caudate must be saved. The caudate lobe is mobilized off the vena cava (Fig. 14.8F). Short hepatic vein branches are ligated and divided to mobilize the left lobe off the vena cava. Large short hepatic veins can be easily taken with an endovascular GIA stapler. Once the mobilization is complete, the caudate lobe and left segment can be retracted lateral to help expose the left and middle hepatic veins (Fig. 14.8G). These can be dissected off the vena cava and marked with a vessel loop. The veins can be controlled and divided either with a vascular GIA stapler or between vascular clamps. The demarcation plane of the right and left lobes should be evident. Using intraoperative ultrasound, the resection plane lateral to the middle hepatic vein can be marked on the surface of the liver. Using a parenchymal transection technique, the liver parenchyma is divided (Fig. 14.8H). Larger vessels encountered in the parenchymal dissection can be taken with a stapler or suture-ligated. Once the parenchymal dissection is complete, the cut surface is cauterized with argon beam coagulation and covered with absorbable fibrin glue. A Pringle maneuver or portal inflow occlusion can be performed during the parenchymal dissection if significant bleeding is encountered during the separation of the liver. A drain is left along the cut surface of the liver at the conclusion of the procedure to monitor for bile duct leak.

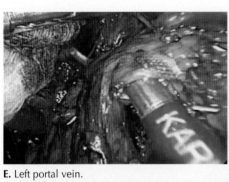

E. Left portal vein.

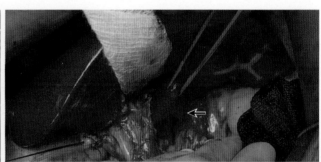

F. Caudate lobe (arrow).

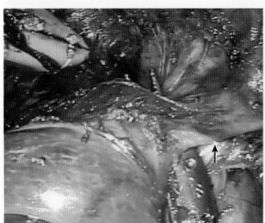

G. Left hepatic vein (arrow). Anatomic variations of middle and left hepatic veins.

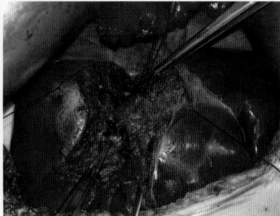

H. Liver parynchema is divided.

FIGURE 14.8 Left hepatectomy (continued).

CENTRAL HEPATECTOMY

Fig. 14.9A and B show large HCC located in the center of the liver. Total vascular isolation is prepared by encircling the infrahepatic and suprahepatic vena cava and inflow and outflow liver structures (Fig. 14.9C and D). Securing vascular control is essential to minimize hemorrhage during parenchymal transection (Fig. 14.9E).

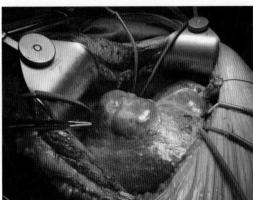

A. Intraoperative view of centrally located HCC.

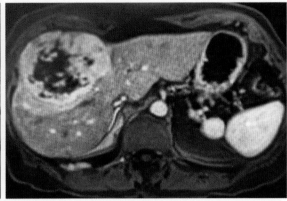

B. Computed tomography (CT) scan showing centrally located HCC.

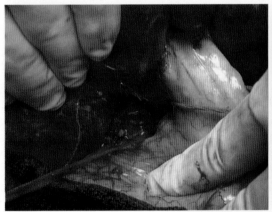

C. Infra-hepatic vena cava and liver hilum encircled.

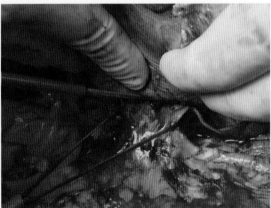

D. Supra-hepatic vena cava, middle and left hepatic veins trunk and right hepatic vein encircled.

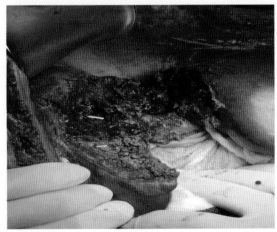

E. Resection bed after central hepatectomy.

FIGURE 14.9 **Central hepatectomy.**

ASSOCIATING LIVER PARTITION AND PORTAL VEIN LIGATION FOR STAGED HEPATECTOMY (ALPPS)

The associating liver partition and portal vein ligation for staged hepatectomy (ALPPS) procedure can be applied to treat colorectal cancer liver metastases (CRLM) when portal vein embolization (PVE) fails to induce sufficient hypertrophy of future liver remnant (FLR) (Fig. 14.10A through D). During first surgical stage, tumor is resected from the lobe less involved, and contralateral portal vein ligation and liver partition are performed to induce enhanced FLR hypertrophy (Fig. 14.10E through H). From 1 to 2 weeks later, completion of hepatectomy is performed by removing the liver lobe carrying the remaining tumor burden (Fig. 14.10I and J).

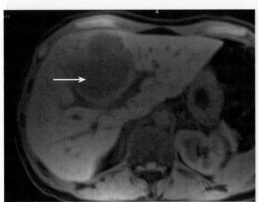

A. Large central metastasis from colorectal cancer (arrow).

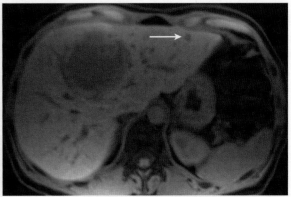

B. Small metastasis in left lateral segment (FLR) (arrow).

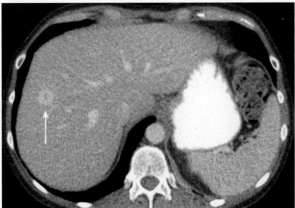

C. Small metastasis in the right lobe (arrow).

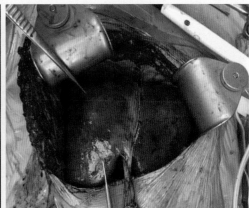

D. Intraoperative view pointing at large centrally located metastasis during first ALPPS step.

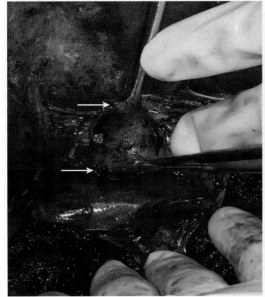

E. Stumps of ligated right anterior and posterior portal veins (arrows) during first ALPPS step.

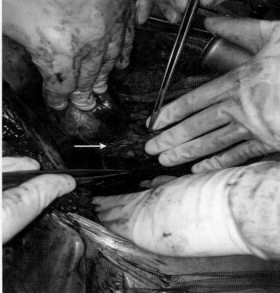

F. Right hepatic artery (RHA) encircled during first ALPPS step to facilitate identification and ligation of RHA during second step.

FIGURE 14.10 **Liver partition and portal vein ligation for stated hepatectomy (ALPPS).**

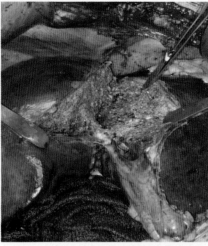

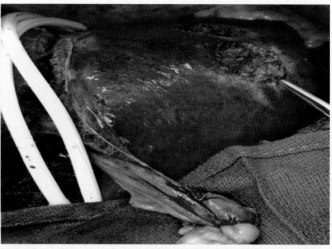

G. Liver partition at level of falciform ligament insertion to interrupt intrahepatic vascular connections during first ALPPS step.

H. Wedge resections performed in the left lateral segment to clear the FLR during first ALPPS step.

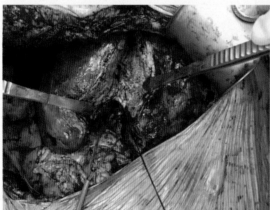

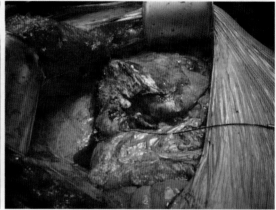

I. Intraoperative view of initial exploration during second ALPPS step 2 weeks later after first step.

J. Finalized ALPPS procedure. Intraoperative view of tumor free and enlarged left lateral segment. Left lateral segment volume increased from 20% to 24% during 6 weeks after right portal vein embolization. As this was considered insufficient future liver volume, ALPPS procedure was attempted. Left lateral segment volume increased from 24% to 31% after 2 weeks of first ALPPS step.

FIGURE 14.10 Liver partition and portal vein ligation for stated hepatectomy (ALPPS) (continued).

SUGGESTED READINGS

Aragon RJ, Solomon NL. Techniques of hepatic resection. J Gastrointest Oncol 2012;3(1): 28–40.

Lang H, de Santibañes E, Schlitt HJ, Malagó M, van Gulik T, Machado MA, Jovine E, Heinrich S, Ettorre GM, Chan A, Hernandez-Alejandro R, Robles Campos R, Sandström P, Linecker M, Clavien PA. 10th Anniversary of ALPPS-lessons learned and quo vadis. Ann Surg 2019;269(1):114–9.

Shinohara H, Mizuno Y, Makino Y. Point of surgical techniques as seen from the anatomy of film—Illustrated surgery. April 6, 2010.

Strasberg SM. Nomenclature of hepatic anatomy and resections: a review of the Brisbane 2000 system. J Hepatobiliary Pancreat Surg 2005;12:351–5.

Distal Pancreatectomy

Valery Vilchez and Toms Augustin

INTRODUCTION

Distal pancreatectomy refers to resection of a portion of the pancreas extending to the left of the superior mesenteric vein-portal vein (SMV-PV) confluence. First described by Billroth in 1884, distal pancreatectomy is performed for various benign and malignant conditions involving the body and tail of the pancreas, the line of transection depending on the location of the pathology, and goals of the resection.

SURGICAL ANATOMY

A key to safety of the procedure is a thorough understanding of the vascular anatomy of the pancreas. The blood supply to the tail of the pancreas is provided by the splenic artery and vein (Fig. 15.1A). The splenic artery arises from the celiac artery and courses along the superior border of the body and tail of the pancreas.

The splenic vein is located on the posterior surface of the pancreas, and as it runs medially, it joins the SMV to form the PV. There are multiple small tributaries that drain posteriorly into the splenic vein (Fig. 15.1B).

The tail of the pancreas terminates in the hilum of the spleen, where a wide array of artery and vein branches exit. Posterior to the spleen is the left kidney and the left adrenal gland.

A. Blood supply of the pancreas

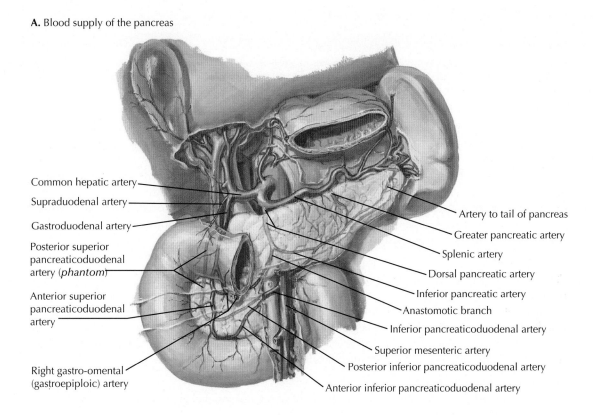

Common hepatic artery

Supraduodenal artery

Gastroduodenal artery

Posterior superior pancreaticoduodenal artery (*phantom*)

Anterior superior pancreaticoduodenal artery

Right gastro-omental (gastroepiploic) artery

Artery to tail of pancreas

Greater pancreatic artery

Splenic artery

Dorsal pancreatic artery

Inferior pancreatic artery

Anastomotic branch

Inferior pancreaticoduodenal artery

Superior mesenteric artery

Posterior inferior pancreaticoduodenal artery

Anterior inferior pancreaticoduodenal artery

B. Venous drainage of spleen showing connection with the inferior mesenteric vein

Left gastric vein

Hepatic portal vein

Right gastric vein

Posterior superior pancreaticoduodenal vein

Superior mesenteric vein

Right gastro-omental (gastroepiploic) vein

Anterior superior pancreaticoduodenal vein

Anterior inferior pancreaticoduodenal vein

Posterior inferior pancreaticoduodenal vein

Splenic vein

Short gastric veins

Left gastro-omental (gastroepiploic) vein

(Great) pancreatic vein

Inferior mesenteric vein

FIGURE 15.1 Blood supply of the pancreas and venous drainage.

SURGICAL APPROACH

Laparoscopic Distal Pancreatectomy

The Dutch distal pancreatic resection group trial (LEOPARD) supported laparoscopic resection as the preferred approach for left-sided tumors confined to the pancreas for improved clinical and quality of life outcomes.

Relative contraindications for the laparoscopic approach include patients with large tumors, tumors involving celiac artery, superior mesenteric artery (SMA), or other large visceral vessels. Post neo-adjuvant status or patients needing resection of adjacent organs may also benefit from an open approach. The presence of pancreatic cancer is not a contraindication, but the oncologic outcome exceeds the importance of the operative approach.

Patient Position

The patient is placed in a supine position, left side 30 degrees elevated with legs apart (supine position is an option). Five ports are placed: 5-mm epigastric port is placed using an optical entry technique and subsequently exchanged for a Nathanson retractor. After insufflation, a 12- to 15-mm supraumbilical port is placed at the midline, a 5- to 12-mm port is placed in the right midclavicular line, a 5-mm trocar in the right midclavicular line subcostal, and a 5-mm port in the right lateral position paraumbilically (Fig. 15.2A).

Mobilization and Dissection

When the procedure is for malignancy, an initial staging laparoscopy is performed. The gastrocolic omentum is divided using an energy device. The short gastric vessels are divided to allow safe retraction of the stomach, regardless of spleen preservation. The stomach is subsequently retracted en-masse with the left lateral segment of the liver (Fig. 15.2B). The lesion is identified, either visually or using intraoperative ultrasound (IOUS). IOUS is especially useful in identifying nonpalpable, nonsurface lesions, detecting multiple lesions and guiding pancreatic transection line.

The inferior margin of the pancreas is next mobilized by incising the peritoneum at the base of the mesocolon. The dissection is carried from right to left, mobilizing the entire inferior edge of the pancreas. Mobilization of the splenic flexure of the colon is then completed. Should the division of the neck of the pancreas be required, then a dissection plane is created along the SMV to create a tunnel posterior to the pancreatic neck. The hepatic artery is identified at the superior margin of the neck, and a lymphadenectomy should commence with the hepatic artery lymph nodes and then proceed to the left to include the celiac, left gastric, and splenic artery lymph nodes. The pancreas can be encircled with a Penrose drain to create a sling to facilitate placement of the gastrointestinal stapler with an appropriate-sized staple height. A graded progressive compression technique is used (Fig. 15.2C). The neck is always divided before division of the splenic vessels.

The splenic artery is divided first, and its dissection is aided by inferior retraction of the divided neck. The artery can be controlled by clips or a stapler after confirmation of a hepatic artery pulse with temporary occlusion. Before the splenic artery is divided, it should be temporarily occluded and pulsations in the proper hepatic artery visualized to ensure that the common hepatic artery (CHA) is not inadvertently ligated. The splenic vein is similarly secured and care is made to preserve the coronary vein. Pancreatic parenchyma should be spared based on lesion location and pathology. An alternative laparoscopic technique is to start at the splenic flexure and proceed in a counterclockwise manner.

Splenic preservation has the advantage of fewer long-term infectious complications and no long-term risk of post-splenectomy sepsis. The splenic vessels are completely spared using Kimura's technique. Once the pancreas is divided and clear of the splenic vessels, the cut edge of the specimen side is retracted and dissected off of the splenic vessels by dividing small branches and tributaries between clips or sutures (Fig. 15.2D).

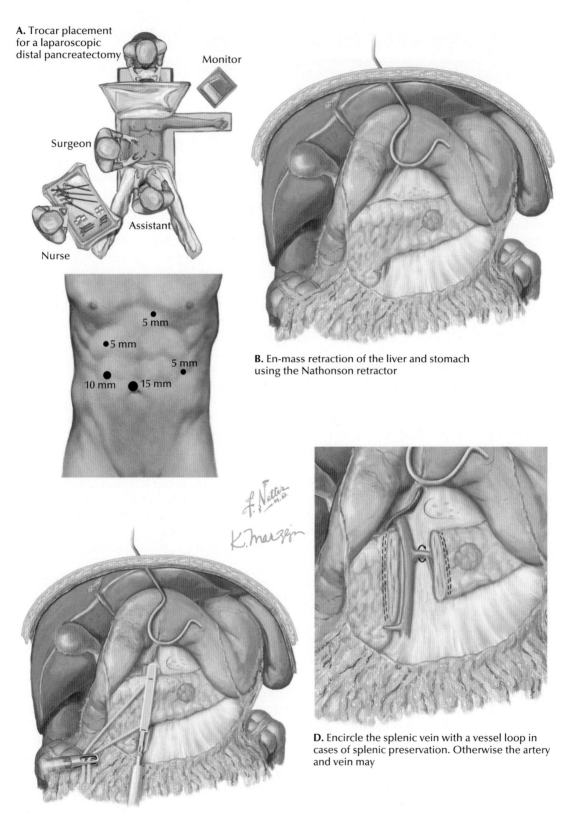

A. Trocar placement for a laparoscopic distal pancreatectomy

Monitor

Surgeon

Assistant

Nurse

5 mm

•5 mm

5 mm

10 mm · 15 mm

B. En-mass retraction of the liver and stomach using the Nathonson retractor

D. Encircle the splenic vein with a vessel loop in cases of splenic preservation. Otherwise the artery and vein may

C. Pancreas division using endomechanical

FIGURE 15.2 Laparoscopic distal pancreatectomy.

Laparoscopic Distal Pancreatectomy (Continued)

When a malignancy is suspected or a technical reason necessitates removal of the spleen, the splenic artery is divided followed by the splenic vein, in that order, with a vascular stapler to prevent any engorgement and bleeding of the spleen that would result from dividing the vein first. The spleen is then mobilized from its attachments as the last step in the operation. Immunization is essential to prevent infections caused by encapsulated bacteria after splenectomy, completed at least 2 weeks before elective surgery and a postoperative booster.

A medial-to-lateral approach is used during the mobilization of the pancreas. When a splenectomy has been performed, the pancreas is separated from the spleen to manually morcellate the spleen for easy extraction of the specimen. The intact specimen is suspended freely in the insufflated abdomen, and the spleen is divided from the tail of the pancreas with an energy device. In the case of malignancy, the specimen is removed en bloc. A surgical drain is placed at the cut end of the pancreas for patients at high risk for fistula.

Open Distal Pancreatectomy

The standard approach is through an upper midline incision from the xiphoid process to the umbilicus.

Open Retrograde Distal Pancreatectomy With Splenectomy

Left to right dissection is the standard open procedure for tumors where the anatomic constraints dictate sacrificing the spleen. The pancreas is approached by opening the lesser sac through the gastrocolic ligament. The short gastric vessels are divided. Dissection along the inferior margin of the pancreas is continued. Careful dissection of the retroperitoneum permits mobilization between the left kidney and the adrenal glands posteriorly and the spleen anteriorly. The vascular attachment at the inferior border of the pancreas between the spleen and the splenic flexure of the colon is divided. Medial dissection is carried to a minimum of 3 cm medial to the mass.

The splenic artery is identified at its origin, traced along the superior border of the pancreas, and divided just distal to its origin. The splenic vein is then isolated and divided just proximal to the confluence with the inferior mesenteric vein. Pancreas transection is determined based on the location of the tumor. The pancreatic parenchyma is divided sharply or with a stapler with suture control of the duct or parenchyma as necessary.

Distal Pancreatectomy With Splenic Preservation

As in the laparoscopic approach, preservation of the splenic artery and vein is favored, and not the Warshaw technique. For adequate exposure to the vessels the pancreas and the spleen are first mobilized en bloc. This requires division of the short gastric vessels and retropancreatic attachments to liberate the pancreas and spleen into the operative field. The pancreas is then dissected free from the vessels lateral to medial beginning at the splenic hilum. This will require securing multiple small venous tributaries and arterial branches. The parenchyma of the pancreas is then divided as previously described. The spleen is returned to its native position and does not require any special fixation to maintain its location.

Radical Antegrade Modular Pancreaticosplenectomy

Resection for pancreatic cancer should include resection with clear margins and regional lymphadenectomy (Fig. 15.3). Radical antegrade modular pancreaticosplenectomy (RAMPS) is a modular technique in which dissection proceeds from medial to lateral, removing all nodal tissue surrounding the body and tail of the pancreas.

After dissection of the gastrocolic omentum and division of the short gastric vessels, the neck of the pancreas is elevated off the SMV and PV. The right gastric artery is divided and the proper hepatic artery is next followed proximally to the CHA and the gastroduodenal artery (GDA). The lymph nodes anterior to the CHA are mobilized, the anterior surface of the PV is exposed, and the tunnel behind the neck of the pancreas is completed. The neck of the pancreas is divided, and the pancreatic duct is oversewn.

The left gastric vein is divided near the lesser curve of the stomach. The splenic artery is ligated and divided close to its origin. The splenic vein is divided and the plane of the dissection now proceeds vertically in the sagittal plane until the SMA is encountered. The periaortic lymph nodes are mobilized and included with the specimen.

If the planned posterior plane of dissection is behind the adrenal, the dissection is carried down the left side of the aorta in the sagittal plane onto the diaphragm. The dissection is continued laterally, usually taking Gerota's fascia off the superior half of the kidney; the inferior mesenteric vein (IMV) is ligated and transected. The left renal artery and vein are identified. The adrenal vein is divided flush with the renal vein. The entire specimen will lift off the posterior muscle layer and can be removed.

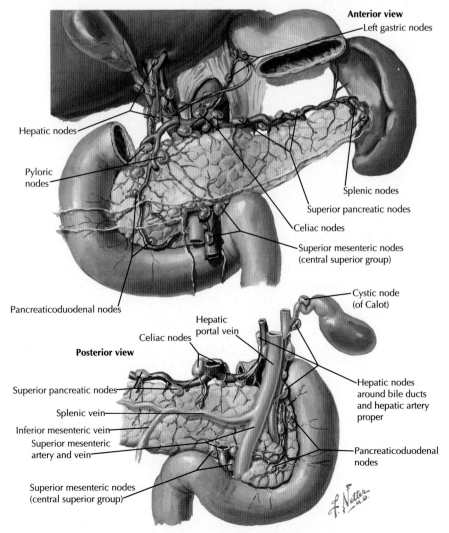

FIGURE 15.3 Lymphatic drainage of the pancreas.

Distal Pancreatectomy and Celiac Axis Resection

The original Lyon Henry Appleby procedure (total gastrectomy and distal pancreatectomy and celiac axis resection [DP-CAR]) achieved a more complete resection of the celiac axis lymph nodes in patients with locally advanced gastric cancer. A modified Appleby, which preserves the stomach, was adopted by Nimura and Fortner in 1976 for pancreatic body and tail adenocarcinoma.

The right-sided approach for accessing the origin of the SMA and evaluating any involvement is used. The most crucial step during surgery is the preservation of the collateral pathways to the CHA from the SMA, namely the inferior pancreaticoduodenal artery and the GDA, to avoid hepatic ischemia. Gastric ischemia can be avoided by preserving both arterial inflow and venous drainage via left/right gastric and right gastroepiploic vessels (Fig. 15.4).

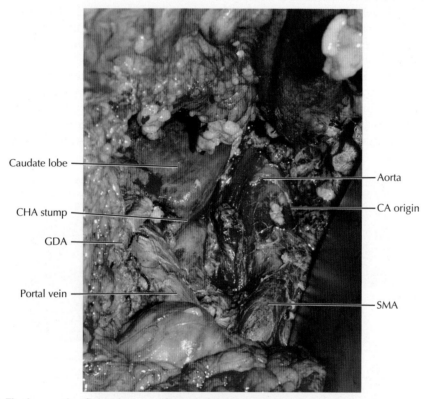

FIG. 15.4 Final operative field after modified Appleby procedure.
The celiac artery has been resected and its origin is oversewn. The entry of the left gastric vein into the reconstructed portal vein is visualized posterior to the common hepatic artery (CHA) stump. *CA,* Celiac artery; *GDA,* gastroduodenal artery; *SMA,* superior mesenteric artery.

SUGGESTED READINGS

De Rooij T, Van Hilst J, Vogel JA, et al. Minimally invasive versus open distal pancreatectomy (LEOPARD): study protocol for randomized controlled trial. Trials 2017 Apr 8;18(1):166.

Dokmak S, Aussilhou B, Ftériche FS, Soubrane O, Sauvanet A. Laparoscopic distal pancreatectomy: surgical technique. J Visc Surg 2019;156:139–45.

Kimura W, Inoue T, Futakawa N, Shinkai H, Han I, Muto T. Spleen-preserving distal pancreatectomy with conservation of the splenic artery and vein. Surgery 1996;120(5):885–90.

Mittal A, de Reuver PR, Shanbhag S, et al. Distal pancreatectomy, splenectomy, and celiac axis resection (DPS-CAR): common hepatic arterial stump pressure should determine the need for arterial reconstruction. Surgery 2015;157:811–7.

Napolitano C, Valvano L, Grillo M. Distal splenopancreatectomy: indications for surgery and technical notes. In: Surgical treatment of pancreatic diseases. Milan: Springer; 2009. p. 321–8.

Strasberg SM, Drebin JA, Linehan D. Radical antegrade modular pancreatosplenectomy. Surgery 2003;133:521–7.

Pancreatoduodenectomy

Kevin El-Hayek and Amit Khithani

▶ VIDEO

16.1 Laparoscopic Pancreaticoduodenectomy

INTRODUCTION

The first pancreatoduodenectomy was described by Kausch in 1909; however, Allen O. Whipple popularized the procedure for pancreatic head adenocarcinoma in 1935 as a two-stage operation with his report of seven cases. The procedure traditionally involves the en bloc removal of the gastric antrum, duodenum, pancreatic head, gallbladder, and bile duct. The pylorus-preserving technique was introduced by Traverso and Longmire in 1978. Pancreatoduodenectomy was previously accompanied by a mortality rate of 20% to 25%. Currently, however, most experienced pancreatic surgery centers report a mortality rate of 3% or less. The morbidity remains high at 20% to 50%, with the most impactful complication being a pancreatic fistula.

The most common indications for pancreatoduodenectomy are periampullary tumors, predominantly cancers of the pancreatic head. Cystic pancreatic neoplasms, particularly intraductal papillary mucinous neoplasms (IPMNs), can have malignant potential and have become an indication for pancreatic resection with greater frequency over the last few decades.

SURGICAL APPROACH

Open Technique

When performed for malignancy, a diagnostic laparoscopy is performed to assess for widespread metastatic disease. After the presence of metastatic disease is ruled out, a laparotomy is performed either through an upper midline incision or a subcostal incision based on the width of the costal margin and body habitus. After a thorough assessment, if the tumor is believed to be unresectable, many surgeons favor palliative biliary and duodenal bypasses.

The dissection begins with mobilization of the hepatic flexure, followed by a generous Kocher maneuver to lyse the lateral retroperitoneal attachments of the duodenum (Fig. 16.1A and B). This maneuver elevates the duodenum and head of the pancreas out of the retroperitoneum. By taking the Kocher maneuver to its fullest extent, the surgeon identifies the inferior vena cava, the left renal vein, the origin of the superior mesenteric artery (SMA), and the superior mesenteric vein (SMV), where it crosses the duodenum and ligament of Treitz. The lesser sac is next explored by dividing the gastrocolic ligament, and the pancreas is exposed. A combination of the Kocher maneuver and division of the gastrocolic ligament includes complete exposure of the pancreatic head with separation of the colonic mesentery from the stomach. The middle colic and the right gastroepiploic veins are next identified. Both of these veins are followed to their point of drainage into the SMV, which represents the groove between the neck of the pancreas and the transverse mesocolon (Fig. 16.1C). The right gastroepiploic vein is divided, the SMV is dissected from the pancreatic neck, and the resectability of the mass from the anterior aspect of the SMV and portal vein is assessed. Blunt dissection may be carried out in this space working gently cephalad, allowing for the development of the plane posterior to the neck of the pancreas and anterior to the SMV. At this point, the surgeon should feel for evidence of a replaced or accessory right hepatic artery, which may lie posterior to the portal vein (Fig. 16.2).

Attention is turned to the hepatoduodenal ligament (Fig. 16.3A and B). First, the right gastric artery is divided. The hepatic artery lymph node (VIIIA) is next identified and excised. This lymph node (LN) is located along the common hepatic artery near the take-off of the gastroduodenal artery (GDA). Removal of this LN not only gives better access to and visualization of the GDA but also facilitates the identification of the suprapancreatic portal vein. Care is taken to identify and preserve a replaced or accessory right hepatic artery. The common hepatic artery and the GDAs are identified, and the GDA is divided (Fig. 16.3C). Before ligating the GDA, the surgeon must be sure that when it is occluded, there is still a pulse in the hepatic artery going to the liver. Loss of that pulse may indicate a median arcuate ligament compression, celiac stenosis, or variant arterial anatomy (see Fig. 16.2). The GDA stump may also be oversewn with 5-0 Prolene.

The gallbladder is next dissected off the gallbladder fossa using a fundus first technique and the junction of the common bile duct (CBD) and cystic duct is identified. The common hepatic duct is identified and encircled with a vessel loop proximal to the cystic duct. The CBD is next dissected off the portal vein, and the superior aspect of the neck of the pancreas is dissected from the portal vein.

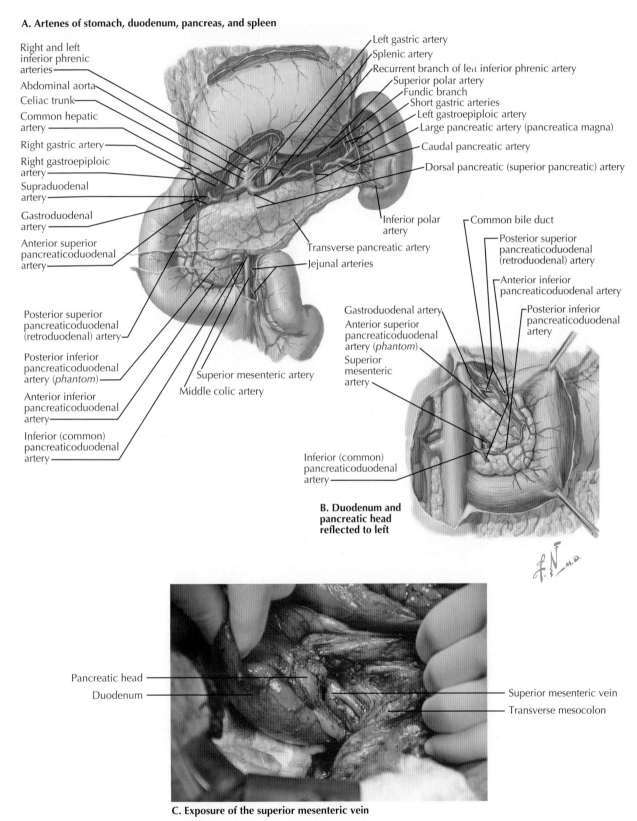

A. Artenes of stomach, duodenum, pancreas, and spleen

Right and left inferior phrenic arteries

Abdominal aorta

Celiac trunk

Common hepatic artery

Right gastric artery

Right gastroepiploic artery

Supraduodenal artery

Gastroduodenal artery

Anterior superior pancreaticoduodenal artery

Posterior superior pancreaticoduodenal (retroduodenal) artery

Posterior inferior pancreaticoduodenal artery (*phantom*)

Anterior inferior pancreaticoduodenal artery

Inferior (common) pancreaticoduodenal artery

Left gastric artery

Splenic artery

Recurrent branch of left inferior phrenic artery

Superior polar artery

Fundic branch

Short gastric arteries

Left gastroepiploic artery

Large pancreatic artery (pancreatica magna)

Caudal pancreatic artery

Dorsal pancreatic (superior pancreatic) artery

Inferior polar artery

Transverse pancreatic artery

Jejunal arteries

Superior mesenteric artery

Middle colic artery

Common bile duct

Posterior superior pancreaticoduodenal (retroduodenal) artery

Anterior inferior pancreaticoduodenal artery

Posterior inferior pancreaticoduodenal artery

Gastroduodenal artery

Anterior superior pancreaticoduodenal artery (*phantom*)

Superior mesenteric artery

Inferior (common) pancreaticoduodenal artery

B. Duodenum and pancreatic head reflected to left

Pancreatic head

Duodenum

Superior mesenteric vein

Transverse mesocolon

C. Exposure of the superior mesenteric vein

FIGURE 16.1 Arterial supply of stomach and duodenum.

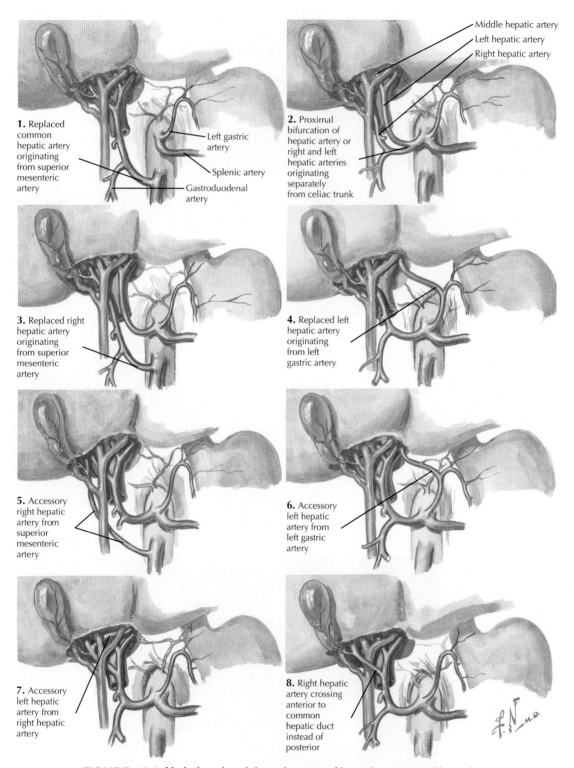

1. Replaced common hepatic artery originating from superior mesenteric artery

Left gastric artery

Splenic artery

Gastroduodenal artery

Middle hepatic artery
Left hepatic artery
Right hepatic artery

2. Proximal bifurcation of hepatic artery or right and left hepatic arteries originating separately from celiac trunk

3. Replaced right hepatic artery originating from superior mesenteric artery

4. Replaced left hepatic artery originating from left gastric artery

5. Accessory right hepatic artery from superior mesenteric artery

6. Accessory left hepatic artery from left gastric artery

7. Accessory left hepatic artery from right hepatic artery

8. Right hepatic artery crossing anterior to common hepatic duct instead of posterior

FIGURE 16.2 Variations in origin and course of hepatic artery and branches.

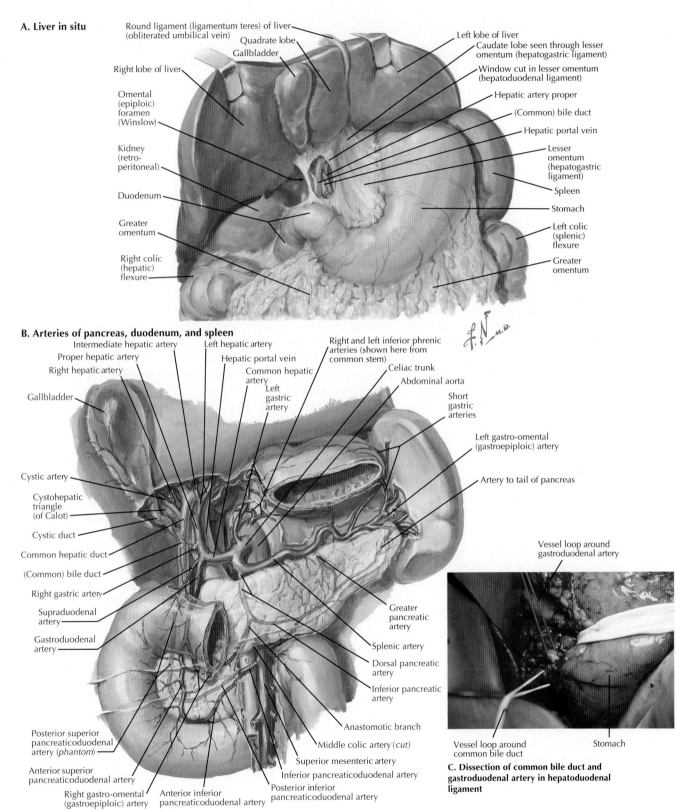

A. Liver in situ

Round ligament (ligamentum teres) of liver (obliterated umbilical vein)

Quadrate lobe

Gallbladder

Right lobe of liver

Omental (epiploic) foramen (Winslow)

Kidney (retro-peritoneal)

Duodenum

Greater omentum

Right colic (hepatic) flexure

Left lobe of liver

Caudate lobe seen through lesser omentum (hepatogastric ligament)

Window cut in lesser omentum (hepatoduodenal ligament)

Hepatic artery proper

(Common) bile duct

Hepatic portal vein

Lesser omentum (hepatogastric ligament)

Spleen

Stomach

Left colic (splenic) flexure

Greater omentum

B. Arteries of pancreas, duodenum, and spleen

Intermediate hepatic artery

Proper hepatic artery

Right hepatic artery

Gallbladder

Cystic artery

Cystohepatic triangle (of Calot)

Cystic duct

Common hepatic duct

(Common) bile duct

Right gastric artery

Supraduodenal artery

Gastroduodenal artery

Posterior superior pancreaticoduodenal artery (*phantom*)

Anterior superior pancreaticoduodenal artery

Right gastro-omental (gastroepiploic) artery

Anterior inferior pancreaticoduodenal artery

Left hepatic artery

Hepatic portal vein

Common hepatic artery

Left gastric artery

Right and left inferior phrenic arteries (shown here from common stem)

Celiac trunk

Abdominal aorta

Short gastric arteries

Left gastro-omental (gastroepiploic) artery

Artery to tail of pancreas

Greater pancreatic artery

Splenic artery

Dorsal pancreatic artery

Inferior pancreatic artery

Anastomotic branch

Middle colic artery (*cut*)

Superior mesenteric artery

Inferior pancreaticoduodenal artery

Posterior inferior pancreaticoduodenal artery

Vessel loop around gastroduodenal artery

Vessel loop around common bile duct

Stomach

C. Dissection of common bile duct and gastroduodenal artery in hepatoduodenal ligament

FIGURE 16.3 **Liver and arterial anatomy of hepatoduodenal ligament for suprapancreatic dissection.**

Open Technique (Continued)

Attention is then turned to the proximal jejunum, which is transected 10 to 15 cm distal to the ligament of Treitz. The ligament of Treitz is dissected, and the distal duodenum is dissected off the retroperitoneum. The distal duodenal and proximal jejunal mesenteries are ligated, and then the bowel is passed underneath the SMA to the right upper quadrant.

The common hepatic duct is then transected sharply while obtaining bile cultures if a preoperative biliary stent was placed. Either the first portion of the duodenum (for a pylorus-preserving pancreatoduodenectomy) or the distal stomach (for a classic pancreatoduodenectomy) is dissected and transected. Next, the right gastroepiploic vessels are divided near the stomach or proximal duodenum. The pancreatic neck is then transected after suture ligating the transverse pancreatic vessels near the neck of the pancreas. A margin may be sent for frozen-section analysis from the pancreatic duct and common hepatic duct, if the indication for resection is a malignancy and the results would alter the extent of resection. If the resection is performed for main duct IPMN, presence of high-grade dysplasia at the margin is assessed and may necessitate total pancreatectomy if unable to achieve a clear margin.

There are few, if any, anterolateral small venous branches off of the portal vein. The posterior superior pancreaticoduodenal vein is reliably identified and ligated (Fig. 16.4A). The uncinate process is then dissected away from the SMA, taking care to ligate the pancreaticoduodenal arteries and in some cases the first jejunal branch to the portal vein. The use of an advanced energy device such as a vessel sealer or ultrasonic scalpel may reduce blood loss during this maneuver. The specimen is oriented and margins inked by the surgeon after removal and the operative field appears as shown in Fig. 16.4B.

Reconstruction is generally done in the following order: pancreas, hepatic duct, then duodenum or stomach. The pancreaticoenteric anastomosis may be done as a pancreaticojejunostomy or a pancreaticogastrostomy. Many high-volume centers prefer a pancreaticojejunostomy, which is typically performed as an end-to-side duct-to-mucosa anastomosis. The Blumgart technique is one such technique of duct to mucosa pancreaticojejunostomy (Fig. 16.5); 5-0 polypropylene or 5-0 PDS (Polydioxanone) interrupted sutures are used to create the duct-to-mucosa pancreaticojejunostomy. Next, the biliary enteric anastomosis is performed typically via an end-to-side hepaticojejunostomy using interrupted or running absorbable sutures. Depending on whether a pylorus-preserving pancreatoduodenectomy is performed, the duodenal/gastric anastomosis is done last. Most surgeons leave one or two drains near the pancreatic and biliary anastomoses, depending on the fistula risk score.

Minimally Invasive Pancreatoduodenectomy

Minimally invasive pancreatoduodenectomy (MI-PD) is increasingly being performed at specialized centers. When combined with enhanced recovery after surgery (ERAS) pathways, an MI-PD may reduce inpatient length of stay, shorten recovery periods, and decrease cost. Various approaches to MI-PD have been described using laparoscopy, robotic surgery, or a hybrid of both techniques.

After a diagnostic laparoscopy, a liver retractor is placed under the left lobe of the liver and the patient is placed in a reverse Trendelenburg position.

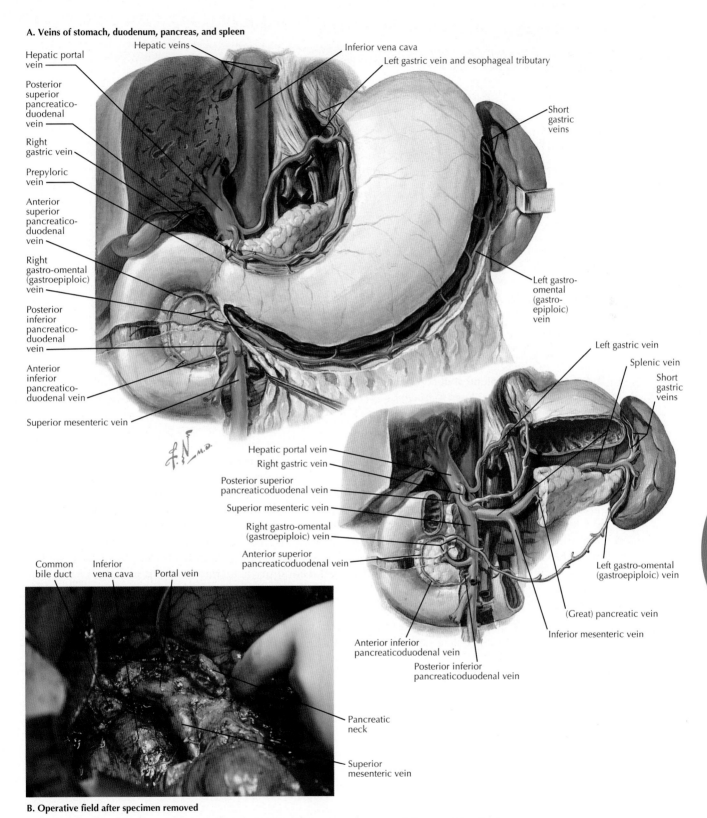

A. Veins of stomach, duodenum, pancreas, and spleen

Hepatic veins

Inferior vena cava

Left gastric vein and esophageal tributary

Hepatic portal vein

Posterior superior pancreatico-duodenal vein

Right gastric vein

Prepyloric vein

Anterior superior pancreatico-duodenal vein

Right gastro-omental (gastroepiploic) vein

Posterior inferior pancreatico-duodenal vein

Anterior inferior pancreatico-duodenal vein

Superior mesenteric vein

Short gastric veins

Left gastro-omental (gastro-epiploic) vein

Left gastric vein

Splenic vein

Short gastric veins

Hepatic portal vein

Right gastric vein

Posterior superior pancreaticoduodenal vein

Superior mesenteric vein

Right gastro-omental (gastroepiploic) vein

Anterior superior pancreaticoduodenal vein

Left gastro-omental (gastroepiploic) vein

(Great) pancreatic vein

Inferior mesenteric vein

Anterior inferior pancreaticoduodenal vein

Posterior inferior pancreaticoduodenal vein

Common bile duct

Inferior vena cava

Portal vein

Pancreatic neck

Superior mesenteric vein

B. Operative field after specimen removed

FIGURE 16.4 Venous anatomy and the resection bed.

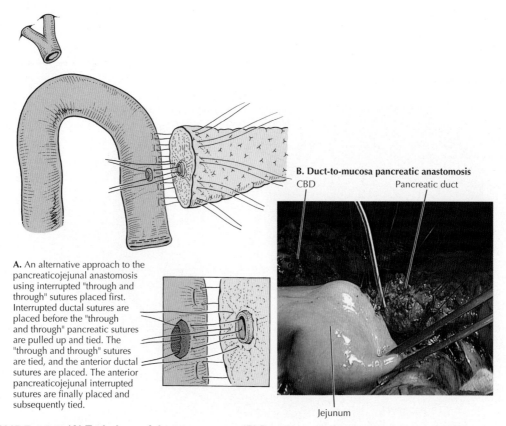

B. Duct-to-mucosa pancreatic anastomosis

CBD   Pancreatic duct

A. An alternative approach to the pancreaticojejunal anastomosis using interrupted "through and through" sutures placed first. Interrupted ductal sutures are placed before the "through and through" pancreatic sutures are pulled up and tied. The "through and through" sutures are tied, and the anterior ductal sutures are placed. The anterior pancreaticojejunal interrupted sutures are finally placed and subsequently tied.

Jejunum

FIGURE 16.5 (A) Technique of duct-to-mucosa. (B) Duct-to-mucosa pancreatic anastomosis.

CBD, Common bile duct. *(A, Reused with permission from Blumgart LH, Corvera CU. Pancreatic and periampullary resection. In Blumgart LH, ed.* Video Atlas: Liver Biliary and Pancreatic Surgery. *Philadelphia: Elsevier; 2010:162–180, Figure 10-13.)*

The resection may be approached by performing a clockwise dissection—that is, initial dissection in the lesser sac and identification of the SMV followed by dissection of the hepatoduodenal ligament followed by transection of the jejunum and dissection of the ligament of Treitz, and finally transection of the pancreatic neck and dissection of the uncinate process. When the hybrid approach is used, the robot is docked for assistance of the reconstruction. An intraoperative ultrasound may be added to compensate for the lack of tactile feedback, especially with the robotic approach, to assess resectability and identify vasculature and variant anatomy. The principles and steps of the procedure are akin to the open technique (a narrated video is included).

SUGGESTED READINGS

Callery MP, Pratt WB, Kent TS, Chaikof EL, Vollmer Jr CM. A prospectively validated clinical risk score accurately predicts pancreatic fistula after pancreatoduodenectomy. J Am Coll Surg 2013;216(1):1–14.

Cameron JL. Rapid exposure of the portal and superior mesenteric veins. Surg Gynecol Obstet 1993;176:395.

Cameron JL, He J. Two thousand consecutive pancreatoduodenectomies. J Am Coll Surg 2015;220(4):530–6.

Giulianotti PC, et al. Operative technique in robotic pancreatoduodenectomy (RPD) at University of Illinois at Chicago (UIC): 17 steps standardized technique. Surg Endosc 2018;32(10):4329–36.

Kausch W. Das carinom de papilla duodeni und seine radikale entfernung. Beltrage sur Klinischen Cirurgie 1912;78:439.

Whipple AO, Parsons WB, Mullins CR. Treatment of carcinoma of the ampulla of vater. Ann Surg 1935;102:763.

Yeo CJ, Cameron JL, Lillemoe KD, et al. Pancreatoduodenectomy with or without distal gastrectomy and extended retroperitoneal lymphadenectomy for periampullary adenocarcinoma. Part 2. Randomized controlled trial evaluating survival, morbidity, and mortality. Ann Surg 2002;236:355.

Splenectomy

Steven Rosenblatt and Robert Naples

▶ VIDEO

17.1 Laparoscopic Splenectomy

INTRODUCTION

The spleen is one of the most commonly injured organs associated with blunt abdominal trauma. Therefore it is not surprising that previously the most common indication for splenectomy was motor vehicle accidents. However, removal of the spleen is not without consequence, as overwhelming post-splenectomy sepsis contributed to increased mortality. Such concerns led to the development of splenic salvage procedures to preserve the immunologic function of the spleen. Because of advances in care-pathways and interventional radiology, most splenic trauma is treated nonoperatively with observation or embolization, and removal of the spleen is now most frequently indicated for patients with benign or malignant hematologic disorders who are not responding to medical therapy. The most common such conditions include immune thrombocytopenic purpura (ITP), autoimmune hemolytic anemia, hereditary spherocytosis, and splenomegaly, in which there is concern for an underlying hematologic malignancy. Other hematologic disorders, such as thrombotic thrombocytopenic purpura (TTP), symptomatic thalassemia, and Felty syndrome, may also require splenectomy. Although still required in some cases, open splenectomy has decreased in favor of minimally invasive approaches, which have been found to safely and effectively reduce pain, hospital stay, and complications.

ANATOMY

A thorough understanding of the anatomy of and surrounding the spleen is crucial for splenectomy (Fig. 17.1). The spleen can vary in size, depending on the underlying pathology. A normal spleen is typically less than 11 cm and weighs between 150 and 200 g; splenomegaly is diagnosed when the weight is greater than 1 kg. Accessory spleens are a common abnormality and occur in approximately 20% of patients. These are usually about 1 cm in size and are most commonly located at the splenic hilum. More than one accessory spleen can be present in a minority of patients. The surgeon must be aware of this because accessory spleens can be missed more commonly with laparoscopy than with an open procedure. Failure to identify an accessory spleen can lead to persistent disease, depending on the diagnosis.

The spleen is located in the left upper quadrant, adjacent to the greater curvature of the stomach, the tail of the pancreas, the left kidney, and the splenic flexure of the colon. Superiorly and laterally, it is bounded by the diaphragm, separating it from the thoracic cavity, and anteriorly it is protected by the ninth through eleventh ribs. The organ is suspended in place by the splenorenal, gastrosplenic, splenocolic, and splenophrenic ligaments. The splenorenal and splenogastric ligaments contain the vascular supply of the spleen, consisting of the splenic and short gastric vessels, respectively. The splenorenal ligament also contains the tail of the pancreas, the only intraperitoneal portion of this organ, which has been found to touch the splenic hilum in approximately 30% of patients and must be protected during splenectomy to prevent a pancreatic fistula.

The vascular supply of the spleen arises from the splenic and short gastric vessels. The splenic artery is a branch of the celiac trunk and travels along the superior border of the pancreas. There is significant variability of this blood supply and there are two main variations. In the distributed type, the artery has a short trunk and separates into multiple branches distal to the splenic hilum. In contrast, the magistral type has a long trunk and divides into multiple branches within 2 cm of the hilum. Normally, there is also a superior polar and an inferior polar artery that arise from the splenic artery. The short gastric arteries originate from the terminal splenic artery, as does the left gastroepiploic artery, and these supply the fundus of the stomach along its greater curvature. The vessels are short in length, variable in number, and course through the gastrosplenic ligament to the gastric fundus. These vessels potentially provide enough blood flow to the spleen independent of the splenic artery. The splenic vein is formed by segmental venous branches from the trabeculae at the hilum. These vessels travels posterior to the superior border of the pancreas to join with the superior mesenteric vein to form the portal vein. The inferior mesenteric vein usually drains into the splenic vein (Fig. 17.2A).

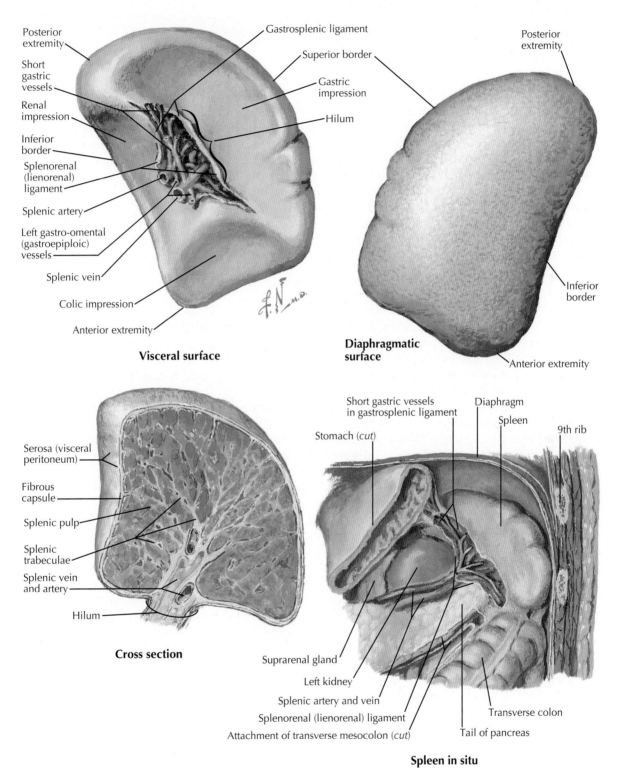

Visceral surface

Posterior extremity
Short gastric vessels
Renal impression
Inferior border
Splenorenal (lienorenal) ligament
Splenic artery
Left gastro-omental (gastroepiploic) vessels
Splenic vein
Colic impression
Anterior extremity

Gastrosplenic ligament
Superior border
Gastric impression
Hilum

Diaphragmatic surface

Posterior extremity
Inferior border
Anterior extremity

Cross section

Serosa (visceral peritoneum)
Fibrous capsule
Splenic pulp
Splenic trabeculae
Splenic vein and artery
Hilum

Spleen in situ

Short gastric vessels in gastrosplenic ligament
Diaphragm
Spleen
9th rib
Stomach (*cut*)
Suprarenal gland
Left kidney
Splenic artery and vein
Splenorenal (lienorenal) ligament
Attachment of transverse mesocolon (*cut*)
Tail of pancreas
Transverse colon

FIGURE 17.1 Spleen and surrounding structures.

SURGICAL PRINCIPLES

Preoperative radiologic imaging can be useful to evaluate the size of the spleen. Normally, before referral to a surgeon for splenectomy, most patients have either undergone an ultrasound or a liver-spleen scan, if not both. In the absence of splenomegaly, such studies do not add much to preoperative planning. However, in a patient with an enlarged spleen, a CT scan can be very helpful to choose the optimal approach (Fig. 17.2B), because the planned technique usually is determined by the size of the spleen, as well as any prior surgery and other medical comorbidities. The laparoscopic approach is optimal for most patients, except those with massive splenomegaly. With large spleens, the hand-assist or open approach is most appropriate. Immunizations for the encapsulated organisms, meningococcus, pneumococcus, and *Haemophilus influenzae* are administered 2 weeks preoperatively to minimize the risk for post-splenectomy sepsis.

LAPAROSCOPIC SURGICAL TECHNIQUE

The patient is placed in a right lateral decubitus position, appropriately secured with a beanbag, and all pressure points are padded. The space between the costal margin and iliac crest is placed at the level of the kidney rest, and the bed is maximally flexed to open this space. Four subcostal ports are used. The first 5-mm port is placed using the 0-degree 5-mm laparoscope and an optical trocar, although an open direct cutdown may be used. The distance of this port from the rib cage depends on the size of the spleen and the body habitus of the patient, because this trocar as well as the others can be placed well away from the costal margin. The camera is then switched over to a 30-degree 5-mm scope. Two further 5-mm trocars are placed a handbreadth away from the initial port. Often the splenocolic ligament must be mobilized to place the fourth trocar. Care must be taken to avoid thermal injury to the splenic flexure of the colon. The use of a 5-mm camera allows continuous change of view, depending on the stage of the procedure.

Initially, a search for accessory spleens is undertaken. After the patient is carefully secured to the operative table, the bed can be rotated and placed into Trendelenburg and reverse Trendelenburg position as needed throughout the case to allow gravity and the weight of the spleen to optimize exposure. Using the energy source, any lateral splenophrenic attachments are taken down, which allows for retraction of the spleen medially and exposure of the splenorenal ligament, which is then incised. Dissection is continued cephalad until the superior pole of the spleen is freed up and the fundus of the stomach is exposed. Attention is then turned to the inferior pole and the spleno-omental attachments are taken down, and any small inferior pole vessels can be controlled with the energy source or clips. The spleen is then retracted laterally with one grasper while another grasper lifts the greater curvature of the stomach, which allows for optimal visualization of the gastrosplenic ligament. The lesser sac is entered, and the intervening short gastric vessels are controlled with the energy source. Care must be maintained to avoid injury to the greater curvature of the stomach or bleeding from the short gastric vessels, because such bleeding may be difficult to control. At this point, the hilum of the spleen is carefully dissected to optimize exposure. Visualization and avoidance of the tail of the pancreas, which abuts the spleen in approximately 30% of all patients, is crucial to avoid a pancreatic leak postoperatively. Although clips are a very reasonable option for the hilar vessels, most use a vascular stapler, which requires upsizing one of the existing ports to a larger trocar. The position of this larger port location depends on anatomy, spleen size, and body habitus.

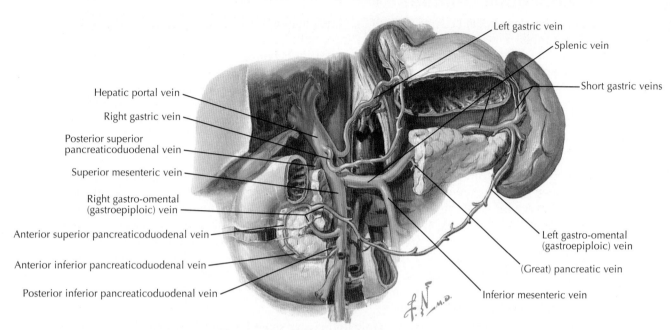

Left gastric vein

Splenic vein

Short gastric veins

Hepatic portal vein

Right gastric vein

Posterior superior pancreaticoduodenal vein

Superior mesenteric vein

Right gastro-omental (gastroepiploic) vein

Anterior superior pancreaticoduodenal vein

Anterior inferior pancreaticoduodenal vein

Posterior inferior pancreaticoduodenal vein

Left gastro-omental (gastroepiploic) vein

(Great) pancreatic vein

Inferior mesenteric vein

A. Venous drainage of spleen showing connection with the inferior mesenteric vein

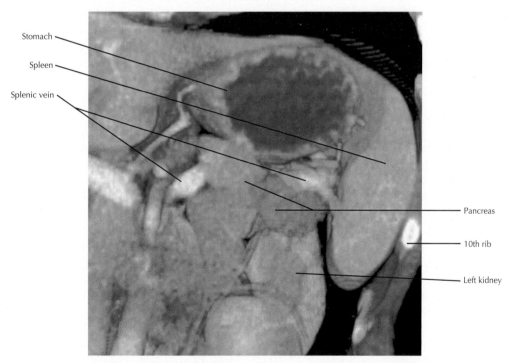

Stomach

Spleen

Splenic vein

Pancreas

10th rib

Left kidney

B. Radiologic imaging can be used to estimate size of the spleen (spleen shown not enlarged)

FIGURE 17.2 Venous anatomy and the resection bed in splenectomy.

(*B, From Weber EC, Vilensky JA, Carmichael JW. Netter's Radiologic Anatomy. Philadelphia: Elsevier; 2008.*)

LAPAROSCOPIC SURGICAL TECHNIQUE (Continued)

The fascial incision should be large enough that one's full forefinger can be placed into the abdomen for eventual morcellation. After the hilum is controlled, a large specimen bag is placed into the abdomen, and the spleen is placed within. The drawstring is brought out through the larger trocar. Using finger fracture and ring forceps, the specimen is removed and sent fresh to pathology. The abdomen is carefully inspected, paying particular attention to the staple line for hemostasis, as well as the greater curvature of the stomach and the controlled short gastric vessels and the transverse and splenic flexure of the colon for any potential injuries. Drains are not routinely used.

HAND-ASSISTED APPROACH

Hand-assisted laparoscopic splenectomy is a very reasonable and useful alternative to the traditional open or laparoscopic approaches. A limited midline incision and special port allows the surgeon to place his or her nondominant hand into the abdomen. Combining the advantages of laparoscopy and open surgery, this technique allows for the tactile sensation, which is not associated with laparoscopy, as well as optimization of exposure and retraction, particularly with large spleens. The technical steps are similar to those described above with the exception that a larger specimen bag is usually necessary.

OPEN APPROACH

At present, the open approach is used mainly for massive splenomegaly, in which exposure and retraction just cannot be obtained with laparoscopy. This technique may also be more appropriate in patients with more complex surgical histories, in which there may exist significant scarring of the left upper quadrant. The steps in laparoscopic splenectomy are truly based on the tenets of the open approach, for which either a midline or left subcostal incision is created with the patient in the supine position. The incision should be large enough to facilitate identification of the surrounding anatomy and to allow for the removal of the spleen.

POSTOPERATIVE CONSIDERATIONS

The potential for splenic vein thrombosis, which can propagate to the portal vein, should be considered in any patient who develops significant postoperative abdominal pain that is not thought to be related to the expected postoperative course. Scheduled postoperative immunizations are given 8 weeks after the operation, and these patients should be counseled about the importance of keeping all scheduled adult immunizations up to date. Last, all such patients should be aware that they should obtain immediate medical attention for any illness characterized by a high fever because of their splenectomized state.

SUGGESTED READINGS

Ahad S, Gonczy C, Advani V, et al. True benefit or selection bias: an analysis of laparoscopic versus open splenectomy from the ACS-NSQIP. Surg Endosc 2013;27(6):1865–71.

Feldman LS. Laparoscopic splenectomy: a standardized approach. Worl J Surg 2011;35(7):1487–95.

Habermalz B, Sauerland S, Decker G, et al. Laparoscopic splenectomy: the clinical practice guidelines of the European Association for Endoscopic Surgery (EAES). Surg Endosc 2008;22(4):821–48.

Iolascon A, Andolfo I, Barcellini W, et al. Recommendations regarding splenectomy in hereditary hemolytic anemias. Haematologica 2017;102(8):1304–13.

McClusky 3rd DA, Skandalakis LJ, Colborn GL, et al. Tribute to a triad: history of splenic anatomy, physiology, and surgery—part 1. World J Surg 1999;23(3):311–25.

Pietrabissa A, Morelli L, Peri A, et al. Laparoscopic treatment of splenomegaly: a case for hand-assisted laparoscopic surgery. Arch Surg 2011;146(7):818–23.

Stassen NA, Bhullar I, Cheng JD, et al. Selective nonoperative management of blunt splenic injury: an eastern association for the surgery of trauma practice management guideline. J Trauma Acute Care Surg 2012;73(5 Suppl. 4):S294–300.

Winslow ER, Brunt LM. Perioperative outcomes of laparoscopic versus open splenectomy: a meta-analysis with an emphasis on complications. Surgery 2003;134(4):647–53.

Organ Transplantation

SECTION EDITOR: Christopher T. Siegel

Liver Transplantation

Giuseppe D'Amico, Cristiano Quintini, and Bijan Eghtesad

INTRODUCTION

Orthotopic liver transplantation (LTX) has become an accepted means for the treatment of end-stage liver disease. Although the technique of LTX has been refined to a relatively standardized approach, the operation remains a formidable surgical challenge. As such, LTX can have numerous technical complications, which can be influenced by recipient pretransplant condition, donor characteristics, and immunologic factors. These risks can be minimized by appropriate ABO matching, donor/recipient size matching, adequate maintenance of donor physiology, graft quality, and procurement technique. LTX today is performed principally with two different techniques: the classic technique with vena cava interposition and the piggyback technique that leaves the native vena cava in situ.

HEPATECTOMY

The "standard incision" for LTX has historically been a bilateral subcostal incision with an upper midline extension to the xiphoid (sometimes called an inverted Y or Mercedes incision) (Fig. 18.1A). Dissection of the hilum of the liver is probably the most important part of the hepatectomy. The essential goal in the hepatectomy is preservation of all the hilar structures, especially the hepatic artery and the portal vein, which will be used to revascularize the liver allograft (Fig. 18.1B). The falciform ligament is divided to the suprahepatic vena cava, and the left triangular ligament is then opened with cautery (Fig. 18.1C and D). The left lateral segment is then retracted up out of the wound and to the right. The gastrohepatic ligament is visualized and requires either cautery division or suture ligation, depending on the extent of the collateral vessels (Fig. 18.1E). If an accessory left hepatic artery is present, it must be ligated and divided. The approach to the hilum can commence either from the right side with dissection of the cystic duct and common bile duct or from the left with dissection of the hepatic artery. The essential issue in either approach is to work close to the hilar plate and to try to preserve as much length of each structure as possible. This approach allows for maximum flexibility for reconstruction at implantation. It is good practice during the dissection of the cystic duct and common bile duct to preserve the surrounding soft tissue so as not to cause damage to the bile duct blood supply. This is important to prevent postoperative bile duct ischemia, necrosis, or stricture formation. The portal vein dissection is usually done after division of the hepatic artery and the bile duct. All the soft tissue around the portal vein should be dissected and removed from the hilar plate to the level of head of the pancreas. The dissection of the right triangular ligament is performed completely with cautery, beginning at the lateral inferior aspect and dividing the ligament carefully to the vena cava (Fig. 18.1F). In cases in which there is an unusual amount of collateral vessels, scarring, or inflammation, this part of the procedure is deferred until after the patient is placed on total venovenous bypass. The right adrenal vein is ligated and divided. At this time, the right lobe is left to fall back into the hepatic fossa, and the left side of the vena cava is exposed by retracting the left lateral segment and the caudate lobe to the right. The peritoneal reflection is opened longitudinally along the vena cava with cautery.

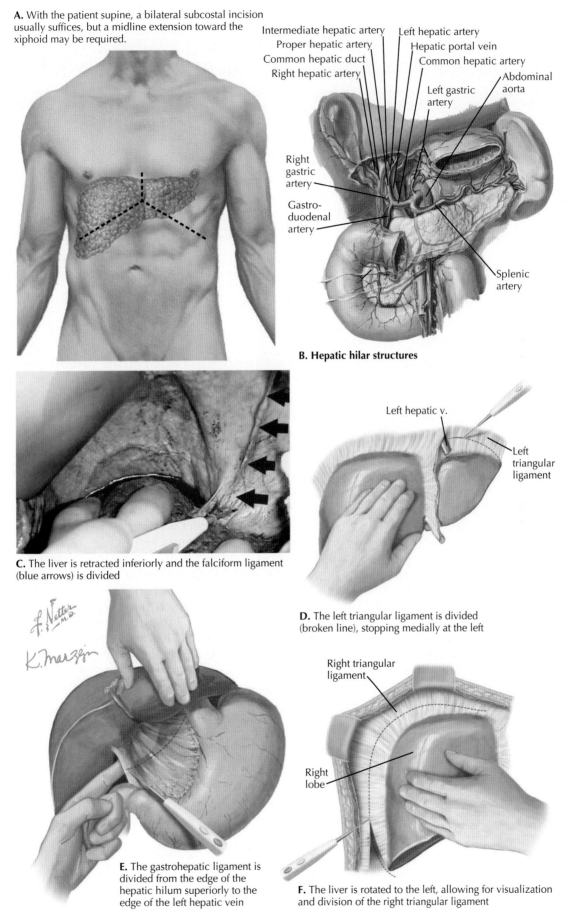

A. With the patient supine, a bilateral subcostal incision usually suffices, but a midline extension toward the xiphoid may be required.

B. Hepatic hilar structures

Intermediate hepatic artery
Proper hepatic artery
Common hepatic duct
Right hepatic artery
Left hepatic artery
Hepatic portal vein
Common hepatic artery
Left gastric artery
Abdominal aorta
Right gastric artery
Gastro-duodenal artery
Splenic artery

C. The liver is retracted inferiorly and the falciform ligament (blue arrows) is divided

Left hepatic v.
Left triangular ligament

D. The left triangular ligament is divided (broken line), stopping medially at the left

Right triangular ligament
Right lobe

E. The gastrohepatic ligament is divided from the edge of the hepatic hilum superiorly to the edge of the left hepatic vein

F. The liver is rotated to the left, allowing for visualization and division of the right triangular ligament

FIGURE 18.1 Hepatectomy.

IMPLANTATION

Orthotopic Liver Transplant (OLT): Standard Technique With and Without Venous-Venous Bypass

At this juncture the patient is prepared for venovenous bypass by cannulation of the femoral vein. Cannulation is performed via the Seldinger technique or by an open cut down in the groin.

The return cannula is inserted by the anesthesia team into the right internal jugular vein. An alternative option is to cut down directly on the axillary vein for cannula placement. Once the cannulas have been introduced and secured, the final dissection of the portal vein is performed. To safely place the portal vein cannula, the portal vein skeletonization is first maximized to obtain the longest possible vessel trunk. A surgical clamp is applied distally to the portal vein at the bifurcation or higher, while the proximal end of the vessel is clamped between fingers. The portal vein is divided as close as possible to the clamp in the porta hepatis (Fig. 18.2A). The wire-reinforced cannula is then inserted and secured in place (Fig. 18.2B). Vascular clamps are now placed on the suprahepatic vena cava and the lower infrahepatic vena cava. The surgeon divides the upper vena cava while taking care to retain as much of the right, middle, and left hepatic veins as possible (Fig. 18.2C). The lower vena cava is then divided, leaving as much inferior vena cava (IVC) as possible. The suprahepatic vena cava is now prepared by opening the right, middle, and left hepatic veins into a common cloaca with the IVC. Corner stitches are placed on the two opposing ends, and a stay suture may be placed in the middle for retraction of the posterior wall (Fig. 18.2D and E).

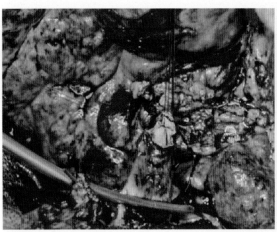

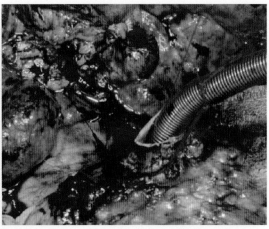

A. To prepare for portal bypass, the portal vein (broken blue line) is clamped proximally and divided as far distally as possible

B. A cannula is placed into the portal vein (PV); a heavy silk tie secures the cannula to the vein

C. Clamps are placed on the suprahepatic and infrahepatic IVC; these structures are divided and the liver is removed

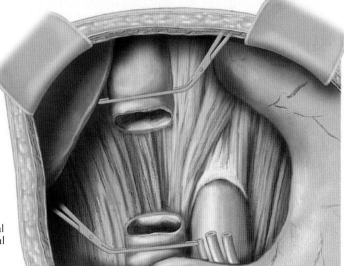

D. The back wall of the suprahepatic caval anastomosis is sutured first, using a vertical mattress technique, followed by an "over and over" stitch for the anterior wall

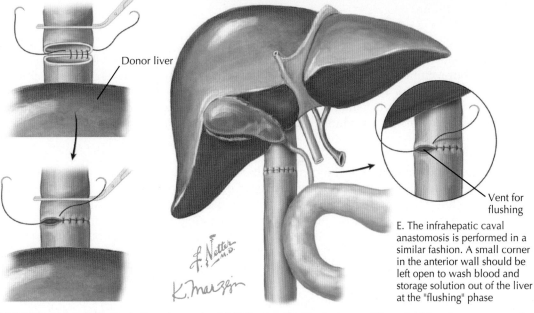

Donor liver

Vent for flushing

E. The infrahepatic caval anastomosis is performed in a similar fashion. A small corner in the anterior wall should be left open to wash blood and storage solution out of the liver at the "flushing" phase

FIGURE 18.2 Orthotopic liver transplant (OLT): standard technique with and without venovenous bypass.

IVC, Inferior vena cava.

Piggyback Technique

The piggyback technique is identical to the standard technique until after the skeletonization of the hepatic hilum is complete. Subsequently, the liver is dissected from the IVC. The accessory hepatic veins are divided. The right hepatic vein is isolated and clamped proximally with a pediatric angled Potts clamp. It is subsequently divided. A German clamp is applied at the common trunk of the left and middle hepatic veins anterior to the vena cava, and the liver is removed from the surgical field. The right, middle, and left hepatic veins are divided as far into the liver as possible. The hepatic veins (right, middle, and left) are usually connected into a common cloaca (Fig. 18.3A). The anastomosis between the recipient hepatic venous cuff and the donor suprahepatic IVC is completed in an end-to-end fashion (Fig. 18.3B). Subsequently, the allograft infrahepatic IVC is ligated or stapled.

Portal Vein

If venovenous bypass is used, the portal bypass cannula is now clamped, and only the systemic venovenous bypass is continued. The cannula is removed from the portal vein, and an atraumatic clamp is carefully placed proximally on the portal vein. In preparation for the portal vein anastomosis, a wet lap sponge is placed between the right hemidiaphragm and the dome of the liver. The right arm of the rib-grip retractor is lowered. The combination of these two maneuvers shortens the distance between the donor and recipient's portal vein stumps. This prevents the possibility of vascular complications from a long portal vein. The portal vein anastomosis is completed end-to-end with running sutures. When the running suture is tied, a generous growth factor is left behind so that the anastomosis can expand at reperfusion and stenosis can be prevented (Fig. 18.3C). There are several methods to reperfuse the liver after portal venous reconstruction: (1) reperfusion through the portal vein with or without vena cava venting, (2) opening of the IVC followed by portal vein reperfusion, and (3) reperfusion through the portal vein and hepatic artery simultaneously. Venting through the intrahepatic IVC with 250 to 400 mL of portal vein blood does ensure washout of the high K+-containing preservation solution.

Hepatic Artery

Successful hepatic artery reconstruction is crucial for graft function, and a variety of methods can be used. In routine cases, a Carrel patch of donor aorta, donor celiac artery, or a branch patch between the donor splenic artery and common hepatic artery is created. This is anastomosed end to end to the recipient common hepatic artery or to a branch patch of the bifurcation between the recipient gastroduodenal and the proper hepatic artery (Fig. 18.3D).

Bile Duct

After the gallbladder is removed, the common duct is shortened proximal to the cystic duct. Usually a lap sponge is placed superior to the liver to better approximate the donor and recipient bile ducts. It is important to prevent redundancy of the bile duct because this can cause biliary obstruction in the postoperative period. The donor cystic duct, if left to preserve common duct length, has to empty freely into the remaining common duct to prevent the development of a mucocele. Mucoceles can compress the duct and cause biliary obstruction. The stump of the donor bile duct is trimmed until arterial bleeding is noted from the edge of the duct. The recipient's duct is opened, explored, and trimmed. The biliary anastomosis is completed with interrupted or running absorbable suture (Fig. 18.3E).

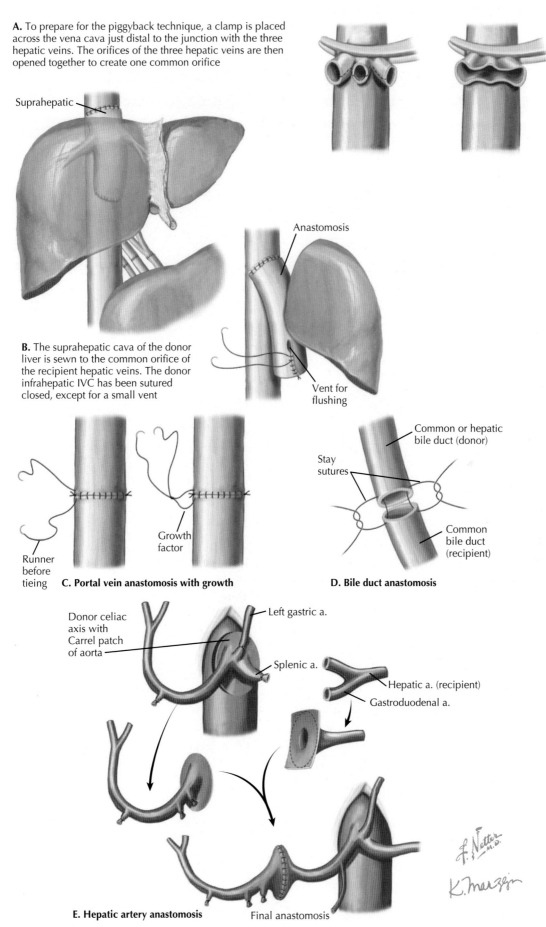

A. To prepare for the piggyback technique, a clamp is placed across the vena cava just distal to the junction with the three hepatic veins. The orifices of the three hepatic veins are then opened together to create one common orifice

Suprahepatic

Anastomosis

B. The suprahepatic cava of the donor liver is sewn to the common orifice of the recipient hepatic veins. The donor infrahepatic IVC has been sutured closed, except for a small vent

Vent for flushing

Growth factor

Runner before tieing

C. Portal vein anastomosis with growth

Common or hepatic bile duct (donor)

Stay sutures

Common bile duct (recipient)

D. Bile duct anastomosis

Donor celiac axis with Carrel patch of aorta

Left gastric a.

Splenic a.

Hepatic a. (recipient)

Gastroduodenal a.

E. Hepatic artery anastomosis

Final anastomosis

FIGURE 18.3 Piggyback technique, portal vein, and hepatic artery.
IVC, Inferior vena cava.

SUGGESTED READINGS

Denmark SW, Shaw BW Jr, Starzl TE, et al. Veno-venous bypass without systemic anticoagulation in canine and human liver transplantation. Surg Forum 1983;34:380–82.

Duffy JP, Hong JC, Farmer DG, et al. Vascular complications of orthotopic liver transplantation: experience in more than 4,200 patients. J Am Coll Surg 2009;208(5):896–903.

Eghtesad B, Kadry Z, Fung J. Technical considerations in liver transplantation: what a hepatologist needs to know (and every surgeon should practice). Liver Transpl 2005;11(8):861–71.

Tzakis A, Todo S, Starzl TE. Orthotopic liver transplantation with preservation of the inferior vena cava. Ann Surg 1989;210(5):649–52.

Living Donor Liver Transplantation

Koji Hashimoto, Choon Hyuck David Kwon, Kazunari Sasaki, Charles Miller,
Keita Okubo, Cristiano Quintini, Teresa Diago-Uso, Masato Fujiki,
Christopher T. Siegel, Amit Nair, and Federico Aucejo

▶ VIDEOS

19.1 Laparoscopic Living Donor Right Hepatectomy
19.2 Open Living Donor Left Hepatectomy

INTRODUCTION

Living donor liver transplant (LDLT) has emerged and is now established as a valuable practice to mitigate the shortage of cadaveric liver grafts. Challenges relate to donor risk and recipient graft function. Preparation for surgery is the most important factor for a successful outcome. The preoperative information about anatomy, volume and function of the graft, and remnant donor liver, along with recipient clinical information, are critical for the optimal surgical strategy.

DONOR ASSESSMENT

Imaging and Liver Volume Calculation

Assessment of a live donor requires imaging studies to determine the liver volume and the vascular and biliary anatomy (Fig. 19.1). Computed tomography (CT) contrast-enhanced multiphasic scan and magnetic resonance image (MRI) are obtained to characterize the donor liver hepatic artery, portal vein, and hepatic vein anatomy. The imaging is also used to estimate the donor liver volume (Fig. 19.2A through D). Magnetic resonance cholangiopancreatography (MRCP) is obtained (Fig. 19.2E) to evaluate the biliary anatomy. MRI/MRCP and CT scan images are fused. At our institution, images are submitted to MeVis distant Services (Bremen, Germany) for volumetric and anatomic analysis. Using MeVis, total and segmental liver volumes are calculated (Fig. 19.3 and 19.4).

Right and left graft volumes/weights are obtained according to the desired transection line and inclusion or exclusion of the middle hepatic vein (see Figs. 19.3B and 19.4C). The left lateral segment and subsegmental volumes are calculated when performing pediatric transplants.

Vascular and biliary anatomy is reconstructed three-dimensionally. Vascular structures and the corresponding territories are color coded, providing visual and quantitative (volume) representation of the liver segments (see Figs. 19.3B and 19.4C).

Assessment of post-transplant venous congestion is crucial when using right lobe grafts. Right lobe grafts (most commonly used in adult-to-adult LDLT) share the venous drainage of the anterior segments (5 and 8) with the left lobe (segment 4a and 4b) through the middle hepatic vein (MHV). Based on imaging, a decision is made to include or exclude the outflow vein from the right lobe graft. In our practice, the MHV is routinely excluded from the right lobe graft for donor safety. The three-dimensional imaging is very important in determining whether segments 5 and 8 veins are reconstructed to avoid graft congestion. Poor graft outflow and portal venous hypertension can be associated with impaired regeneration and small-for-size syndrome.

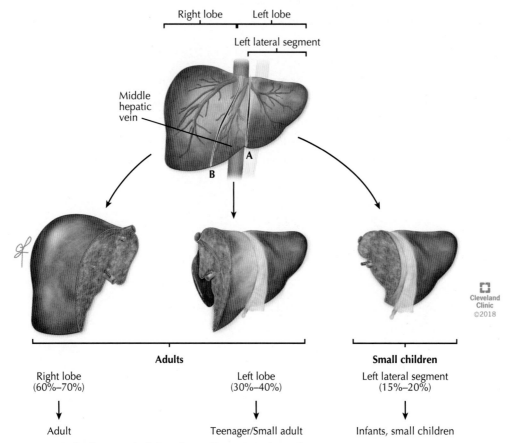

FIGURE 19.1 Graft types in living donor liver transplantation.

(Reprinted with permission, Cleveland Clinic Center for Medical Art & Photography © 2018-2019. All Rights Reserved)

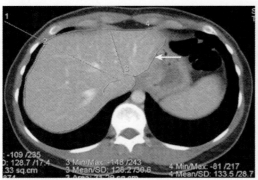

A. CT displaying liver volumes. Left lateral segment (arrow)

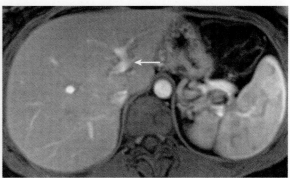

B. MRI showing left portal vein (arrow)

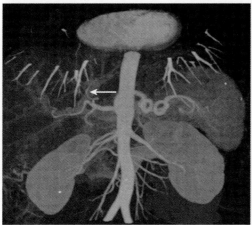

C. Tridimensional reconstruction of hepatic arterial anatomy. Arrow pointing at left hepatic artery

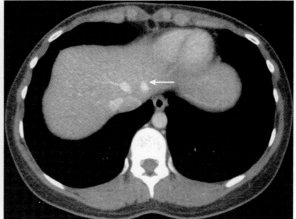

D. Hepatic veins. Arrow pointing at left hepatic vein

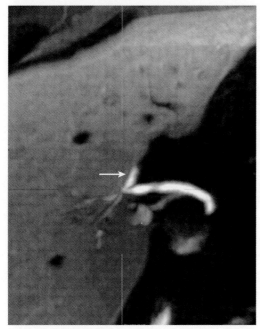

E. MRCP showing biliary anatomy. Trifurcation of right anterior, right posterior and left hepatic ducts. Arrow pointing at left hepatic duct

FIGURE 19.2 **Left lateral segment graft.**

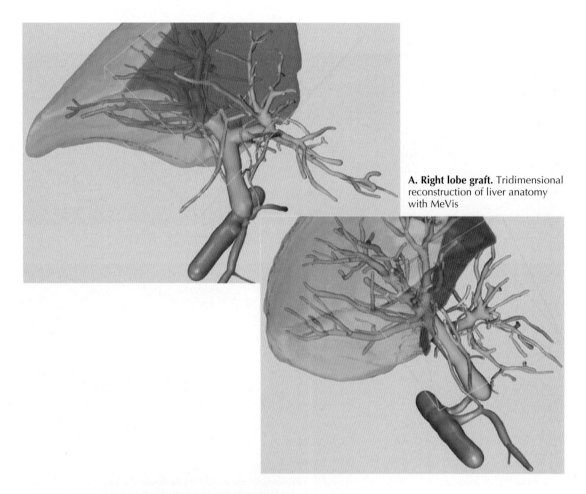

A. Right lobe graft. Tridimensional reconstruction of liver anatomy with MeVis

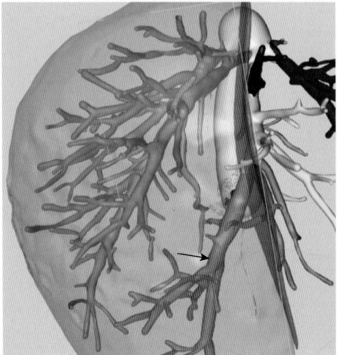

Plane 1, Right lobe graft without MHV
Plane 1, Right lobe graft without MHV, HV territories in graft (volumes)

	Territory	Volume	Relative (%)
	HV1	3 ml	< 1.0
	inf.HV	8 ml	< 1.0
	MV4a	1 ml	< 1.0
	MV4a_4b_8	11 ml	1.1
	MV4a_8	10 ml	1.0
	MV4b_5_8	213 ml	21.7
	MV4bs	2 ml	< 1.0
	MV8p	5 ml	< 1.0
	MV8s	266 ml	27.1
	RHV	463 ml	47.1
	Total	**982 ml**	**100**

Minimal deviations can be caused by rounding errors.

B. Right lobe graft. Hepatic vein anatomy. Segment 5 vein (arrow). Table shows volume estimates of territories drained by veins of medial segments.

FIGURE 19.3 **Right lobe graft (reconstructions using MeVis software).**

MHV, Middle hepatic vein; *RHV,* right hepatic vein.

(MeVis Distant Services, MeVis Medical Solutions AG, Bremen, Germany.)

A. Left lobe graft. Tridimensional reconstruction of liver anatomy with MeVis. Hepatic artery anatomy in orange, portal vein anatomy in blue, and biliary anatomy in green.

B. Hepatic vein anatomy. MeVis reconstruction.

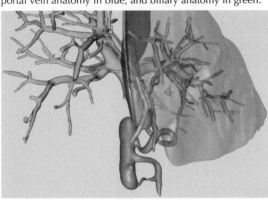

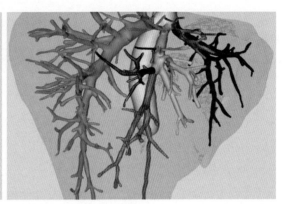

C. MeVis volume calculation of left lobe graft, donor right lobe volume remnant, and graft recipient body weight ratio.

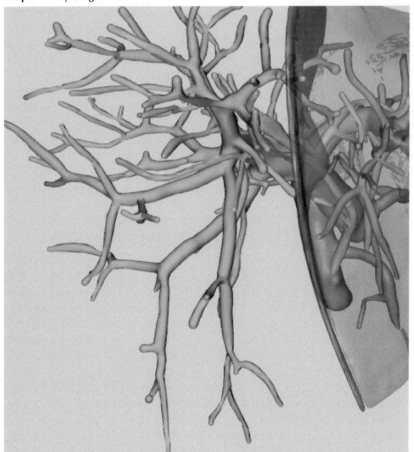

Plane 2, Left lobe graft with MHV

Plane 2, Left lobe graft with MHV (volumes)

	Territory	Volume	Relative (%)
	Plane	16 ml	1.0
	Graft	583 ml	35.7
	Remnant	1035 ml	63.3
	Total	**1634 ml**	**100**

The estimated graft weight is about 531 g.

Key figures

Ratio	Based on	Value
Graft Recipient Body Weight Ratio	Estimated Graft Weight	0.79
Graft Recipient Body Weight Ratio	Graft Volume	0.87
Graft to SLV Ratio	Estimated Graft Weight	0.44
Graft to SLV Ratio	Graft Volume	0.48

Minimal deviations can be caused by rounding errors.

FIGURE 19.4 **Left lobe graft and hepatic vein anatomy (reconstructions using MeVis software).**
SLV, Standard liver volume.
(MeVis Distant Services, MeVis Medical Solutions AG, Bremen, Germany.)

TECHNICAL ASPECTS OF SURGERY

Minimal blood loss during parenchymal transection is fundamental. To that end, low central venous pressure along with meticulous dissection are required. Different energy devices can be used; however, ultrasonic dissector may be preferred to allow for fine dissection and minimal blood loss (Fig. 19.5A, B, and C).

Intraoperative liver ultrasound to find the trajectory of the middle hepatic vein and localization of segments 5 and 8 veins is performed. Additionally, clamping of inflow to the lobe induces ischemic demarcation to guide marking the line of parenchymal transection (Fig. 19.5C).

When a right lobe graft is procured, reconstruction of middle segments veins 5 and 8 should be performed to avoid congestion. Similarly, venoplasty of the right hepatic vein should be considered to improve the outflow (Fig. 19.5D).

When a left lobe graft is procured, the caudate lobe is preferably included. Fig. 19.6A shows a dissected left hepatic artery and left portal vein. Fig. 19.6B shows caudate lobe dissection off the vena cava to be included in the left lobe graft. Similarly to the right lobe graft, venoplasty of left lobe outflow is recommended to avoid graft congestion and outflow impairment (Fig. 19.6C and D).

Bile duct transection is a critical step of the operation. Intraoperative cholangiography is performed to display biliary anatomy and to localize the point of bile duct transection (Fig. 19.7).

GRAFT TYPE

There are essentially three types of grafts that can be used in LDLT: the left lateral segment (segments II and III), the left lobe (segments I through IV) with the middle hepatic vein, and the right lobe (segments V through VIII) without the middle hepatic vein (see Fig. 19.1). The left lateral segment graft is usually used for children. The left lobe graft is usually used for teenagers or small adults. The right lobe is the largest graft, accounting for 60% to 70% of the whole liver and is usually used for adults.

There are two important concepts to determine the type of grafts used in LDLT. The future liver remnant (FLR) is the proportion of remaining liver that will remain in the donor after the graft is surgically removed. An FLR of 30% to 35% is considered to be an acceptable lower limit to prevent postoperative liver failure in the donor. The graft-to-recipient body weight ratio (GRWR) is the ratio of graft weight to recipient body weight. The conservative lower limit of GRWR to avoid liver graft failure is considered to be 0.8%. In pediatric cases of recipient body weight less than 5 kg, a reduced left lateral segment graft is used to avoid large-for-size syndrome.

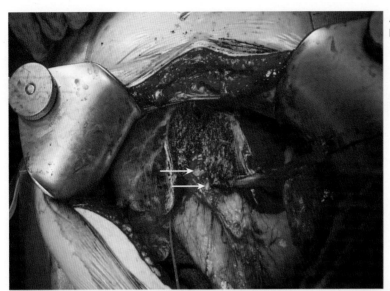

A. Split liver. Arrows pointing at left portal vein and left hepatic artery

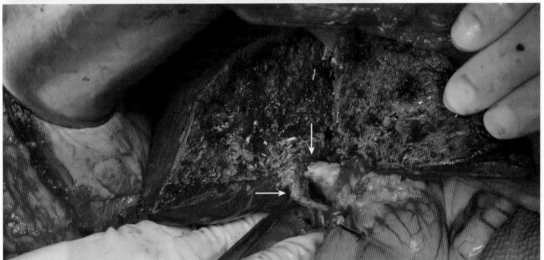

B. Right lobe graft. Right portal vein and right hepatic artery

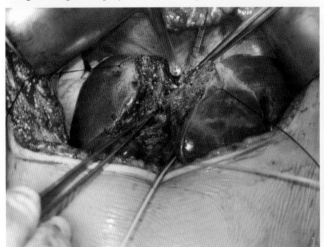

C. Forceps pointing at segments 5 and 8 veins

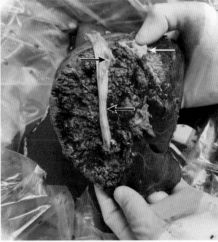

D. Right lobe graft. Reconstruction of segments 5 and 8 veins with cadaveric iliac vein graft during bench table (black arrows) to improve outflow and avoid congestion of segments 5 and 8. Right hepatic vein after venotomy and plasty with cadaveric vein patch to enlarge outflow orifice (white arrow).

FIGURE 19.5 Technical aspects of surgery.

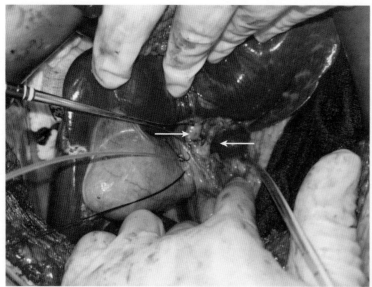

A. Hilar dissection. Left portal vein and left hepatic artery (arrows)

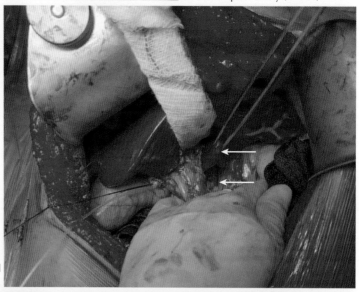

B. Caudate lobe mobilized from vena cava (arrows)

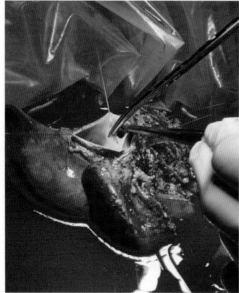

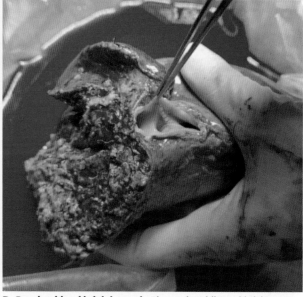

C. Bench table of left lobe graft. Plasty of middle and left hepatic veins to enhance graft outflow.

D. Bench table of left lobe graft. Plasty of middle and left hepatic veins completed.

FIGURE 19.6 **Technical aspects of surgery (continued).**

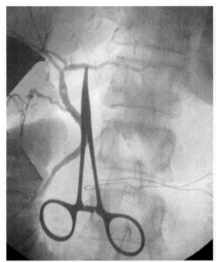

A. Intraoperative cholangiogram localizing the left hepatic duct before transection

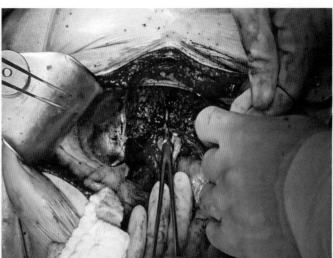

B. Transection of left hepatic duct

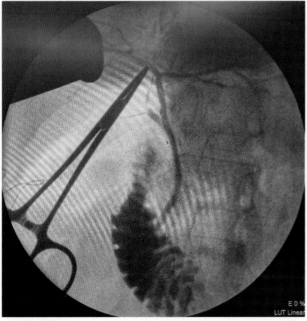

C. Intraoperative cholangiogram localizing the right hepatic duct before transection

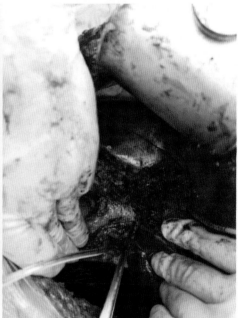

D. Forceps pointing at left hepatic duct

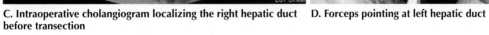

FIGURE 19.7 Technical aspects of surgery (continued).

RECIPIENT SURGICAL TECHNIQUE

There are several differences in performing a hepatectomy when comparing liver transplants from living donors and deceased donors. In LDLT, the donor vessels and bile duct are shorter and smaller than deceased donor liver transplant, so it is important to leave longer distal branches of the liver hilar structures including the hepatic artery, portal vein, and bile duct. Tissue dissection around the recipient bile duct should be minimized to avoid suboptimal vascular supply to the stump of the recipient bile duct. In LDLT, the recipient hepatectomy must be done as a piggyback transplant, leaving the native vena cava intact, because the living donor graft does not have vena cava.

For left lobe implantation, all three hepatic veins of the recipient are joined, similar to the piggyback implantation of a deceased donor liver transplant using a whole liver graft (Fig. 19.8A, B, and C). After the portal vein anastomosis, the graft liver is re-perfused. The hepatic artery anastomosis frequently requires a microsurgical technique because of its small size (2 to 3 mm). Generally, the left lobe graft has a single hepatic vein (the common channel of the left and middle hepatic veins), a single left portal vein, and a single left hepatic bile duct.

For right lobe implantation, the vena cava including the stump of the right hepatic vein is vertically clamped, and a caudal cavotomy is made to widen the venous anastomosis (Fig. 19.8D). Biliary reconstruction in LDLT is usually done with choledochocholedochostomy (duct-to-duct anastomosis). Generally the right lobe graft has multiple hepatic veins and hepatic ducts to be reconstructed.

In pediatric cases using the left lateral segment graft, venous outflow can be maximized by making a triangular vena caval orifice in the recipient (Fig. 19.8E). This technique was first described in 1988 but remains the gold standard of outflow venous reconstruction in pediatric partial grafting.

It is extremely important to optimize graft inflow and outflow to achieve good outcomes in LDLT. Graft congestion resulting from suboptimal venous outflow decreases functional graft size and causes graft failure because of small-for-size syndrome. Equally important is to actively control graft inflow. In size-mismatch LDLT, a small graft receives excessive portal flow, resulting in arterial spasm via a hepatic arterial buffer response. Splenic artery ligation is most frequently used as graft inflow modulation, but the effect of portal flow reduction is not always as much as expected. Splenectomy is more effective as inflow modulation but less frequently used because of the risk of blood loss, portal vein thrombosis, and post-splenectomy sepsis. A portosystemic shunt can also be used, but there is an increased risk of portal steal resulting in graft hypoperfusion.

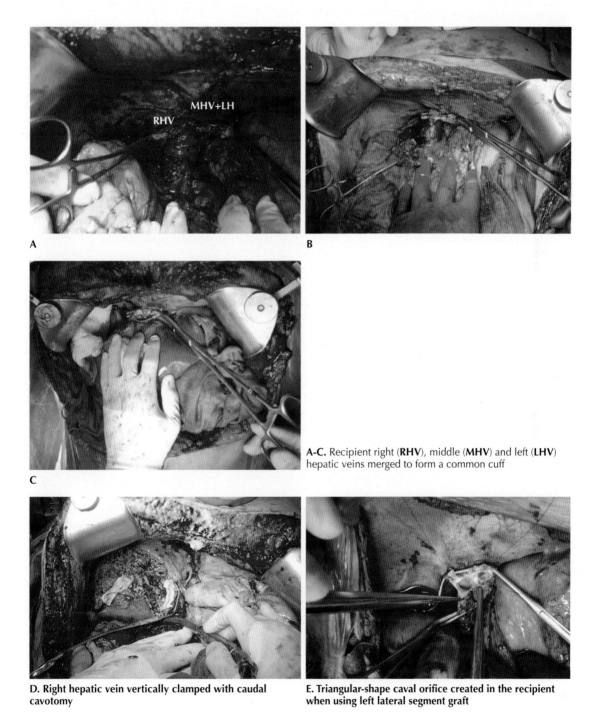

A-C. Recipient right (**RHV**), middle (**MHV**) and left (**LHV**) hepatic veins merged to form a common cuff

D. Right hepatic vein vertically clamped with caudal cavotomy

E. Triangular-shape caval orifice created in the recipient when using left lateral segment graft

FIGURE 19.8 **Recipient surgical technique.**

SUGGESTED READINGS

Akamatsu N, Sugawara Y, Kaneko J, Sano K, Imamura H, Kokudo N, et al. Effects of middle hepatic vein reconstruction on right liver graft regeneration. Transplantation 2003;76(5): 832–7.

Florman S, Miller CM. Live donor liver transplantation. Liver Transpl 2006;12(4):499–510.

Kelly DM, Demetris AJ, Fung JJ, Marcos A, Zhu Y, Subbotin V, et al. Porcine partial liver transplantation: a novel model of the "small-for-size" liver graft. Liver Transpl 2004;10(2): 253–63.

Lee S, Park K, Hwang S, Lee Y, Choi D, Kim K, et al. Congestion of right liver graft in living donor liver transplantation. Transplantation 2001;71(6):812–4.

Pomposelli JJ, Tongyoo A, Wald C, Pomfret EA. Variability of standard liver volume estimation versus software-assisted total liver volume measurement. Liver Transpl 2012;18(9):1083–92.

Quintini C, Aucejo F, Hashimoto K, Zein N, Miller C. State of the art and future developments for surgical planning in LDLT. Curr Transpl Rep 2014;1:35–42.

Roll GR, Parekh JR, Parker WF, Siegler M, Pomfret EA, Ascher NL, et al. Left hepatectomy versus right hepatectomy for living donor liver transplantation: shifting the risk from the donor to the recipient. Liver Transpl 2013; 19(5):472–81. *This review summarizes the most relevant aspects inherent to LDLT regarding the surgical risk for both donor and recipient according to the utilization of right lobe vs left lobe grafts.*

Shinohara H, Mizuno Y, Makino Y. Point of surgical techniques as seen from the anatomy of film—Illustrated surgery. April 6, 2010.

Tsang LL, Chen CL, Huang TL, Chen TY, Wang CC, Ou HY, et al. Preoperative imaging evaluation of potential living liver donors: reasons for exclusion from donation in adult living donor liver transplantation. Transplant Proc 2008;40(8):2460–2.

Yonemura Y, Taketomi A, Soejima Y, Yoshizumi T, Uchiyama H, Gion T, et al. Validity of preoperative volumetric analysis of congestion volume in living donor liver transplantation using three-dimensional computed tomography. Liver Transpl 2005;11(12):1556–62.

Intestinal and Multivisceral Transplantation

Masato Fujiki and Kareem Abu-Elmagd

▶ **VIDEOS**

20.1 Intestinal Graft Procurement
20.2 Multivisceral Transplantation

INTRODUCTION

All different types of visceral organ transplants containing small bowel can be categorized into three main prototypes: isolated intestinal, liver-intestinal, and multivisceral transplantations. The proper understanding of vascular anatomy is necessary to procure these different types of visceral allografts in donor surgery. Pancreas and intestinal allografts can be procured by dividing the superior mesenteric artery distal to the origin of the inferior pancreaticoduodenal artery. Division distal to the inferior pancreaticoduodenal artery is performed to maintain sufficient arterial flow to the head of the pancreas.

Recipient surgery is initiated with removal of the diseased native organs followed by vascular reconstruction and implantation of the new organs. Interposition arterial and venous grafts are commonly used for implantation of isolated intestinal allografts. In the case of a composite visceral graft (liver-intestine and multivisceral graft), both the celiac and superior mesenteric arteries are retrieved and constructed with donor aortic conduit. The venous outflow is established with portal or systemic drainage of the intestinal allograft and with hepatic venous reconstruction for composite visceral allografts. Foregut reconstruction is part of multivisceral transplantation. The residual native stomach or abdominal esophagus is anastomosed to the anterior wall of the allograft stomach with a pyloroplasty performed as a drainage procedure. With a liver-intestinal transplant, the very proximal allograft jejunum is anastomosed to the retained short segment of the native jejunum. Reconstruction of the hind gut is established with anastomosis to the recipient residual colorectal segment with creation of a chimney ileostomy or simple loop ileostomy.

NOMENCLATURE

Because of improved outcomes and increased practicality, visceral transplantation has been successfully used to treat patients with different varieties of irreversible gastrointestinal failure. All different types of en bloc, abdominal visceral organ transplants containing small bowel can be categorized into three main prototypes: isolated intestinal, liver-intestinal, and multivisceral.

Although the small intestine is the central core of a visceral allograft, the term *multivisceral* is distinctive nomenclature for stomach-containing visceral allografts. Among multivisceral transplants, "full" contains a liver allograft, whereas "modified" does not (Fig. 20.1). Secondary organs include colon and the pancreaticoduodenal complex with or without a spleen. The colon can be retained with any three types of visceral allografts.

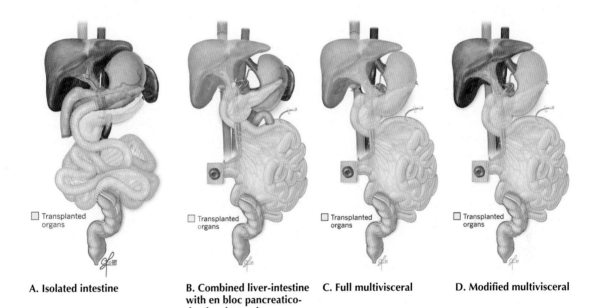

A. Isolated intestine

B. Combined liver-intestine
with en bloc pancreatico-
duodenal complex

C. Full multivisceral

D. Modified multivisceral

FIGURE 20.1 The different visceral allografts.

(Reprinted with permission, Cleveland Clinic Center for Medical Art & Photography © 2018–2019. All Rights Reserved.)

DONOR SURGERY

Isolated Intestinal Graft

Because of the increasing gap between organ donation and demand, organ procurement requires multiple-organ retrievals for separate recipients waiting for liver, pancreas, and intestinal allografts. A detailed understanding of vascular anatomy is necessary to procure pancreas and intestinal allografts from the same donor.

The proximal jejunum is transected at the ligament of Treitz after ligation and division of the inferior mesenteric vein. At this juncture, the intestine is attached to the donor only by the superior mesenteric vascular pedicle, containing the superior mesenteric artery (SMA) and vein (SMV) (Fig. 20.2A). These vessels are exposed by transversely dividing the anterior peritoneal sheath of the mesenteric root, distal to the level of the ligated middle colic vessels. When the pancreas is procured for a separate recipient, the inferior pancreaticoduodenal artery must be preserved for the pancreatic graft. The inferior pancreaticoduodenal artery originates just proximal to the origin of the middle colic artery (Video 20.1; Fig. 20.2A). Because the gastroduodenal artery is transected when donor liver grafts are procured, injury to the inferior pancreaticoduodenal artery will devascularize the head of the pancreas. To maintain sufficient arterial flow to the head of the pancreas, the SMA is therefore divided distal to the origin of inferior pancreaticoduodenal artery. Because the first few jejunal arterial branches may originate from the origin of the SMA to the inferior pancreaticoduodenal artery, these proximal jejunal branches may have to be sacrificed. When the pancreas is not procured, the numerous small venous and arterial pancreatic branches in the head of the pancreas and uncinate process can be divided to obtain more length of the main SMA trunk of mesenteric vessels (Fig. 20.2B and C). Further meticulous dissection leads to the splenomesenteric confluence of the portal vein. After the cross clamp and cold flush infusion, the SMA will be transected at its root, and the SMV will be transected at the splenomesenteric confluence.

Multivisceral Graft

En bloc dissection of the liver, stomach, duodenum, intestine, pancreas, and spleen from the diaphragm and retroperitoneum is performed. The graft to be retrieved can be modified according to the patient's need with exclusion of the liver (modified multivisceral graft). After the diaphragmatic crura are divided, the abdominal esophagus is stapled. A long segment of thoracic and abdominal aorta is retrieved in continuity with a Carrel patch containing the celiac axis and the SMA (Fig. 20.2D). The combined liver-intestine organ is procured in the same manner as en bloc multivisceral retrieval, including preservation of the pancreaticoduodenal axis to maintain continuity of the gastrointestinal tract and the integrity of axial blood supply. The only difference is the exclusion of the stomach, which occurs either during the organ procurement or during the back table organ preparation.

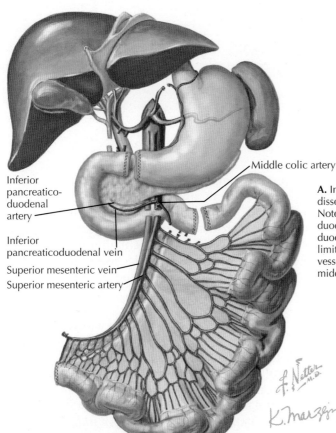

Middle colic artery

Inferior
pancreatico-
duodenal
artery

Inferior
pancreaticoduodenal vein

Superior mesenteric vein

Superior mesenteric artery

A. In situ separation of the intestinal graft and dissection of the superior mesenteric pedicle. Note preservation of both the inferior pancreatico-duodenal artery (IPDA) and inferior pancreatico-duodenal vein (IPDV) with the pancreatic graft by limiting the dissection of the superior mesenteric vessels (SMV, SMA) below the level of the ligated middle colic artery (MCA).

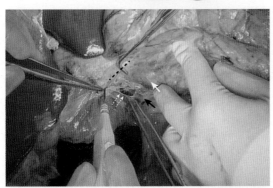

B. Superior mesenteric vein (SMV) of high bifurcation type. During intestine organ procurement, the mesentery was rotated clockwise to expose the back of mesentery. White arrow indicates the large SMV branch. Black arrow indicates another large branch that drains several branches (dotted arrows) from uncinate process of the pancreas. Dashed black line indicates cutting line of SMV when pancreas is not used to procure intestinal graft.

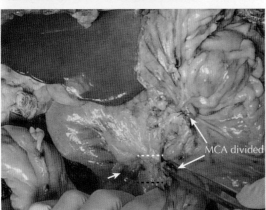

MCA divided

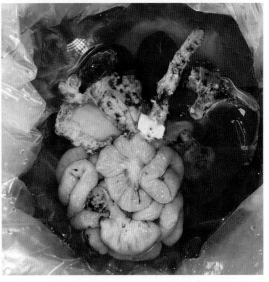

C. Right colon was mobilized and middle colic artery (MCA) was divided to access "the hilum" of superior mesenteric vessels. Dashed black line indicates cutting line of SMV when pancreas and intestine are procured for separate recipients. Dashed white line indicates cuttling line of SMV when pancreas is not procured.

D. The posterior view of full multivisceral graft with a long segment of thoracic and abdominal aorta retrieved in continuity with a Carrel patch containing celiac artery and superior mesenteric artery.

FIGURE 20.2 Donor surgery.

RECIPIENT SURGERY

Removal of the recipient's diseased organs precedes implantation of the new organs and is based on the underlying visceral pathology. The commonly used piecemeal evisceration technique consists of completion of a total enterectomy, subtotal gastrectomy, and hepatectomy for multivisceral transplant recipients. The native pancreaticoduodenal complex or the splenic compartment is preserved in those who undergo multivisceral transplantation when feasible. The spleen and pancreas are left, if possible, to reduce the risk of infection, post-transplant lymphoid proliferative disorder, and diabetes. Vascular reconstruction using interposition vessel grafts is performed in the recipient and/or at the back table (Fig. 20.3A, B, and C) after removal of the diseased organs.

Arterial Inflow

During an isolated intestine transplant, the iliac or carotid arterial graft is anastomosed to the native aorta in an end-to-side fashion. The arterial graft is anastomosed to the SMA of the intestinal graft. For a composite visceral graft, the celiac and the superior mesenteric artery are retrieved and constructed on a single Carrel patch. The Carrel patch is then anastomosed on the back table to a donor aortic conduit (Fig. 20.3D). Before implantation of the visceral organ transplant grafts, another donor aortic conduit is anastomosed to the recipient supraceliac or infrarenal aorta in an end-to-side manner. Accordingly, the arterial anastomosis is completed to the multivisceral organ graft with an anastomosis to both aortic conduits in an end-to-end manner.

Venous Outflow

Venous outflow for an isolated intestinal graft can be established with either portal or systemic drainage. The iliac vein is commonly used as an interposition graft in an end-to-end or end-to-side manner to the recipient portal vein in the hepatic hilum or to the SMV. Systemic drainage to the vena cava can be obtained with an interposition venous graft to the recipient infrarenal vena cava, renal, or iliac veins. Venous outflow of liver-contained visceral allografts is created between recipient and donor vena cava frequently using a piggyback technique (Video 20.2). With combined liver-intestinal transplantation, a portocaval shunt is created to decompress the remaining native organs, including the stomach and pancreaticoduodenal complex.

Restoration of Gastrointestinal Continuity

The gastrointestinal reconstruction is commonly dictated by the surgical anatomy of the retained native gut organs and the type of visceral allograft. Foregut reconstruction is part of multivisceral transplantation. The residual native stomach or abdominal esophagus is anastomosed to the anterior wall of the allograft stomach, and a pyloroplasty is performed as a drainage procedure. In recipients of liver-intestinal allografts and those with preserved pancreaticoduodenal complex, midgut reconstruction is required to restore continuity between the native and transplanted gut. With liver-intestinal transplant, the very proximal allograft jejunum is anastomosed to the retained short segment of the native jejunum. A piggyback duodenoduodenal reconstruction is performed when there is retained duodenum. Reconstruction of the hind gut is performed with anastomosis in the recipient to the residual colorectal segment with creation of a chimney ileostomy or a simple loop ileostomy. Patients with a previous proctocolectomy receive an end ileostomy.

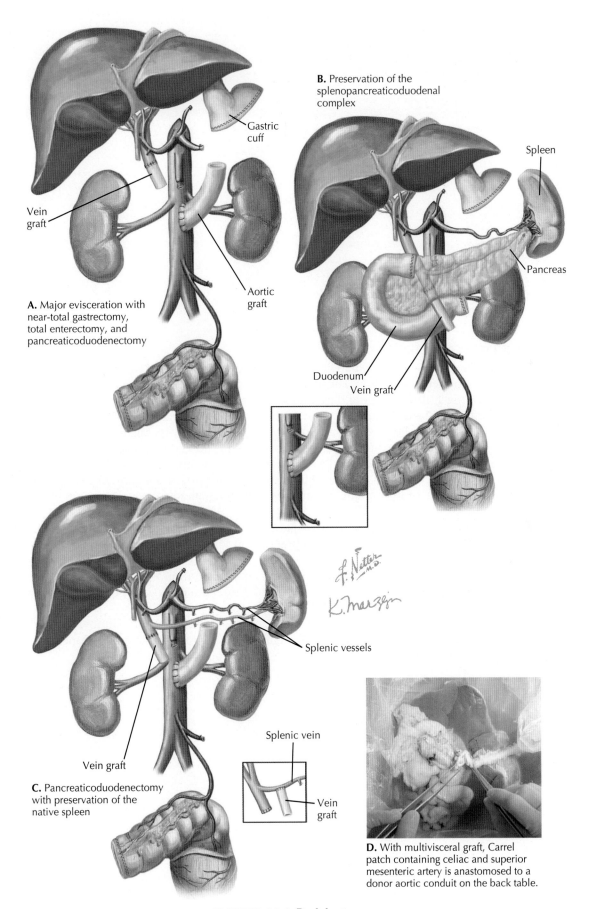

Gastric cuff

Vein graft

Aortic graft

A. Major evisceration with near-total gastrectomy, total enterectomy, and pancreaticoduodenectomy

B. Preservation of the splenopancreaticoduodenal complex

Spleen

Pancreas

Duodenum

Vein graft

Splenic vessels

Vein graft

C. Pancreaticoduodenectomy with preservation of the native spleen

Splenic vein

Vein graft

D. With multivisceral graft, Carrel patch containing celiac and superior mesenteric artery is anastomosed to a donor aortic conduit on the back table.

FIGURE 20.3 Recipient surgery.

SUGGESTED READINGS

Abu-Elmagd K. The concept of gut rehabilitation and the future of visceral transplantation. Nat Rev Gastroenterol Hepatol 2015;12:108–20.

Abu-Elmagd K, Fung J, Bueno J, et al. Logistics and technique for procurement of intestinal, pancreatic and hepatic grafts from the same donor. Ann Surg 2000;232:680–7.

Abu-Elmagd K, Khanna A, Fujiki M, et al. Surgery for gut failureto-reconstruction and allo-transplantation. In: Fazio V, Church JM, Delaney CP, Kiran RP, editors. Current therapy in colon and rectal surgery. Philadelphia, PA: Elsevier, Inc.; 2017. pp. 372–84.

Abu-Elmagd KM, Costa G, Bond G, et al. Five hundred intestinal and multivisceral transplantations at a single center: major advances with new challenges. Ann Surg 2009;250:567–81.

Cruz RJ, Costa G, Bond G, et al. Modified "liver-sparing" multivisceral transplant with preserved native spleen, pancreas, and duodenum: technique and long-term outcome. J Gastrointest Surg 2010;14:1709–21.

Cruz RJ, Costa G, Bond GJ, et al. Modified multivisceral transplantation with spleen-preserving pancreaticoduodenectomy for patients with familial adenomatous polyposis "Gardner's syndrome". Transplant 2011;91:1417–23.

Fujiki M, Hashimoto H, Khanna A, Quintini C, Costa G, Abu-Elmagd K. Technical innovation and visceral transplantation. In: Subramaniam K, Sakai T, editors. Anesthesia and perioperative care for organ transplantation. New York: Springer; 2017. pp. 497–511.

Kidney Transplantation

Eric T. Miller, David A. Goldfarb, and Alvin C. Wee

 VIDEO

21.1 Kidney Transplantation

INTRODUCTION

Kidney transplantation is a multidimensional operation that involves early and ongoing evaluation of the intended kidney recipient. When an appropriately cross-matched kidney becomes available, the kidney is procured in a manner that preserves arterial, venous, and periureteral tissues. The donor and recipient anatomy is then carefully examined to determine the exact surgical approach during transplantation. Multiple options for both vascular and ureteral anastomoses are at the surgeon's disposal and are what makes each case unique and specific to a donor–recipient pair. A complete and thorough understanding of the renal and retroperitoneal anatomy are of the utmost importance to achieve successful kidney transplantation.

PREOPERATIVE PLANNING AND CONSIDERATION

The favored and optimal location for kidney transplantation is the iliac fossa. The iliac vessels are in juxtaposition to the urinary bladder, facilitating revascularization and urinary drainage for the majority of cases. Although a donor kidney from either side may be placed into either fossa, the left kidney will always have the collecting system in a superior position and be readily accessible if placed into the right iliac fossa. This fact is similar for a right donor kidney placed on the left iliac fossa. A direct ureteroneocystostomy is used for most cases; however, in circumstances with a small defunctionalized bladder, ureteroureterostomy may be preferable (Fig. 21.1). When the iliac vessels are unsuitable for use secondary to prior surgery or severe iliac artery calcification, a more proximal location on the aorta or the inferior vena cava (IVC) may be used, including an orthotopic position after native nephrectomy. In such cases, the ureter may be anastomosed using an end-to-end uretero-ureterostomy.

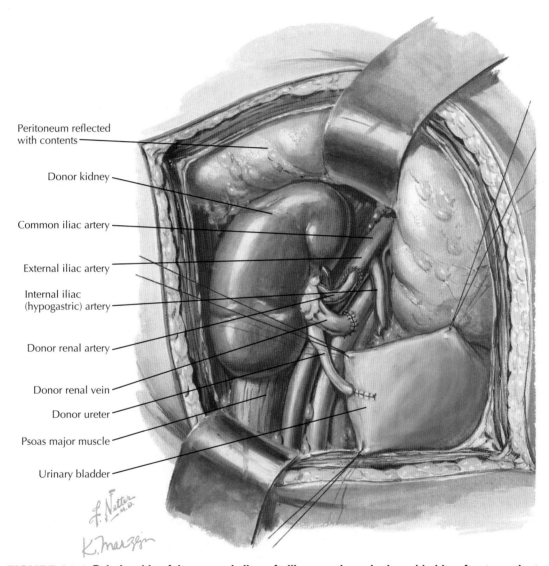

Peritoneum reflected with contents

Donor kidney

Common iliac artery

External iliac artery

Internal iliac (hypogastric) artery

Donor renal artery

Donor renal vein

Donor ureter

Psoas major muscle

Urinary bladder

FIGURE 21.1 **Relationship of donor renal allograft, iliac vessels, and urinary bladder after transplantation into the right iliac fossa.**

PROCUREMENT AND PREPARATION OF KIDNEY ALLOGRAFT ON THE BACKTABLE

During procurement, it is important to recognize the potential for variations in renal vascular anatomy and to maintain the integrity of all arteries and veins to the kidney (Fig. 21.2A and B). These are end vessels, and loss of arteries will result in a loss of an entire renal parenchymal segment (Fig. 21.2C). Dominant veins must be preserved, but small-caliber veins can be sacrificed because collateral circulation is established through the vasa rectae. In the transplant kidney, the ureteral blood supply originates entirely from the renal hilum and becomes progressively more ischemic with distance from the hilum. It is important to preserve tissues bounded by the renal hilum, ureter, and lower pole of the kidney. Furthermore, it is important for the procurement surgeon to avoid extensive dissection around the transplant ureter because it may compromise ureteral blood supply.

The donor kidney requires preparation before transplantation. Perinephric fat is removed and all vessels are mobilized to allow for well-positioned anastomoses without kinking. In deceased donors, multiple arteries in close proximity may be preserved on a common Carrel patch. For arteries more widely separated, independent anastomoses may be performed with or without a patch. In living donor kidneys with multiple arteries, independent anastomoses are usually performed. In select cases of two equal-size arteries, a conjoined anastomosis may be performed. When anastomotic sites for inflow are limited, an end-to-side anastomosis of a smaller renal artery to the dominant renal artery may be required, which allows for a single anastomosis to the inflow source. In deceased donor kidneys, the right renal vein and inferior vena cava usually require reconstruction. By closing the suprarenal IVC and infrarenal IVC, with either sutures or a stapling device, the surgeon may use the ostia from the left renal vein for the outflow anastomosis. Alternatively, the suprarenal IVC can be closed in a way that fashions an L-shaped extension of the infrarenal IVC, which can be used for the outflow anastomosis.

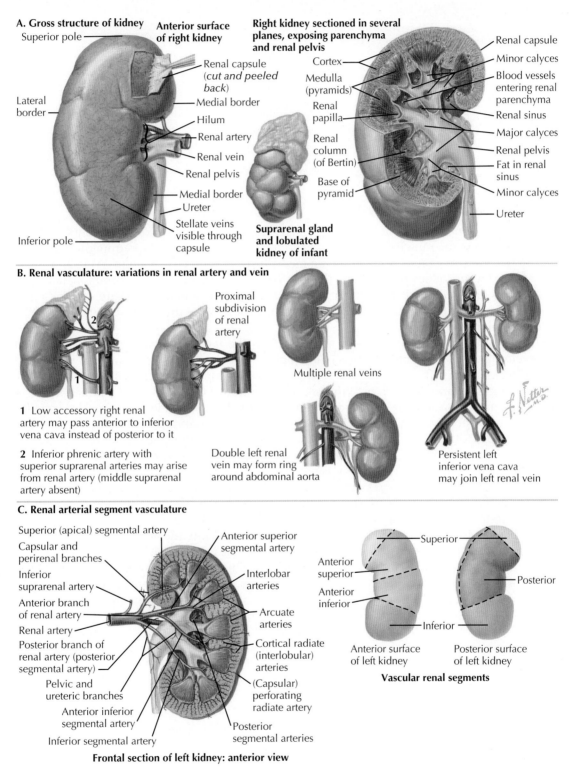

A. Gross structure of kidney

Superior pole

Lateral border

Inferior pole

Anterior surface of right kidney

Renal capsule (*cut and peeled back*)

Medial border

Hilum

Renal artery

Renal vein

Renal pelvis

Medial border

Ureter

Stellate veins visible through capsule

Suprarenal gland and lobulated kidney of infant

Right kidney sectioned in several planes, exposing parenchyma and renal pelvis

Cortex

Medulla (pyramids)

Renal papilla

Renal column (of Bertin)

Base of pyramid

Renal capsule

Minor calyces

Blood vessels entering renal parenchyma

Renal sinus

Major calyces

Renal pelvis

Fat in renal sinus

Minor calyces

Ureter

B. Renal vasculature: variations in renal artery and vein

Proximal subdivision of renal artery

Multiple renal veins

1 Low accessory right renal artery may pass anterior to inferior vena cava instead of posterior to it

2 Inferior phrenic artery with superior suprarenal arteries may arise from renal artery (middle suprarenal artery absent)

Double left renal vein may form ring around abdominal aorta

Persistent left inferior vena cava may join left renal vein

C. Renal arterial segment vasculature

Superior (apical) segmental artery

Capsular and perirenal branches

Inferior suprarenal artery

Anterior branch of renal artery

Renal artery

Posterior branch of renal artery (posterior segmental artery)

Pelvic and ureteric branches

Anterior inferior segmental artery

Inferior segmental artery

Anterior superior segmental artery

Interlobar arteries

Arcuate arteries

Cortical radiate (interlobular) arteries

(Capsular) perforating radiate artery

Posterior segmental arteries

Frontal section of left kidney: anterior view

Superior

Anterior superior

Anterior inferior

Inferior

Posterior

Anterior surface of left kidney

Posterior surface of left kidney

Vascular renal segments

FIGURE 21.2 Variations in renal vasculature and renal arterial segment vasculature.

KIDNEY TRANSPLANTATION

A Gibson incision is used to access the iliac fossa (Fig. 21.3AB). The external oblique fascia is divided to access the muscles just lateral to the rectus. At this point, the retroperitoneum can be entered, sweeping the intact peritoneum medially off the anterior abdominal wall and creating a space for the kidney that includes the iliac vessels. Dissection can be accommodated more cephalad as required. A self-retaining retractor is deployed to maintain exposure, ensuring that no pressure is exerted directly on the psoas major muscle because this can result in a postoperative femoral neuropathy.

The external iliac artery and vein are dissected. The large lymphatic trunks are divided between silk ties to prevent formation of a lymphocele. Other investing tissues can be divided using electrocautery. It is important to recognize the position of the genitofemoral nerve as it courses along the anterior surface of the psoas major muscle (Fig. 21.3C and D). The kidney is simulated into the wound in its final resting position to identify the ideal locations for vascular anastomoses. The iliac vein is controlled with a clamp, and a carefully calibrated venotomy is created (Fig. 21.4A). The end-to-side anastomosis is constructed using a permanent running monofilament suture (Fig. 21.4B). The artery is clamped and the arteriotomy is created (Fig. 21.4C). The anastomosis is performed using a permanent running monofilament suture (Fig. 21.4D). When both anastomoses are completed, the clamps are removed (venous first, then arterial) and the kidney is reperfused. Careful inspection of the vascular anastomoses and the kidney surface is performed and meticulous hemostasis is achieved.

The bladder is then expanded by infusing a saline solution into the bladder. This can be done using a pre-placed three-way bladder irrigation system. The ureter is trimmed to an appropriate length and spatulated (Fig. 21.4E). Refluxing or nonrefluxing techniques may be used for the donor ureter to recipient bladder ureteroneocystostomy (Fig. 21.4F). Absorbable suture is critical because use of a nonabsorbable suture may result in bladder stone formation.

The kidney is positioned in the retroperitoneum to avoid kinking of the donor renal vessels. A drain may be deployed in the deep wound, in the subcutaneous space, or both, at the surgeon's discretion. The fascial layers are closed in anatomic fashion, and the skin is approximated to conclude the case.

Making the Gibson Incision

A. Gibson incision

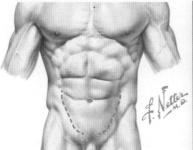

B. Left lower quadrant Gibson incision

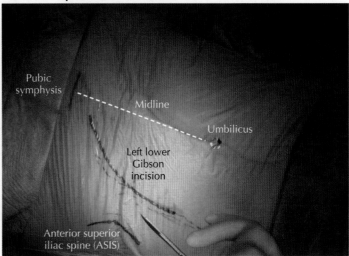

Pubic symphysis

Midline

Umbilicus

Left lower Gibson incision

Anterior superior iliac spine (ASIS)

Preparation of right iliac fossa in preparation for renal allograft placement and anastomosis

C. Pelvic vascular anatomy

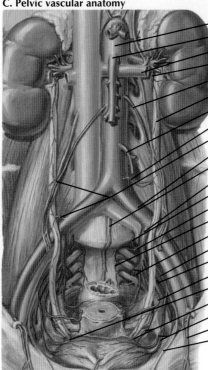

Abdominal aorta
Superior mesenteric artery
Renal artery and vein
Ureteric branch from renal artery
Ovarian artery
Ureter
Inferior mesenteric artery (*cut*)
Ureteric branch from aorta
Ureteric branches from ovarian and common iliac arteries
Common iliac artery
Median sacral artery
Internal iliac artery
Iliolumbar artery
Superior gluteal artery
Lateral sacral artery
Inferior gluteal and internal pudendal arteries
Umbilical artery (patent part)
Obturator artery
Uterine artery
Ureteric branch from superior vesical artery
Inferior vesical artery and ureteric branch
Superior vesical arteries
Inferior epigastric artery
Medial umbilical ligament

D. Anatomy of the right iliac fossa

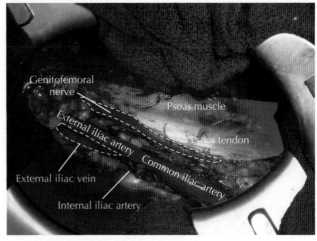

Genitofemoral nerve

Psoas muscle

External iliac artery

Psoas tendon

External iliac vein

Common iliac artery

Internal iliac artery

FIGURE 21.3 Kidney transplantation.

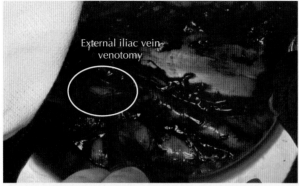
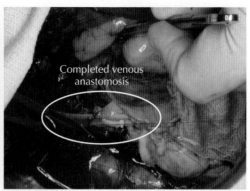

A. A venotomy is made in preparation for end-to-side donor renal vein to external iliac vein anastomosis.

B. Completed end-to-side venous anastomosis.

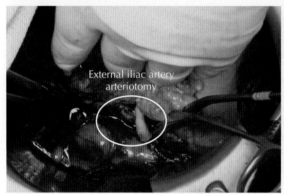
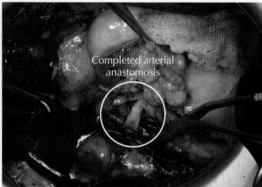

C. An arteriotomy is made in preparation for end-to-side donor renal artery to external iliac artery anastomosis.

D. Completed end-to-side arterial anastomosis.

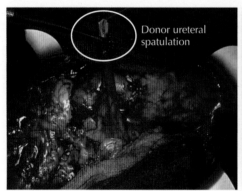
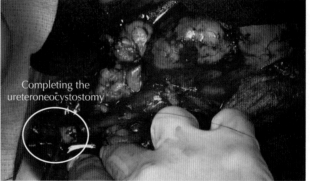

E. Donor ureter spatulation in preparation for ureteral anastomosis.

F. Ureteral anastomosis completed as a direct ureteroneocystostomy.

FIGURE 21.4 Kidney transplantation (continued).

SUGGESTED READINGS

Englesbe M. Operative techniques in transplantation surgery. Wolters Kluwer; 2014.

Goldfarb DA, Flechner SM, Modlin CS. Chapter 11. Renal transplantation. In: Novick AC, Jones JS, editors. Operative urology at the cleveland clinic. Totowa, NJ. 2006. pp. 121–32.

Knechtle SJ. Kidney transplantation—principles and practice. 7th ed. Saunders Elsevier; 2014.

Shoskes DA. Kidney and pancreas transplantation: practical guide. Kidney transplant recipient surgery. Humana Press; 2011.

Pancreas and Kidney Transplantation

Eric T. Miller and Venkatesh Krishnamurthi

 VIDEO

22.1 Simultaneous Pancreas and Kidney Transplantation

PREOPERATIVE PLANNING AND CONSIDERATION

Pancreas transplantation is currently a therapeutic option for patients with type 1 diabetes mellitus and, in selected circumstances, those with type 2 diabetes mellitus. The primary goal of the procedure is to replace insulin that is otherwise absent as a result of islet cell loss from the native pancreas. There are three possible scenarios for pancreas transplantation, including simultaneous pancreas and kidney transplant (SPK), pancreas after kidney transplant (PAK), and pancreas transplant alone (PTA). SPK is the most common procedure performed and has the best pancreas graft survival rates. Although the risks of the SPK operation include those related to chronic immunosuppression, as well as the inherent morbidity and mortality of the surgery, the benefits of the transplant include freedom from exogenous insulin, superior blood glucose control compared with all other insulin replacement strategies, no further need for dietary restrictions, and decreased progression, or potential improvement in, secondary diabetic complications (i.e., neuropathy and cardiovascular disease).

Aside from ABO blood group compatibility and negative human leukocyte antigen cross-matching, the next most important factor when considering a potential *recipient* for pancreas transplantation is the presence and/or extent of underlying coronary artery disease. Patients with diabetes mellitus often have comorbid diseases, including hypertension, hyperlipidemia, and peripheral vascular disease. To avoid life-threatening complications during or after a surgery, a thorough cardiac and possible vascular surgery evaluation is critical before listing for transplantation.

Appropriate organ *donor* selection limits complications such as bowel anastomotic leaks and vascular thrombotic events. The preferred donor age ranges from 10 to 45 years old. When potential donors are considered, graft outcomes are generally better from donors with traumatic cause of death in contrast to donor death secondary to cerebrovascular disease. Donor size is critical and ideally greater than 45 kg to avoid issues related to small donor vessels at time of Y-graft reconstruction. A *donor* BMI less than 30 is favored to prevent transplanting pancreata with high proportions of fatty intrusion, which has been shown to increase rates of graft thrombosis, pancreatitis, worsened ischemia reperfusion injury, and higher rates of postoperative infection. There are many additional factors involved in choosing the appropriate recipient and donor pair; however, a full list of criteria is beyond the scope of this chapter.

SIMULTANEOUS PANCREAS AND KIDNEY TRANSPLANTATION
Incision, Exposure, and Preparation for Implantation

A midline intraperitoneal incision following the linea alba is made and extends from the xiphoid to the pubic symphysis. Postoperative pain is minimized with this approach because it avoids splitting of the rectus abdominis muscles, as well as the thoracoabdominal, subcostal, and ilio-hypogastric nerves.

Once the fascia is fully incised, the peritoneum is identified and entered, and a self-retaining retractor is placed to maintain adequate exposure to the peritoneal cavity. The right lower quadrant posterior peritoneum is incised along the white line of Toldt. The right ascending colon and small bowel are mobilized from right to left to expose the retroperitoneal vasculature. The external iliac vessels, the common iliac vessels, and the distal IVC are exposed in preparation for combined kidney and pancreas implantation in the right iliac fossa and right retroperitoneum.

Vascular targets for the kidney transplant are exposed with circumferential dissection and isolation of the right external iliac vein and artery. Our preferred method of pancreatic venous drainage is via a systemic route, so vascular targets for the pancreas transplant are developed with circumferential dissection and isolation of the common iliac artery and inferiormost segment of the inferior vena cava. Finally, the right ureter of the native kidney is carefully mobilized and will later demarcate a line of separation between the pancreas allograft medially and the kidney allograft laterally (Fig. 22.1A).

A final step in preparation for pancreas transplantation involves anastomosis of a 4- to 5-cm segment of a donor artery interposition graft to the common iliac artery. After end-to-side anastomosis, a temporary clamp is placed on the interposition graft, and blood flow is returned to the distal pelvic and lower extremity vasculature (Fig. 22.1B and C).

KIDNEY TRANSPLANTATION

In general, there are few differences in anatomic and surgical principles presented in the chapter on standard kidney transplantation. The largest notable difference is that after simultaneous kidney and pancreas transplantation, the donor kidney allograft occupies a space that communicates with the peritoneal cavity. Because of this, the retroperitoneal pocket that is produced in a standard kidney transplant is not present; therefore the operating surgeon must perform a nephropexy after implantation to affix the kidney to the lateral wall of the iliac fossa to prevent twisting of the kidney on its vascular pedicle. Furthermore, the kidney is placed in a position that is lateral to the native ureter, which allows for adequate space for the pancreas allograft in the ipsilateral retroperitoneum. Please refer to Chapter 21 on kidney transplantation for further details.

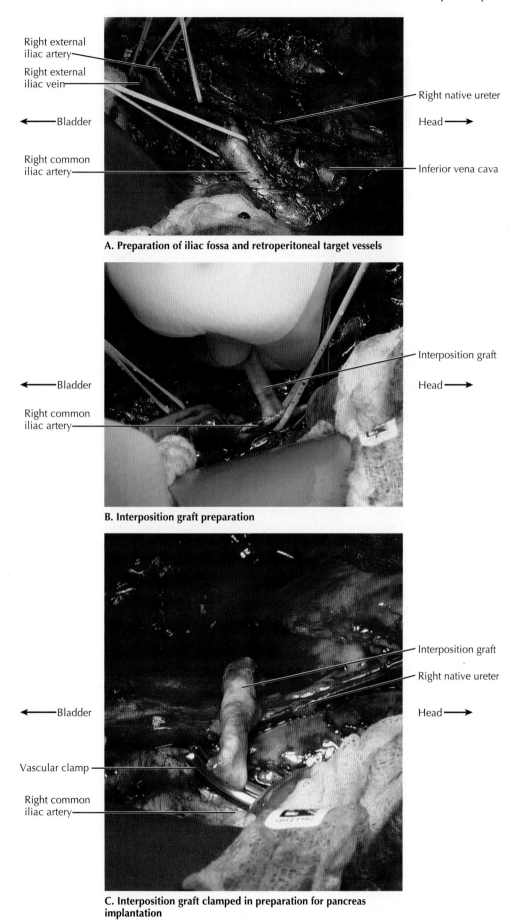

A. Preparation of iliac fossa and retroperitoneal target vessels

B. Interposition graft preparation

C. Interposition graft clamped in preparation for pancreas implantation

FIGURE 22.1 Placement of donor arterial interposition graft on recipient common iliac artery.

Bench Preparation of the Pancreas Allograft

During bench preparation, the pancreas allograft is kept entirely immersed in cold organ preservation solution. Bench preparation begins with meticulous inspection of the pancreas and attached segment of the duodenum. The allograft parenchyma must have a consistency that is easily pliable and a dull orange color and must lack major injury to the pancreatic parenchyma (Figs. 22.2 and 22.3). The duodenum and donor vessels must be inspected for evidence of injury and appropriate length.

During initial procurement, the spleen remains attached to the pancreas and must be removed with careful suture ligation of perforating splenic vessels. An appreciation of portal vein anatomy in the pancreas is important to develop a length of portal vein that extends 2 cm beyond the surface of the gland. This length is achieved by dividing and ligating branches of the anterior superior pancreaticoduodenal vein on the right and the left gastric or coronary vein on the left. The small bowel vascular mesenteric root, which was stapled and cut during procurement, is reinforced with thick, nonabsorbable monofilament suture to ensure hemostasis at time of reperfusion. The donor duodenal segment is further dissected and stapled again to ensure that the distal and proximal ends contain adequate perfusion via retrograde flow from the inferior pancreaticoduodenal artery. Specifically, the proximal duodenum is trimmed to about the level of the gastroduodenal artery and the distal segment approximately 2 cm from the uncinate process of the donor pancreas (Fig. 22.4).

The final step in bench preparation involves reconstruction of the donor superior mesenteric artery (SMA) and splenic artery. This is achieved by using a donor arterial graft composed of the deceased donor iliac artery bifurcation "Y-graft" (see Fig. 22.4). The Y-graft is oriented along the SMA and splenic artery, whereby in most cases the internal iliac artery is sewn to the splenic artery and the external iliac artery is sewn to the SMA, both in end-to-end fashion. The Y-graft allows for a single extended length arterial graft that can be anastomosed to the previously placed interposition graft on the common iliac artery.

A. Veins of stomach, duodenum, pancreas, and spleen

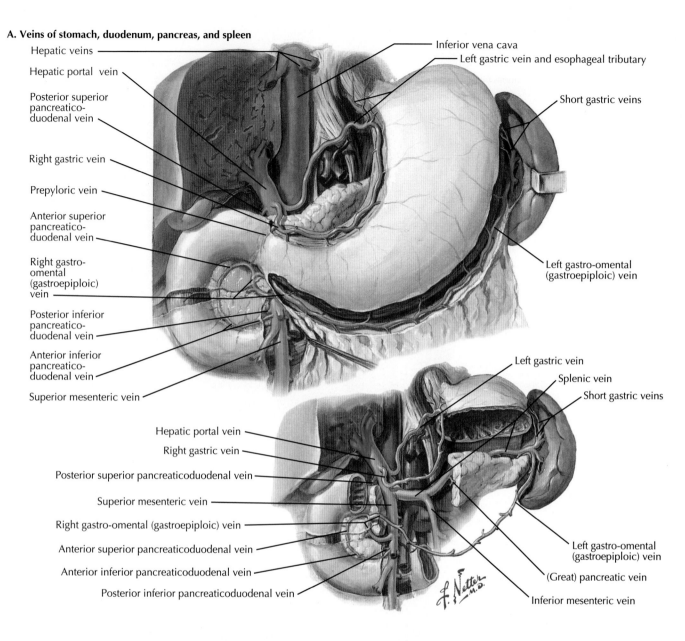

Hepatic veins

Hepatic portal vein

Posterior superior pancreatico-duodenal vein

Right gastric vein

Prepyloric vein

Anterior superior pancreatico-duodenal vein

Right gastro-omental (gastroepiploic) vein

Posterior inferior pancreatico-duodenal vein

Anterior inferior pancreatico-duodenal vein

Superior mesenteric vein

Inferior vena cava

Left gastric vein and esophageal tributary

Short gastric veins

Left gastro-omental (gastroepiploic) vein

Hepatic portal vein

Right gastric vein

Posterior superior pancreaticoduodenal vein

Superior mesenteric vein

Right gastro-omental (gastroepiploic) vein

Anterior superior pancreaticoduodenal vein

Anterior inferior pancreaticoduodenal vein

Posterior inferior pancreaticoduodenal vein

Left gastric vein

Splenic vein

Short gastric veins

Left gastro-omental (gastroepiploic) vein

(Great) pancreatic vein

Inferior mesenteric vein

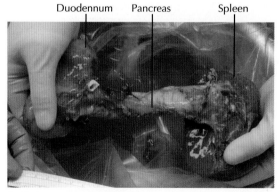

Duodennum   Pancreas   Spleen

B. *El vivo* **pancreas allograft**

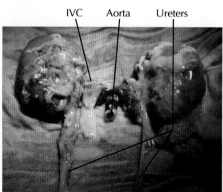

IVC   Aorta   Ureters

C. *El vivo* **kidney allograft**

FIGURE 22.2 Preparation of pancreas and kidney at time of procurement.

Duodenum and head of pancreas reflected to left

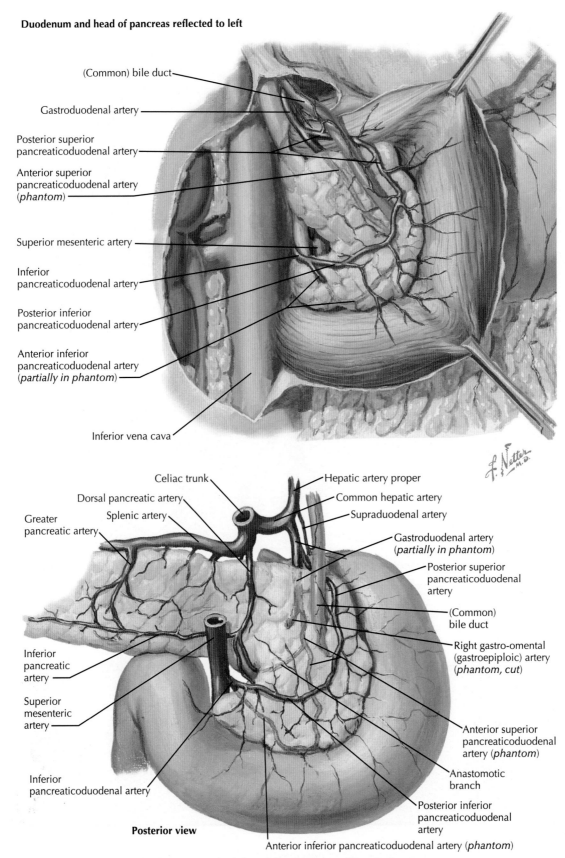

(Common) bile duct

Gastroduodenal artery

Posterior superior pancreaticoduodenal artery

Anterior superior pancreaticoduodenal artery (*phantom*)

Superior mesenteric artery

Inferior pancreaticoduodenal artery

Posterior inferior pancreaticoduodenal artery

Anterior inferior pancreaticoduodenal artery (*partially in phantom*)

Inferior vena cava

Celiac trunk

Dorsal pancreatic artery

Greater pancreatic artery

Splenic artery

Hepatic artery proper

Common hepatic artery

Supraduodenal artery

Gastroduodenal artery (*partially in phantom*)

Posterior superior pancreaticoduodenal artery

(Common) bile duct

Right gastro-omental (gastroepiploic) artery (*phantom, cut*)

Inferior pancreatic artery

Superior mesenteric artery

Inferior pancreaticoduodenal artery

Anterior superior pancreaticoduodenal artery (*phantom*)

Anastomotic branch

Posterior inferior pancreaticoduodenal artery

Posterior view

Anterior inferior pancreaticoduodenal artery (*phantom*)

FIGURE 22.3 Arteries of duodenum and head of pancreas.

Anterior view

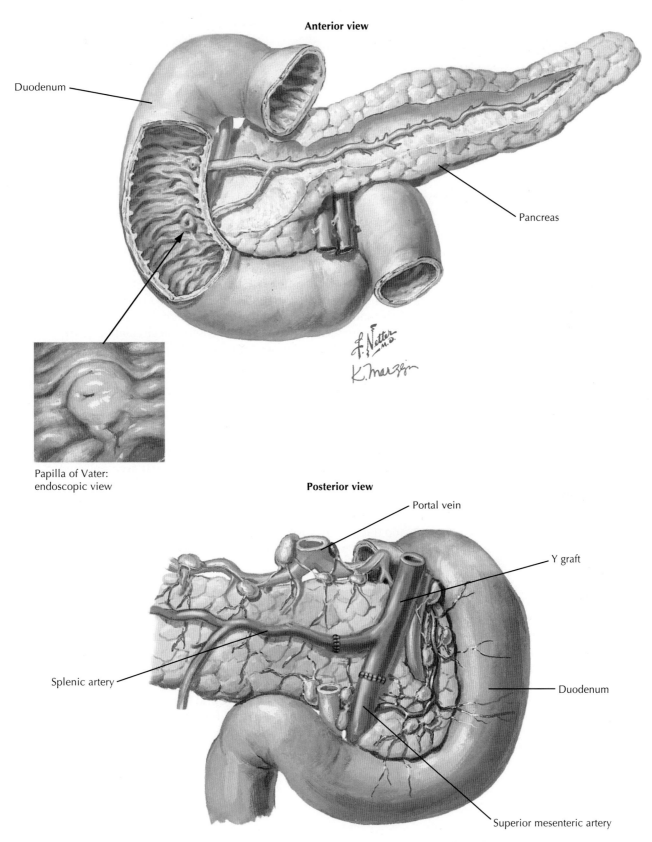

Duodenum

Pancreas

Papilla of Vater:
endoscopic view

Posterior view

Portal vein

Y graft

Splenic artery

Duodenum

Superior mesenteric artery

FIGURE 22.4 Arterial reconstruction for pancreas allograft.

REVASCULARIZATION AND REPERFUSION

When the kidney transplantation is complete, the pancreas is then brought to the operative field and wrapped in an ice-cold sterile pad. As mentioned, our center's preferred method of venous drainage is via a systemic route to the inferior vena cava, thus the pancreas allograft is positioned medial to the native ureter in the retroperitoneum and adjacent to the prepared IVC and iliac interposition graft. The recipient's IVC is clamped, and the allograft portal vein is sewn to the distal IVC in end-to-side fashion using nonabsorbable monofilament suture (Fig. 22.5A). The common iliac artery segment of the donor Y-graft is sewn to the common iliac interposition graft in end-to-end fashion (Fig. 22.5B). The vascular clamps are released and circulation to the pancreas is restored (Fig. 22.5C). The ice blanket is removed and the allograft is inspected for hemostasis and adequate perfusion.

PANCREAS EXOCRINE DUCT MANAGEMENT VIA DUODENOJEJUNOSTOMY

There are two methods for exocrine drainage, mainly bladder drainage and enteric drainage. The majority of transplant centers now use enteric drainage because of the high rate of urologic and metabolic complications that arise with bladder drainage. Enteric drainage is accomplished by positioning a loop of the recipient's jejunum adjacent to and in line with the donor duodenum. A hand-sewn anastomosis is performed between the donor duodenum and the recipient jejunum (Fig. 22.5D). The potential posteriorly positioned "trap-door" between the donor duodenum, head of the pancreas, and the posterior retroperitoneum is closed with interrupted sutures in order to prevent herniation and incarceration of bowel loops behind the pancreas transplant.

ABDOMINAL LAVAGE AND CLOSURE

Once the kidney and pancreas allografts have been carefully inspected for adequate perfusion and hemostasis, copious sterile saline irrigation is applied to the entire peritoneal space. The large and small bowel loops are inspected and then returned to their orthotopic position. The surgical retractor is removed, and the edges of the abdominal wall are repositioned adjacent to each other in preparation for closure (Fig. 22.5E). The fascial edges are then closed with a combination of interrupted and running monofilament sutures. The wound is irrigated and the skin is then closed with monofilament suture. The patient is admitted for inpatient hospitalization and monitoring to ensure graft function, as measured by daily decrease in serum creatinine and near immediate normalization of serum glucose levels.

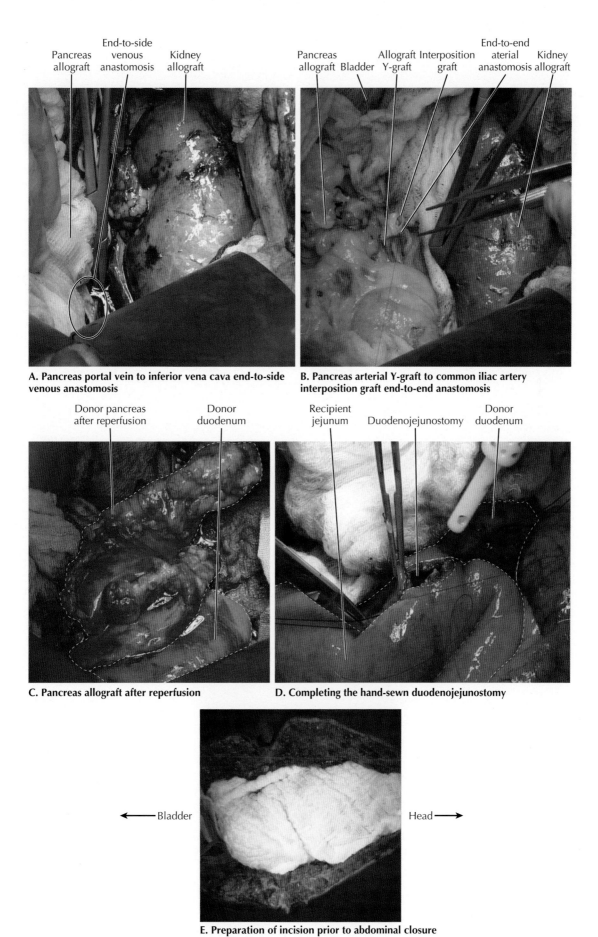

A. Pancreas portal vein to inferior vena cava end-to-side venous anastomosis

B. Pancreas arterial Y-graft to common iliac artery interposition graft end-to-end anastomosis

C. Pancreas allograft after reperfusion

D. Completing the hand-sewn duodenojejunostomy

E. Preparation of incision prior to abdominal closure

FIGURE 22.5 **Fundamental maneuvers in pancreas allograft transplantation.**

SUGGESTED READINGS

Dean PG, Kudva YC, Stegall MD. Long-term benefits of pancreas transplantation. Curr Opin Organ Transplant 2008;13(1):85–90. https://doi.org/10.1097/MOT.0b013e3282f2fd7f.

Dean PG, Kukla A, Stegall MD, Kudva YC. Pancreas transplantation. BMJ 2017;357:j1321. https://doi.org/10.1136/bmj.j1321.

Senaratne NV, Norris JM. Bladder vs enteric drainage following pancreatic transplantation: how best to support graft survival? A best evidence topic. Int J Surg 2015;22:149–52. https://doi.org/10.1016/j.ijsu.2015.08.072. Epub 2015 Sep 3.

Siskind E, Amodu L, Liu C, et al. A comparison of portal venous versus systemic venous drainage in pancreas transplantation. HPB (Oxford) 2019;21(2):195–203. https://doi.org/10.1016/j.hpb.2018.07.018. Epub 2018 Aug 28.

Wee AC, Krishnamurthi V. Chapter 12: Pancreas transplantation: surgical techniques. In: Kidney and pancreas transplantation: practical guide. Humana Press; 2011.

Laparoscopic Donor Nephrectomy

Eric T. Miller and Alvin C. Wee

▶ VIDEO

23.1 Left Laparoscopic Donor Nephrectomy

INTRODUCTION

A donor nephrectomy is an operation that allows for safe removal of a patient's kidney in such a way that permits and optimizes transplantation into an appropriately matched recipient. The surgical procedure must be done in an efficient and reliable manner to minimize, or completely eliminate, any problematic complications that may arise in the donor and recipient pair. A thorough and complete understanding of the key anatomic structures, in addition to surrounding contents, is important to ensure success in every case.

PREOPERATIVE PLANNING

The donor nephrectomy is one the few operations in medicine in which the patient accepts the risks of the procedure with no potential gain in his or her own physical health or well-being. A thorough understanding of the risks is therefore paramount in every preoperative counseling session. After an extensive medical and psychologic evaluation, as dictated by the American Society of Transplant Surgeons, the patient is seen and examined by the donor surgeon. A thorough history should be conducted, which focuses on existing health conditions, and a systematic examination of the abdomen and pelvis should be performed. All potential intraoperative complications, including vascular and surrounding visceral injuries, must be reviewed and discussed.

Once the patient has been deemed an appropriate surgical candidate, one of the most important components of the evaluation includes assessment of the kidney vasculature via cross-sectional imaging. A contrast-enhanced helical computed tomography scan of the abdomen, with venous and arterial phases, offers excellent visualization of the vasculature (Fig. 23.1A) and will help predict variations in vascular anatomy (Fig. 23.1B). Given the potential for serious harm, a detailed understanding of the anatomy is key to completing each case with precision and the expectation of a perfect outcome.

OPERATIVE TECHNIQUES (LEFT LAPAROSCOPIC DONOR NEPHRECTOMY)

Patient Positioning and Establishing Abdominal Access

An integral first step in the laparoscopic donor nephrectomy is proper patient preparation and positioning. After induction of general anesthesia, an indwelling bladder drainage catheter and orogastric tube are placed. A horizontal mark is made in the suprapubic region two fingerbreadths above the pubic symphysis in preparation for donor kidney extraction through a Pfannenstiel incision. The dependent hip, knees, axilla, and ankles are padded and the patient is repositioned to the 70- to 90-degree semi-lateral decubitus position with the side of donor nephrectomy in the upward position. With the patient's iliac crest at the level of the break in the table, the table is flexed to maximize distance between the subcostal margin and the iliac crest. The dependent knee is flexed and the upper leg is kept straight with ample padding between thighs and lower extremities. The arms are secured with tape to a double arm board. Once the position is optimized, the patient is secured to the table across the chest and hip. The surgical field is then prepped and draped in sterile fashion to include the abdomen from the xiphoid process to the pubic symphysis.

Before laparoscopic port placement, key landmarks include the xiphoid process, the subcostal margin, the umbilicus, the iliac crest, and the pubic symphysis. A 12-mm incision is made in a vertical plane at or near the inferior level of the umbilicus and in a horizontal plane halfway between the iliac crest and the abdominal midline. A Veress insufflation needle is introduced through the first incision and pneumoperitoneum is established after puncturing the peritoneum. The Veress needle is exchanged for a 12-mm trocar. Two additional trocars are visualized and placed in a cumulative vector triangulated with the renal hilum at or near the level of the lateral tip of the 11th rib. Port placement differs slightly from patient to patient and must be adjusted based on anatomy and body habitus.

A. Preoperative contrast-enhanced abdominal computed tomography scan in coronal (top) and axial (bottom) planes

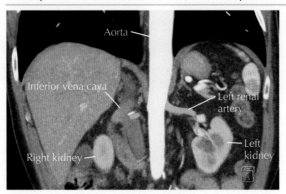

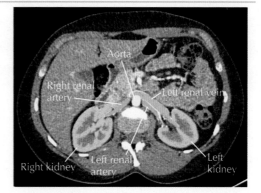

B. Renal vasculature - variations in renal artery and vein variations in renal artery and vein

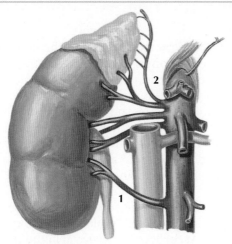

1. Low accessory right renal artery may pass anterior to inferior vena cava instead of posterior to it

2. Inferior phrenic artery with superior suprarenal arteries may arise from renal artery (middle suprarenal artery absent)

Double left renal vein may form ring around abdominal aorta

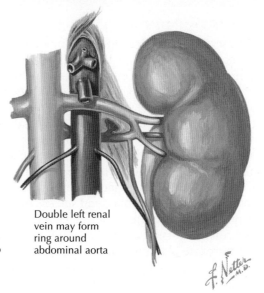

Proximal subdivision of renal artery

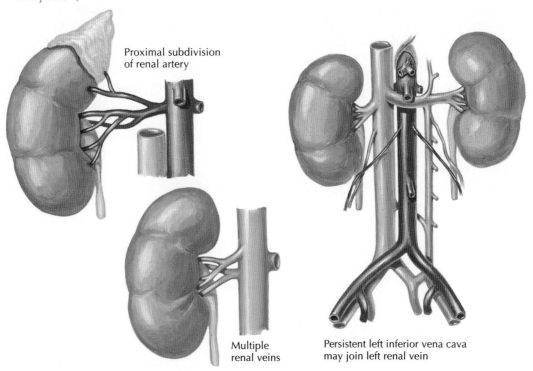

Multiple renal veins

Persistent left inferior vena cava may join left renal vein

FIGURE 23.1 Preoperative planning.

Operative Approach

The dissection of the left donor kidney operation begins with mobilization of the descending large bowel. Adhesions to the anterior abdominal wall are often encountered at the splenic flexure in the left upper quadrant and must be lysed before incising the posterior peritoneum. A nearly bloodless plane is encountered between the light yellow fat of Gerota's fascia and the more dark orange fat of the large bowel mesentery. The dissection is continued superiorly above the upper pole of the donor kidney, which allows for medial mobilization of the spleen and tail of the pancreas. Large bowel mobilization is continued inferiorly to the level of the bifurcation of the ipsilateral iliac vessels. This more inferior dissection allows for adequate ureteral length in the recipient operation. The large bowel is optimally mobilized when the left adrenal gland, left renal vein, and left gonadal vein come into view.

With the bowel, pancreas, and spleen fully mobilized, the next step involves identifying and isolating the ureter. The ureter takes a more lateral to medial path in relation to the gonadal vessels on its course from the renal hilum to the pelvis. At the level of the renal hilum the ureter is more lateral to the gonadal vein, crosses paths with the gonadal vessels near the kidney's lower pole, and then runs medially along the psoas muscle before passing into the pelvis as it crosses the bifurcation of the common iliac artery (Fig. 23.2A). Understanding this anatomic principle allows the surgeon to reliably locate the ureter slightly medial to the gonadal vein at the inferior location of the psoas muscle. The ureter and gonadal vein are identified and then lifted together as a complex. With continued upward traction, a combination of blunt and electrocautery dissection allows for separation of the posterior and lateral attachments of the donor kidney from the bed of the psoas muscle. The primary blood supply of the ureter originates from the renal artery proximally, the gonadal arteries and aorta at the level of the mid-ureter, and from the common and internal iliac more distally (Fig. 23.3). Ureteral blood supply is optimized by ensuring that an adequate sheath of periureteral and perigonadal tissue is maintained around the ureteral and gonadal vessel complex.

With continued dissection the lower pole is elevated to place gentle tension on the renal hilar vessels, optimizing visualization of the renal hilum (see Fig. 23.2B). The left gonadal vein can be seen entering the inferior border of the left renal vein and is ligated. Single or sometimes multiple lumbar vein branches enter the posterior renal vein and must be ligated to optimize donor vein length.

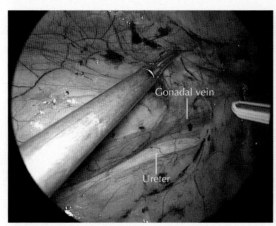

A. Relationship of the ureter to the gonadal vein

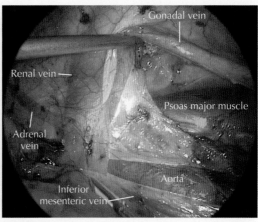

B. Elevation of the lower pole reveals the donor renal vein and surrounding structures

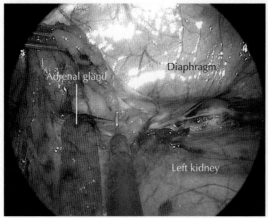

C. The left adrenal gland is positioned superiorly and medially to the left kidney

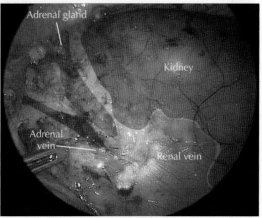

D. The left adrenal vein is seen draining into the left renal vein

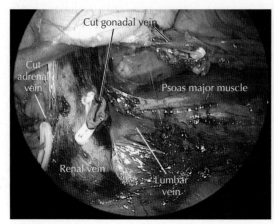

E. Lumbar veins are often encountered draining into the posterior renal vein

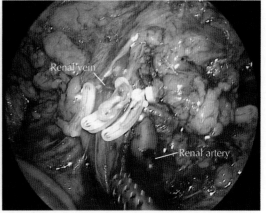

F. Intraoperative view of hilum in preparation for final ligation

FIGURE 23.2 Important intraoperative landmarks.

Operative Approach (Continued)

Dissection of the fibrous attachment along the course of the renal hilar vessels allows for isolation and visualization of the primary renal vessels. The renal artery is most easily identified by following the course of the aorta in the cephalad direction and in a vector coursing between the main renal vein and any lumbar veins if present. To optimize donor length on the artery, the artery is completely cleared of its adventitial fibrous attachments down to the branch point of the aorta. The renal vein is then cleared of circumferential attachments down to the medial interaortocaval region. To prevent catastrophic injury, it is important to recognize the relation of the left renal vein as it passes beneath the superior mesenteric artery on its course to the left kidney (see Fig. 23.1B). The primary renal artery and vein are sufficiently prepared for final ligation when they are circumferentially cleared of all surrounding tissue.

Attention is now turned toward the more cephalad border of the renal vein and adrenal gland. The adrenal vein is identified at its entrance into the renal vein and then carefully skeletonized. Ligation of adrenal vein then allows for identification of a plane between the adrenal gland and the upper pole of the kidney (see Fig. 23.2C and D). An abundance of small veins and arterial branches course along the inferior border of the adrenal gland, thus careful attention toward hemostasis is important. Once a plane is fully developed, the adrenal gland is pulled in the medial direction, and the psoas muscle should come into view behind the upper pole of the kidney.

In preparation for rapid and careful extraction of the donor kidney, the laparoscopic instruments are removed and a 7- to 8-cm horizontal Pfannenstiel incision is made in open fashion and carried through the rectus fascia, just down to the level of the peritoneum at midline.

The laparoscopic instruments are returned to the abdomen, and the ureter is sharply divided at the level of the bifurcation of the common iliac artery. The gonadal vessels are ligated at a similar level. The lateral attachments between the donor kidney and body wall are divided with electrocautery. At this point, the only remaining attachments are the vessels of the donor kidney (see Fig. 23.2E and F).

The kidney is elevated to optimize and maximize length to the renal vessels. An endovascular stapler and a surgical clip are deployed across the renal artery as near to the aorta as safely possible. The renal artery is transected above this staple line and clip. An endovascular stapler and a surgical clip are deployed across the renal vein as near to the interaortocaval region as safely possible. The renal vein is transected above the staple line and clip.

The peritoneum is incised at the previously developed Pfannenstiel incision. The hand of a second surgeon is introduced into the peritoneal cavity, and the donor kidney is retrieved under direct laparoscopic vision. The kidney is immediately handed to the recipient surgeon and flushed with cold preservation solution. The fascia of the Pfannenstiel incision is closed and the abdomen is reinsufflated. Careful inspection ensures adequate hemostasis. Additional port sites are closed after removal of all laparoscopic trocars.

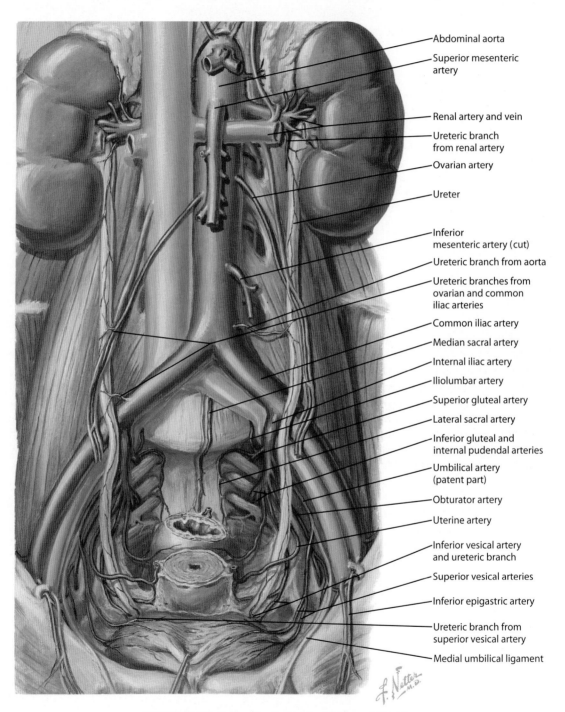

Abdominal aorta

Superior mesenteric artery

Renal artery and vein

Ureteric branch from renal artery

Ovarian artery

Ureter

Inferior mesenteric artery (cut)

Ureteric branch from aorta

Ureteric branches from ovarian and common iliac arteries

Common iliac artery

Median sacral artery

Internal iliac artery

Iliolumbar artery

Superior gluteal artery

Lateral sacral artery

Inferior gluteal and internal pudendal arteries

Umbilical artery (patent part)

Obturator artery

Uterine artery

Inferior vesical artery and ureteric branch

Superior vesical arteries

Inferior epigastric artery

Ureteric branch from superior vesical artery

Medial umbilical ligament

FIGURE 23.3 Blood supply of ureters and bladder.

SUGGESTED READINGS

Ratner LE, Ciseck LJ, Moore RG, Cigarroa FG, Kaufman HS, Kavoussi LR. Laparoscopic live donor nephrectomy. Transplantation 1995;60(9):1047–9.

Ratner LE, Montgomery RA, Kavoussi LR. Laparoscopic live donor nephrectomy: a review of the first five years. Urol Clin North Am 2001;28(4):709–19. Review.

Su LM, Ratner LE, Montgomery RA, Jarrett TW, Trock BJ, Sinkov V, et al. Laparoscopic live donor nephrectomy: trends in donor and recipient morbidity. Ann Surg 2004;240(2):358–63.

Tan H, Orloff M, Marcos A, et al. Laparoscopic live-donor nephrectomy: development of a new standard in renal transplantation. Graft 2002;5:405–16.

Deceased Donor Organ Recovery

Teresa Diago-Uso and Bijan Eghtesad

INTRODUCTION

Organ transplantation is the only viable lifesaving option for many patients with end-stage organ failure. The progress in transplant procedures and post-transplant care has resulted in decreased morbidity and mortality after transplantation. More patients with end-stage organ failure are now being placed on the waiting list, resulting in more need for lifesaving organs.

The sources of organs are either from living donors, which are discussed in another chapter, or deceased donors, defined as donation from those with neurologic criteria or brain-dead donors (DBD), and donation with cardiocirculatory criteria or donation after cardiac death donors (DCD). In this section we discuss organ recovery from deceased donors and focus on the process and procedures to safely recover abdominal organs for transplantation.

ABDOMINAL ORGAN RECOVERY

After the initial evaluation of the donor and confirmatory tests for brain death, and after obtaining consent for donation, the donor is brought to the operating room for recovery of assigned organs.

A long midline incision is made from the suprasternal notch to the symphysis pubis. The sternum is split with a sternal saw. After control of sternal bleeding, a sternal retractor is placed to open the sternum, and a Balfour retractor is placed to open the abdominal cavity. At this point, thoracic and abdominal recovery teams can work simultaneously on both sides of the diaphragm (Fig. 24.1A and B).

After the initial exploration for possible pathology, the umbilical ligament is divided between 0-silk ties, and the falciform ligament is divided to the level of the suprahepatic inferior vena cava (IVC). The left triangular ligament is divided to the level of left hepatic vein and IVC, taking care not to injure the stomach. The right triangular ligament is divided and the attachments between the right lobe of the liver and retroperitoneum are divided to the level of right hepatic vein. At this point, the retrohepatic IVC and adrenal gland can be visualized.

It is good practice to dissect the lower abdominal aorta and prepare it for cannulation (see Fig. 24.1A, C–E). In cases of donor instability, there may be a need to cannulate and flush the organs in an immediate fashion. It is also important to dissect and isolate the supraceliac aorta because it may not be possible to cross-clamp the thoracic aorta at the time the organs are flushed with the preservative solution. For isolation of the supraceliac aorta, the diaphragmatic muscles of the crura are divided longitudinally and the aorta is visualized. After dissection, the aorta can be isolated with umbilical tape should the need arise to clamp the aorta below the diaphragm.

The practice of recovery of abdominal organs can be different in transplant programs. Accordingly, the two methods of initial dissection of the recovery are called classic/standard, or rapid, technique.

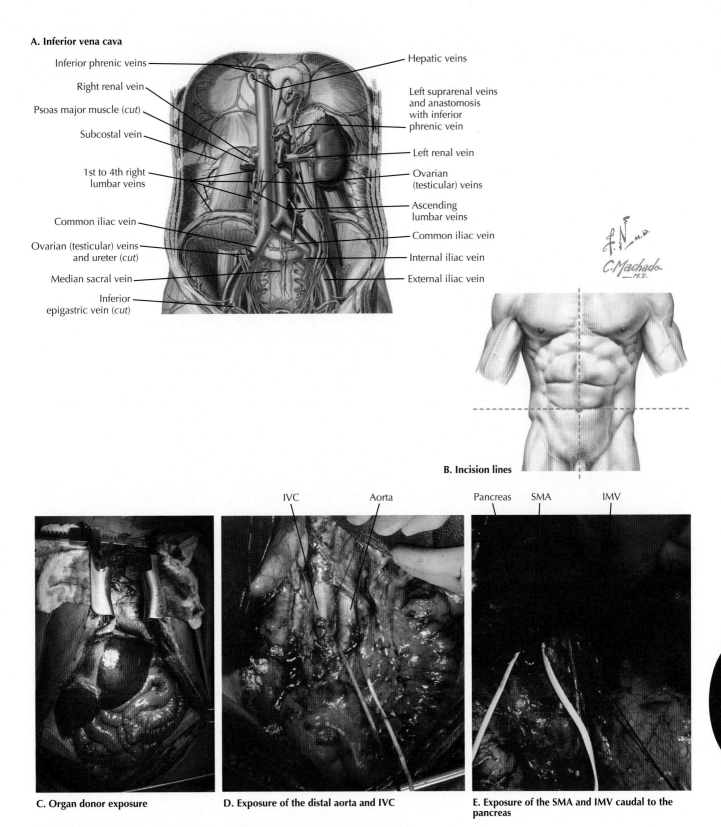

A. Inferior vena cava

Inferior phrenic veins

Right renal vein

Psoas major muscle (*cut*)

Subcostal vein

1st to 4th right lumbar veins

Common iliac vein

Ovarian (testicular) veins and ureter (*cut*)

Median sacral vein

Inferior epigastric vein (*cut*)

Hepatic veins

Left suprarenal veins and anastomosis with inferior phrenic vein

Left renal vein

Ovarian (testicular) veins

Ascending lumbar veins

Common iliac vein

Internal iliac vein

External iliac vein

B. Incision lines

IVC   Aorta   Pancreas   SMA   IMV

C. Organ donor exposure

D. Exposure of the distal aorta and IVC

E. Exposure of the SMA and IMV caudal to the pancreas

FIGURE 24.1 Abdominal anatomy and organ procurement exposures.

IMV, Inferior mesenteric vein; *IVC,* inferior vena cava; *SMA,* superior mesenteric artery.

STANDARD TECHNIQUE

After isolation of the liver from surrounding ligaments, the dissection is focused on the gastro-hepatic ligament. There is an 18% chance for the presence of an accessory or left hepatic artery originating from the left gastric artery (Fig. 24.2). This should be isolated and preserved. The rest of the ligament is divided. Both the hilum of the liver and the posterior hilum (the area behind the portal vein and bile duct) are inspected for an arterial pulse. Presence of a pulse in the posterior hilum can signify the presence of an accessory or replaced right hepatic artery or a completely replaced hepatic artery originating from superior mesenteric artery (SMA) (see Fig. 24.2). Care should be taken not to damage this artery at the time of recovery. The bile duct is isolated and divided close to the duodenal wall. Devascularization of the bile duct by dissection from its surrounding tissue should be avoided. The hepatic artery and gastroduodenal artery are isolated and evaluated for a pulse. The portal vein is also isolated and skeletonized. Dissection of the left gastric artery and splenic artery to the celiac artery can be done at this time or preferably during the "cold dissection" after the organs are flushed. Dissection of the splenic artery before cross-clamping is helpful when the pancreas is being recovered as well. This can minimize the risk of damaging these arteries in a cold and pulseless environment. The liver is dissected and ready to be removed after flushing the abdominal organs with preservative solution.

Dissection is continued by medial mobilization of the right colon and duodenum to expose the right kidney and ureter. Next, the left colon is mobilized off the left kidney and ureter. The IVC and abdominal aorta are exposed to the level of the renal vessels and the origin of the superior mesenteric artery from the aorta.

RAPID TECHNIQUE

Use of this technique minimizes the dissection until after the organs are flushed with preservation solution and cooled with ice. This is a good technique for unstable donors and for DCD donors. Some transplant centers prefer to perform all donations in this fashion. After the initial quick evaluation of organs, the lower abdominal aortal is dissected and a cannula placed for the cold flush. Cross-clamping is performed either on the supraceliac aorta or descending thoracic aorta, and venting is done by cutting the suprailiac IVC or, preferably, the supradiaphragmatic IVC in the pericardium. After the organs are flushed with the cold preservation solution, the abdominal cavity is packed with ice for external cooling. This is followed by regular dissection and recovery of all the organs. This is the most preferred method for organ recovery in DCD donors.

Flushing of intra-abdominal organs and cross-clamping of the aorta should be synchronized with the thoracic team. There should be a mutual agreement about where and when to cross-clamp the aorta and whether the IVC is to be vented in the supradiaphragmatic space and pericardium.

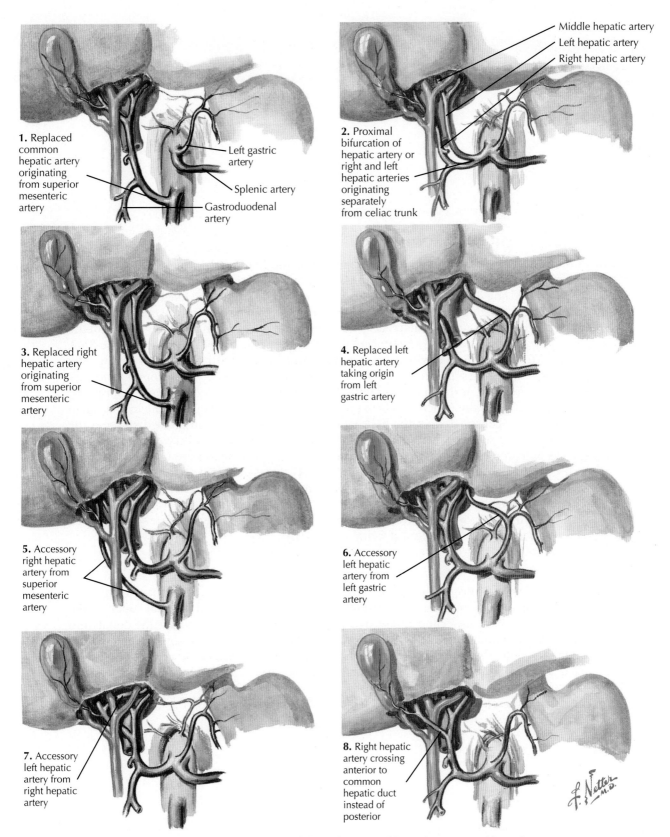

FIGURE 24.2 Variations in origin and course of hepatic artery and branches.

RECOVERY OF THE LIVER

After the dissection of the duodenohepatic ligament, the left gastric artery is dissected and divided at the level of lesser curvature of stomach and followed to the celiac artery. The splenic artery is followed and divided close to its origin from the celiac artery. The length of the remaining splenic artery depends on whether the pancreas is being recovered. In case of the latter, the splenic artery is divided close to the celiac artery with a margin. This enables safe closure of the artery on the proximal side. The superior mesenteric artery is followed to the aorta. The SMA and celiac artery are removed with a patch of abdominal aorta, with care not to damage the origin of the renal arteries. It is important to inspect for and preserve any superior polar arteries to the kidneys from the aorta. In cases in which there is an arterial branch to the liver originating from the SMA and the pancreas is being recovered, the arterial branch to the liver is taken at the SMA and reconstructed on the back table. The portal vein is then divided either at the level of splenic and superior mesenteric vein if there is no pancreas recovery or, in the case of a pancreas procurement, the mid-portion of the portal vein. This spares enough portal vein to be used with the pancreas graft for transplant. The IVC above the renal veins is divided at this point. The suprahepatic IVC and part of the diaphragm attached to the liver are excised with the liver to be subsequently dissected on the back table. After removal of the liver from the donor, it is flushed with preservative solution through the portal vein and hepatic artery and packed on ice to be transferred to the donor hospital (Fig. 24.3A).

RECOVERY OF PANCREAS

Most of the pancreatic dissection can be done before the cross-clamp as standard technique. The duodenum and pancreas are recovered together with the spleen and vascular supply to the pancreas. As part of the dissection and recovery process, some programs irrigate the duodenum with a cleansing solution such as betadine, before transecting it at the postpyloric and duodenojejunal junction. The pancreas is then separated from attachments to the transverse colon, stomach, and omentum with care not to damage the splenic vein and artery coursing alongside the pancreas.

The pancreas is removed with the spleen attached to its tail (Fig. 24.3B).

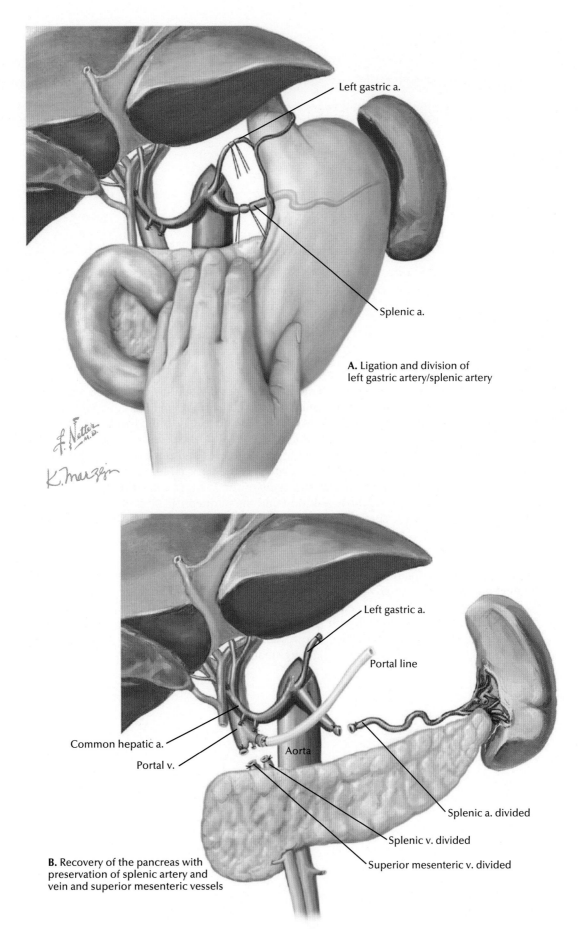

A. Ligation and division of left gastric artery/splenic artery

B. Recovery of the pancreas with preservation of splenic artery and vein and superior mesenteric vessels

FIGURE 24.3 Recovery of the liver and pancreas.

RECOVERY OF KIDNEYS

Kidneys are the last organs to be removed. The ureters are divided distally in the pelvis with preservation of the surrounding retroperitoneal tissue, which may include gonadal veins and small arteries supplying the ureter (Fig. 24.4A). These are dissected to the level of kidneys.

The aorta and IVC are also dissected en bloc to the level of renal vessels (Fig. 24.4B). The kidneys are then dissected from the colon and other structures and removed with the ureters, aorta, and the IVC. They are subsequently separated on the back table. Some surgeons prefer to do the dissection and separation in situ and remove the kidneys individually. The kidneys are then flushed with more preservative solution and the perinephric fat is removed to ensure there is no pathology present. The kidneys are then packed on ice and prepared for transport.

RECOVERY OF ILIAC VESSELS FOR GRAFT

After recovery of all the organs, the iliac vessels are removed for use as potential vascular grafts for the liver and pancreas. Removal of iliac arteries and veins should be done with care not to damage these vessels. These vessels can be indispensable when needed as conduit in the recipient. The vessels should be removed with the perivascular tissues and lymphatics to minimize potential damage to the vessels. If needed, the vessels are prepared on the back table by removing all extraneous tissue and repairing or ligating small branches from the vessels.

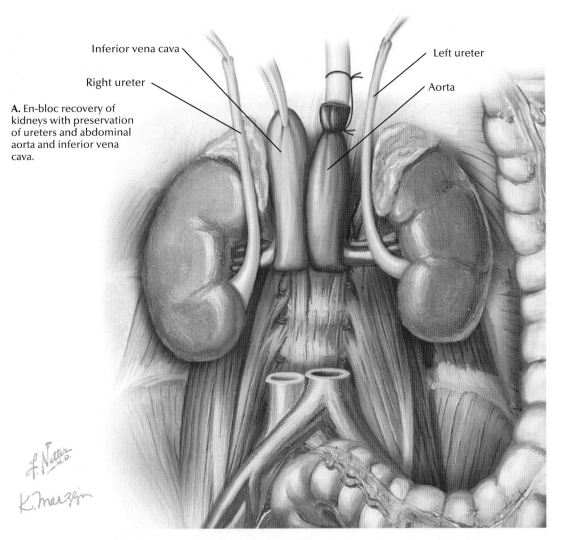

Inferior vena cava

Right ureter

Left ureter

Aorta

A. En-bloc recovery of kidneys with preservation of ureters and abdominal aorta and inferior vena cava.

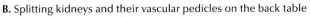

B. Splitting kidneys and their vascular pedicles on the back table

Left kidney

Aorta

Inferior vena cava

Right kidney

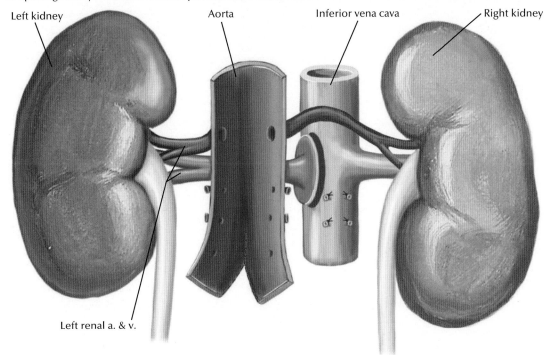

Left renal a. & v.

FIGURE 24.4 Recovery of kidneys.

SUGGESTED READINGS

Miller C, Mazzaferro V, Makowka L, et al. Rapid flush technique for donor hepatectomy: safety and efficacy of an improved method of liver recovery for transplantation. Transplant Proc 1988;20(1 suppl 1):948–50.

Rosenthal JT, Shaw BW Jr, Hardesty RL, et al. Principles of multiple organ procurement from cadaver donors. Ann Surg 1983;198(5):617–21.

Starzl TE, Hakala TR, Shaw BW Jr, et al. A flexible procedure for multiple cadaveric organ procurement. Surg Gynecol Obstet 1984;158(3):223–30.

Lower Gastrointestinal

SECTION EDITOR: Scott R. Steele

Appendectomy

Michael A. Valente

 VIDEO

25.1 Appendectomy

INTRODUCTION

The first recorded appendectomy was performed by Claudius Amyand in December 1735. Since that time, it has become the standard of care for the treatment of acute appendicitis because of its efficacy and low morbidity. The term *appendectomy* was first coined by pathological anatomist Reginald Fitz in 1886, in which he described the clinical features of acute appendicitis and advocated for early surgical treatment. Appendicitis is a worldwide disease, which in the United States carries a 1 in 15 lifetime risk, with approximately 300,000 appendectomies performed each year.

Appendectomy is the most common emergency operation in the United States and throughout the world. Because of its frequency, a thorough knowledge of the diagnostic evaluation, preoperative considerations, operative decision making, anatomic variations, and various operative techniques for appendectomy is critical for every abdominal surgeon.

ANATOMIC PRINCIPLES OF PHYSICAL EXAMINATION AND DIAGNOSIS

There is considerable variation in the clinical presentation of appendicitis. The "classic" patient experiences several hours of periumbilical pain that migrates to the right lower quadrant (RLQ) of the abdomen, usually in association with anorexia. The migration of the pain is mediated by the separate innervation of visceral and parietal peritoneum. Appendiceal obstruction and inflammation, which occur early in the disease process, cause appendiceal swelling and stretching of the visceral peritoneum. This irritation of the visceral peritoneum results in activation of autonomic afferent nerves of the superior mesenteric ganglion at the level of thoracic spinal level 10, which results in a nonspecific, poorly localized epigastric or periumbilical pain (Fig. 25.1). Ileus, nausea, anorexia, and diarrhea may also be mediated in this manner. Once inflammation reaches the parietal surface of the peritoneum (e.g., through inflammation or perforation), somatic sensory fibers create more localized pain in the RLQ, with findings of localized peritonitis involving abdominal wall rigidity, distention, and hyperesthesia.

Physical examination of the patient with appendicitis may further localize inflammation and determine the stage of the diagnosis. Severe tenderness in the RLQ is typical. Well-recognized and reproducible signs include RLQ pain upon palpation of the left abdomen (i.e., Rovsing sign) and internal rotation of the right hip, resulting in the motion of deep pelvic musculature, which can cause pain in the case of pelvic appendicitis (i.e., obturator sign). Pain with extension of the right hip is caused by motion of the psoas muscle posterior to the cecum (i.e., psoas sign) (Fig. 25.2A).

Although the diagnosis of appendicitis may often be made with physical examination alone, computed tomography (CT) has been used increasingly for the evaluation of patients with appendiceal pathology because of its high sensitivity and specificity. Coronal and sagittal reconstructions provide excellent anatomic detail that is useful in surgical planning (Fig. 25.2B and C).

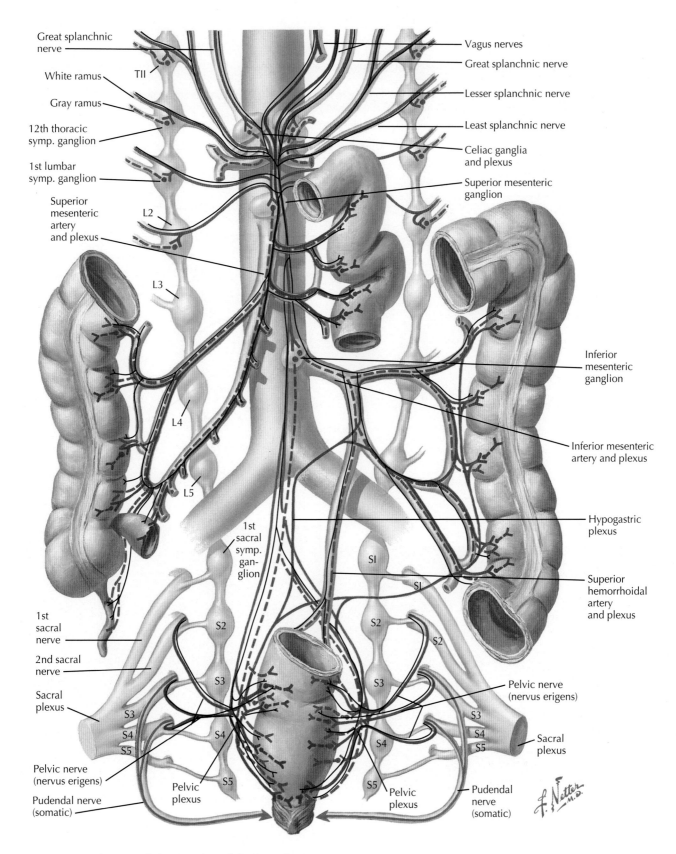

FIGURE 25.1 Autonomic innervation of the intestine.

Symp., Sympathetic; *T11,* 11th thoracic.

A. Cross-sectional anatomy at the sacral promontory

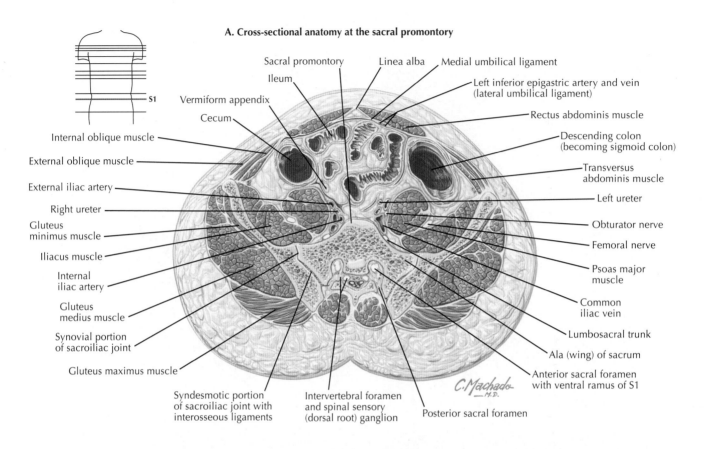

- Sacral promontory
- Linea alba
- Medial umbilical ligament
- Ileum
- Left inferior epigastric artery and vein (lateral umbilical ligament)
- Vermiform appendix
- Rectus abdominis muscle
- Cecum
- Descending colon (becoming sigmoid colon)
- Internal oblique muscle
- Transversus abdominis muscle
- External oblique muscle
- Left ureter
- External iliac artery
- Obturator nerve
- Right ureter
- Femoral nerve
- Gluteus minimus muscle
- Psoas major muscle
- Iliacus muscle
- Internal iliac artery
- Common iliac vein
- Gluteus medius muscle
- Lumbosacral trunk
- Synovial portion of sacroiliac joint
- Ala (wing) of sacrum
- Gluteus maximus muscle
- Anterior sacral foramen with ventral ramus of S1
- Syndesmotic portion of sacroiliac joint with interosseous ligaments
- Intervertebral foramen and spinal sensory (dorsal root) ganglion
- Posterior sacral foramen

C. Machado
_M.D._

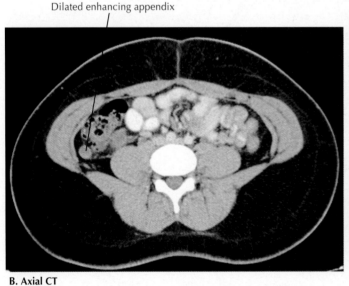

Dilated enhancing appendix

B. Axial CT

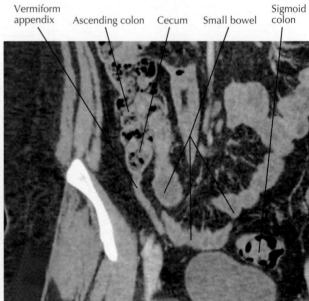

- Vermiform appendix
- Ascending colon
- Cecum
- Small bowel
- Sigmoid colon

C. Oblique coronal reconstruction, abdominal CT

FIGURE 25.2 Cross-sectional periappendicular anatomy.
CT, Computed tomography; *S1,* 1st sacral vertebra.

SURGICAL PRINCIPLES

Operative Anatomy

The vermiform (L. vermis, wormlike) appendix is a blind intestinal diverticulum (5 to 10 cm in length), which arises from the posteromedial aspect of the cecal base (Fig. 25.3). The position of the appendix is variable, with more than half located in the retrocecal location (Fig. 25.4). The appendix receives its blood supply from the appendiceal artery, a terminal branch of the ileocolic pedicle, which is supplied by the superior mesenteric artery. The appendiceal artery often travels posterior to the terminal ileum and into the mesoappendix, but the surgeon must be aware of the many variations of the appendicular and cecal arterial supply (Fig. 25.5).

The terminal ileum joins the cecum at the ileocecal valve and generally lies medial to the appendiceal base (Fig. 25.6A). The right ureter lies within the retroperitoneum and is usually located medial to the appendix. Its location must be considered when dissection in the region is performed, especially when there is an intense inflammatory reaction or abscess/phlegmon or a retrocecal location. The appendix often courses over the right external iliac vessels into the pelvis (Fig. 25.6B). Laparoscopically, relational anatomy must be conceptualized because wide visualization is more limited; Fig. 25.7 shows a laparoscopic depiction as well an intraoperative image of the relevant anatomy.

Identification of the appendiceal base and full resection of the entire length of the appendix are critical to avoid partial appendectomy, or retained appendiceal fecolith. Complete appendectomy prevents recurrent infection of the appendiceal stump and decreases the likelihood of having a stump blowout with resultant abscess or fistula formation. Additionally, ligation of the appendiceal stump in an area of healthy tissue away from inflammation is necessary to ensure safe closure of the cecal base. Full dissection of the appendix along its course, followed by firm but atraumatic traction on the appendix, can aid in directing dissection to allow visualization of the base of the appendix. Before division, the terminal ileum, base of the cecum, and retroperitoneum should be identified and preserved (see Fig. 25.6A).

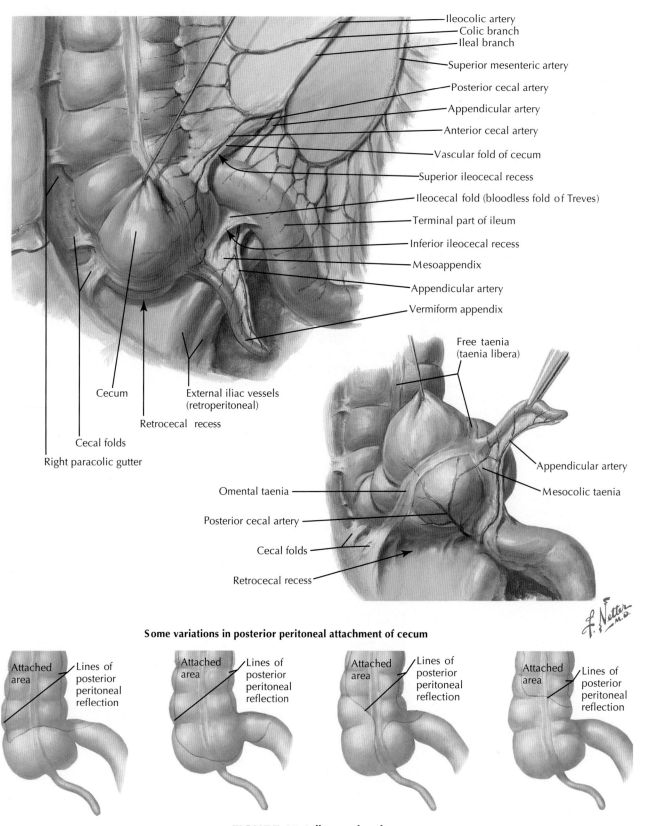

Ileocolic artery
Colic branch
Ileal branch
Superior mesenteric artery
Posterior cecal artery
Appendicular artery
Anterior cecal artery
Vascular fold of cecum
Superior ileocecal recess
Ileocecal fold (bloodless fold of Treves)
Terminal part of ileum
Inferior ileocecal recess
Mesoappendix
Appendicular artery
Vermiform appendix

Cecum
External iliac vessels
(retroperitoneal)
Retrocecal recess
Cecal folds
Right paracolic gutter

Free taenia
(taenia libera)
Appendicular artery
Mesocolic taenia
Omental taenia
Posterior cecal artery
Cecal folds
Retrocecal recess

Some variations in posterior peritoneal attachment of cecum

Attached area — Lines of posterior peritoneal reflection

Attached area — Lines of posterior peritoneal reflection

Attached area — Lines of posterior peritoneal reflection

Attached area — Lines of posterior peritoneal reflection

FIGURE 25.3 Ileocecal region.

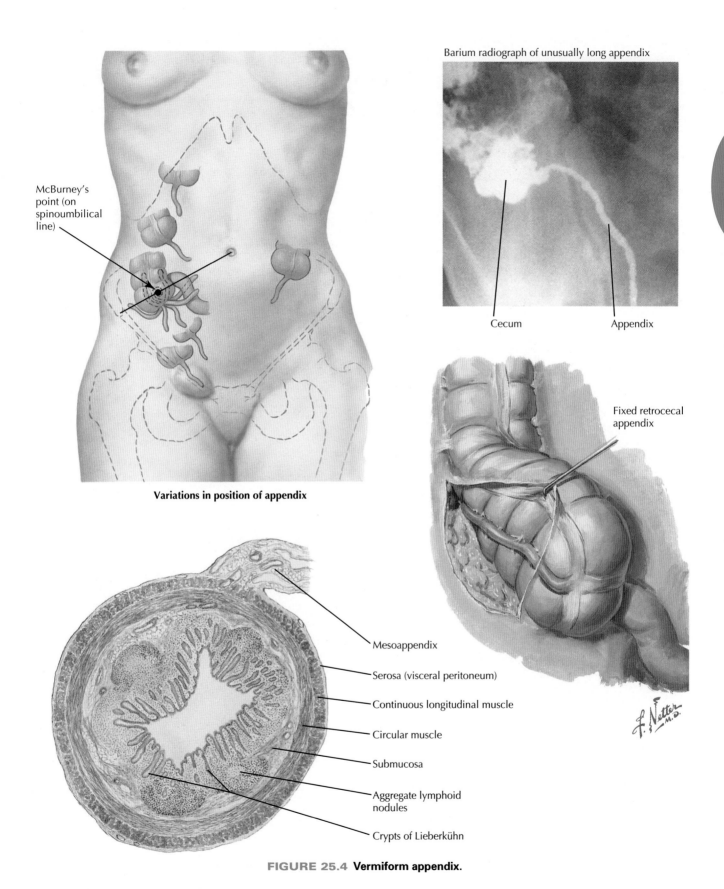

McBurney's point (on spinoumbilical line)

Variations in position of appendix

Barium radiograph of unusually long appendix

Cecum   Appendix

Fixed retrocecal appendix

Mesoappendix

Serosa (visceral peritoneum)

Continuous longitudinal muscle

Circular muscle

Submucosa

Aggregate lymphoid nodules

Crypts of Lieberkühn

FIGURE 25.4 Vermiform appendix.

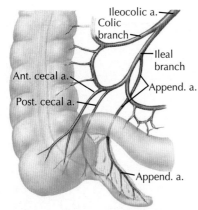

Anterior cecal and posterior cecal arteries originate from arcade between colic and ileal branches of ileocolic appendicular artery from ileal branch

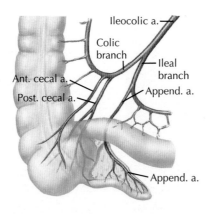

Anterior cecal and posterior cecal arteries originate from colic branch; appendicular artery from ileal branch of ileocolic artery

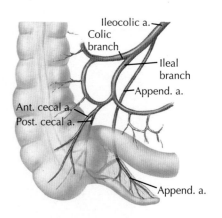

Anterior cecal and posterior cecal arteries have common origin from arcade; appendicular artery from ileocolic artery proper

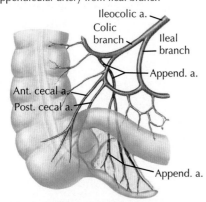

Anterior cecal and posterior cecal arteries originate from arcade between colic and ileal branches of ileocolic artery; appendicular artery from colic branch bifurcates high

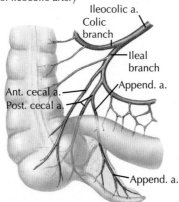

Anterior cecal and posterior cecal arteries originate from ileal branch of ileocolic artery; appendicular artery from posterior cecal

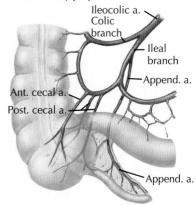

Anterior cecal and two posterior cecal arteries originate from arcade; appendicular artery from ileal branch of ileocolic artery

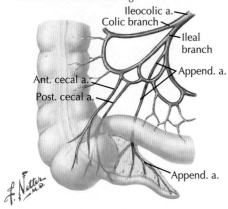

Multiple arcades between ileal branch and colic branch of ileocolic artery. Anterior cecal and posterior cecal originate from these arcades; appendicular artery from ileal branch

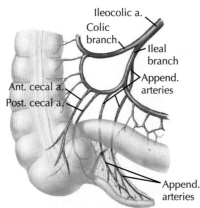

Anterior cecal and posterior cecal arteries originate from arcade between colic and ileal branches of ileocolic artery; two appendicular arteries, one deriving from arcade, the other from ileal branch, are present

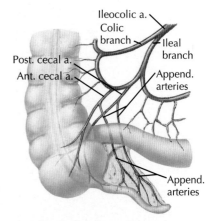

Anterior cecal and posterior cecal arteries originate from arcade; two appendicular arteries, one deriving from anterior cecal, the other from posterior cecal, are present

FIGURE 25.5 Variations in cecal and appendicular arteries.

A. Ileocecal region

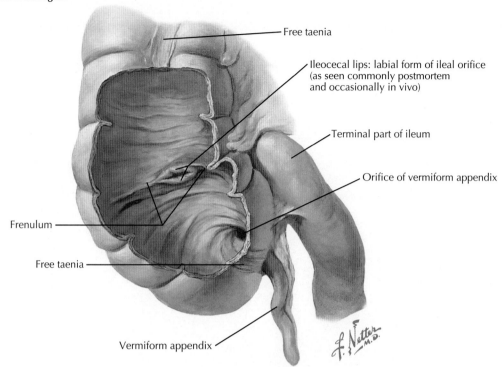

Free taenia

Ileocecal lips: labial form of ileal orifice (as seen commonly postmortem and occasionally in vivo)

Terminal part of ileum

Orifice of vermiform appendix

Frenulum

Free taenia

Vermiform appendix

B. Iliac vessels

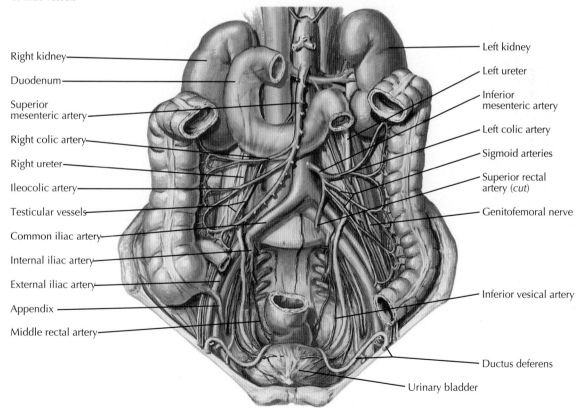

Right kidney

Duodenum

Superior mesenteric artery

Right colic artery

Right ureter

Ileocolic artery

Testicular vessels

Common iliac artery

Internal iliac artery

External iliac artery

Appendix

Middle rectal artery

Left kidney

Left ureter

Inferior mesenteric artery

Left colic artery

Sigmoid arteries

Superior rectal artery (*cut*)

Genitofemoral nerve

Inferior vesical artery

Ductus deferens

Urinary bladder

FIGURE 25.6 Ileocecal region and iliac vessels.

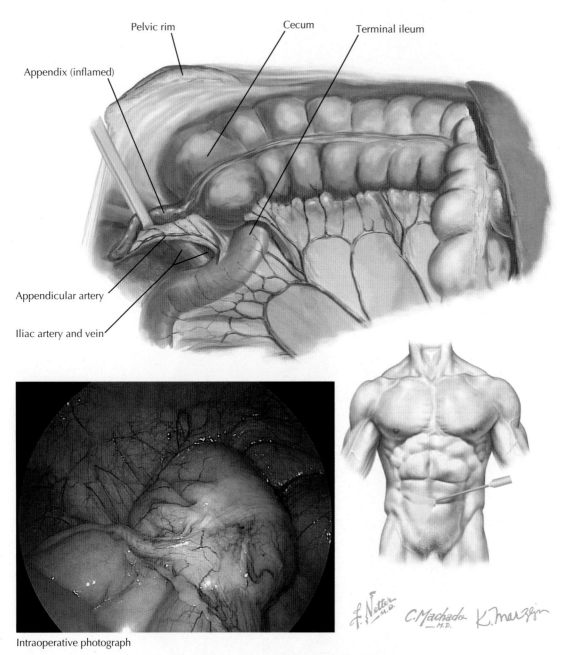

Pelvic rim

Cecum

Terminal ileum

Appendix (inflamed)

Appendicular artery

Iliac artery and vein

Intraoperative photograph

FIGURE 25.7 Right lower quadrant anatomy: laparoscopic view.

Anatomic Principles of Exposure

When the laparoscopic approach is used, placing the patient in a left-side down and Trendelenburg position aids visualization by employing gravity to retract the intestinal structures away from the RLQ and cecum. The small intestine can be manipulated manually into the left upper quadrant to prevent injury and aid in visualization. The greater omentum often wraps the ileocecal area, localizing the infectious process to the RLQ. Blunt dissection using an atraumatic laparoscopic instrument with gentle traction can mobilize the omentum away from the cecum, revealing the appendix. The challenges of dissection in appendectomy are typically related to inflammatory changes that make the appendix adherent to inflamed surrounding tissues. Again, blunt dissection in this setting is most effective for safely separating inflamed tissues.

In the open setting, incision length and type should allow adequate visualization of the critical anatomy. The choice of incision should be based on the patient's body habitus, previous surgical sites, physical examination findings, preoperative imaging, and surgeon preference. Use of small, handheld Richardson or appendiceal retractors is standard practice when an RLQ *Rocky-Davis* (transverse) or *McBurney* (oblique) incision is used. Retrocecal appendicitis may also be approached in this manner, although a somewhat longer incision is often required to mobilize the cecum adequately for appendectomy. When the surgeon uses an open approach, patients with perforated appendicitis, generalized peritonitis, or those with suspected neoplastic processes may be best approached with the use of a standard midline laparotomy.

SURGICAL TECHNIQUE

Laparoscopic Approach

Midline umbilical access is accomplished by using the open Hassan technique, and pneumoperitoneum is established. Next, using laparoscopic assistance and avoiding the inferior epigastric vessels, the surgeon places a 12-mm port in the left lower quadrant, which allows use of a stapling device and provides an aperture for specimen removal at the conclusion of the procedure. A third suprapubic port offers a good cosmetic option but is not always appropriate, depending on the patient's anatomy. Alternative approaches include use of a periumbilical port for stapling and specimen removal.

The patient is placed in the Trendelenburg position, and the operating table is tilted with the right side up. This arrangement facilitates exposure of the RLQ. Initial exploration includes retraction of the omentum, evaluation for abscesses or collections, and evaluation of the adnexal structures.

The tip of the appendix is identified and dissected free from the periappendiceal structures, which can include the adnexa, gonadal vessels, and ureter. Once freed, the appendix is grasped and elevated by using an atraumatic grasper. An aperture in the mesoappendix is created bluntly at its base along the wall of the appendix using a fine dissector. This window is widened to admit a bowel grasper to identify the cecal-appendiceal junction clearly. The mesoappendix is then ligated with a vascular stapler or an energy device, or alternatively the appendiceal artery may be dissected, clipped, and sharply transected. A suture loop or laparoscopic tissue stapler is then used to ligate or divide the appendiceal base. This step of the procedure is performed at a site where tissue quality is healthy. If there is any doubt about tissue quality, the stapler may be applied slightly onto the base of the cecum. If a portion of the cecum is to be removed, the surgeon must take extra care to ensure there is adequate distance from the ileocecal valve to avoid narrowing the entrance of the ileum into the colon (see Fig. 25.6A).

The appendix is placed in a specimen bag and removed through the 12-mm port in the left lower quadrant. Any abscess or fluid collections can be irrigated before closure. If needed, a closed-suction drain can be left in place at the site of an abscess.

Open Technique

A standardized incision for appendectomy has never been established, and therefore each patient's incision should be approached on a case-by-case basis. An open incision is traditionally made at McBurney's point, located one-third the distance between the anterior superior iliac spine and the umbilicus (on the spinoumbilical line) (see Fig. 25.4). This area generally corresponds to the location of the base of the appendix. Subcutaneous tissues are opened to the level of the external oblique muscle by using electrocautery, and its fascia is incised parallel to its fibers. External oblique fibers run inferomedially and are separated along their length, exposing the internal oblique muscle and then the transversus abdominis muscle. These muscles also are preserved and separated through blunt retraction along their length. The peritoneum is opened sharply, with caution taken to avoid injury to underlying viscera. Occasionally, the incision must be extended medially toward the rectus abdominus muscle, which can be transected if necessary.

The RLQ is explored to identify the pathology. A finger sweep can be used to identify an inflamed appendix, which typically feels firm and indurated, revealing its location. Alternatively, identification of the decussation of the three taenia coli (omentum, mesocolic, libera taeniae) can be used to identify the base of the appendix (see Fig. 25.3). The appendix should be followed to the tip to ensure complete resection. In the case of a retrocecal appendix, the cecum may have to be mobilized laterally at the white line of Toldt for adequate exposure (see Fig. 25.4).

After identification and mobilization, the base of the cecum and appendix can be gently grasped with a gauze pad and pulled up into the wound. Consideration for the use of a self-retaining wound protector is encouraged. While holding traction on the appendiceal tip with the aid of a moist sponge or Babcock clamp, the surgeon sequentially divides the mesoappendix and appendiceal artery from distal to proximal to the base, freeing the appendix to be drawn out to length. Mesenteric attachments should be taken with fine clamps and ties to avoid hemorrhage when the mesentery retracts into the abdominal cavity.

Once the appendiceal base is visible, the appendix is clamped at its base; an absorbable tie is used to ligate the base. It is divided sharply distal to the tie, and the appendix is passed off the field and sent for pathological review. Alternatively, the use of a mechanical stapling device can be employed to remove the appendix.

Some surgeons invert the appendiceal stump by using a purse-string suture or Lembert-type sutures to bury the stump. Additionally, the use of electrocautery can be used on the stump to ensure no appendiceal mucosa is left behind. Although the necessity of these maneuvers has not been proven to be beneficial, these adjunct steps may be used, provided that the tissue quality of the cecum is appropriately pliant.

The peritoneum is closed with a running absorbable suture, and then the internal oblique and transversus muscles are closed in either running or interrupted fashion, followed by closure of the external oblique. If significant purulence or gangrenous changes are found during the operation, consideration can be made to leave the skin incision open to avoid postoperative wound infection.

SUGGESTED READINGS

Cameron JL. Current surgical therapy. 12th ed. St. Louis: Mosby; 2011. p. 219–23.

Morris KT, Kavanagh M, Hansen P, et al. The rational use of computed tomography scans in the diagnosis of appendicitis. Am J Surg 2002;183(5):547.

Sauerland S, Lefering R, Neugebauer EA. Laparoscopic versus open surgery for suspected appendicitis. Cochrane Database Syst Rev 2004:CD001546.

Wei HB, Huang JL, Zheng ZH, et al. Laparoscopic versus open appendectomy: a prospective randomized comparison. Surg Endosc 2010;24(2):266–9.

Abdominal Wall Marking and Stoma Site Selection

Barbara J. Hocevar, Judith Landis-Erdman, and James S. Wu

INTRODUCTION

Intestinal stomas serve as the end of the gastrointestinal tract, protect distal anastomoses, and relieve obstruction. Small intestinal stomas frequently are used in the management of inflammatory bowel disease, familial adenomatous polyposis, motility disorders, and colorectal cancer. Colostomies are used in the treatment of colorectal cancer, diverticulitis, rectal atresia, Hirschsprung disease, and trauma.

STOMA SITE SELECTION

The optimal stoma site for an ileostomy typically would be in the right lower quadrant below the umbilicus on the summit of the infraumbilical fat mound and lateral to the midline, but within the confines of the rectus sheath. A stoma siting disc has been included in the illustrations (Fig. 26.1A and B). For a left colostomy, the left lower quadrant would be preferable. Education by a wound, ostomy, and continence (WOC) nurse can assuage many concerns about life with a stoma. Ideally, stoma sites have characteristics listed in Box 26.1. An ileostomy located at a satisfactory site is shown in Fig. 26.1C.

Techniques used for stoma site selection follow. Fig. 26.1D shows a right lower quadrant ileostomy site that has been marked with water-fast ink (X). Its position in between the midline and the lateral border of the rectus is ensured by gentle palpation. A siting disc encompasses the area around the stoma that must be flat.

Sites are chosen both in the supine and upright positions. Sites that on original marking in the supine position look perfect may prove to be unusable if they disappear into a skin crease when the patient is upright. For example, a patient (Fig. 26.2) was seen preoperatively for loop ileostomy marking. A skin crease compromised the initially selected stoma site. An alternative lower site was chosen. The remarked site then was checked with the patient sitting. The final site was marked with an India ink tattoo.

In some cases, it is not clear what type of stoma will be needed. In this instance, multiple stoma sites are selected as depicted in Fig. 26.3A.

In general, a pouching system can be maintained without changing from 3 to 7 days, depending on the volume and liquidity of the effluent. Potential adverse consequences of poor stoma site selection are listed in Box 26.2. Examples of stomas located at poor sites are shown in Fig. 26.3B through E.

SUMMARY

Stomas are created commonly in colorectal surgical practice. Ostomy placement at sites that can accommodate a pouching system and that are visible and accessible will help make postoperative stoma management easier for the patient and the surgeon. The adverse consequences of poor stoma site selection may have a significant negative impact on a patient's quality of life and ability to work. Proper preoperative stoma site selection and education may prevent some of these problems.

Box 26.1   Ideal Stoma Site Characteristics

Flat or smooth surface large enough to accommodate a pouching system
On the summit of the infraumbilical fat mound
Through the center of the rectus sheath to provide even supportive tissue around the stoma
Adequately avoiding the umbilicus, skin creases, scars, and bony prominences
Visible and accessible

Box 26.2 . Adverse Consequences of Suboptimal Stoma Site Selection

Leakage
Skin irritation and eroded tissue
Pain
Malodor
Inability to work
Need for reoperation(s)
Social isolation because of fear of leakage and odor
Financial burden of equipment replacement, reoperation, and time away from work

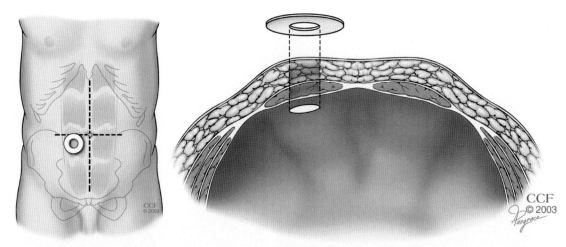

A. Four possible stoma sites, one in each quadrant surrounding the umbilicus, are defined using midline and transverse dotted lines. A stoma siting disc approximates the area needed for the ostomy and the surrounding skin barrier adhesive.

B. The stoma site is located over the rectus sheath. Different size stoma siting discs are available. The siting disc size chosen is based on the width of the patient's rectus sheath.

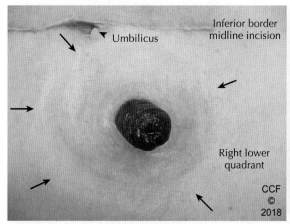

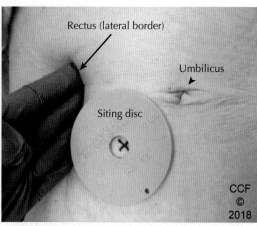

C. Right lower quadrant ileostomy. The ostomy and the peristomal skin are healthy. The border of the appliance is marked with arrows. The umbilicus is identified by an arrowhead. The ileostomy protrudes above the skin surface with a gentle inferiorly directed spout.

D. Ileostomy stoma site selection. The lateral border of the rectus muscle is defined by palpation. A siting disc is used to select a site with an appropriate 2- to 3-inch area of flat skin. The site is marked in the center of this area using water-fast ink.

FIGURE 26.1 Stoma site selection.

(Reprinted with permission, Cleveland Clinic Center for Medical Art & Photography © 2019. All Rights Reserved.)

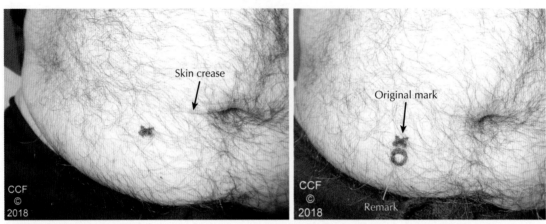

A. The initial stoma site mark selected (X) is too close to a skin crease

B. An alternative site is remarked inferiorly (O)

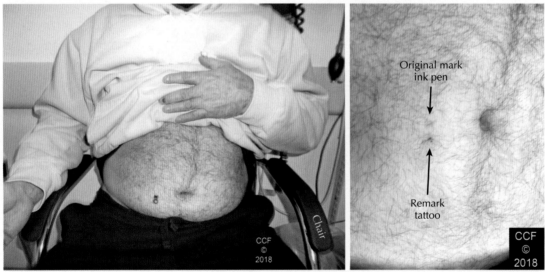

C. The sites are reexamined with the patient sitting upright in a chair

D. The remarked site is tattooed with India ink

FIGURE 26.2 Stoma site selection (continued).

(Reprinted with permission, Cleveland Clinic Center for Medical Art & Photography © 2019. All Rights Reserved.)

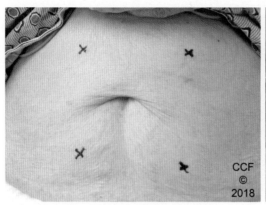

A. For this patient, in whom either ileostomy or colostomy might be selected, stoma sites were preselected in all four quadrants.

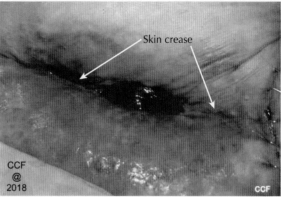

B. An ileostomy located in a skin crease (arrows). Maintaining an appliance for a normal period of time is impossible. The surrounding skin is macerated and shows partial-thickness tissue loss.

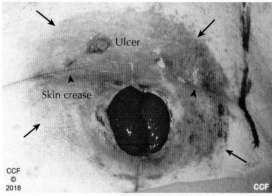

C. The skin surrounding a stoma located adjacent to a skin crease (arrowheads) is inflamed and ulcerated (arrows). Maintaining a pouching system proved difficult.

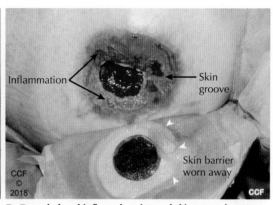

D. Denuded and inflamed peristomal skin around a stoma located in skin groove. The underside of the skin barrier is worn away from stool leaking under the pouching system (arrowheads) and corresponds to the area of skin damage.

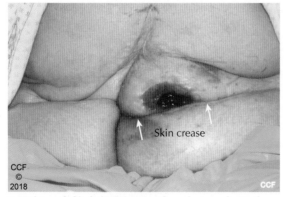

E. Peristomal skin irritation around a colostomy located close to a natural skin crease (arrows).

FIGURE 26.3 Stoma site selection and adverse consequences of poor stoma site selection.
(Reprinted with permission, Cleveland Clinic Center for Medical Art & Photography © 2019. All Rights Reserved.)

SUGGESTED READINGS

Fazio VW, Church JM, Wu JS. Atlas of intestinal stomas. NY: Springer; 2012.

Marking discs: Marlen Manufacturing & Development Co., 5150 Richmond Road Bedford, OH 44146, U.S.A.

Turnbull Jr RB, Weakley FL. Atlas of intestinal stomas. St. Louis: CV Mosby Company; 1967.

Wound Ostomy, Continence Nurses Society™. WOCN® Society and ASCRS Position Statement on Preoperative Stoma Site Marking for Patients Undergoing Colostomy or Ileostomy Surgery. NJ: Mt. Laurel; 2014.

Right Colectomy

Bradley J. Champagne

 VIDEO

27.1 Right Colectomy

INTRODUCTION

A right colectomy is performed to treat a variety of pathologies. Common indications include an unresectable polyp, colon cancer, and Crohn's disease of the terminal ileum. Ischemia, volvulus, and malignant lesions of the appendix or terminal ileum may also be indications. Resection of the terminal ileum and cecum is common to all these procedures. The distal extent of the right hemicolectomy varies, depending on the indication, oncologic principles, and adequacy of perfusion to the right or transverse colon. Laparoscopic approaches are the current standard of care, and with careful patient selection and precise operative technique, this approach improves patient recovery, using smaller incisions with a resulting decrease in patient discomfort and shorter hospital stay.

SUPERFICIAL ANATOMY AND TOPOGRAPHIC LANDMARKS

Before making an incision, either laparoscopic or open, the surgeon must understand the relationship between surface anatomy and the abdominal anatomy (Fig. 27.1A). For example, in the morbidly obese patient, surface anatomy such as the location of the umbilicus may be greatly altered. The umbilicus may reach down to the pubis and overlie a large pannus, which may distort normal relationships with internal anatomy. Additionally, in elderly patients, the cecum is often in the right upper quadrant as the lateral connective tissue loses its integrity over time.

The right colon is attached by its retroperitoneal and lateral attachments, the ileocolic and middle colic arteries. Attachments at the middle colic and lesser sac are typically the most tethered portion of the operation, often making isolation of the middle colic vessels the most difficult part of the case (Fig. 27.1B). For this reason, and the fact the transverse mesocolon is often short, laparoscopic extraction incisions can be made over the middle colic arteries.

The middle colic arteries typically lie approximately midway between the xiphoid process and the umbilicus in a non-obese patient. The inferior extent of the procedure (i.e., inferior dissection of terminal ileum and cecum) is typically only centimeters below the umbilicus and medial to the anterior superior iliac spine. Therefore, an open right colectomy can often be performed through a relatively small periumbilical midline or right-sided transverse incision in a thin patient.

ANATOMIC APPROACH TO RIGHT COLECTOMY

Different surgical approaches to the right colon have been described and include medial-to-lateral, lateral-to-medial, inferior-to-superior, and superior-to-inferior. Varying the approach can allow for a safe, oncologically appropriate operation, depending on body habitus and pathology.

Positioning and Port Placement

The patient can often be placed in a supine position; however, if the location of the tumor is unclear preoperatively or there is concern for more extensive disease (e.g., ileosigmoid fistula in a patient with Crohn's disease), the lithotomy position can prove beneficial to permit access to the anus. Both arms should be tucked at the patient's side with appropriate padding. In some cases, if the patient is obese, only one arm can be tucked safely. In these instances, the left arm should be tucked preferentially to allow for the surgeon to stand at the patient's left side. The hands and fingers should be padded and positioned with the thumbs up in a neutral position to reduce the risk of injury. A Foley catheter and orogastric tube should be placed, along with appropriate antibiotics given before skin incision.

The abdomen is prepped and draped after general anesthesia is induced. The operating surgeon stands on the left side of the patient with the assistant on the patient's right for abdominal entry. The assistant can then move to the left side, next to the surgeon, for the remainder of the operation.

Our preference is to perform a modified Hasson approach for abdominal entry. A 1-cm vertical incision is made, and the linea alba is identified. Kocher clamps are used to grasp each side of the midline, and cautery is used to open the fascia. A Kelly clamp is used to open the peritoneum bluntly, and a 10-mm port is introduced. Once this is placed, the abdomen is insufflated to 12 to 15 mm Hg with carbon dioxide, and a 10-mm scope with a 30-degree angulation is used to survey the abdomen. A 5-mm trocar is placed in the left lower quadrant 2 to 3 cm medial and superior to the anterior superior iliac spine. This is performed under direct vision with avoidance of the inferior epigastric vessels. A second 5-mm trocar is placed in the left upper quadrant one handbreadth cranially. An additional 5-mm right lower quadrant port is inserted to aide in retraction, when needed.

A. Right colectomy

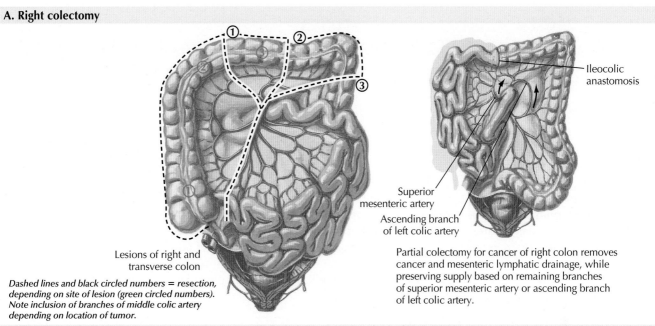

Lesions of right and
transverse colon

*Dashed lines and black circled numbers = resection,
depending on site of lesion (green circled numbers).
Note inclusion of branches of middle colic artery
depending on location of tumor.*

Partial colectomy for cancer of right colon removes
cancer and mesenteric lymphatic drainage, while
preserving supply based on remaining branches
of superior mesenteric artery or ascending branch
of left colic artery.

B. Arteries of the colon

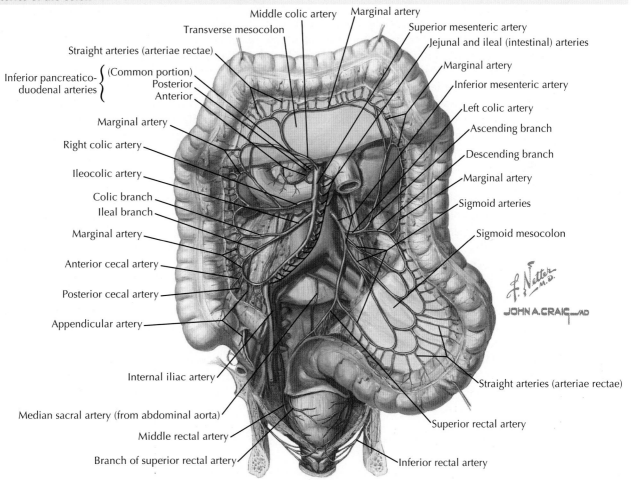

FIGURE 27.1 Right colectomy and arteries of the colon.

Medial-to-Lateral

Many surgeons prefer a medial-to-lateral approach for a laparoscopic surgery and often for an open right colectomy. This provides several benefits: the vessels are taken early in the operation, decreasing stretch and torque, and providing ligation before manipulation of the tumor in the patient with malignancy. In addition, this approach demonstrates the location of the duodenum early in the surgery.

The medial-to-lateral approach is more difficult in patients with thickened Crohn's mesentery; often the mesentery is extremely difficult to mobilize and resect and requires the use of Kelly clamps and suture ligatures. In these patients, the lateral dissection is performed early in the operation, and having obtained greater mobilization of the colon, ligation of the ileocolic vessels can safely be performed.

Identification of Ileocolic Vessels

To expose the ileocolic vessels, the small bowel must be swept to the left side or into the pelvis so that the mesentery lies flat. Grasping and lifting the mesentery just proximal to the ileocolic valve tents the ileocolic artery (ICA), even in heavy patients. Care should be taken to avoid tearing the mesenteric fat, which may result in blood loss that may obscure the operative view. A single vessel is noted extending from the superior mesenteric artery (SMA) to the ileocolic junction. Scoring the peritoneum just below this fullness, usually with electrocautery or a bipolar device, allows isolation of the pedicle. An avascular space exists below the vessel. In oncologic resections, this isolation should occur closer to and parallel to the SMA, including the lymphatic vessels, to obtain a complete mesocolic excision. If performed too distally along the ICA, many branches to the ileum will be noted as the arcades are encountered, and dissection will be more tedious.

Once the avascular plane is identified, dissection can be carried posterior to the mesentery in a superior, medial, and lateral direction within this avascular space, elevating the posterior fascia of the mesocolon off Toldt's fascia as it lies on the retroperitoneum. Borders of the space will be the mesentery of the right colon superiorly (i.e., ceiling), attachments of the colon to the liver cephalad, and Toldt's fascia laterally and posteriorly, as the retroperitoneum forms the floor of the space (Fig. 27.2).

Just lateral to the origin of the ileocolic vessels, care must be taken to prevent injury to the duodenum, which lies close to the SMA-ICA junction. Just above the duodenum, a subtle change in fat identifies the head of the pancreas, which should also be preserved. In fact, the plane anterior to the head of the pancreas mobilizes the transverse colon mesentery to complete the medial dissection for a right colectomy. Reaching the liver superiorly, the pancreas medially, and the white line of Toldt laterally facilitates later dissection (see Fig. 27.2). Once the duodenum has been identified and the proximal ICA has been isolated, this can be transected just distal to the SMA. Means of transection include energy device, clips, staplers, and ties.

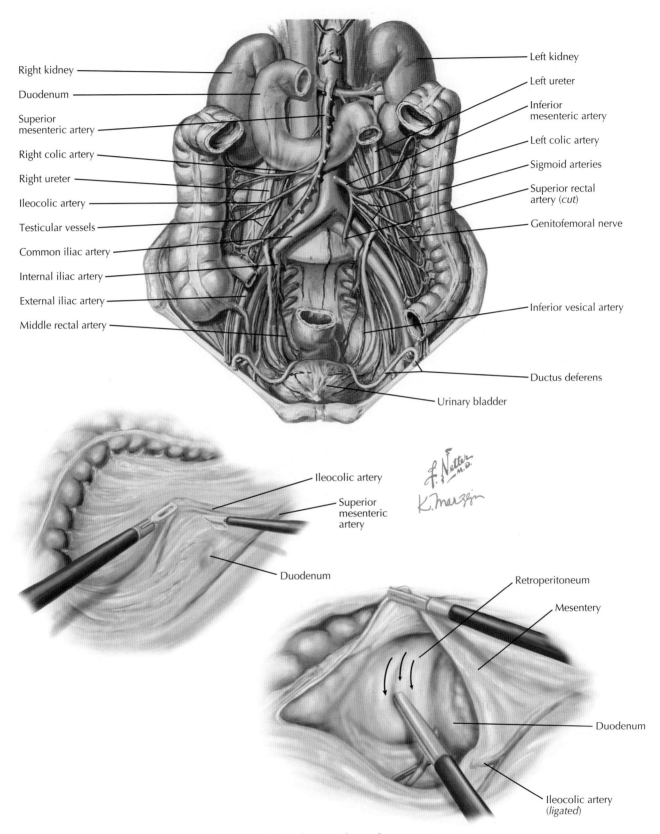

Right kidney

Duodenum

Superior
mesenteric artery

Right colic artery

Right ureter

Ileocolic artery

Testicular vessels

Common iliac artery

Internal iliac artery

External iliac artery

Middle rectal artery

Left kidney

Left ureter

Inferior
mesenteric artery

Left colic artery

Sigmoid arteries

Superior rectal
artery (*cut*)

Genitofemoral nerve

Inferior vesical artery

Ductus deferens

Urinary bladder

Ileocolic artery

Superior
mesenteric
artery

Duodenum

Retroperitoneum

Mesentery

Duodenum

Ileocolic artery
(*ligated*)

FIGURE 27.2 Retroperitoneal structures.

Variation in Arteries of Right Colon

Many textbooks demonstrate a distinct ICA and right and middle colic vessels, but arterial variation is common in this location. Often, the right colic artery (RCA) is either a branch from the ICA or not found at all. If a high ligation of the ICA is performed, the RCA may not have to be transected again. If it is a separate branch of the SMA, the RCA will also have to be transected as a high or "proximal" ligation if the operation is performed for oncologic reasons (Fig. 27.3).

Middle Colic Vessels

The middle colic anatomy is often varied. From a single vessel to more than five branches may extend from the SMA in this location. The level of transection will depend on oncologic principles (see Fig. 27.1A). If a tumor is located at the hepatic flexure or proximal transverse colon, it may be necessary to resect all the branches with a high ligation. However, for a typical right hemicolectomy, only the right branch is resected. This provides additional lymphatic information with the specimen as well as important mobility to the transverse colon.

In addition to isolating and transecting the vessels, it is important to free the mesentery extending to the bowel wall. If surgery is performed laparoscopically, torque and tension may be applied while exteriorizing the bowel. Cleaning the mesentery close to the bowel margin minimizes the risk of tension and prevents unnecessary bleeding. The marginal vessel is not divided until the specimen is removed so that pulsatile flow can be confirmed.

Omentum and Lesser Sac

To mobilize the transverse colon for an anastomosis and perform a *complete hemicolectomy,* the lesser sac must be entered. Anatomically, the easiest place to enter the lesser sac is toward the midline, where layers of the omentum and lesser sac are fused. A subtle change in color or texture of fat differentiates extraneous epiploic and colonic adipose tissue from the omentum. Typically, an avascular plane close to the colon can be identified and entered. As a general rule, for benign disease the dissection can be performed by separating the omentum off the transverse colon, whereas for hepatic flexure or transverse colon cancers, the omentum is resected en bloc with the colon.

Full dissection is ensured by visualization of the posterior aspect of the stomach, with gastroepiploic branches on the superior aspect of the stomach when elevated. The lesser sac should still be entered medially to the pathology, to ensure full mobilization. A branch of the venous drainage from the gastroepiploic vein to the colon mesentery is often noted toward the midline and may have to be transected to prevent injury.

After the lesser sac has been entered, if a full mobilization of the retroperitoneum has occurred, a thin purple plane will be noted as the hepatic flexure is approached. This will be the only remaining layer between the previous medial dissection and the hepatic flexure. Opening this layer will complete the dissection and facilitate identification of planes.

When approaching the line of Toldt from a superior approach, the surgical instruments must stay close to the colon just inside the white line, unless necessary for oncologic margins. If lateral to the line of Toldt, it is easy to migrate into the retroperitoneum and behind the kidney. Staying immediately on the colon side of the line of Toldt will help prevent entering the incorrect plane. Dissection is typically continued inferiorly to the cecum, just inside the line of Toldt, but preserving the fascia propria of the mesocolon.

Inferior Dissection

The inferior approach to the cecum, appendix, and terminal ileum creates a potential risk to the gonadal vessels and ureter. A thin, filmy plane separates the natural attachments from the retroperitoneum and must be carefully dissected. The ureter crosses the iliac vessels medial to the gonadal vessels, just inferior to the cecum or ileum. Identification of the ureter within the pelvis and following it back to the dissection plane can prevent injury. Once this plane has been entered, dissection should continue to ensure adequate mobility of the ileum for the anastomosis. If necessary, dissection of the small bowel mesentery off the retroperitoneum can continue all the way to the duodenum, without transection of any vessels.

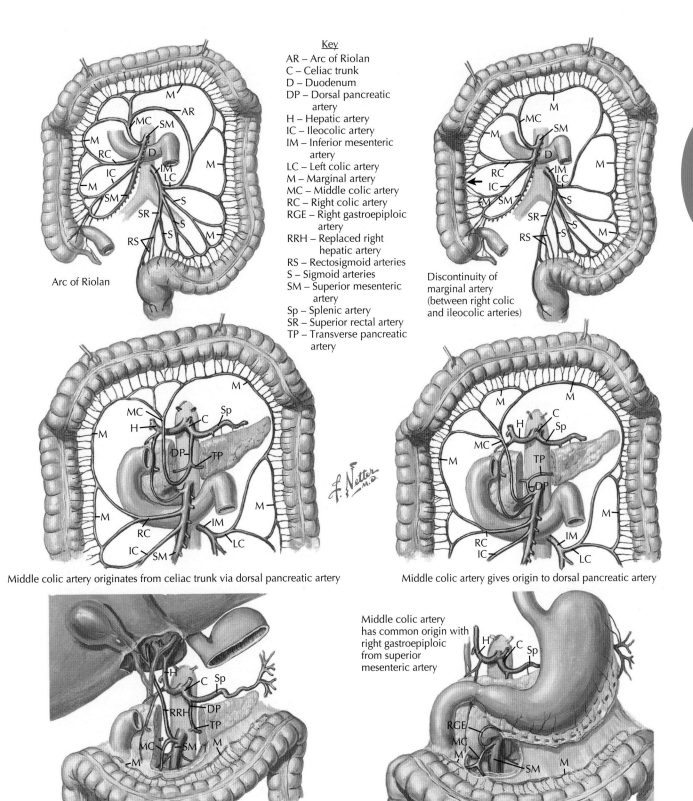

Key
AR – Arc of Riolan
C – Celiac trunk
D – Duodenum
DP – Dorsal pancreatic artery
H – Hepatic artery
IC – Ileocolic artery
IM – Inferior mesenteric artery
LC – Left colic artery
M – Marginal artery
MC – Middle colic artery
RC – Right colic artery
RGE – Right gastroepiploic artery
RRH – Replaced right hepatic artery
RS – Rectosigmoid arteries
S – Sigmoid arteries
SM – Superior mesenteric artery
Sp – Splenic artery
SR – Superior rectal artery
TP – Transverse pancreatic artery

Arc of Riolan

Discontinuity of marginal artery (between right colic and ileocolic arteries)

Middle colic artery originates from celiac trunk via dorsal pancreatic artery

Middle colic artery gives origin to dorsal pancreatic artery

Middle colic artery originates from or with replaced right hepatic artery (from sup. mesenteric a.)

Middle colic artery has common origin with right gastroepiploic from superior mesenteric artery

FIGURE 27.3 Variations in vascular anatomy of right colon.

Extracorporeal Anastomosis

The bowel should be grasped with a ratcheted grasper, pneumoperitoneum relieved, and the umbilical port removed. The umbilical incision should be extended vertically to approximately 4 cm to allow evisceration of the bowel, using a wound protector. The right colon is grasped using a Babcock clamp externally and exteriorized. Care should be taken to ensure that the mesentery is not twisted when eviscerating the bowel. The orientation of the small bowel must be confirmed several times before the actual anastomosis to preserve the anatomic clockwise rotation of the mesentery.

The terminal ileum is evaluated and divided at a site of healthy, well-perfused bowel. A linear cutting stapler is used to divide the bowel. The transverse colon is then inspected. The site of division should occur where the bowel is healthy and well perfused. Division of the mesentery and resulting pulsatile bleeding is performed to confirm good perfusion. A linear cutting stapler can be used to divide the transverse colon. Before an anastomosis is performed, both ends of the bowel should be assessed again for viability. Perfusion to the colon side should be evaluated with confirmation of arterial marginal vessel bleeding. Either a hand-sewn or stapled anastomosis may be performed. Our preference is to perform a stapled anastomosis in most situations. A hand-sewn technique may be considered in situations in which staplers may be ill advised, such as poor tissues in Crohn's disease. Enterotomies are made on the antimesenteric ends of the ileum and transverse colon, and a linear cutting stapler (i.e., GIA) is placed inside to align them in a side-to-side fashion. The linear stapler is inserted, ensuring that the mesentery is not caught in the staple line during alignment. After the first firing of the stapler, the bowel lumen is assessed for bleeding. The bowel opening is then aligned to mismatch the first staple firing, and a second TA linear stapler is used to close the ends of the bowel (an additional GIA linear staple load may be used).

To avoid the potential mesenteric "twist" and use fewer staple firings, a "Barcelona" anastomosis may also be used. In this technique, the mesentery of the bowel is divided up to the points of proximal and distal resection initially. An enterotomy and colotomy are performed on the antimesenteric portion of the small bowel and colon, respectively. The linear GIA stapler is advanced into these openings and fired along the antimesenteric border of the bowel, after ensuring the remaining mesentery is out of the way. The common enterotomy is then closed and the specimen transected with a second firing of a TA linear stapler or hand sewn.

INTRACORPOREAL ANASTOMOSIS

After laparoscopic transection of the vessels and mobilization of the bowel, the transverse colon and terminal ileum are transected using the laparoscopic linear cutting stapler. The specimen is placed in an EndoCatch bag over the liver to maximize working space. The transverse colon and ileum are then aligned in a side-to-side fashion, and a stay suture is placed on the antimesenteric border about 15 cm away from the stapled ends. An enterotomy and colotomy are made on the antimesenteric border of each piece of bowel near the staple line using the cautery. A second stay suture is then placed at the enterotomy site closest to the staple line. An endoscopic linear cutting stapler is then fed into the enterotomy carefully, ensuring that the mesentery is free underneath. This stapler is fired to create the side-to-side anastomosis. A free suture is then used to suture the enterotomy site closed in a running fashion. A second continuous suture line is then performed in a running fashion using seromuscular bites using the stay sutures to help manipulate the bowel. The umbilical incision is then extended to extract the specimen, or a Pfannenstiel incision may be used.

SUGGESTED READINGS

Delaney CP, Lawrence J, Keller DS, Champagne BJ, Senagore AJ. Operative techniques in laparoscopic colorectal surgery. 2nd ed. Philadelphia, PA: Lippincott Williams & Wilkins; 2013.

Mancino AT. Laparoscopic colectomy. In: Scott-Conner CEH, editor. The SAGES manual: fundamentals of laparoscopy, thoracoscopy and GI endoscopy. 2nd ed. New York: Springer; 2006.

Okuda J, Tanigawa N. Right colectomy. In: Milson JW, Bohm B, Nakajima K, editors. Laparoscopic colorectal surgery. New York: Springer; 2006.

Scott-Conner CEH. Right colectomy for cancer. In: Chaissin's operative strategy in general surgery: an expositive atlas. 3rd ed. New York: Springer; 2002.

Sonoda T. Laparoscopic medial to lateral. In: Wexner SD, Fleshman JW, editors. Colon and rectal surgery: abdominal operations. Philadelphia: Lippincott, Williams & Wilkins; 2012.

Left and Sigmoid Colectomy

Christopher Mascarenhas and Mathew F. Kalady

▶ VIDEO

28.1 Left and Sigmoid Colectomy

INTRODUCTION

Left colectomy or hemi-colectomy is a resection of the colon within the territory supplied by the left branch of the middle colic artery and the inferior mesenteric artery within the embryologic partitioning of the hindgut. Common indications include neoplasia of the distal transverse colon descending or sigmoid colon; segmental ischemia; or occasionally diffuse diverticulitis. Sigmoid colectomy involves resection of the portion of the colon supplied by the sigmoid arterial cascade and superior rectal (i.e., superior hemorrhoidal artery) artery. This is the portion of the inferior mesenteric artery that lies distal to the takeoff of the left colic artery.

SURGICAL PRINCIPLES

The pattern of left colonic resection is defined by the indication for surgery, the need to facilitate a tension-free colocolonic anastomosis, the disease process, and the blood supply. The most common indication for isolated left colonic resection is *neoplasia*. In this case, a radical lymphadenectomy guided by high vascular ligation is necessary for treatment and staging. Because the pattern of lymphatic drainage for the colon follows that of the arterial supply, the inclusion of the mesocolic envelope containing the inferior mesenteric artery (IMA) and its branches, with ligation of the IMA close to its origin, ensures adequate lymphadenectomy.

Other indications for left-sided colonic resection include diverticular disease, ischemia, Crohn's disease, sigmoid volvulus, rectal prolapse, and secondary involvement in non-colonic processes, such as ovarian carcinoma. None of these conditions mandate high ligation of the IMA, and it may be acceptable to ligate only the relevant arterial branches to the resected portion of the colon, as long as a tension-free anastomosis can be created and the remaining portions of bowel have excellent blood supply.

A high ligation of the IMA in conjunction with ligation of the inferior mesenteric vein at the inferior border of the pancreas, lateral to the jejunum, usually provides enough laxity of the remaining colon to allow the new colon conduit to reach into the pelvis for a tension-free anastomosis.

ANATOMY FOR PREOPERATIVE IMAGING

For colonic carcinoma, computed tomography (CT) of the chest, abdomen, and pelvis provides preoperative staging of the disease. CT includes identification of distant metastases, gross local lymph node involvement, and local invasion of the primary tumor (Fig. 28.1A). Full colonoscopic evaluation helps confirm the location of the lesion within the colon, and placement of a tattoo is preferred to help localize the tumor intraoperatively, particularly in laparoscopic cases in which tactile sensation is limited. For benign disease, CT and colonoscopy may help to identify pathological features, such as the extent of Crohn's disease or ischemia, that may affect approach and extent of dissection.

SURFACE ANATOMY, INCISION, AND PORT PLACEMENT

Left colectomy may be performed as either an open or a laparoscopic procedure. For either approach, the patient should be in the Lloyd-Davis position, supine, with the buttocks at the distal edge of the table to allow easy access to the anal canal for introduction of a stapler or scope as needed. The legs should be slightly flexed in the horizontal position and held in leg supports. For a laparoscopic approach, the patient is secured with gel pad or bean bag or pink pad, taking care to pad all pressure points, in anticipation of an extreme head-down/up and right lateral tilt position.

A number of different port configurations have been described; our preferred approach is shown in Fig. 28.1B. Open left hemicolectomy may be performed through either a midline or a left transverse incision. Additionally a Pfannenstiel with a superior left "hockey stick" extension has been described.

A. Preoperative computed tomographic imaging

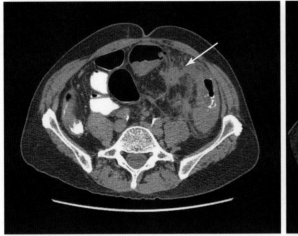

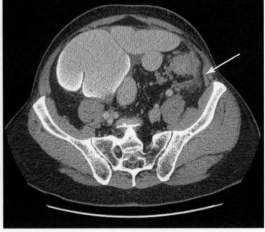

Thicken sigmoid secondary to diverticular disease with marked inflammatory fat stranding

Sigmoid descending junction obstructing carcinoma with dilated proximal large and small bowel

B. Key landmarks of the surface anatomy of the anterolateral abdominal wall

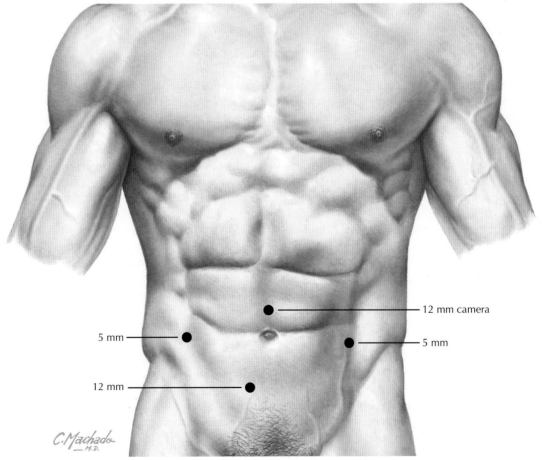

12 mm camera

5 mm

5 mm

12 mm

● Standard laparoscopic port placement

FIGURE 28.1 Laparoscopic port placement.

PROCEDURAL STEPS

As with all colorectal resections, the basic tenants of the operation include mobilization of the bowel; identification, isolation, and division of the vascular supply; resection of the bowel segment; and anastomosis. Once this is completed, the left-sided anastomosis should be evaluated with a leak test that often involves direct endoscopic examination. For a left colonic resection, the sigmoid and descending colon, splenic flexure, proximal rectum, and distal transverse colon require mobilization. Knowledge of the blood supply, the autonomic nerves, and the lymphatic drainage, as well as the colon's relationship to the spleen, pancreas, kidney, and ureter, is required for successful completion of the left hemicolectomy and sigmoid colectomy (Figs. 28.2 and 28.3).

VASCULAR ANATOMY

The anatomy of the vascular supply to the colon is demonstrated in Fig. 28.2.

The arterial blood supply to the left colon is derived from the IMA, which is the most distal of the three midline branches of the abdominal aorta. The ascending left colic or left colic artery is the first branch of the IMA. This supplies the descending colon and the splenic flexure, via the marginal artery of Drummond. The marginal artery joins the middle colic branch of the superior mesenteric artery in the mid-transverse colon (see Fig. 28.2A). The arterial supply to the splenic flexure is subject to a great degree of variability (Fig. 28.4A). The marginal artery may be augmented by a second arcade, located more proximally in the mesocolon, known as the *arc of Riolan*. Also, the marginal artery of Drummond and the arc of Riolan (i.e., meandering mesenteric artery) may be absent. Therefore, if the IMA and its branches have been ligated, it is essential to assess the vascularity of the colon at the proximal resection margin intraoperatively to ensure an adequate blood supply to the anastomosis. Distally, branches of the IMA supply the sigmoid colon and vary greatly in number. The IMA proceeds to pass over the pelvic brim and thereby changes its name to the superior rectal artery, at which point it bifurcates and supplies the majority of the rectum.

Venous drainage of the left colon and hindgut is through tributaries of the inferior mesenteric vein (IMV) (see Fig. 28.2B). The IMV lies in the base of the left mesocolon and passes posterior to the lower border of the pancreas, just lateral to the 4th portion of the duodenum. Under the pancreas, the IMV joins the splenic vein and superior mesenteric vein to form the portal vein. The IMV is significant in colorectal disease because it tethers the left colon, and high ligation is necessary for full left colon mobilization. Division of the IMV 2 to 3 cm below the inferior border of the pancreas provides several inches of extra mobility, often assisting the creation of a tension-free anastomosis (Fig. 28.4B and C).

A. Arteries of large intestine. Note the proximity of the left ureter to the IMA trunk and branches at the pelvic brim.

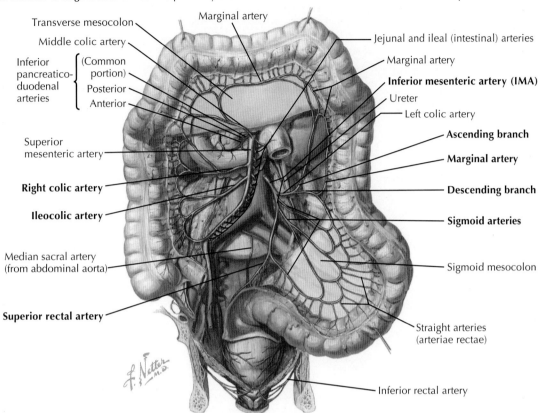

Transverse mesocolon

Middle colic artery

Inferior pancreatico-duodenal arteries { (Common portion) / Posterior / Anterior

Superior mesenteric artery

Right colic artery

Ileocolic artery

Median sacral artery (from abdominal aorta)

Superior rectal artery

Marginal artery

Jejunal and ileal (intestinal) arteries

Marginal artery

Inferior mesenteric artery (IMA)

Ureter

Left colic artery

Ascending branch

Marginal artery

Descending branch

Sigmoid arteries

Sigmoid mesocolon

Straight arteries (arteriae rectae)

Inferior rectal artery

B. Veins of large intestine. Note the proximity of the IMV to the lateral border of the fourth part of the duodenum and the inferior border of the body of the pancreas.

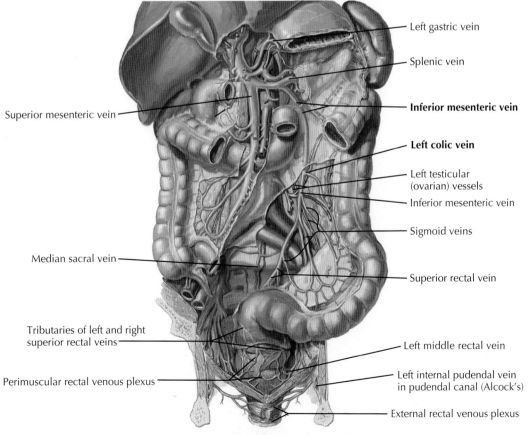

Superior mesenteric vein

Median sacral vein

Tributaries of left and right superior rectal veins

Perimuscular rectal venous plexus

Left gastric vein

Splenic vein

Inferior mesenteric vein

Left colic vein

Left testicular (ovarian) vessels

Inferior mesenteric vein

Sigmoid veins

Superior rectal vein

Left middle rectal vein

Left internal pudendal vein in pudendal canal (Alcock's)

External rectal venous plexus

FIGURE 28.2 Vascular supply to colon.

A. Left-sided resection pattern. Shaded area denotes extent of intended lymph node harvest.

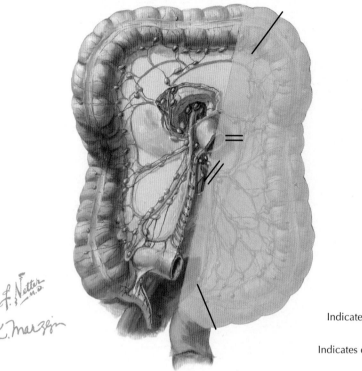

=
Indicates point of ligation

——
Indicates division of the colon

B. Margins and level of division of the blood vessels for a sigmoid colectomy.

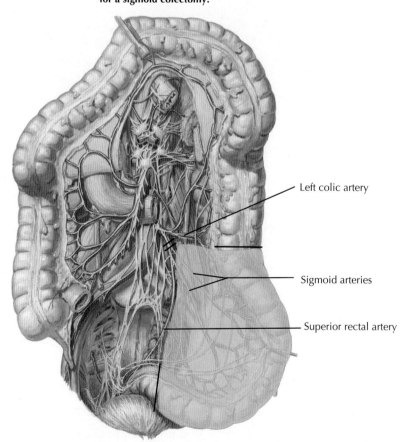

Left colic artery

Sigmoid arteries

Superior rectal artery

FIGURE 28.3 Left and sigmoid resection pattern; autonomic nerves and lymphatic drainage to colon.

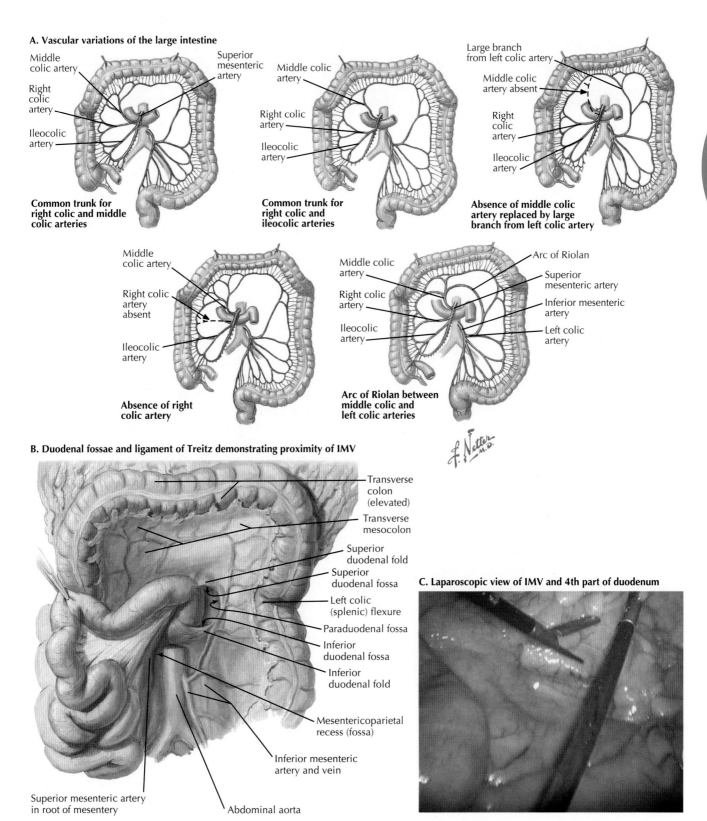

A. Vascular variations of the large intestine

Middle colic artery
Right colic artery
Ileocolic artery
Superior mesenteric artery

Common trunk for right colic and middle colic arteries

Middle colic artery
Right colic artery
Ileocolic artery

Common trunk for right colic and ileocolic arteries

Large branch from left colic artery
Middle colic artery absent
Right colic artery
Ileocolic artery

Absence of middle colic artery replaced by large branch from left colic artery

Middle colic artery
Right colic artery absent
Ileocolic artery

Absence of right colic artery

Middle colic artery
Right colic artery
Ileocolic artery
Arc of Riolan
Superior mesenteric artery
Inferior mesenteric artery
Left colic artery

Arc of Riolan between middle colic and left colic arteries

F. Netter M.D.

B. Duodenal fossae and ligament of Treitz demonstrating proximity of IMV

Transverse colon (elevated)
Transverse mesocolon
Superior duodenal fold
Superior duodenal fossa
Left colic (splenic) flexure
Paraduodenal fossa
Inferior duodenal fossa
Inferior duodenal fold
Mesentericoparietal recess (fossa)
Inferior mesenteric artery and vein
Superior mesenteric artery in root of mesentery
Abdominal aorta

C. Laparoscopic view of IMV and 4th part of duodenum

FIGURE 28.4 Vascular variations in colon; duodenal anatomy.
IMV, Inferior mesenteric vein.

IDENTIFICATION AND ISOLATION OF THE VASCULAR PEDICLE

The IMA may be dissected from a medial or lateral approach. Our preference is a medial approach laparoscopically. With a medial-to-lateral approach, the peritoneum is opened at the sacral promontory, and dissection proceeds cephalad toward the base of the IMA. The left ureter must be identified and kept in a retroperitoneal location, avoiding injury. At the base of the IMA, the peritoneum overlying and inferior to the IMA is carefully opened and the vessel is mobilized, as the autonomic nerves are noted and preserved. This approach allows the origin of the IMA to be encircled before division (Fig. 28.5A). Rather than aiming for flush ligation at its origin, a 1- to 2-cm length of the IMA should be preserved to ensure that the superior hypogastric plexus of the autonomic nervous system is not inadvertently damaged where it encircles the IMA (see Fig. 28.5A). For malignant disease, dissection closer to the origin may be required for an adequate lymphadenectomy, particularly if there are grossly abnormal lymph nodes in that area. For tumors of the left colon or sigmoid colon, the IMA should be divided proximal to the takeoff of the left colic artery (i.e., high ligation; see surgical principles earlier) to ensure a full lymphadenectomy. In case of sigmoid colectomy for benign conditions, dividing the sigmoid artery branches alone may be adequate, with preservation of the superior hemorrhoidal artery.

While preparing for vascular ligation, surgeons must note important structures to avoid injury. The colon mesentery can be mobilized medially off the retroperitoneum. From a lateral approach, Toldt's fascia is identified and carefully preserved. The left gonadal vessels, left ureter, and para-aortic autonomic nerves are posterior to this layer and should therefore be protected when the dissection is in the correct plane. The white line of Toldt indicates the reflection of the parietal and visceral peritoneum. The peritoneum should be incised just inside this line (Fig. 28.5B). The sigmoid mesocolon is then elevated from the retroperitoneum under slight tension, and medial mobilization continues.

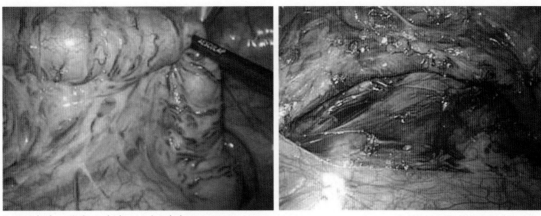

A. IMA before (*left*) and after (*right*) skeletonization

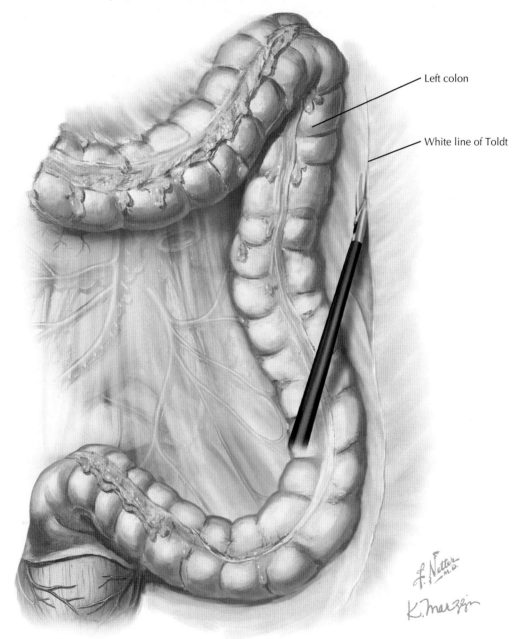

Left colon

White line of Toldt

B. Dissection along the white line of Toldt

FIGURE 28.5 Left hemicolectomy: skeletonization and white line of Toldt.

SPLENIC FLEXURE

Although the splenic flexure is not mobilized routinely by all surgeons for a sigmoid colectomy, it is usually required to create adequate length for a colorectal anastomosis, particularly in malignant disease and certainly when a full left colon resection is performed. Furthermore, the splenic flexure may have to be resected in cases of ischemia or for tumors of the splenic flexure. The flexure may be mobilized from a medial, lateral, or inferior approach, each of which may be used in laparoscopic or open surgery. Often, successful mobilization requires the use of a combination of approaches, allowing the surgeon to make progress from different angles until the entire flexure is released.

Starting at the mid-transverse colon, the greater omentum is elevated superiorly, demonstrating the avascular plane between the omentum and transverse colon. At its left lateral extent, the omentum often exhibits adhesions to the splenic flexure and the capsule of the spleen. Traction on the flexure may cause inadvertent trauma to the spleen. This complication may be mitigated by superior/cephalad retraction of the greater omentum in the midline and commencing dissection in the mid-transverse colon. Opening this plane medially provides entry to the lesser sac, identified by visualization of the posterior wall of the stomach, and exposes the superior aspect of the transverse mesocolon (Fig. 28.6A). As with the lateral descending and sigmoid mobilization, there is a line of reflection between the parietal and visceral peritoneum. This line is less easy to see than the white line of Toldt but is present nevertheless (Fig. 28.6B). The peritoneum must again be incised just above this line of reflection (closer to the colon). Mobilization too far from the retroperitoneum (too close to the colon) makes a defect through the mesentery of the colon. During mobilization, attention must be paid to the jejunum, which is often only a layer of peritoneum away from the area of dissection. Superior mobilization is complete when the colon to the left of the midline is fully freed from its superior attachments.

Full mobilization of the splenic flexure requires division of the IMV. The inferior approach to the splenic flexure uses this as the starting point. With the transverse colon retracted superiorly and the small bowel retracted to the patient's right, the fourth part of the duodenum and ligament of Treitz are visualized (see Figs. 28.4B and C and 28.6C). This approach exposes the IMV inferior to the vessel passing posterior to the pancreas. Once this has been divided, with Toldt's fascia identified, mobilization of the proximal descending colon continues from medial-to-lateral, through the mesocolon to the left lateral side wall. The retroperitoneum, gonadal vessels, and ureter are protected deep to the dissection, and the mesocolon and colon are preserved anteriorly.

Toldt's fascia continues superiorly, posterior to the body of the pancreas. Therefore, at the inferior border of the pancreas, the surgeon must cease to use this as the plane of dissection and instead release the transverse mesocolon from the anterior surface of the pancreas. This is most readily achieved toward the tail of the pancreas. In doing so, the lesser sac is entered. The lateral attachments are then divided, and the greater omentum is freed from the colon as previously described.

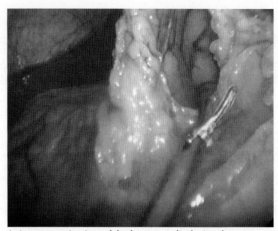

A. Laparoscopic view of the lesser sac displaying the transverse colon, posterior wall of the stomach, greater omentum, and left lobe of the liver

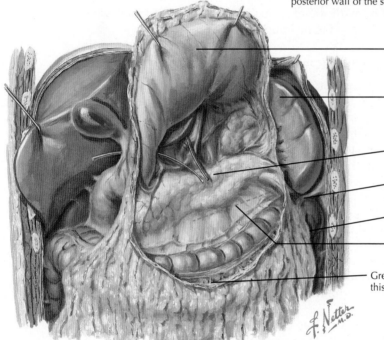

Posterior wall of stomach (*reflected*)

Spleen

Pancreas

Omental adhesions to spleen, abdominal side wall, and splenic flexure of colon

Splenic flexure

Dotted line denoting point of incision in the peritoneal covering of the transverse mesocolon

Greater omentum incised; in operative surgery this is freed from the colon and reflected

- - - - - Transverse mesocolic reflection

B. Omental bursa (stomach reflected). Attachments of greater omentum and splenic flexure and spleen as well as pancreas. Note the dotted line indicates the line of incision in the visceral peritoneum of the transverse mesocolic reflection to allow full mobilization of the splenic flexure and distal transverse colon.

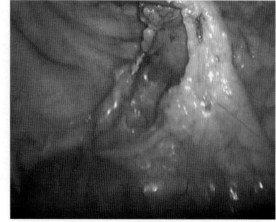

C. IMV skeletonized and clipped prior to division

FIGURE 28.6 Dissection of the splenic flexure, lesser sac, and IMV.
IMV, Inferior mesenteric vein.

SIGMOID AND DESCENDING COLON

The left colon, as a part of the hindgut, originated as a midline structure. Through developmental rotation, however, the left colon has come to reside on the left side of the abdominal cavity, with the descending colon/mesocolon adherent to the parietal peritoneum overlying the retroperitoneum. The junction of the visceral peritoneum and retroperitoneum is known as the white line of Toldt. Dissection at this junction mobilizes the mesocolon and restores the left colon to the midline after meeting up with the previous medial-to-lateral mobilization of the sigmoid colon performed while mobilizing and dividing the IMA.

UPPER MESORECTAL MOBILIZATION AND ANASTOMOSIS

The principles of choosing the proximal level of transection are ensuring that there is at least a proximal 5-cm margin in cancer cases and that the colon at the proposed line of transection reaches down to the rectal stump without any tension and is well perfused. It is therefore recommended to check for an adequate pulse in the marginal artery at the level of division of the colon, most commonly by sharply dividing the marginal artery between clamps, and open the proximal clamp and observe blood flow at the time of specimen removal.

In a left hemicolectomy and sigmoid colectomy, the distal level of transection is usually the rectosigmoid junction, and no rectum is usually resected, provided a 5-cm distal margin is obtained in patients undergoing an oncologic resection. However, it is often necessary to mobilize the proximal rectum to facilitate transanal passage of the circular stapling device to the top of the rectal stump for a stapled anastomosis. This approach is covered in detail in Chapter 30.

Once an adequate distal margin has been obtained and the mesentery cleared circumferentially at the point for division, the rectum may be transected. The specimen is removed from the field, generally through a left lower quadrant muscle-splitting incision, or a Pfannenstiel incision.

The colorectal anastomosis is now created. Using an end-to-end anastomotic (EEA) stapler is preferred, but it could be hand sewn. It is critical to ensure at this stage that there is no twisting of the mesentery of the colon brought down to the rectal stump (by tracing the cut edge of the mesentery to the retroperitoneum) and that no small bowel has crept up beneath the colon. Finally, after creation of the anastomosis, the donuts are inspected to confirm that they are complete, and a flexible sigmoidoscopy is performed after clamping the bowel atraumatically and placing the anastomosis under water to inspect the anastomosis and help with an air leak test.

SUGGESTED READINGS

Farquharson M, Moran B. Farquharson's textbook of operative general surgery. 9th ed. Philadelphia; 2005.

Kirk RM, Winslet MC. Essential general surgical operations. 2nd ed. New York: Churchill Livingston; 2007.

Sinnatamby CS. Last's anatomy: regional and applied. 12th ed. New York: Churchill Livingstone; 2011.

Transverse Colectomy

David R. Rosen and Jeremy M. Lipman

INTRODUCTION

Transverse colectomy, in isolation, is an uncommon procedure. Potential indications for transverse colectomy include transverse colon cancer, segmental inflammatory bowel disease, and segmental transverse colon ischemia. In contrast, mobilization and resection of the transverse colon—in total or segmental—is commonly performed as a component of a right, left, subtotal, or total colectomy. Familiarity with the potential anatomic variability of this part of the colon, along with knowledge and expertise regarding the different surgical approaches, is critical.

SURGICAL PRINCIPLES

Transverse colectomy requires detailed knowledge of the vascular supply of the colon, the anatomy of the hepatic and splenic flexures, and the relationship of the omentum to the colon and stomach. The goal of the operation is to resect the transverse colon and create a tension-free, well-vascularized bowel anastomosis. The procedure usually involves the following steps:

1. Mobilization of hepatic flexure
2. Mobilization of splenic flexure
3. Mobilization of the greater omentum, either off the transverse colon or en bloc with it
4. Division of middle colic artery and vein
5. Proximal division of the colon
6. Distal division of the colon
7. Re-anastomosis of the divided bowel

The particular order of completing steps 1 to 4 is usually dictated by the operative approach, although it is often easiest to perform the division of the middle colic vessels after the colon and omentum have been completely mobilized.

ANATOMY FOR TRANSVERSE COLECTOMY

Hepatic Flexure

The *hepatic flexure* is the anatomic name for the bend in the colon as it transitions from the ascending colon to the transverse colon. The intraoperative photograph demonstrates the hepatic flexure in situ (Fig. 29.1A, B, and C). The liver is cephalad and the right kidney is posterior. When mobilizing from a right-sided lateral approach, the surgeon mobilizes the ascending colon from its lateral attachments at the white line of Toldt. As the right hemicolon is retracted inferiorly and medially, the gastrocolic ligament is exposed and divided moving medially (Fig. 29.1D). It is important to identify the gallbladder because it can be densely adherent to the omentum, transverse colon, or gastrocolic ligament. As dissection proceeds medially, the duodenum is exposed and preserved posteriorly with the retroperitoneum (Fig. 29.1E). If not already performed from a medial dissection of the right colon, the duodenum and pancreas are bluntly mobilized posteriorly off the transverse colon mesentery (Fig. 29.1F).

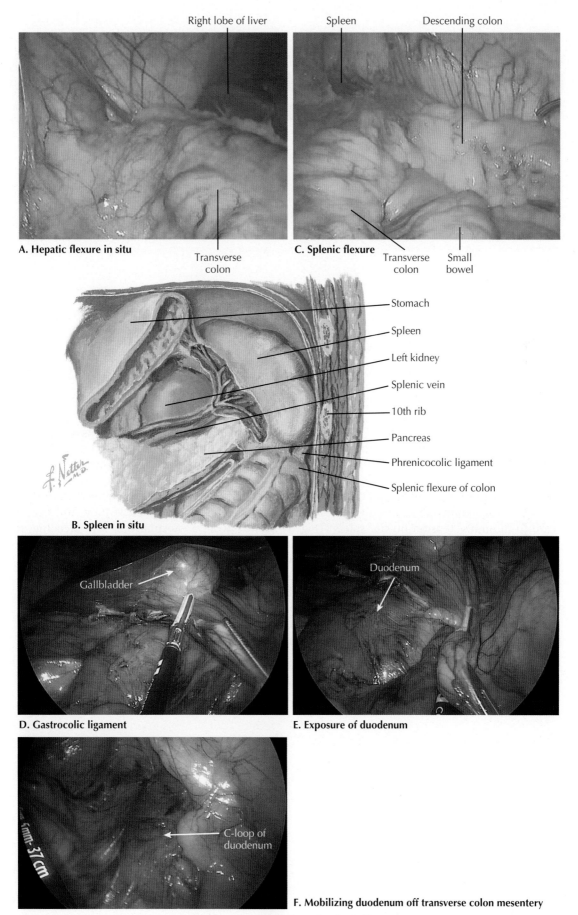

Right lobe of liver

Spleen Descending colon

A. Hepatic flexure in situ

Transverse colon

C. Splenic flexure

Transverse colon Small bowel

Stomach

Spleen

Left kidney

Splenic vein

10th rib

Pancreas

Phrenicocolic ligament

Splenic flexure of colon

B. Spleen in situ

Gallbladder

Duodenum

D. Gastrocolic ligament

E. Exposure of duodenum

C-loop of duodenum

F. Mobilizing duodenum off transverse colon mesentery

FIGURE 29.1 Hepatic and splenic flexures.

Splenic Flexure

The splenic flexure of the colon is the bend in the bowel where the distal transverse colon transitions to the descending colon. When the surgeon is mobilizing from a left-sided lateral approach, the avascular lateral attachments of the descending colon to the retroperitoneum must be divided along the white line of Toldt. The left hemicolon is retracted medially and inferiorly, exposing the splenocolic ligament, the lateral attachments at the splenic flexure (Fig. 29.2A). These attachments are divided, avoiding Gerota's fascia of the left kidney, and taking care to minimize tension on the spleen (Fig. 29.2B) to avoid a capsular tear and bleeding. If not already performed from a medial dissection of the left colon, posterior attachments to the descending colon, splenic flexure, and mesocolon must be freed to provide adequate mobilization of the splenic flexure. The omentum is then retracted superiorly and anteriorly while the transverse colon is retracted inferiorly. This will expose a window through which to access the lesser sac (Fig. 29.2C). Even minimal traction on the splenic flexure can cause a splenic capsule tear; therefore, great care and attention to detail are critical. As a general rule, the spleen should never move because of excessive traction on any attachment.

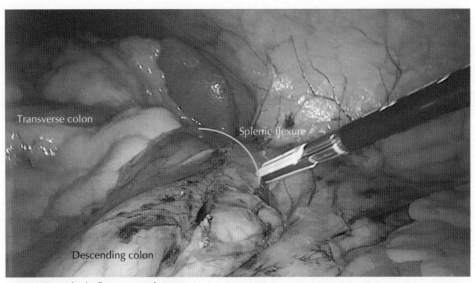

A. Exposing splenic flexure attachments

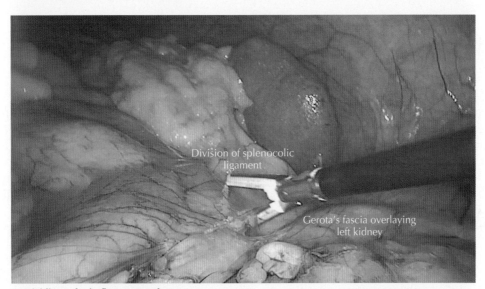

B. Dividing splenic flexure attachments

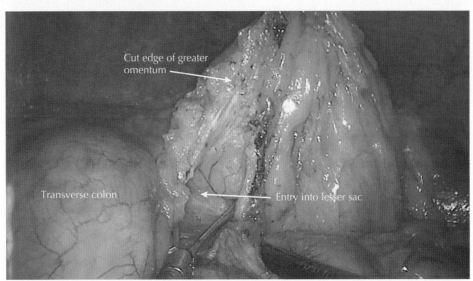

C. Accessing the lesser sac

FIGURE 29.2 **Splenic flexure.**

Relationships of Greater Omentum to Transverse Colon and Stomach

The surgeon must decide whether the clinical setting requires preservation of the omentum; it is often easier to leave it attached to the transverse colon and resect it with the specimen, and it is mandatory in patients with a tumor in either flexure or in the transverse colon itself. In patients having surgery for a benign indication, before dissecting the mesentery of the transverse colon, the surgeon may prefer to dissect the omentum from the colon. Performing this step before mesenteric dissection completely opens the lesser sac and provides better exposure and control of the mesenteric vessels.

The omentum originates from the greater curvature of the stomach and continues anteriorly and caudad anterior to the transverse colon. If the omentum is preserved, it should be separately dissected from its attachments to the transverse colon by dissecting along the avascular plane between the two (Fig. 29.3A). If the omentum is to be resected, the gastroepiploic artery, which runs parallel to the greater curve of the stomach, is preserved, while its branches into the omentum require ligation (Fig. 29.3C). The stomach is reflected cephalad to provide entry to the lesser sac (Fig. 29.3B, C, and D). Regardless of whether the omentum is to be preserved or resected, once the lesser sac is entered, the mobilization is complete when the posterior wall of the stomach is clearly visualized, and the origin of the mesentery of the transverse colon becomes visible along the anterior border of the pancreas.

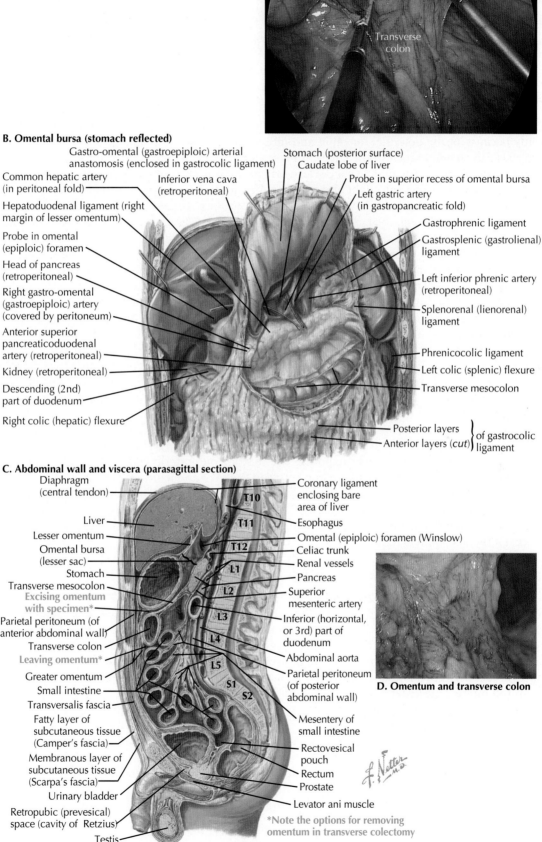

A. Dividing omentum off of transverse colon

Greater omentum

Transverse colon

B. Omental bursa (stomach reflected)

Gastro-omental (gastroepiploic) arterial anastomosis (enclosed in gastrocolic ligament)

Stomach (posterior surface)

Caudate lobe of liver

Common hepatic artery (in peritoneal fold)

Inferior vena cava (retroperitoneal)

Probe in superior recess of omental bursa

Left gastric artery (in gastropancreatic fold)

Hepatoduodenal ligament (right margin of lesser omentum)

Gastrophrenic ligament

Gastrosplenic (gastrolienal) ligament

Probe in omental (epiploic) foramen

Head of pancreas (retroperitoneal)

Left inferior phrenic artery (retroperitoneal)

Right gastro-omental (gastroepiploic) artery (covered by peritoneum)

Splenorenal (lienorenal) ligament

Anterior superior pancreaticoduodenal artery (retroperitoneal)

Phrenicocolic ligament

Kidney (retroperitoneal)

Left colic (splenic) flexure

Descending (2nd) part of duodenum

Transverse mesocolon

Right colic (hepatic) flexure

Posterior layers

Anterior layers (*cut*)

} of gastrocolic ligament

C. Abdominal wall and viscera (parasagittal section)

Diaphragm (central tendon)

Coronary ligament enclosing bare area of liver

T10

Liver

T11

Esophagus

Lesser omentum

Omental (epiploic) foramen (Winslow)

Omental bursa (lesser sac)

T12

Celiac trunk

Stomach

Renal vessels

L1

Transverse mesocolon

Pancreas

Excising omentum with specimen*

L2

Superior mesenteric artery

Parietal peritoneum (of anterior abdominal wall)

L3

Inferior (horizontal, or 3rd) part of duodenum

Transverse colon

L4

Abdominal aorta

Leaving omentum*

Greater omentum

L5

Parietal peritoneum (of posterior abdominal wall)

Small intestine

S1

D. Omentum and transverse colon

Transversalis fascia

S2

Fatty layer of subcutaneous tissue (Camper's fascia)

Mesentery of small intestine

Membranous layer of subcutaneous tissue (Scarpa's fascia)

Rectovesical pouch

Urinary bladder

Rectum

Prostate

Retropubic (prevesical) space (cavity of Retzius)

Levator ani muscle

*Note the options for removing omentum in transverse colectomy

Testis

FIGURE 29.3 Greater omentum and stomach.

Transverse Mesocolon: Middle Colic Artery and Vein

Division of the middle colic artery and vein are the most difficult aspect of a transverse colectomy because of the potential for rapid and difficult-to-control hemorrhage. The middle colic artery is the second branch of the superior mesenteric artery (SMA), after the inferior pancreaticoduodenal artery. The middle colic artery originates from the right lateral aspect of the SMA and classically bifurcates into right and left branches, although as many as five different variations to this branching pattern have been noted. The classic arrangement of arteries to the large intestine is shown in Fig. 29.4. Although called the *middle colic artery*, it is generally oriented more to the patient's right than in the middle (Fig. 29.5A, B, and C).

When the surgeon is dividing the transverse mesocolon from the right via a laparoscopic or minimally invasive approach, a grasper is swept posterior to the cut edge of the colonic mesentery and lifted anteriorly (Fig. 29.5D). This will draw the transverse colon mesentery and middle colic artery distribution anteriorly and leave the superior mesenteric artery safely posterior (Fig. 29.5B). Dissection then proceeds across the transverse colon mesentery (Fig. 29.5E). The duodenojejunal junction will come into view and must be avoided (Fig. 29.5F).

When the surgeon mobilizes the transverse mesocolon from the left, the transverse colon and mesentery are again lifted anteriorly. The transverse colon mesentery is dissected off the inferior border of the pancreas in a lateral to medial direction until the middle colic vessels are encountered and subsequently divided. Again, the duodenojejunal junction must be identified and preserved.

Alternatively, the transverse colon can be approached in a mesenteric fashion. After the operating table is positioned to the right with reverse Trendelenburg, the distal transverse colon mesentery is retracted anteriorly, exposing the inferior mesenteric vein and duodenojejunal junction (Fig. 29.5G). The avascular plane between the IMV and jejunum is opened. Dissection continues laterally and superiorly, taking care to continue the dissection anterior to the tail of the pancreas until the lesser sac is entered. This approach will allow complete division of the mesentery of the splenic flexure. The middle colic vessels can then be taken as described above from a left-sided approach.

COMPLETION OF TRANSVERSE COLECTOMY

Once both flexures are mobilized, and the omentum dissected and the middle colic artery and vein ligated, the bowel is divided to create a tension-free, well-vascularized anastomosis. As previously stated, usually this involves an extended right, left, or total colectomy and is infrequently performed as an isolated procedure. It is important to understand the vascular anatomy of the colon to know where the perfusion lies relative to the new anastomosis. For example, in an extended right or subtotal colectomy, the distal colonic segment will be perfused retrograde from the inferior mesenteric artery via the marginal artery of Drummond. In an extended left colectomy, the proximal colonic segment will be perfused either by remaining branches of the right branch of the middle colic artery or from the ileocolic pedicle. Sharply dividing the marginal artery at the point of bowel transection and evaluating for pulsatile blood flow before ligation can ensure adequacy of perfusion to these segments. In the rare setting where a true transverse colectomy is performed, it would be wise to consider performing an end-to-end hand-sewn anastomosis. A stapled side-to-side, functional end-to-end anastomosis or end-to-side anastomosis is possible but may create more tension than an end-to-end anastomosis.

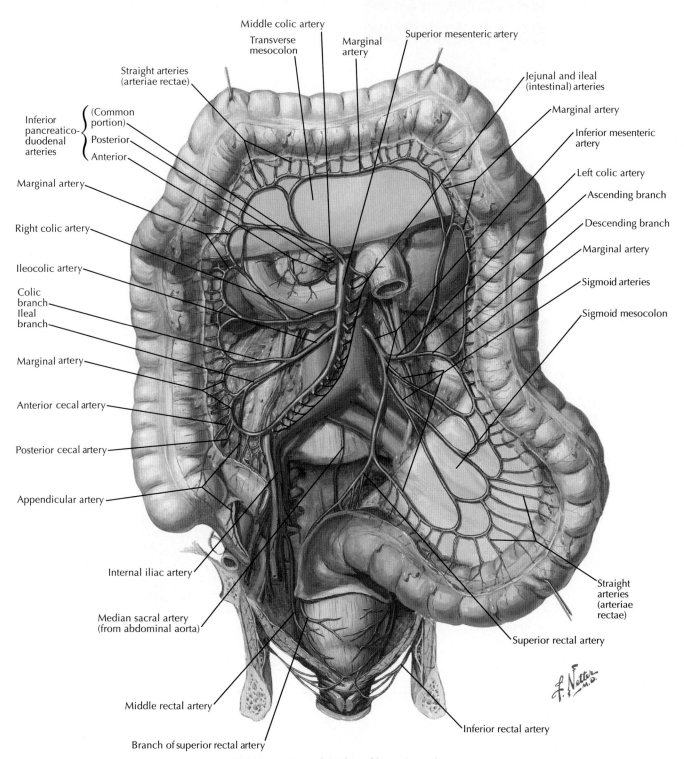

Middle colic artery

Transverse mesocolon

Marginal artery

Superior mesenteric artery

Straight arteries (arteriae rectae)

Jejunal and ileal (intestinal) arteries

Marginal artery

Inferior mesenteric artery

Inferior pancreatico-duodenal arteries
{ (Common portion)
Posterior
Anterior

Left colic artery

Ascending branch

Descending branch

Marginal artery

Marginal artery

Sigmoid arteries

Right colic artery

Sigmoid mesocolon

Ileocolic artery

Colic branch
Ileal branch

Marginal artery

Anterior cecal artery

Posterior cecal artery

Appendicular artery

Straight arteries (arteriae rectae)

Internal iliac artery

Superior rectal artery

Median sacral artery (from abdominal aorta)

Middle rectal artery

Inferior rectal artery

Branch of superior rectal artery

FIGURE 29.4 Arteries of large intestine.

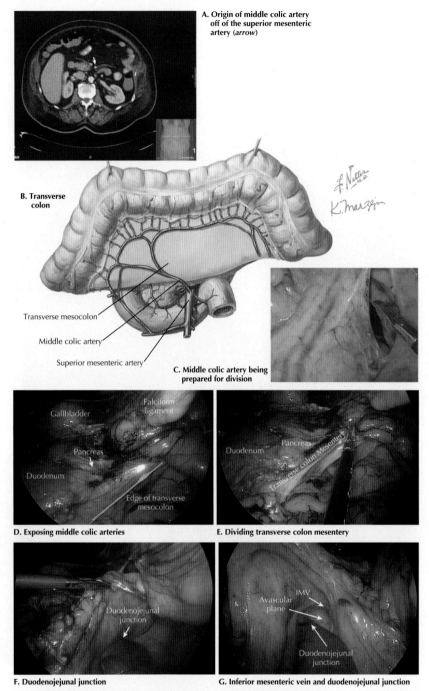

FIGURE 29.5 Transverse mesocolon: middle colic artery and vein.

IMV, Inferior mesenteric vein.

SUGGESTED READINGS

Chitra R. Clinically relevant variations of the coeliac trunk. Singapore Med J 2010;51(3):216–9.

Garcia-Ruiz A, Milsom JW, Ludwig KA, Marchesa P. Right colonic arterial anatomy: implications for laparoscopic surgery. Dis Colon Rectum 1996;39(8):906–11.

Gerber SA, Rybalko VY, Bigelow CE, et al. Preferential attachment of peritoneal tumor metastases to omental immune aggregates and possible role of a unique vascular microenvironment in metastatic survival and growth. Am J Pathol 2006;169(5):1739–52.

Lawrance RJ, Loizidou M, Cooper AJ, Alexander P, Taylor I. Importance of the omentum in the development of intraabdominal metastasis. Br J Surg 1991;78(1):117–9.

McGory ML, Zingmond DS, Sekeris E, Ko CK. The significance of inadvertent splenectomy during colorectal cancer resection. Arch Surgery 2007;142(7):668–74.

Low Anterior Resection With Total Mesorectal Excision and Anastomosis

Vladimir Bolshinsky and Conor P. Delaney

▶ VIDEO

30.1 Low Anterior Resection With Total Mesorectal Excision and Anastomosis

INTRODUCTION

Colorectal cancer is the second most common tumor in men and women in the Western world. Tumors occur most frequently in the rectum and sigmoid colon and are usually treated by resection and primary anastomosis. Surgery is the mainstay of therapy, and patients with positive nodal disease also require adjuvant chemotherapy. Some additional patients require radiation treatment preoperatively.

Rectal cancer is a more challenging surgical problem than colon cancer, and its management is more complex. Since Miles' initial description of abdominoperineal resection in 1925, the main change in approach occurred when Dixon described the technique of anterior resection and re-anastomosis for tumors of the upper rectum and distal sigmoid. The surgical principles involve wide resection of the rectum, including the entire investing fascia with the enclosed mesentery of the rectum. The results of total mesorectal excision (TME) indicate that complete excision with clear radial margins is important and that local recurrence rates much lower than 10% can be achieved with good surgical technique.

SURGICAL PRINCIPLES

The current standards of care for patients with low rectal cancer include complete excision of the rectum and surrounding mesorectum, ideally ensuring a minimal distal margin of 1 to 2 cm before a coloanal anastomosis is performed, although this is subject to anatomy, tumor location, and tumor differentiation. In general, this procedure is performed in conjunction with a high ligation of the inferior mesenteric artery and vein and mobilization of the splenic flexure. The autonomic nerves are carefully protected. Patients with colon or middle or upper rectal cancer require a minimum 5-cm proximal and distal margin, with at least 12 lymph nodes being harvested in the mesocolic excision.

ANATOMY FOR PREOPERATIVE IMAGING

Preoperative imaging of rectal cancer is extremely important and helps define tumors that may threaten the circumferential resection margin, therefore requiring preoperative chemoradiation. Both sagittal and coronal views are obtained, and magnetic resonance imaging (MRI) is used more frequently because of the high-quality resolution obtained (Figs. 30.1 and 30.2). Ultrasound is also used in the assessment of rectal cancer and can provide excellent results for T staging (tumor infiltration), particularly of early T-stage lesions.

ANATOMY FOR COLONIC MOBILIZATION AND DISSECTION

The anatomy of the vascular supply to the colon is demonstrated in Fig. 30.3. A knowledge of these vessels, the autonomic nerves, and the ureters is required before the surgeon begins the steps of the procedure (Figs. 30.4 and 30.5).

Median (sagittal) section

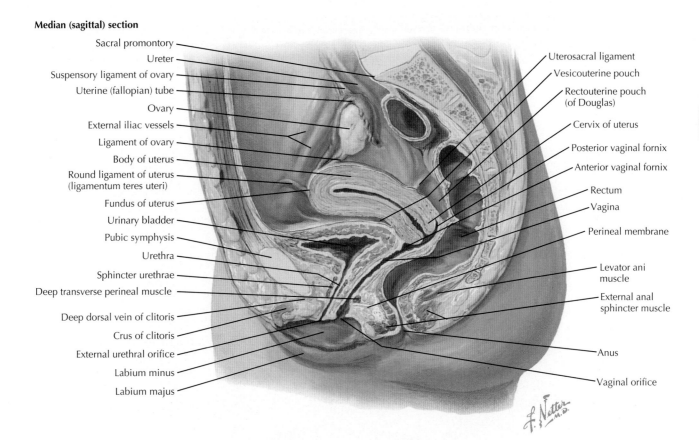

Sacral promontory
Ureter
Suspensory ligament of ovary
Uterine (fallopian) tube
Ovary
External iliac vessels
Ligament of ovary
Body of uterus
Round ligament of uterus (ligamentum teres uteri)
Fundus of uterus
Urinary bladder
Pubic symphysis
Urethra
Sphincter urethrae
Deep transverse perineal muscle
Deep dorsal vein of clitoris
Crus of clitoris
External urethral orifice
Labium minus
Labium majus

Uterosacral ligament
Vesicouterine pouch
Rectouterine pouch (of Douglas)
Cervix of uterus
Posterior vaginal fornix
Anterior vaginal fornix
Rectum
Vagina
Perineal membrane
Levator ani muscle
External anal sphincter muscle
Anus
Vaginal orifice

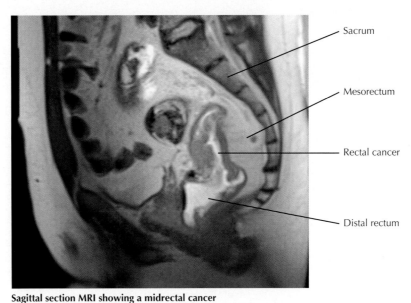

Sacrum
Mesorectum
Rectal cancer
Distal rectum

Sagittal section MRI showing a midrectal cancer

FIGURE 30.1 Pelvic viscera and perineum: female.

Female: superior view (peritoneum and loose areolar tissue removed)

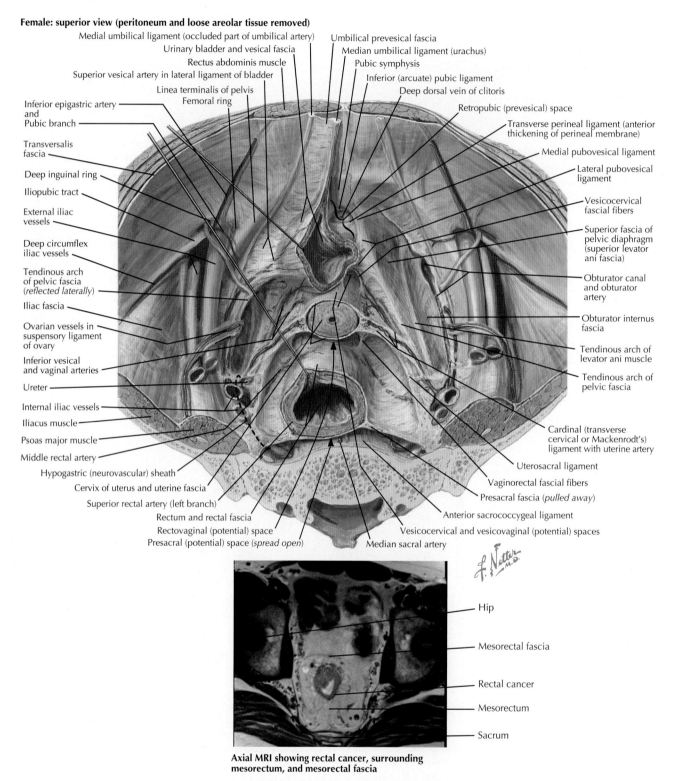

Medial umbilical ligament (occluded part of umbilical artery)
Urinary bladder and vesical fascia
Rectus abdominis muscle
Superior vesical artery in lateral ligament of bladder
Linea terminalis of pelvis
Femoral ring
Inferior epigastric artery and Pubic branch
Transversalis fascia
Deep inguinal ring
Iliopubic tract
External iliac vessels
Deep circumflex iliac vessels
Tendinous arch of pelvic fascia (*reflected laterally*)
Iliac fascia
Ovarian vessels in suspensory ligament of ovary
Inferior vesical and vaginal arteries
Ureter
Internal iliac vessels
Iliacus muscle
Psoas major muscle
Middle rectal artery
Hypogastric (neurovascular) sheath
Cervix of uterus and uterine fascia
Superior rectal artery (left branch)
Rectum and rectal fascia
Rectovaginal (potential) space
Presacral (potential) space (*spread open*)

Umbilical prevesical fascia
Median umbilical ligament (urachus)
Pubic symphysis
Inferior (arcuate) pubic ligament
Deep dorsal vein of clitoris
Retropubic (prevesical) space
Transverse perineal ligament (anterior thickening of perineal membrane)
Medial pubovesical ligament
Lateral pubovesical ligament
Vesicocervical fascial fibers
Superior fascia of pelvic diaphragm (superior levator ani fascia)
Obturator canal and obturator artery
Obturator internus fascia
Tendinous arch of levator ani muscle
Tendinous arch of pelvic fascia
Cardinal (transverse cervical or Mackenrodt's) ligament with uterine artery
Uterosacral ligament
Vaginorectal fascial fibers
Presacral fascia (*pulled away*)
Anterior sacrococcygeal ligament
Vesicocervical and vesicovaginal (potential) spaces
Median sacral artery

F. Netter M.D.

Hip
Mesorectal fascia
Rectal cancer
Mesorectum
Sacrum

Axial MRI showing rectal cancer, surrounding mesorectum, and mesorectal fascia

FIGURE 30.2 Endopelvic fascia and potential spaces: female.

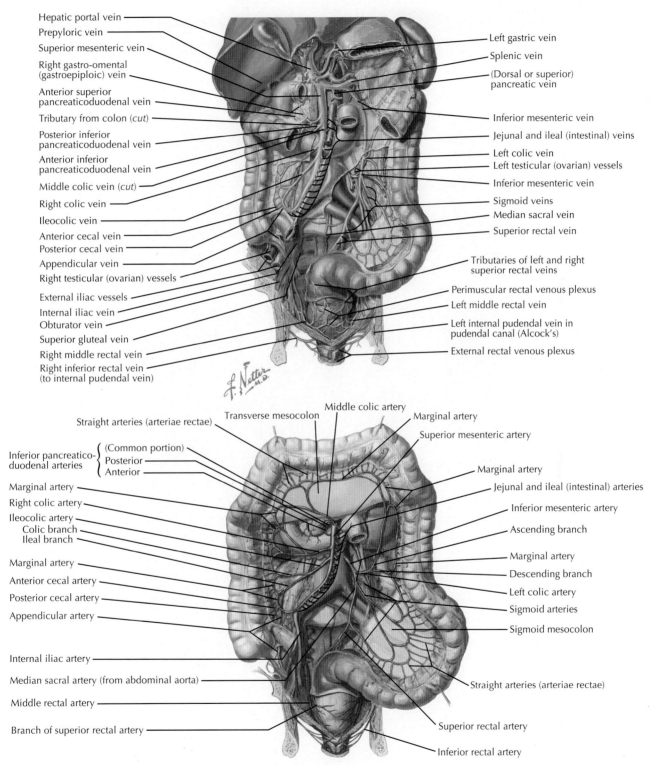

Hepatic portal vein
Prepyloric vein
Superior mesenteric vein
Right gastro-omental (gastroepiploic) vein
Anterior superior pancreaticoduodenal vein
Tributary from colon (cut)
Posterior inferior pancreaticoduodenal vein
Anterior inferior pancreaticoduodenal vein
Middle colic vein (cut)
Right colic vein
Ileocolic vein
Anterior cecal vein
Posterior cecal vein
Appendicular vein
Right testicular (ovarian) vessels
External iliac vessels
Internal iliac vein
Obturator vein
Superior gluteal vein
Right middle rectal vein
Right inferior rectal vein (to internal pudendal vein)

Left gastric vein
Splenic vein
(Dorsal or superior) pancreatic vein
Inferior mesenteric vein
Jejunal and ileal (intestinal) veins
Left colic vein
Left testicular (ovarian) vessels
Inferior mesenteric vein
Sigmoid veins
Median sacral vein
Superior rectal vein
Tributaries of left and right superior rectal veins
Perimuscular rectal venous plexus
Left middle rectal vein
Left internal pudendal vein in pudendal canal (Alcock's)
External rectal venous plexus

Straight arteries (arteriae rectae)
Transverse mesocolon
Middle colic artery
Marginal artery
Superior mesenteric artery
Inferior pancreatico-duodenal arteries { (Common portion) Posterior Anterior
Marginal artery
Right colic artery
Ileocolic artery
Colic branch
Ileal branch
Marginal artery
Anterior cecal artery
Posterior cecal artery
Appendicular artery
Internal iliac artery
Median sacral artery (from abdominal aorta)
Middle rectal artery
Branch of superior rectal artery

Marginal artery
Jejunal and ileal (intestinal) arteries
Inferior mesenteric artery
Ascending branch
Marginal artery
Descending branch
Left colic artery
Sigmoid arteries
Sigmoid mesocolon
Straight arteries (arteriae rectae)
Superior rectal artery
Inferior rectal artery

FIGURE 30.3 Arteries and veins of colon and rectum.

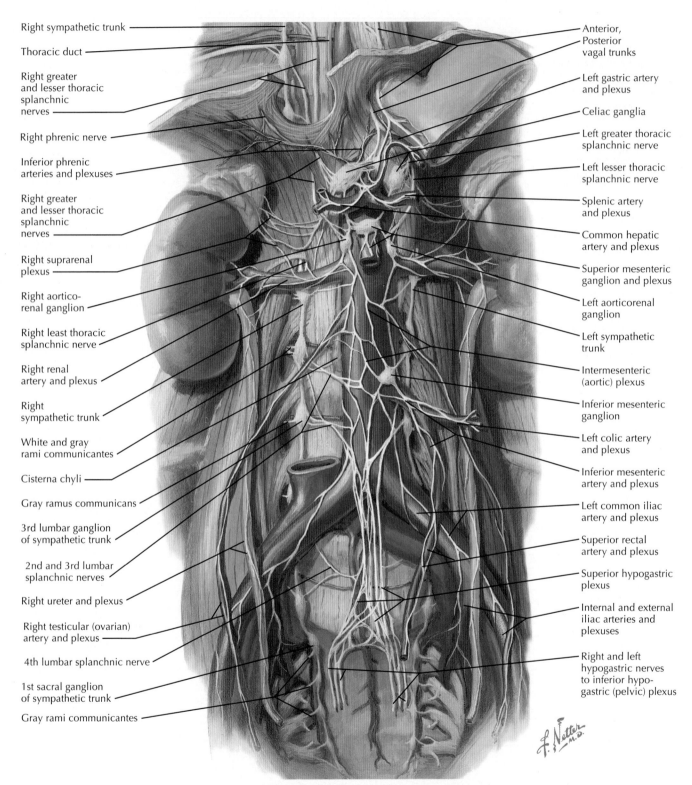

Right sympathetic trunk

Thoracic duct

Right greater and lesser thoracic splanchnic nerves

Right phrenic nerve

Inferior phrenic arteries and plexuses

Right greater and lesser thoracic splanchnic nerves

Right suprarenal plexus

Right aortico-renal ganglion

Right least thoracic splanchnic nerve

Right renal artery and plexus

Right sympathetic trunk

White and gray rami communicantes

Cisterna chyli

Gray ramus communicans

3rd lumbar ganglion of sympathetic trunk

2nd and 3rd lumbar splanchnic nerves

Right ureter and plexus

Right testicular (ovarian) artery and plexus

4th lumbar splanchnic nerve

1st sacral ganglion of sympathetic trunk

Gray rami communicantes

Anterior, Posterior vagal trunks

Left gastric artery and plexus

Celiac ganglia

Left greater thoracic splanchnic nerve

Left lesser thoracic splanchnic nerve

Splenic artery and plexus

Common hepatic artery and plexus

Superior mesenteric ganglion and plexus

Left aorticorenal ganglion

Left sympathetic trunk

Intermesenteric (aortic) plexus

Inferior mesenteric ganglion

Left colic artery and plexus

Inferior mesenteric artery and plexus

Left common iliac artery and plexus

Superior rectal artery and plexus

Superior hypogastric plexus

Internal and external iliac arteries and plexuses

Right and left hypogastric nerves to inferior hypo-gastric (pelvic) plexus

FIGURE 30.4 Autonomic nerves and ganglia of abdomen.

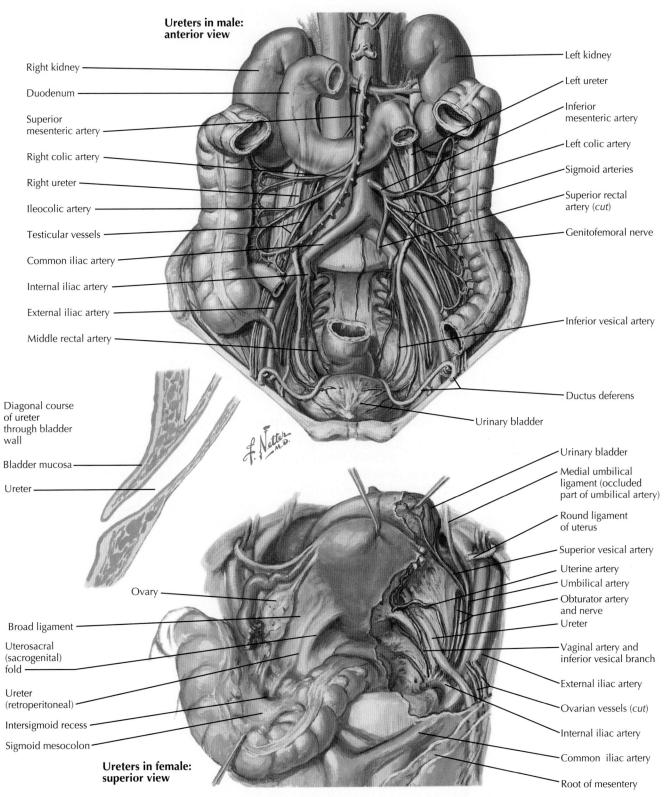

Ureters in male: anterior view

Right kidney

Duodenum

Superior mesenteric artery

Right colic artery

Right ureter

Ileocolic artery

Testicular vessels

Common iliac artery

Internal iliac artery

External iliac artery

Middle rectal artery

Left kidney

Left ureter

Inferior mesenteric artery

Left colic artery

Sigmoid arteries

Superior rectal artery (cut)

Genitofemoral nerve

Inferior vesical artery

Ductus deferens

Urinary bladder

Diagonal course of ureter through bladder wall

Bladder mucosa

Ureter

Urinary bladder

Medial umbilical ligament (occluded part of umbilical artery)

Round ligament of uterus

Superior vesical artery

Uterine artery

Umbilical artery

Obturator artery and nerve

Ureter

Vaginal artery and inferior vesical branch

External iliac artery

Ovarian vessels (cut)

Internal iliac artery

Common iliac artery

Root of mesentery

Ovary

Broad ligament

Uterosacral (sacrogenital) fold

Ureter (retroperitoneal)

Intersigmoid recess

Sigmoid mesocolon

Ureters in female: superior view

FIGURE 30.5 Anatomic relations of ureters: male and female.

Inferior Mesenteric Artery and Vein: Anterior View

The sigmoid colon may be mobilized starting on the medial or the lateral side. When the correct planes are defined, Toldt's fascia is carefully preserved and remains as a parietal layer over the retroperitoneum. The ureters and para-aortic autonomic nerves are by definition posterior to this layer. The mesentery of the distal sigmoid is then elevated from the retroperitoneum under slight tension. The peritoneum to the right of the inferior mesenteric artery (IMA) is opened parallel to the vessel, allowing the index finger of the left hand to encircle the origin of the IMA (Fig. 30.6).

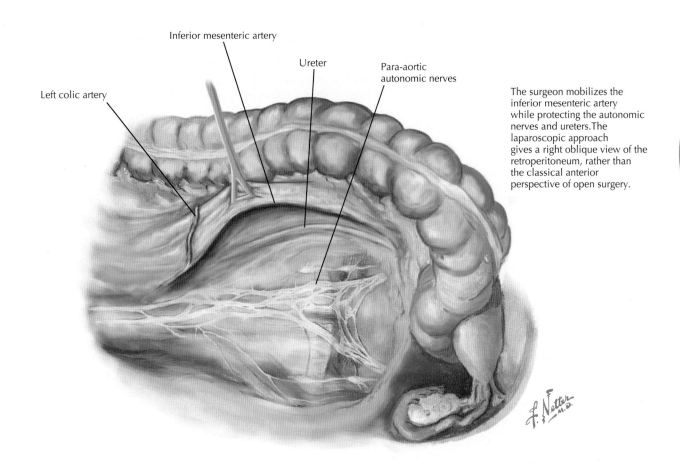

Left colic artery — Inferior mesenteric artery — Ureter — Para-aortic autonomic nerves

The surgeon mobilizes the inferior mesenteric artery while protecting the autonomic nerves and ureters. The laparoscopic approach gives a right oblique view of the retroperitoneum, rather than the classical anterior perspective of open surgery.

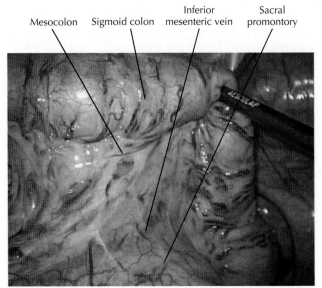

Mesocolon   Sigmoid colon   Inferior mesenteric vein   Sacral promontory

Inferior mesenteric vein can be seen deep to the peritoneum, while the rectosigmoid junction is stretched anteriorly to place it under tension.

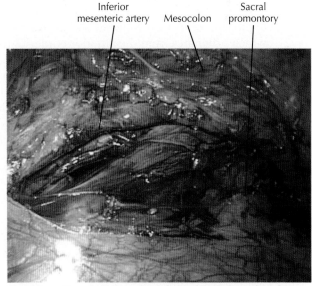

Inferior mesenteric artery   Mesocolon   Sacral promontory

Once the peritoneum is opened, parallel and posterior to the inferior mesenteric artery, the autonomic nerves are swept posteriorly and protected. The left ureter can be seen behind and lateral to the artery.

FIGURE 30.6 Inferior mesenteric artery.

Inferior Mesenteric Artery and Vein: Medial Oblique View

The same anatomy is approached differently in laparoscopic surgery. The position of the camera means that the perspective of the vessels is from a much more oblique view. Nevertheless, the same structures can be observed. When the IMA is divided, this is performed 1 cm distal to its origin to protect the para-aortic autonomic nerves, and just proximal to the left colic artery. The left colic artery is then divided close to the IMA, thereby preserving the collateral circulation to the left colic to maximize blood flow to the segment of bowel that will be used as the neorectum (Fig. 30.7).

Splenic Flexure

Although the splenic flexure is not mobilized routinely by all surgeons, this is an important and frequently necessary skill. The flexure can be mobilized from a medial, lateral, or inferior approach. Entry to the lesser sac exposes the superior aspect of the transverse mesocolon, which originates from the anterior border of the pancreas. Mobilization too far from the retroperitoneum (too close to the colon) creates a defect through the mesentery of the colon. While the surgeon is mobilizing the flexure, care must be paid to the jejunum, which is often only a few cell layers away in thin patients (through the mesentery) from the area of dissection.

The greater omentum is then elevated superiorly, demonstrating the avascular plane between this and the transverse colon. This plane is opened, mobilizing the splenic flexure so that the colon to the left of the midline is fully freed from its attachments. At this stage the colon is tethered by the inferior mesenteric vein (IMV) as it enters the splenic vein behind the pancreas. The IMV is divided just below the pancreas, giving several extra inches of length to allow the descending colon to reach into the pelvis (see Fig. 30.7).

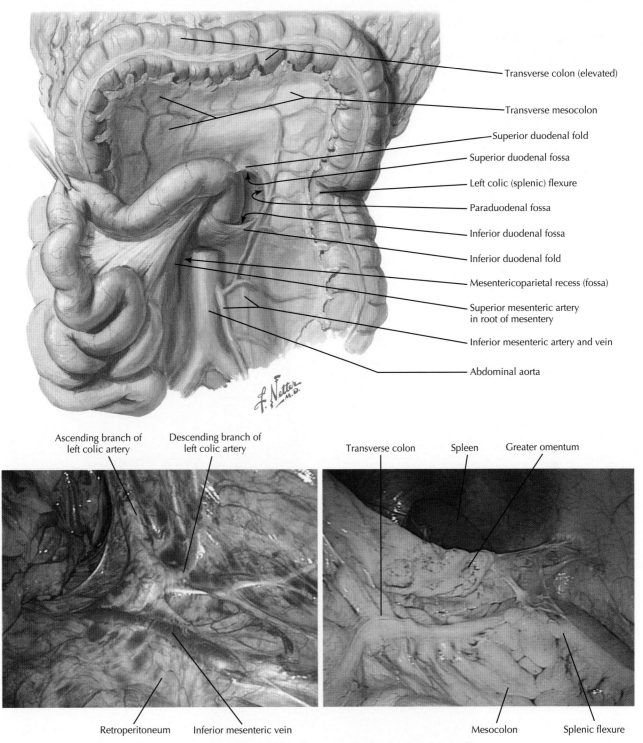

Transverse colon (elevated)

Transverse mesocolon

Superior duodenal fold

Superior duodenal fossa

Left colic (splenic) flexure

Paraduodenal fossa

Inferior duodenal fossa

Inferior duodenal fold

Mesentericoparietal recess (fossa)

Superior mesenteric artery
in root of mesentery

Inferior mesenteric artery and vein

Abdominal aorta

Ascending branch of
left colic artery

Descending branch of
left colic artery

Transverse colon   Spleen   Greater omentum

Retroperitoneum   Inferior mesenteric vein

Mesocolon   Splenic flexure

The splenic flexure is mobilized to obtain adequate reach for a colorectal anastomosis. The operative photographs
demonstrate the view of the splenic flexure lying in the retroperitoneum before mobilization.

FIGURE 30.7 Inferior mesenteric vein and splenic flexure.

Upper Mesorectum: Posterior Mesorectal Anatomy

The anatomy of the dissection of the upper rectum is demonstrated in Fig. 30.6, along with the pelvic autonomic nerve anatomy. Dissection commences behind the rectum, staying between the plane of the parietal peritoneum (Toldt's fascia) and the investing fascial layer of the mesorectum. The initial dissection is in the midline posteriorly and continues down to the level of the levator muscles, demonstrating the bilobed appearance of the intact mesorectum. Adequate traction and countertraction of tissues assists in demonstration of the correct anatomic planes. Dissection continues laterally on both sides until the rectum becomes tethered by the anterior peritoneal attachments at the pouch of Douglas (Fig. 30.8).

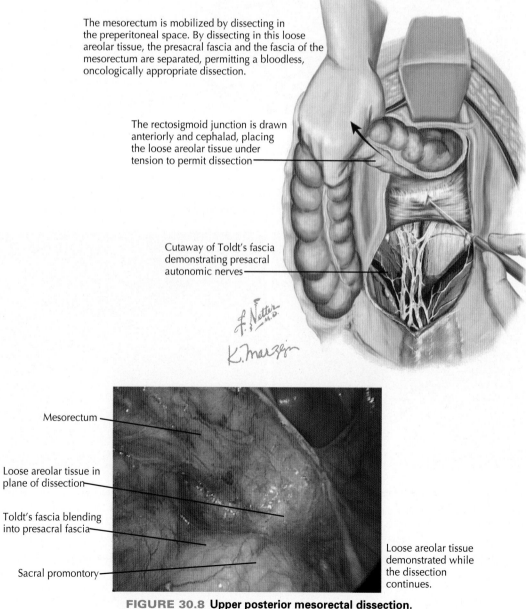

The mesorectum is mobilized by dissecting in the preperitoneal space. By dissecting in this loose areolar tissue, the presacral fascia and the fascia of the mesorectum are separated, permitting a bloodless, oncologically appropriate dissection.

The rectosigmoid junction is drawn anteriorly and cephalad, placing the loose areolar tissue under tension to permit dissection

Cutaway of Toldt's fascia demonstrating presacral autonomic nerves

Mesorectum

Loose areolar tissue in plane of dissection

Toldt's fascia blending into presacral fascia

Sacral promontory

Loose areolar tissue demonstrated while the dissection continues.

FIGURE 30.8 Upper posterior mesorectal dissection.

Lower Mesorectum: Anterior Mesorectal Anatomy

The bladder or uterus is then drawn anteriorly, and cautery is used to continue the lateral dissection anteriorly, opening the peritoneum immediately behind Denonvilliers' fascia. The dissection then continues distally until the levators are seen to curve distally into the anal canal, protecting the anterolateral neurovascular bundles (Fig. 30.9). The posterior and lateral dissection can now be completed down to the level of the anal canal, facilitated by the anterior dissection, improving mobility.

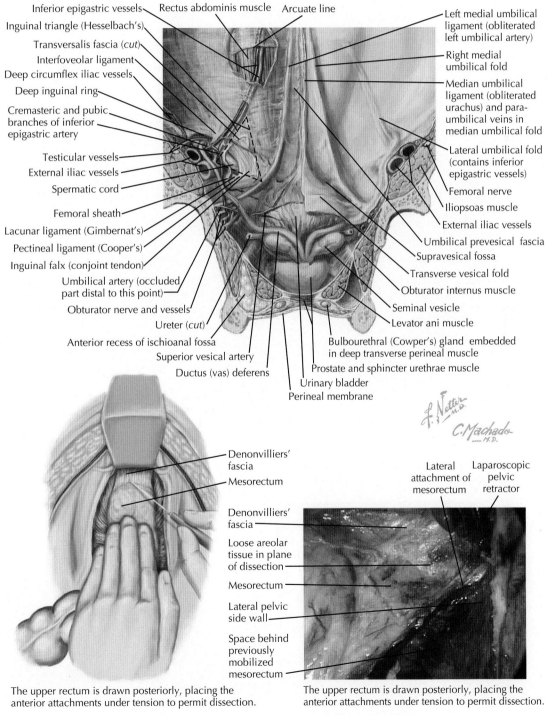

The upper rectum is drawn posteriorly, placing the anterior attachments under tension to permit dissection.

The upper rectum is drawn posteriorly, placing the anterior attachments under tension to permit dissection.

FIGURE 30.9 Lower anterior mesorectal dissection.

Rectal Transection From Above

Once an adequate distal margin has been obtained, the rectum may be transected below the level of the tumor, usually at the anorectal junction. At this level there is no mesorectum to divide, and a stapler usually fits easily around the rectum. The specimen is amputated and removed from the field. This approach leaves a transverse staple line that can be easily seen from above, sitting just into the upper anal canal within the sling of the levators, ready for a stapled coloanal anastomosis (Fig. 30.10). Perineal pressure can facilitate appropriate stapler placement in the distal pelvis.

Superior view

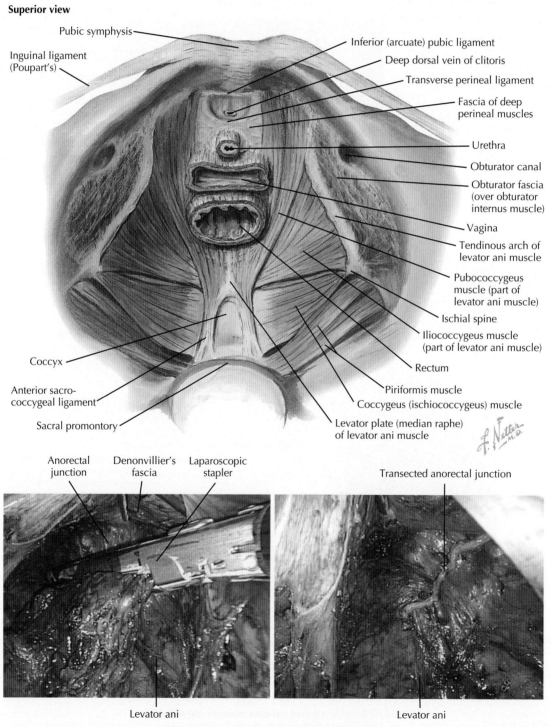

FIGURE 30.10 **Stapled rectal transection.**

Rectal Transection From Below

Some patients have insufficient distal margin for a stapled anastomosis, usually for tumors within 2 cm from the dentate line. In these cases, the intra-abdominal dissection proceeds as previously described until the anal canal is reached. At this stage the surgeon moves to the perineum. An operating anoscope is used to visualize the dentate line, which is incised circumferentially with cautery. The dissection is continued to the internal sphincter, which is transected circumferentially. An intersphincteric dissection is then performed, joining the prior plane of dissection from above (Fig. 30.11). The anastomosis between the neorectum and the anal canal may then be sutured or stapled. A defunctioning proximal ostomy is usually created to mitigate potential complications of anastomotic leak.

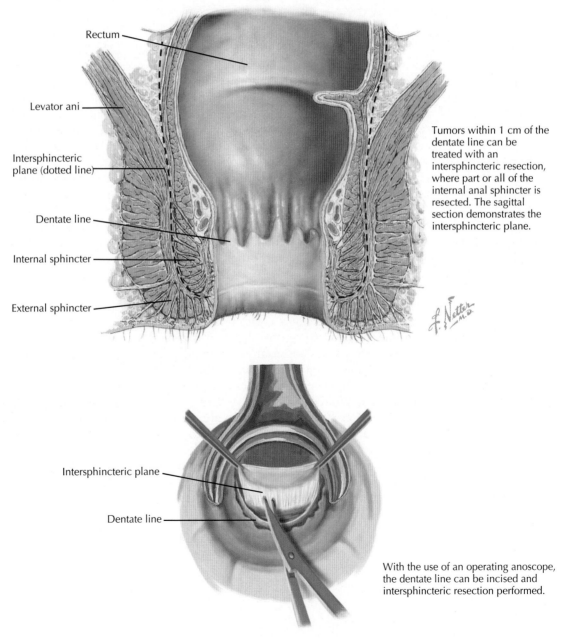

Rectum

Levator ani

Intersphincteric plane (dotted line)

Dentate line

Internal sphincter

External sphincter

Tumors within 1 cm of the dentate line can be treated with an intersphincteric resection, where part or all of the internal anal sphincter is resected. The sagittal section demonstrates the intersphincteric plane.

Intersphincteric plane

Dentate line

With the use of an operating anoscope, the dentate line can be incised and intersphincteric resection performed.

FIGURE 30.11 **Intersphincteric transanal transection of rectum.**

TRANSANAL MESORECTAL DISSECTION

Developments in minimally invasive surgical technology now permit surgeons to dissect further proximally after transecting the rectum from below, now called transanal total mesorectal excision (taTME). Indeed, much or all of the mesorectal mobilization can be accomplished from this approach, which is becoming favored by many surgeons. The surgical principles of achieving a complete resection margin (CRM) are maintained, with a theoretical improvement in the identification of critical anatomic structures. This approach can be particularly useful for patients with unfavorable characteristics, such as obesity, male gender, and a narrow pelvis.

Similar to the section on transection from below, after identification of an appropriate distal margin, a purse-string suture is placed to occlude the rectal lumen, and the taTME dissection is commenced via a circumferential full-thickness proctotomy just distal to the purse string. The dissection is commenced at the posterior quadrant. A plane of dissection can be created just lateral to the rectococcygeal fibers. These fibers are then divided to gain access to the space between the leaves of the presacral fascia (Fig. 30.12A). As the dissection progresses cranially, the surgeon needs to be cognizant of sacral angulation as well as the retrosacral fascial attachment at the level of S3 *(diagram sagittal)*. Misidentification of these structures can lead to bleeding from the pelvic venous plexus.

Once the posterior plane has been defined, the dissection is commenced at the anterior quadrant. Two windows can be created anterolaterally and connected by dividing the recto-urethralis fibers (see Fig. 30.12A). These fibers typically tether the rectum to the prostate in males. The neurovascular bundle of Walsh can be identified anterolaterally (10 and 2 o'clock position). The correct plane of dissection is posterior to this bundle, and failure to recognize the pulsatile vessels increases the chance of a prostatic and urethral injury.

Lateral dissection is typically commenced after anterior and posterior mobilization. Adipose pillars are seen at the level of the midrectum that may appear to be connected to the pelvic sidewall by loose areolar tissue (Fig. 30.12B). This loose areolar tissue is misleading, and lateral dissection in an incorrect plane at this point may lead to catastrophic injuries of the pelvic sidewall.

After circumferential mobilization, the perineal and abdominal dissections are connected. taTME can be performed independently or as part of a two-team approach. An anastomosis is typically performed with a circular stapler.

A. Sagittal female pelvis

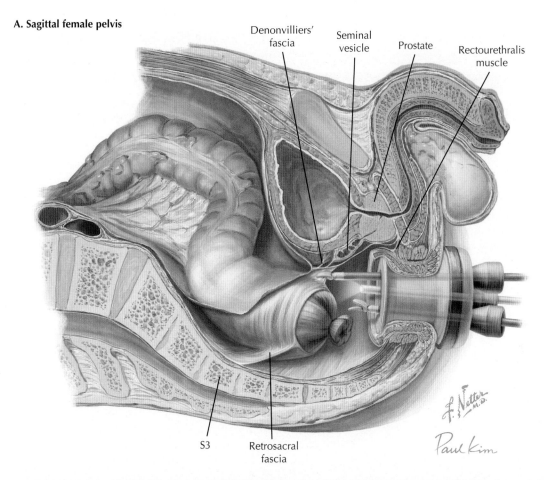

Denonvilliers' fascia

Seminal vesicle

Prostate

Rectourethralis muscle

S3

Retrosacral fascia

B. Image demonstrating the lateral "adipose" pillars and the correct vs incorrect plane of lateral dissection.

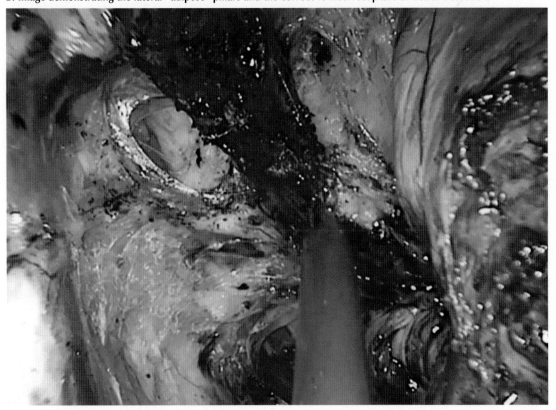

FIGURE 30.12 (A) Sagittal view of taTME device in place performing distal dissection. (B) Transanal TME view of lateral pillars during the taTME dissection.

SUGGESTED READING

Delaney CP. Low anterior resection. In: Operative techniques in general surgery. Philadelphia: Saunders; 2003. p. 214–23.

Abdominoperineal Resection

Stefan D. Holubar and Hermann Kessler

INTRODUCTION

Abdominoperineal resection (APR) is most often employed for lower-third rectal cancers, rare low pelvic tumors, and other low pelvic cancers requiring pelvic exenteration with involvement of the sphincters. Tumors above the levator muscles and inflammatory bowel diseases (IBD) can typically be treated with sphincter-sparing restorative and nonrestorative intersphincteric proctectomy. Patients with anal squamous cell carcinoma with persistent or recurrent disease despite, or who have contraindication to, definitive chemoradiation with Nigro protocol, are also candidates for APR. Occasionally, patients with severe fistulizing perianal Crohn's disease require an APR, often with myocutaneous flap reconstruction. This chapter describes a standardized approach to resection of the rectum and anal sphincter complex.

PRINCIPLES OF PREOPERATIVE EVALUATION

Dedicated workup typically starts with a baseline full colonoscopy. The operating surgeon's examination includes a digital rectal examination and flexible and/or rigid proctoscopy to confirm tumor location, mobility, or IBD disease extent and to assess feasibility of a sphincter-sparing approach (Fig. 31.1A). Proctoscopy also allows the surgeon to tattoo the distal edge of the tumor in case of a complete clinical response for future identification. In women, bimanual/vaginal examination, and occasionally vaginoscopy, may help assess for local invasion, and surgeons should have a low threshold for performing an examination under anesthesia. Computed tomographic (CT) scanning of the chest, abdomen, and pelvis is done to survey for metastatic disease.

For both malignant and benign disease, pelvic magnetic resonance imaging (MRI) is now standard, providing a more complete and less operator-dependent visualization of the extent of the tumor in the pelvis (Fig. 31.1B). Pelvic MRI is exceptionally accurate in predicting involvement of the circumferential radial margin (CRM) and the degree of involvement of the pelvic side wall, sacrum, or anterior organs. Pelvic MRI is also useful in anteriorly based tumors, because it identifies local involvement of the vagina, distal ureters, prostate, seminal vesicles, or urinary bladder, indicating a need for exenteration. Conversely, in locally advanced prostate or gynecologic cancers, it identifies noncolorectal tumors that are invading the sphincters. Endorectal ultrasound is also used for local staging to assess the need for preoperative chemoradiation (Fig. 31.1C) in those unable to obtain pelvic MRI and for early stage tumors.

Patients with locally advanced rectal cancer, particularly those with clinical stage II or stage III, are treated with long-course preoperative radiochemotherapy, and surgery is performed 10 to 12 weeks after cessation of radiation. Before surgery, the patient evaluated and the eventual stoma site is marked by enterostomal therapy, and the surgeon will reassess the tumor with proctoscopy, noting the response to radiochemotherapy. Some patients initially not thought to be candidates for a low anterior resection occasionally may be "down-staged" and determined to be suitable for sphincter-sparing procedures when assessed after neoadjuvant therapy. Caution should be used in determining the extent of resection necessary, lest microscopic islands of cancer at the leading edge of the tumor be left behind; microscopic deposits are frequently seen in deep specimens despite clear mucosa. If the surgeon anticipates the need for perineal flap reconstruction (see below), a plastic surgeon should be consulted early to avoid delays in operative scheduling.

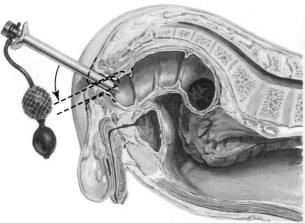

A. Rigid proctoscopy. Performed on all patients with rectal tumors. Location from anal verge should be noted as well as location and tumor characteristics prior to neoadjuvant or surgical therapy.

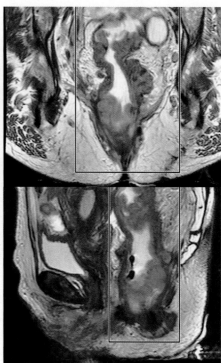

B. Magnetic resonance imaging of rectal cancer.

C. Endorectal ultrasonography. A digital exam can determine tumor characteristics, local invasion, and fixation of tumor. Anatomic location of the tumor can help to predict possible invasion into prostate or vagina anteriorly, side wall or coccyx posteriorly. It is very important to determine invasion of the levator muscles distally prior to therapy. Endorectal ultrasound can stage the tumor infiltration (T stage) as well as presence or absence of pathological nodes. These findings will determine whether the patient is a candidate for surgical therapy or neoadjuvant chemoradiation.

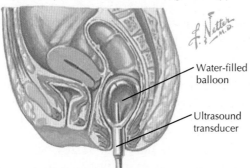

Water-filled balloon

Ultrasound transducer

Endorectal ultrasonography assesses depth of tumor penetration and degree of perirectal involvement

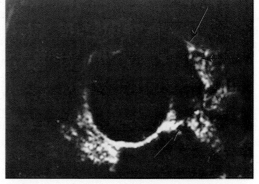

Ultrasonogram. Rectal tumor invades perirectal fat

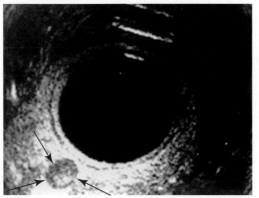

Ultrasonogram. Rectal tumor and involvement of perirectal lymph nodes (arrows)

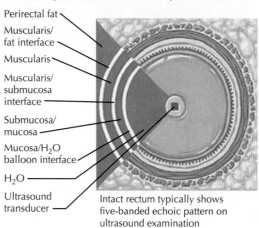

Perirectal fat

Muscularis/ fat interface

Muscularis

Muscularis/ submucosa interface

Submucosa/ mucosa

Mucosa/H_2O balloon interface

H_2O

Ultrasound transducer

Intact rectum typically shows five-banded echoic pattern on ultrasound examination

FIGURE 31.1 Proctoscopy and endorectal ultrasonography.

ANATOMIC APPROACH TO LEFT COLON MOBILIZATION

The modern approach to rectal cancer may be through an open, laparoscopic, robotic, trans-anal, or hybrid approach. Regardless of the method chosen, following standard oncologic principles such as total mesorectal excision (TME) remain the same. However, if a vertical rectus abdominis musculocutaneous (VRAM) flap is planned, open surgery may be preferred.

The left colon is mobilized either from a medial-to-lateral or lateral-to-medial fashion. The lateral mobilization occurs medial to the white line of Toldt (in the avascular plane between Gerota's fascia), preserving the mesocolic fascia. This approach allows a bloodless mobilization of the sigmoid and descending colon to the midline, even as far as entering the presacral space. The left gonadal vein and ureter are usually readily identified and protected throughout the dissection as they lie posterior to Toldt's fascia, which is kept intact over the retroperitoneum. If difficult to find, dissection either proximally toward the kidney or distally into the pelvis can assist in identifying the ureter. Further, if this is anticipated, prophylactic or intraoperative ureteral stent placement may be helpful.

The mobilization is extended to the root of the mesocolon, and the inferior mesenteric artery (IMA) is identified at its takeoff from the aorta (Fig. 31.2A). The hypogastric plexus (sympathetic fibers), which lie posterior to the IMA, are protected by keeping close to the back wall of the IMA, and if necessary, carefully sweeping the nerve branches posteriorly away from the vessel (Fig. 31.2B). The IMA is isolated, ligated, and divided. The left colic artery and the inferior mesenteric vein are divided and ligated at the level of the IMA (Fig. 31.2C). The mesentery is then divided perpendicularly to the level of the marginal artery, just proximal to the first sigmoidal branch, and pulsatile arterial flow in the marginal artery is confirmed by sharp transection and re-ligation. Unlike in low anterior resection, where extra length is needed for a tension-free colorectal anastomosis, mobilization of the splenic flexure is not required unless the patient is morbidly obese and extra length is needed for stoma construction.

A. Arteries of the large intestine and rectum. For rectal tumors, a high ligation of the inferior mesenteric artery at its takeoff from the aorta is performed. The left colic artery may be preserved. The dissection is carried out to the marginal artery proximal to the first sigmoidal branch.

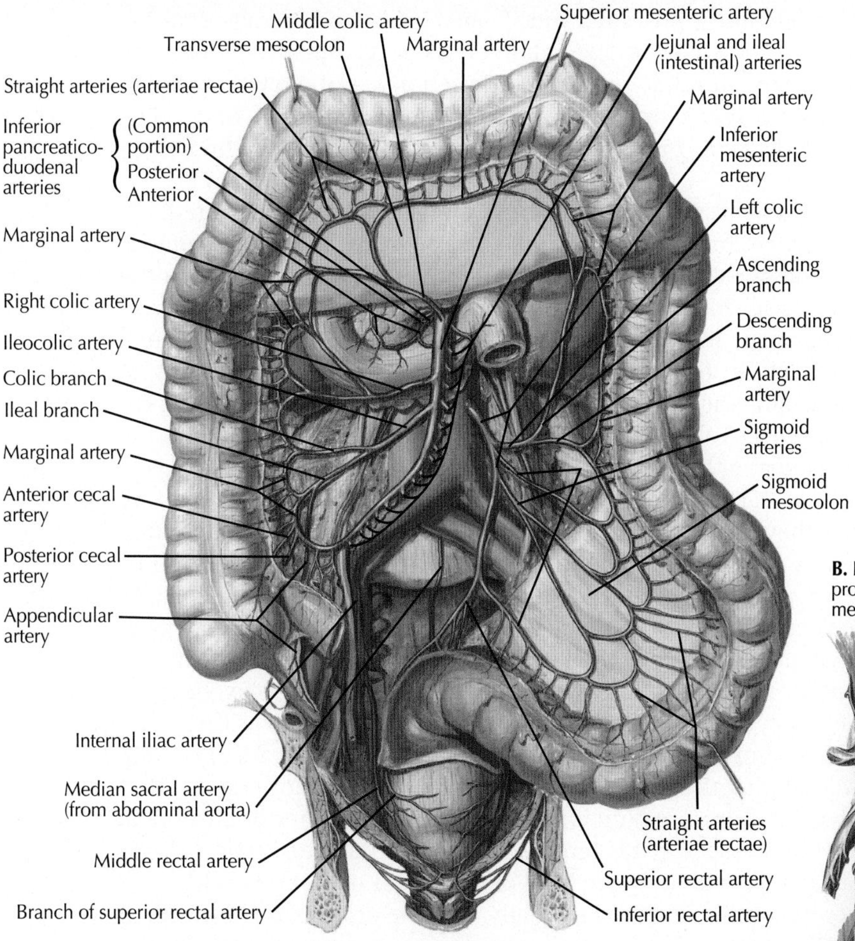

Middle colic artery
Superior mesenteric artery
Transverse mesocolon
Marginal artery
Jejunal and ileal (intestinal) arteries
Straight arteries (arteriae rectae)
Marginal artery
Inferior pancreatico-duodenal arteries
(Common portion)
Posterior
Anterior
Inferior mesenteric artery
Left colic artery
Marginal artery
Ascending branch
Right colic artery
Descending branch
Ileocolic artery
Marginal artery
Colic branch
Sigmoid arteries
Ileal branch
Marginal artery
Sigmoid mesocolon
Anterior cecal artery
Posterior cecal artery
Appendicular artery
Internal iliac artery
Median sacral artery (from abdominal aorta)
Middle rectal artery
Straight arteries (arteriae rectae)
Superior rectal artery
Branch of superior rectal artery
Inferior rectal artery

B. Nerves of the rectum and pelvis. Note the close proximity of the sympathetic plexus to the inferior mesenteric artery.

Inferior mesenteric ganglion, artery, and plexus
Hypogastric nerves
5th lumbar splanchnic nerve
Sacral splanchnic nerves (sympathetic)
Gray rami communicantes
Inferior hypogastric (pelvic) plexus
Pelvic splanchnic nerves (parasympathetic)
Obturator nerve and artery
Piriformis muscle
Ductus deferens and plexus
Gluteus maximus muscle and sacro-tuberous ligament
Vesical plexus
Coccygeus (ischio-coccygeus) muscle and sacrospinous ligament
Rectal plexus
Prostatic plexus
Pudendal nerve
Levator ani muscle
Cavernous nerves of penis
Inferior anal (rectal) nerve
Perineal nerve
Posterior scrotal nerves
Dorsal nerve of penis

Inferior mesenteric artery at takeoff from aorta
Inferior mesenteric vein

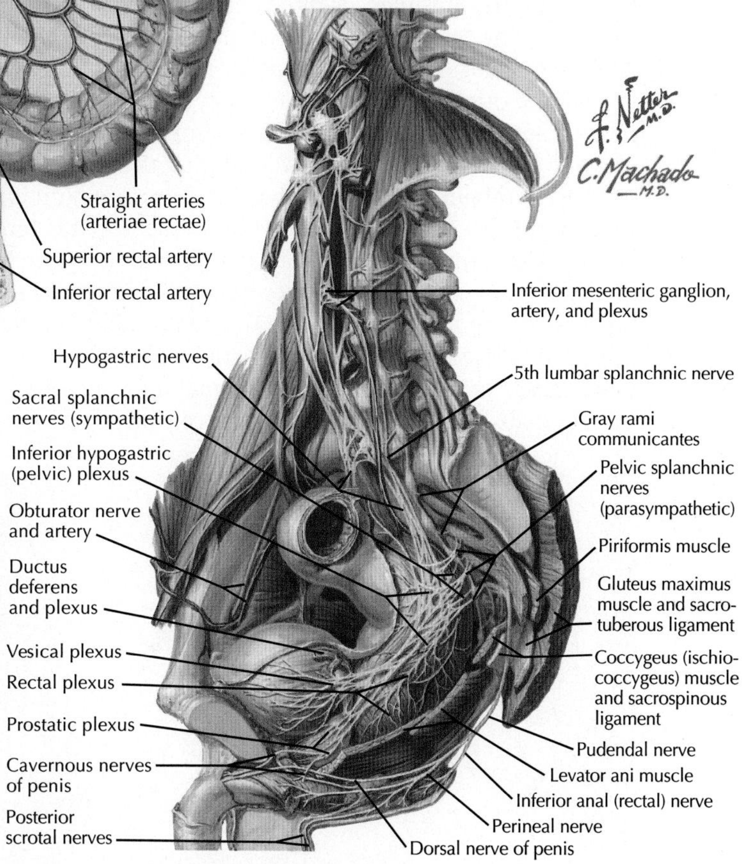

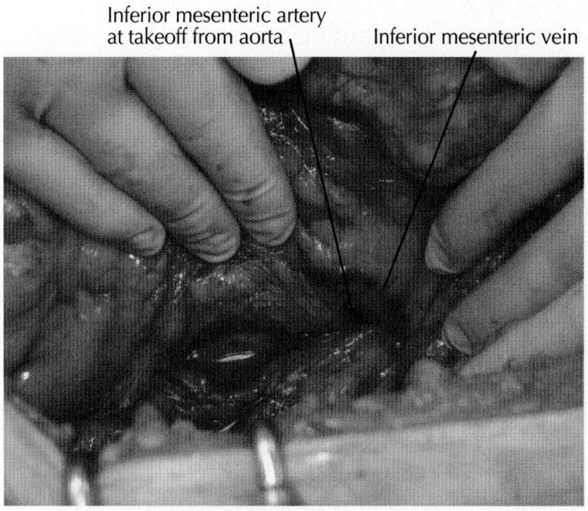

C. Arteries and veins of the left colon.

FIGURE 31.2 Arteries and nerves of pelvis and rectum.

APPROACH FOR RECTAL DISSECTION

The patient is placed in the Trendelenburg position, and if open or hybrid, a self-retaining retractor is placed. In both minimally invasive and open approaches, it is helpful to elevate the uterus by placing a suture in the uterine fundus, retracting it anteriorly, and pexying through the abdominal wall in laparoscopic surgery, or to the self-retaining retractor if open (Fig. 31.3A). In open surgical cases, the dissection is greatly facilitated by the use of lighted, deep pelvic retractors and headlights.

The pelvic dissection usually commences posteriorly, then laterally, and finally anteriorly. Mobilization of the rectum and its investing mesorectum and fascia begins behind the inferior mesenteric vessels, at the level of the sacral promontory in the loose areolar tissue between the mesorectal fascia and the presacral fascia. Posterior dissection may be facilitated by lifting the rectosigmoid junction anterior and cephalad, and the avascular plane can be identified and entered, anterior to the nerves. The right and left hypogastric nerves (i.e., first division of the pelvic nerves) are identified and swept posterolaterally; they are carefully avoided, and in fact most easily protected, by keeping them behind an intact Toldt's fascia. The posterior dissection continues to the pelvic floor with the use of electrocautery or large Harrington-type scissors (Fig. 31.3B), but importantly avoiding blunt dissection. Unless an extended resection is being performed, the ureters are generally easily protected because they lie deep to the endopelvic fascia in the retroperitoneum. Nevertheless, the ureters' location is verified throughout the dissection (Fig. 31.3C). Posteriorly, the dissection continues in the avascular plane until Waldeyer's rectosacral fascia is reached. As the dissection continues, its direction will tilt more anteriorly, above the level of the coccyx (Fig. 31.3D). In the "classic" APR, dissection continues to the levator hiatus, whereas in a "cylindrical" APR for oncologic purposes, the pelvic dissection stops at the level of the tip of the coccyx, near the level of the origin of the levators. The cylindrical APR follows similar TME principles as the mesorectum naturally tapers above the levators, and the surgeon should avoid "coning in," resulting in a narrow waist, which may compromise the circumferential margin of the tumor (Fig. 31.3E).

The lateral peritoneum overlying the mesorectum is scored down to the anterior peritoneal reflection (Fig. 31.3F). Laterally, the presacral parasympathetic nerves (i.e., *nervi erigentes*) can be seen along the pelvic side wall at approximately the level of the lateral stalks and middle rectal arteries (Fig. 31.3G). The mesorectum is retracted medially, and the dissection is continued bilaterally. The *nervi erigentes* are allowed to fall laterally as the dissection proceeds, continuing until the pelvic floor and levators are reached. In most cases, the mesorectal fascia and endopelvic fascia are carefully separated, maintaining an avascular plane. The middle rectal vessels are often absent, and the dissection is completely bloodless.

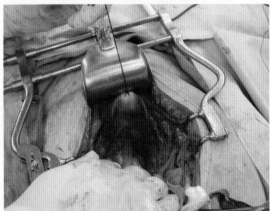
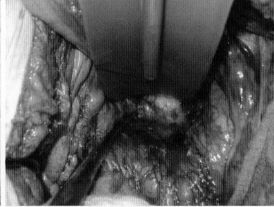

A. Uterus retracted anteriorly by suture attached to self-retaining retractor

B. IMA retraction anteriorly and starting dissection in the proper mesorectal plane identifying the hypogastric nerves. Lighted deep pelvic retractor facilitates dissection.

FIGURE 31.3 Approach for rectal dissection. *IMA,* Inferior mesenteric artery.

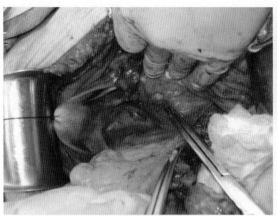

C. Mesorectal peritoneum scored bilaterally

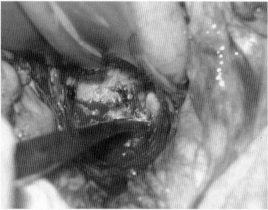

D. View into the pelvis, localization of the right ureter prior to dissection

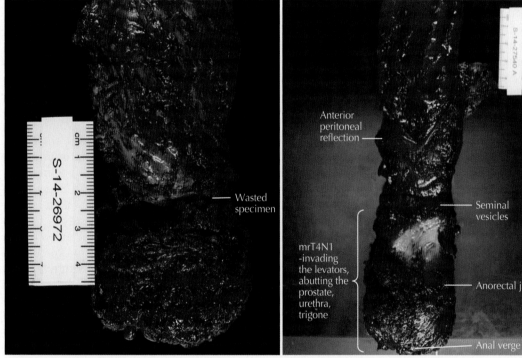

E. Specimen from a traditional and cylindrical APR

Wasted specimen

Anterior peritoneal reflection

Seminal vesicles

mrT4N1 -invading the levators, abutting the prostate, urethra, trigone

Anorectal jxn

Anal verge

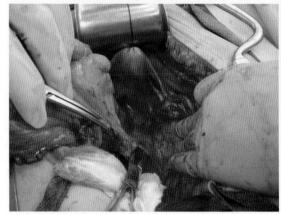

F. Completion of posterior dissection to the pelvic floor, showing pelvic floor/levators

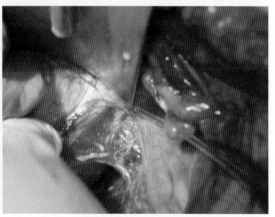

G. Lateral attachments with the nervi erigentes at border of mesorectum

FIGURE 31.3 Approach for rectal dissection—cont'd.

APPROACH FOR RECTAL DISSECTION (Continued)

Finally, the anterior dissection is performed. The peritoneum in the cul-de-sac is scored just anterior to the fold at the peritoneal reflection. Denonvilliers' fascia is typically reflected posteriorly to keep the mesorectum intact on the specimen, particularly staying anterior to Denonvilliers' fascia in case of anterior tumors. The surgeon must keep in mind the location of the pelvic plexus of nerves that overlies the seminal vesicles (SV) anteriorly in the male. It is important to avoid skeletonizing the vesicles to prevent nerve injury. Also to avoid injury, the proximity of the ureters to the apex of the SV must be considered (Fig. 31.4). The anterior dissection continues as far distally as possible, even to the pelvic floor and into the anal canal, because this is the same plane that is entered from below, and it facilitates the distal dissection. In women with a bulky, anteriorly based tumor, en bloc posterior vaginectomy may be necessary, which may then require flap reconstruction depending on the amount of tissue taken.

After the abdominal dissection is completed, two options exist for the perineal dissection. Typically, the patient's legs can be moved to high lithotomy position and the perineal dissection completed with the surgeon seated between the legs. Alternatively, the stoma can be created, the abdomen closed, and the stoma matured, followed by subsequent turning of the patient to the prone jackknife position. Each approach has its proponents.

Regardless of positioning, the margins of dissection are determined by anatomy and tumor location. In general, the posterior margin is determined by palpation of the coccyx, the lateral margins by palpation of the ischial tuberosities, and the anterior margin by the urethra in the male and the posterior vaginal wall in the female. As previously noted, posterior vaginectomy is typically performed for any bulky, anteriorly based lesion.

After outlining margins, the skin is scored. The amount of skin that must be taken is typically not great, and usually the anal verge suffices, except with a malignant fistulae, fungating tumors, recurrent disease, or squamous lesions. The pelvic dissection may be aided by the placement of everting sutures or a Lone Star–type retractor. The dissection is continued until the ischiorectal fossa is entered circumferentially (Fig. 31.5A). Usually, the posterior dissection is performed first because it has the clearest landmarks. The anococcygeal ligament is divided and the dissection proceeds to join the abdominal dissection, just anterior to the coccyx unless an en bloc coccygectomy is required. The surgeon then continues the lateral dissection, dividing the lateral origin of the levator muscles in cancer cases, maintaining an "extra-levator" plane. A finger is placed in the patient's pelvis and hooked behind the levators, and cautery is used to divide the left and right muscles (Fig. 31.5B).

The anterior dissection is finally undertaken, taking great care to observe and follow anatomic planes, although this is not always easy. In the male patient, the urethra is noted by palpation of the Foley catheter, and great care is taken to avoid injury. In the female patient, a finger in the vagina can help to define the anterior rectovaginal septal plane. In cylindrical APRs, the dissection continues higher up to meet the extent of pelvic dissection from above, resulting in a specimen without narrowing. After the dissection is completed circumferentially, the specimen is delivered through the perineum and carefully examined for adequacy of the CRM (Fig. 31.5C) and intactness of the TME specimen.

Closure of the perineum is accomplished in layers with absorbable sutures. Generous bites are taken from the remaining ischiorectal fat. A deep layer is placed in the subcutaneous fat. In cases in which a partial posterior vaginectomy is required, the vagina can usually be closed in a tubular fashion, although somewhat narrowed. The perineum is then closed with interrupted vertical mattress sutures, beginning at the introitus (Fig. 31.5D). In the case of a larger perineal defects, or cylindrical APR, additional perineal reconstruction may be required. Options including absorbable mesh for the deep layer with either flap skin closure, posterior thigh (gluteal) flaps, anterolateral thigh (ALT) flaps, or vertical rectus abdominis flaps.

Note the location of the tip of the seminal vesicle in relation to the ureter and its entrance into the bladder. The pelvic plexus of nerves is immediately overlying the seminal vesicles and the prostate.

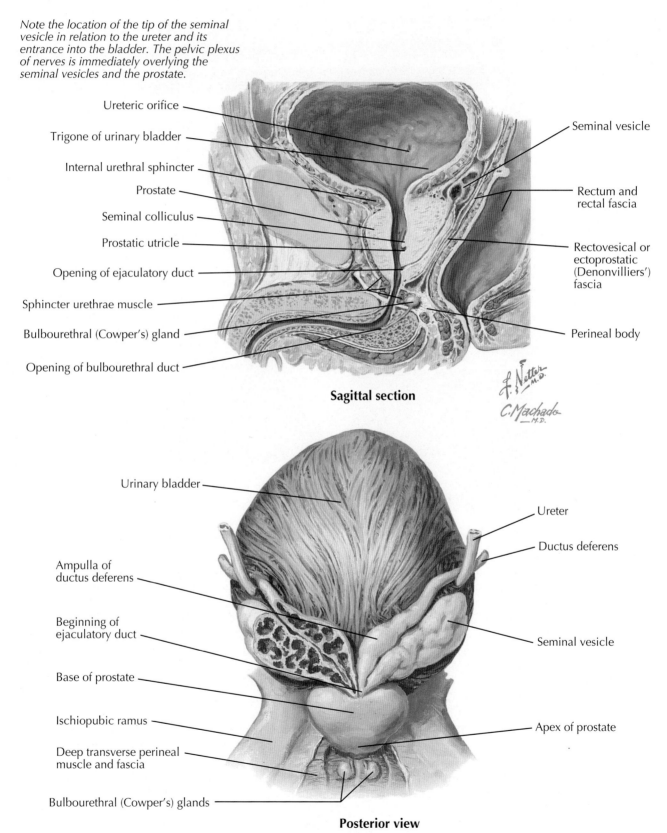

Ureteric orifice

Trigone of urinary bladder

Internal urethral sphincter

Prostate

Seminal colliculus

Prostatic utricle

Opening of ejaculatory duct

Sphincter urethrae muscle

Bulbourethral (Cowper's) gland

Opening of bulbourethral duct

Seminal vesicle

Rectum and rectal fascia

Rectovesical or ectoprostatic (Denonvilliers') fascia

Perineal body

Sagittal section

Urinary bladder

Ampulla of ductus deferens

Beginning of ejaculatory duct

Base of prostate

Ischiopubic ramus

Deep transverse perineal muscle and fascia

Bulbourethral (Cowper's) glands

Ureter

Ductus deferens

Seminal vesicle

Apex of prostate

Posterior view

FIGURE 31.4 **Prostate and seminal vesicles.**

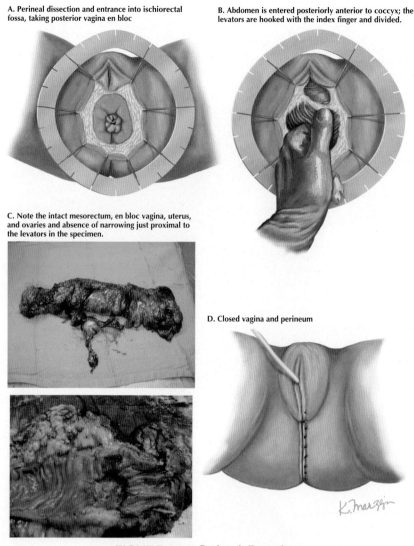

A. Perineal dissection and entrance into ischiorectal fossa, taking posterior vagina en bloc

B. Abdomen is entered posteriorly anterior to coccyx; the levators are hooked with the index finger and divided.

C. Note the intact mesorectum, en bloc vagina, uterus, and ovaries and absence of narrowing just proximal to the levators in the specimen.

D. Closed vagina and perineum

FIGURE 31.5 Perineal dissection.

SUGGESTED READINGS

Fleshman J, Branda ME, Sargent DJ, et al. Disease-free survival and local recurrence for laparoscopic resection compared with open resection of stage II to III rectal cancer: follow-up results of the ACOSOG Z6051 randomized controlled trial. Ann Surg 2018. https://doi.org/10.1097/SLA.0000000000003002. [Epub ahead of print].

Han JG, Want ZJ, Wei GH, et al. Randomized clinical trial of conventional versus cylindrical abdominoperineal resection for locally advanced lower rectal cancer. Am J Surg 2012;204:274–82.

Heald RJ, Santiago I, Pares O, et al. The perfect total mesorectal excision obviates the need for anything else in the management of most rectal cancers. Clin Colon Rectal Surg 2017;30(5):324–32.

Lindsetmo RO, Delaney CP. A standardized technique for laparoscopic rectal resection. J Gastrointest Surg 2009;13(11):2059–63.

Miskovic D, Ahmed J, Bissett-Amess R, et al. European consensus on the standardisation of robotic total mesorectal excision for rectal cancer. Colorectal Dis 2018. https://doi.org/10.1111/codi.14502. [Epub ahead of print].

PelvEx Collaborative. Surgical and survival outcomes following pelvic exenteration for locally advanced primary rectal cancer: results from an international collaboration. Ann Surg 2019;269(2):315–21.

Perry WB, Connaughton JC. Abdominoperineal resection: how is it done and what are the results? Clin Colon Rectal Surg 2007;20(3):213–20.

Stelzner S, Hellmich G, Schubert C, et al. Short-term outcome of extra-levator abdominoperineal excision for rectal cancer. Int J Colorectal Dis 2011;26:919–25.

West NP, Anderin C, Smith KJ, Holm T, et al. Multicentre experience with extralevator abdominoperineal excision for low rectal cancer. Br J Surg 2010;97(4):588–99.

Hemorrhoids and Hemorrhoidectomy

Massarat Zutshi

INTRODUCTION

"Doctor, I have hemorrhoids" is a common complaint. The majority of these complaints are not truly hemorrhoids but other benign conditions; some may hide a more threatening diagnosis, such as anal cancer. Evaluating each patient based on his or her symptoms is important to avoid missing a condition that may require further management. Management of symptomatic hemorrhoids requires an in-depth understanding of the anorectal anatomy for successful treatment and to avoid complications.

ANATOMY OF HEMORRHOIDS

Hemorrhoids are normally occurring vascular cushions found within the anal canal. They are described as being predominately at three anatomic locations in the anal canal (i.e., in left lateral, right anterolateral, and right posterolateral columns) (Fig. 32.1A). However, in reality, this is not always the case, and they often are more circumferential. Their location is around the dentate line, which is an anatomic landmark that divides the anal canal based on the epithelial lining and nerve supply. The region above the dentate line is insensate, whereas that below is supplied by nerve endings that perceive pain. This is an important landmark to consider when treatment is planned. Hemorrhoids are found in the submucosal layer and are considered *sinusoids* because they typically have no muscular wall. They are suspended in the anal canal by the muscle of Treitz, which is a submucosal extension of the conjoined longitudinal ligament.

Anatomically, hemorrhoids are classified as internal or external. *Internal hemorrhoids* are located proximal to the dentate line and have visceral innervation; therefore, the most common presentation is painless bleeding. Because they are close to the anal transitional zone (ATZ), internal hemorrhoids can be covered by columnar, squamous, or basaloid cells. *External hemorrhoids* are located in the distal third of the anal canal and are covered by anoderm (i.e., squamous epithelium). Because of the somatic innervation of external hemorrhoids, patients who have these are more likely to be seen with pain when these are inflamed, and interventional treatment will require some form of anesthesia (Fig. 32.1B).

Hemorrhoids are thought to enhance anal continence and may contribute 15% to 20% of resting anal canal pressure. They also provide complete closure of the anus, enhancing control of defecation. In addition to making important contributions to the maintenance of continence through pressure phenomena, hemorrhoids also relay important sensory data regarding the composition (gas, liquid, stool) of intrarectal contents. Hence it may be important to make note of this, especially in patients who have low sensation in the rectum and anal area, such as spinal cord injury patients, in whom internal sphincter tone and hemorrhoid function may be the only factors contributing to continence.

The central causative pathway for the development of hemorrhoidal pathology is an associated increase in intraabdominal pressure. This increase may be secondary to straining, constipation, or obesity. Other etiologic factors can include diarrhea, pregnancy, and ascites. Aging is also associated with dysfunction of the supporting smooth muscle tissue, resulting in prolapse of hemorrhoidal tissues.

Hemorrhoids are normal structures and thus are treated only if they become symptomatic. Common complaints include bleeding, pain, prolapse, and swelling. After nonoperative measures have failed, treatment is largely applied on the basis of size and symptomatology. Internal hemorrhoids classically are categorized as grade 1, with enlargement, but no prolapse outside the anal canal; grade 2, with prolapse through the anal canal on straining, but with spontaneous reduction; grade 3, manual reduction required; or grade 4, hemorrhoids cannot be reduced into the anal canal.

First-degree hemorrhoidal disease can usually be treated with nonsurgical measures. The primary goal is to decrease straining with bowel movements and thus reduce the intra-abdominal pressure transmitted to the hemorrhoidal vessels. Larger hemorrhoids may present with prolapse of the mucosal lining with or without bleeding. Irritation of the external hemorrhoid may cause pain/itching. The mainstay of nonoperative hemorrhoidal treatment is aimed at keeping the stool soft and consists of increased fiber and water consumption.

Patients with second-degree hemorrhoids can be offered a trial of nonsurgical management, although a number of these measures may fail and require procedural intervention. Third- and fourth-degree hemorrhoids generally require surgery.

A. Anatomy of hemorrhoids

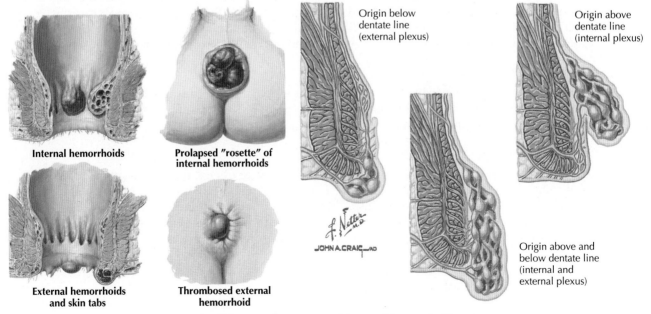

Left lateral

Right posterior

Right anterior

Usual position of internal hemorrhoids, or anal cushions

External hemorrhoidal plexus

Internal hemorrhoidal plexus

Dentate line

Rectosigmoid junction

Fibers of taenia spread out to form longitudinal muscle layer of rectum

Sigmoid colon

Free taenia (taenia libera)

Fibers from longitudinal muscle join circular muscle layer

Window cut in longitudinal muscle layer to expose underlying vasculature

Circular muscle layer

Levator ani muscle

Deep
Superficial
Subcutaneous } Parts* of external anal sphincter muscle

Fibrous septum

Corrugator cutis ani muscle

Anterior view

Perianal skin

Parts variable and often indistinct

B. Types of hemorrhoids

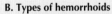

Internal hemorrhoids

Prolapsed "rosette" of internal hemorrhoids

Origin below dentate line (external plexus)

Origin above dentate line (internal plexus)

External hemorrhoids and skin tabs

Thrombosed external hemorrhoid

Origin above and below dentate line (internal and external plexus)

FIGURE 32.1 **Anatomy and types of hemorrhoids.**

MINOR PROCEDURES

Common office procedures in the management of patients with symptomatic hemorrhoids include rubber band ligation, infrared coagulation, bipolar diathermy, sclerotherapy, and cryotherapy. All these techniques rely on some form of tissue destruction, which then results in fixation of the remaining hemorrhoidal tissues.

Rubber Band Ligation

Rubber band ligation is the most frequently used procedure in the United States. This technique is most often used to address first- and second-degree hemorrhoids, although third-degree hemorrhoids can occasionally be treated with this technique as well. The rubber band causes necrosis of the intervening tissue over the course of 7 to 10 days and is passed in the patient's stool. The resultant ulcer and scar are thought to cause a local "pexy" of the surrounding tissue. The most common of the many implements available for application of the rubber bands is a *suction ligator,* which allows the surgeon to draw in the hemorrhoidal tissue and apply the rubber band with one hand (Fig. 32.2A). Other devices require that the operator grasp the hemorrhoidal pedicle with a long forceps and apply the rubber band with the other hand (Fig. 32.2B and C). The most important visual factor is application of the band above the dentate line. Questioning the patient about pain and sensation before applying the band may prevent application of the band at an incorrect site.

Hemorrhoidal banding controls bleeding in more than 90% of cases. Complications are rare but include vasovagal response, pain, bleeding, and pelvic sepsis. Pelvic sepsis may rarely result from perforation by incorporation of the distal rectal wall into the band. Classically, the combination of pain, urinary retention, and fever after banding should raise suspicion of pelvic sepsis.

HET Bipolar System

The HET Bipolar System (Medtronic, St. Paul, MN) is a bipolar diathermy applied to the hemorrhoid above the dentate line. The advantage of this procedure is that multiple hemorrhoids may be treated. The disadvantage is that smaller hemorrhoids are hard to grasp within the forceps.

Sclerotherapy

Sclerotherapy involves injection of a sclerosing agent such as phenol in almond oil or hypertonic saline in the submucosa and not into the hemorrhoid (Fig. 32.2D). This procedure is done in the office or at the bedside. When using the phenol in almond oil, a large-bore needle is recommended. Alternatively, this procedure can be done through a colonoscopy or a sigmoidoscope using hypertonic saline as is done in treatment of esophageal varices.

A. Rubber band ligation using the suction ligator. The figure shows the correct placement of the suction apparatus.

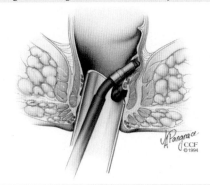

B. Ligature of internal hemorrhoids

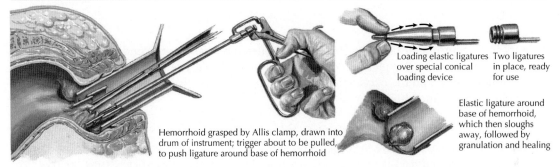

Hemorrhoid grasped by Allis clamp, drawn into drum of instrument; trigger about to be pulled, to push ligature around base of hemorrhoid

Loading elastic ligatures over special conical loading device

Two ligatures in place, ready for use

Elastic ligature around base of hemorrhoid, which then sloughs away, followed by granulation and healing

C. Surgical management of internal hemorrhoids: Elastic ligation technique

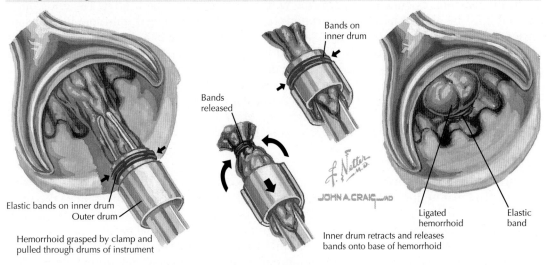

Elastic bands on inner drum
Outer drum

Hemorrhoid grasped by clamp and pulled through drums of instrument

Bands released

Bands on inner drum

Inner drum retracts and releases bands onto base of hemorrhoid

Ligated hemorrhoid

Elastic band

D. Sclerotherapy. Injection into the submucosa and not into the hemorrhoid

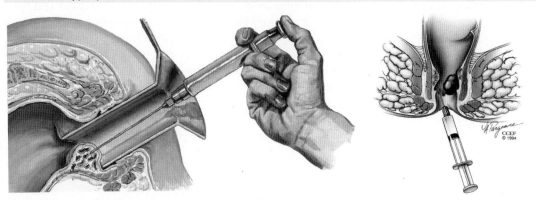

FIGURE 32.2 Office procedures for hemorrhoids.

(Parts A and D reprinted with permission, Cleveland Clinic Center for Medical Art & Photography © 1994–2019. All Rights Reserved.)

SURGICAL OPTIONS

Patients for whom medical or nonsurgical therapies have failed are candidates for operative procedures such as the Doppler-guided hemorrhoidal arterial ligation and mucopexy, stapled hemorrhoidectomy, and the excisional hemorrhoidectomy. Typically, these patients have third- or fourth-degree hemorrhoids.

Doppler-Guided Hemorrhoidal Arterial Ligation and Mucopexy

This procedure is usually done for prolapsing third-degree hemorrhoids. Clinically the hemorrhoids that can be reduced in the office with few skin tags are most successfully treated. The procedure is done under general anesthesia and involves a Doppler-guided hemorrhoidal arterial ligation system, essentially an anoscope with a Doppler attachment on it. The anoscope is inserted into the anal canal after lubrication; based on Doppler signal, multiple ligations are carried out starting at the patient's right lateral position and going in a circumferential pattern. The anoscope is then pulled out by 1 cm, and this process is repeated. All ligations are done using 2-0 polyglycolic acid sutures. Subsequently, the areas of prolapse are evaluated and a mucopexy (or a rectoanal repair) is carried out, which entails suturing higher than the previous ligations and then running the stitch up to the dentate line of the prolapsed segment. The suture is then tied such that the knot pushes the tissue inside the anal canal. Approximately three areas are ligated in this fashion, each using 2-0 polyglycolic acid suture (Fig. 32.3A).

Stapled Hemorrhoidopexy

This procedure involves using a circular stapler to excise approximately 1 cm of the mucosa that lies proximal to the dentate line. The premise is that there is a disconnection of the hemorrhoidal vessels, leading to decrease in the size of the hemorrhoid and therefore treating the symptoms, and that the resection "pexies" the remaining hemorrhoidal tissue.

This requires general anesthesia. A specialized anoscope that is half-circle in diameter is inserted into the anal canal, and a circumferential suture using 2-0 polypropylene is taken about 4 cm above the dentate line. The stapler is then inserted into the anal canal, and the suture is pulled around the head of this taper and tightened. The stapler is then closed and fired, excising the mucosa and stapling the cut ends. Any bleeding site is taken care of by oversewing the area with 2-0 polyglycolic acid sutures or electrocautery (Fig. 32.3B).

This technique is associated with less pain and analgesic use but has higher rates of recurrence and residual prolapse. The most common complication of stapled hemorrhoidopexy is bleeding. Other rare complications include rectal perforation, pelvic sepsis, and chronic pain syndrome.

A. Doppler-guided hemorrhoidal ligation

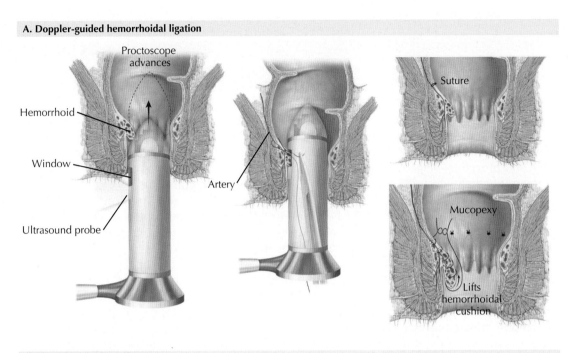

B. Stapled hemorrhoidectomy

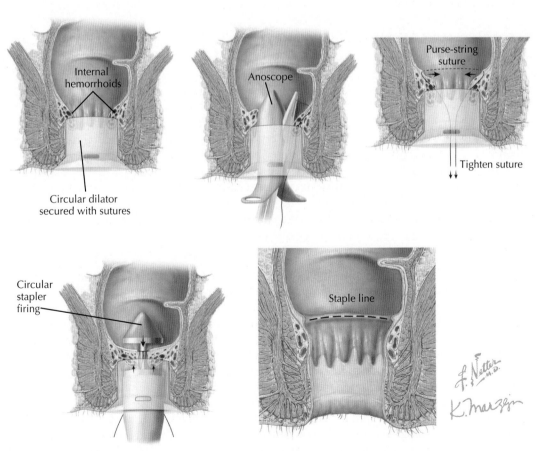

FIGURE 32.3 (A) Techniques of Doppler-guided hemorrhoidal ligation and mucopexy. (B) Stapled hemorrhoidopexy.

Excisional Hemorrhoidectomy

This is usually performed for fourth-degree hemorrhoids or third-degree hemorrhoids with a large external component or skin tags. This procedure involves excising the skin and mucosa overlying the hemorrhoid and the hemorrhoid pedicle. The most common procedures are the Ferguson procedure (Fig. 32.4A), which involves suture-closing the wound; and the Milligan-Morgan hemorrhoidectomy, which leaves the wounds open to granulate.

The procedure is usually performed under general anesthesia, although conscious sedation with an anal block is effective. A Hill-Ferguson or an operating anoscope is placed in the anal canal. An ellipse of anoderm is raised and dissected back toward the anal canal. The hemorrhoids are then raised off the anal sphincters. During this dissection it is important to separate the hemorrhoidal tissue from the internal sphincter without damaging the latter. After completion, the procedure is repeated on any further hemorrhoid columns that require removal.

The Ferguson technique is frequently used in the United States. After removal of the hemorrhoidal tissues, the base of the hemorrhoid is suture-ligated, and the anal mucosa/anoderm are reapproximated using a running absorbable stitch. The Milligan-Morgan technique is used primarily in the United Kingdom. The defect is left open and allowed to granulate inward over 4 to 8 weeks. When resecting more than one column, a minimum of 1 cm of anoderm should be preserved between excision sites to avoid anal stenosis.

STRANGULATED HEMORRHOIDS

Prolapsed and strangulated (or incarcerated) hemorrhoids are third- or fourth-degree hemorrhoids that become thrombosed because of acute on chronic prolapse and resultant swelling. Patients typically have severe anal pain and sometimes urinary retention. Physical examination typically reveals thrombosis of the internal and external hemorrhoids, with or without evidence of necrosis (Fig. 32.4B), and a moderate amount of edema.

Patients can usually be managed with emergent excisional hemorrhoidectomy. If there is evidence of tissue necrosis, all nonviable tissue should be excised and the incision left open. In poor candidates for surgical intervention, the anoderm can be infiltrated with local anesthesia. The anesthesia causes the internal sphincter to relax, and the internal hemorrhoids can be reduced with gentle massage. External thrombectomies and multiple rubber band ligations of the internal hemorrhoids can be performed as an alternative to excisional hemorrhoidectomy.

THROMBOSED EXTERNAL HEMORRHOIDS

The external portion of the hemorrhoid can form a clot and become large and very painful. Patients commonly have a bump or lump in the anal area usually after lifting weights or doing something strenuous, although this can occur without any activity. If seen within 4 to 5 days of the onset, pain can be relieved by enucleation of the clot and the roofing of the thrombosed hemorrhoid (Fig. 32.5). It is recommended that the hemorrhoid be removed and not simply "stabbing" the overlying skin and expressing the clot—this has been shown to lead to a higher rate of recurrence. This is done in the office setting under local anesthetic. After the base of the hemorrhoid is numbed, an elliptical excision is taken to de-roof the hemorrhoid, and the clot is evacuated. This procedure is typically not done beyond 5 days, because most patients will have resolving symptoms by then, and the clot can be allowed to resolve on its own. Classically warm sitz baths and nonopioid analgesics are adequate. Conservative management using nitrates or calcium channel blockers, lidocaine jelly, and keeping the patient's stools soft is indicated. The pain usually subsides within a few weeks whether or not a surgical treatment is offered.

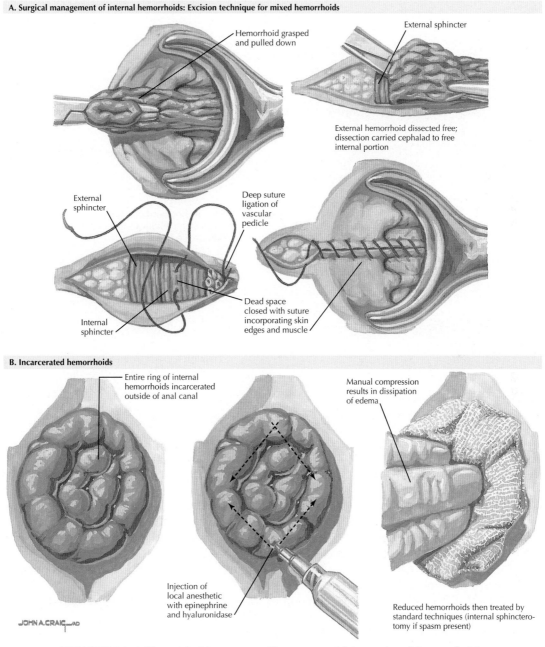

A. Surgical management of internal hemorrhoids: Excision technique for mixed hemorrhoids

Hemorrhoid grasped and pulled down

External sphincter

External hemorrhoid dissected free; dissection carried cephalad to free internal portion

External sphincter

Deep suture ligation of vascular pedicle

Internal sphincter

Dead space closed with suture incorporating skin edges and muscle

B. Incarcerated hemorrhoids

Entire ring of internal hemorrhoids incarcerated outside of anal canal

Manual compression results in dissipation of edema

Injection of local anesthetic with epinephrine and hyaluronidase

Reduced hemorrhoids then treated by standard techniques (internal sphincterotomy if spasm present)

JOHN A. CRAIG—AD

FIGURE 32.4 Hemorrhoidectomy and incarcerated (strangulated) hemorrhoids.

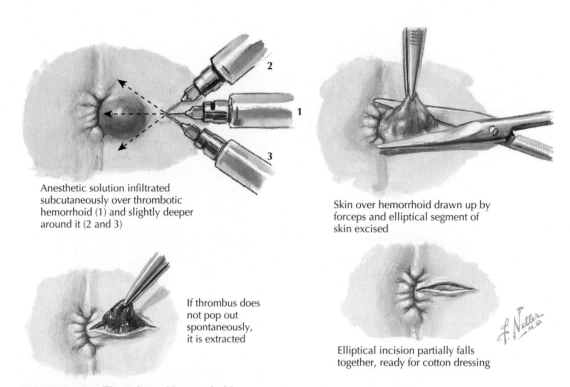

Anesthetic solution infiltrated subcutaneously over thrombotic hemorrhoid (1) and slightly deeper around it (2 and 3)

Skin over hemorrhoid drawn up by forceps and elliptical segment of skin excised

If thrombus does not pop out spontaneously, it is extracted

Elliptical incision partially falls together, ready for cotton dressing

FIGURE 32.5 Thrombosed hemorrhoids.
De-roofing of a thrombosed hemorrhoid with excision of the underlying clot.

SUGGESTED READINGS

Hemorrhoids. In Bailey HR. et al., eds. Colorectal Surgery, Philadelphia: Elsevier/Saunders;2013:95–116.

Hemorrhoids: anatomy, physiology, concerns and treatment. In Coughlin O, Page M., eds. Anorectal Disease: Contemporary Management, New York: Springer; 2016:225–42.

Lestar B, Pennickx F, Kerremans R. The composition of anal basal pressure: an in vivo and in vitro study in man. Int J Colorectal Dis 1989;4:118–22.

Milligan ET, Morgan CN, Jones LE. Surgical anatomy of the anal canal and the operative treatment of hemorrhoids. Lancet 1937;2:119–24.

Ratto C, Donisi L, Parello A, et al. Evaluation of transanal hemorrhoidal dearterialization as a minimally invasive therapeutic approach to hemorrhoids. Dis Colon Rectum 2010;53:803.

Schubert MC, Sridhar S, Schade RR, Wexner SD. What every gastroenterologist needs to know about common anorectal disorders. World J Gastroenterol 2009;15(26):3201–9.

Su MY, Chiu CT, Wu CS, et al. Endoscopic hemorrhoidal ligation of symptomatic internal hemorrhoids. Gastrointestinal Endosc 2003;58:871–4.

Szmulowicz UM, Gurland B, Garofalo T, Zutshi M. Doppler-guided hemorrhoidal artery ligation: the experience of a single institution. J Gastrointest Surg 2011;15(5):803–8.

Thomson WH. The nature of haemorrhoids. Br J Surg 1975;62:542–52.

Perianal Abscess and Fistula in Ano

James M. Church

INTRODUCTION

Perianal sepsis is a common problem that can be handled simply and successfully if treatment is based on an understanding of its anatomy and pathophysiology. The anatomy of the anus and the surrounding areas of the pelvis and perineum is complex, and sepsis in the area can be complex also. The aim of this chapter is to explain perianal sepsis in the context of anatomy and to describe the way in which treatments are determined by this relationship.

ANATOMY AND PATHOGENESIS

Most cases of perianal sepsis begin in an anal gland. Up to 10 of these glands are distributed around the anus, with each main duct passing from the gland opening at the base of an anal crypt through the internal sphincter into the intersphincteric space. Here the branches of the gland are dispersed. Anal crypts are located at the dentate line, at the proximal extent of the squamous epithelium of the mid–anal canal. These crypts form the lowest end of the anal columns of Morgagni, which extend vertically, cephalad from the dentate line through the anal transitional epithelium into the rectum (Fig. 33.1). Abuse of anal function that occurs with straining at stool and frequent defecation can cause edema of the anoderm and potentially block the openings of the anal glands.

Pressure within the anal canal tends to be highest front and back, making the anterior and posterior midlines the common places for deep mucosal splits that lead to fissures, and for blocked anal glands that lead to abscesses and fistulas. A blocked anal gland means that gland secretions accumulate and are then prone to bacterial overgrowth, gland rupture, and sepsis. Sometimes the blocked duct clears and the sepsis can settle, but if this does not happen, the increasing septic pressure enlarges the abscess and forces it through the perianal tissues along lines of least resistance. At some time in this evolution the patient will be aware of a constant and increasing pain. As the sepsis worsens, the pain will become increasingly severe, and if the abscess has become more superficial, a lump may be palpable. Sometimes an abscess will start to drain through the gland duct back into the anus (this can often be seen during a careful anoscopy, the bead of pus showing the position of the infected gland); however, spontaneous drainage through the skin is common.

Geographic anatomy of anorectum

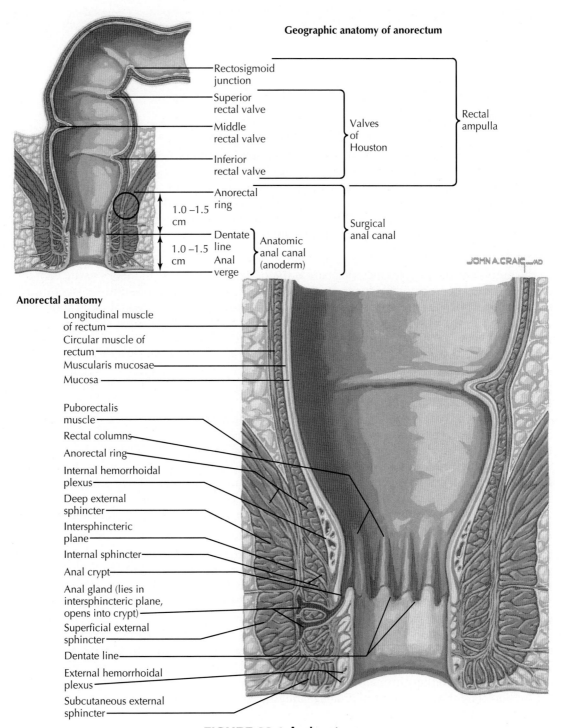

Rectosigmoid junction

Superior rectal valve

Middle rectal valve

Inferior rectal valve

Anorectal ring

Dentate line

Anal verge

1.0 –1.5 cm

1.0 –1.5 cm

Valves of Houston

Rectal ampulla

Surgical anal canal

Anatomic anal canal (anoderm)

JOHN A. CRAIG—MD

Anorectal anatomy

Longitudinal muscle of rectum

Circular muscle of rectum

Muscularis mucosae

Mucosa

Puborectalis muscle

Rectal columns

Anorectal ring

Internal hemorrhoidal plexus

Deep external sphincter

Intersphincteric plane

Internal sphincter

Anal crypt

Anal gland (lies in intersphincteric plane, opens into crypt)

Superficial external sphincter

Dentate line

External hemorrhoidal plexus

Subcutaneous external sphincter

FIGURE 33.1 Anal anatomy.

PERIANAL ABSCESS

Describing the Abscess and Its Treatment by Its Location

There are a variety of directions in which worsening perianal sepsis can extend, and this is reflected in its categorization, summarized in Fig. 33.2. The categories reflect the spaces around the anus and extraperitoneal rectum, where increasing pressure of sepsis causes expansion of the abscess. The path of the sepsis in the formation of an abscess determines the track of the fistula that results from the sepsis, if that is the patient's fate. Therefore the site of the abscess can determine the classification of the fistula (Table 33.1).

Perianal

At the bottom of the intersphincteric plane is the perianal space: subcutaneous tissue containing the external hemorrhoidal plexus. In it, fibers of the longitudinal rectal muscle pass through the lowest part of the external sphincter and attach it to the skin (corrugator cutis ani). If the sepsis passes downward in the intersphincteric plane, it will reach the subcutaneous perianal space and, being somewhat contained by the muscular and fibrous septa, will form an easily detectable abscess. This is the most common type of perianal abscess and is easily diagnosed on examination as a discrete lump that is erythematous, tender, and sometimes fluctuant. Fluctuance is a useful sign, because it shows where the pus is trying to exit through the skin and is the target for incisional drainage.

Depending on the size and depth of the cavity, the abscess can be unroofed or drained with or without an appropriately sized mushroom drain. If used, a drain is removed in 7 to 10 days. Packing is discouraged, because it must be changed daily and is painful. About 30% of patients develop an anal fistula, which will be either low transsphincteric or subcutaneous. Recent data suggest that postdrainage treatment with ciprofloxacin and metronidazole for a week can minimize fistula formation. In addition, searching gently for a fistula at the time of abscess drainage can allow seton drainage or fistulotomy, as appropriate, and prevention of later complications.

Intersphincteric

In an intersphincteric abscess, the infected anal gland forms an abscess in the intersphincteric plane, but it is detected before it has tracked in any direction. It is not usually visible on external examination but can sometimes be palpated or seen on anoscopy (usually with the patient under anesthetic). Pure intersphincteric abscesses are clinically uncommon because there is no external lump. In this respect they are like sepsis in the deep postanal space. Severe constant anal pain is an indication for examination under anesthetic, during which time pus can often be expressed through the anal gland. This offers the opportunity to drain the abscess by opening the gland. Otherwise, drainage can be done as indicated by the position of the pus and the nearest point of access, either through the perianal skin, the anoderm of the anal canal, or through the ischiorectal fossa. The point of drainage and the track used to access the abscess determine the anatomy of any resulting fistula.

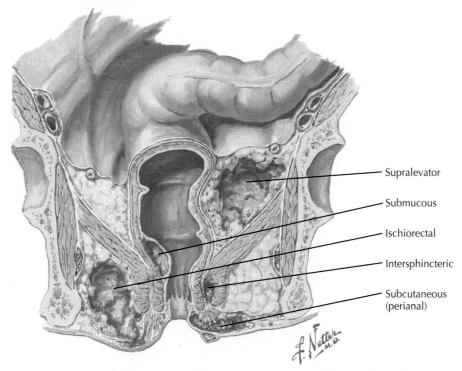

FIGURE 33.2 Spaces around the rectum and anus where abscesses develop.

Table 33.1   Likely Category of Fistula Depending on the Location of the Abscess

Abscess	Fistula
Perianal	Intersphincteric/Low trans-sphincteric
Ischiorectal	Trans-sphincteric
Submucosal	Subcutaneous
Intersphincteric	Intersphincteric/trans-sphincteric, depending on how it is drained
Supralevator	Suprasphincteric
Extrasphincteric	Usually iatrogenic

Ischiorectal

The external anal sphincter is the medial border of the ischiorectal space (and the anterior border of the deep postanal space) (Fig. 33.3A). If sepsis extends from the intersphincteric space laterally through the internal sphincter, it will reach this large, fat-filled space, which offers little resistance to the development of an abscess. An expanding abscess can also spread circumferentially around the anus in this plane and present as a horseshoe. The degree to which this happens depends on the unique bacterial flora causing the infection and the patient's innate ability to contain them. Ischiorectal abscesses can be very large and distort the buttock. If treatment is delayed, there may be systemic symptoms. On examination there is not usually an obvious point of fluctuance, although a general swelling is seen. The most erythematous area is the best target for drainage, and the presence of pus can be confirmed by aspiration with a large-bore needle. In some cases, drainage can be done in the office under local anesthesia, but a more effective and comfortable option is under general anesthetic in the operating room. Ischiorectal abscesses are deeper than perianal abscesses and so unroofing is not a good option. With the patient asleep, the size of the cavity can be assessed with an instrument or a finger, a counter-incision made at the edge of the cavity, and a drain placed through and through. If there is no tracking, a mushroom drain is inserted, as large as is necessary to ensure free drainage of the pus (Fig. 33.3B). Depending on the size of the abscess, the drain can be removed in 10 to 14 days or downsized to a smaller one if necessary.

HORSESHOE ABSCESS

A deep horseshoe abscess usually originates from an infected posterior midline anal crypt. The sepsis extends posteriorly into the deep postanal space and then spreads laterally into the ischiorectal spaces, often detected as a tender mass on the lateral aspect of the perineum. Drainage of the pus through the most obvious point of sepsis leads to a deep cavity that communicates across the midline in the deep postanal space to the other side of the perineum. A midline incision is made behind anus, entering the deep postanal space, and each "arm" of the fistula is controlled by a large seton-type drain (usually a Penrose drain) placed between the midline counterincision and the lateral incision. Probing through the midline incision will often find the internal opening of the fistula and allow a seton to be passed from the incision to the infected crypt along the transsphincteric track. The "modified Hanley Procedure," which involves widely opening the deep postanal space and an extensive sphincterotomy, has been recommended for treatment of horseshoe abscesses. A less radical technique of insertion of an effective seton into the fistula track without division of muscle is preferred, and a delayed advancement flap repair of the internal opening.

SUPRALEVATOR ABSCESS

Supralevator abscess results from a spread of the intersphincteric infection upward above the levator muscle, or spread of pelvic sepsis downward to the pelvic floor. This deep sepsis causes pelvic pain and systemic symptoms of infection and is discovered on imaging and/or examination under anesthesia. Drainage can be accomplished through the rectum or through the buttock, depending on the anatomy of the abscess. Imaging or colonoscopy can diagnose or exclude associated pelvic sepsis.

A. Deep postanal space

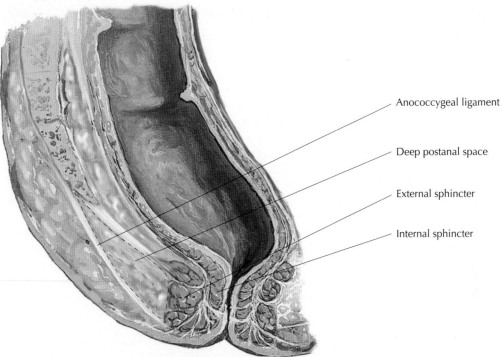

Anococcygeal ligament

Deep postanal space

External sphincter

Internal sphincter

B. Catheter drainage of perirectal abscesses

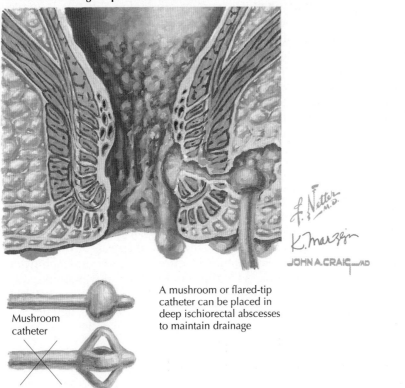

A mushroom or flared-tip catheter can be placed in deep ischiorectal abscesses to maintain drainage

Mushroom catheter

Malecot catheter
(allows ingrowth of fibrous tissue, making removal difficult)

FIGURE 33.3 (A) Deep postanal space. (B) Mushroom catheter drainage of ischiorectal abscess.

GENERAL PRINCIPLES OF TREATMENT FOR PERIANAL ABSCESSES

1. Effective drainage: Make a big enough hole to let the pus flow out freely, and make sure that the skin edges of the drainage incision will not heal together before the abscess cavity is healed. This means excising skin edges and a complete unroofing of superficial cavities. Deep cavities can be treated with a drain that is as large as possible. The site of drainage is at the site of fluctuance, or at the most medial edge of the abscess if fluctuance is not obvious.
2. Antibiotics are needed in patients prone to sepsis (patients with diabetes or on chemotherapy), and a case can be made for their routine use to prevent fistula.
3. Packing should not be needed, but follow up in 7 to 10 days to reassess the abscess.
4. Recurrent or nonhealing abscess suggests there may be a fistula.
5. If the patient is under general anesthesia, you can gently search for a fistula at the time of drainage of the abscess. An obvious fistula may be gently probed and a seton inserted, or a fistulotomy performed if the track is superficial.

ANAL FISTULA

Pathogenesis and Presentation

An anal fistula is an abnormal communication between the inside of the anus and the perianal/perineal skin or the vaginal mucosa. The most common cause of anal fistula is cryptoglandular sepsis, and fistulas evolve from a perianal abscess. When a perianal abscess drains, there is potentially a track that connects the duct of the infected anal gland with the exit hole of the sepsis. Sometimes the track heals, usually proximally by the gland opening. If the gland opening does not heal, bacteria from inside the rectum enter the gland and perpetuate sepsis, which decompresses through the opening that has been created for drainage. If the external part of the track heals or narrows, increasing pressure within the proximal track causes a recurrent abscess, or spread of the sepsis outside the track. Sometimes new external openings are created. Anal fistulas generally present as recurrent perianal abscesses, or abscesses that never heal but continue to drain.

Classification

Anal fistulas have an internal opening at the infected anal crypt, a track, and one or more external openings. In cryptoglandular sepsis the internal opening is usually at the crypt in the posterior or anterior midline (see Goodsall's rule, Fig. 33.4A). They are classified according to the anatomy of their track, which is determined by the path of spread of the sepsis from the infected gland opening through the internal sphincter muscle into the intersphincteric space and from there to the skin or vagina. Table 33.1 and Fig. 33.4B list the anatomic types of fistula. Classification of the anatomy of anal fistulas is clinically important because it defines the relationship of the tract to the internal and external anal sphincter muscles, and determines the most appropriate choice of treatment.

Superficial or Subcutaneous Fistula

The track passes either submucosally or subcutaneously from the internal opening to an external opening near the anal verge. It is easily treated by a simple fistulotomy. Place a probe through the track, make sure there is no muscle superficial to the probe, and cut down onto the probe. Do not remove the granulating base of the fistula, but trim any overhanging edges.

A. Goodsall-Salmon's rule

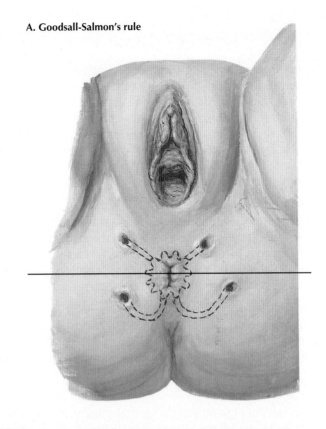

B. Types of anorectal fistula

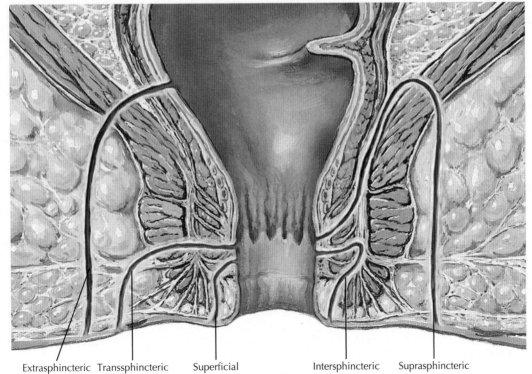

Extrasphincteric Transsphincteric   Superficial   Intersphincteric   Suprasphincteric

FIGURE 33.4 **Anatomy of anal fistulas.**

Intersphincteric

The track passes from the internal opening through the internal sphincter muscle to the intersphincteric groove. It then descends down the intersphincteric plane to an external opening in the perianal skin. The track therefore contains a variable amount of internal anal sphincter, and decisions about treatment are made depending on how much sphincter is included. Options are fistulotomy (for minimal or no muscle), delayed sphincterotomy with cutting seton (for <1 cm of muscle), and insertion of a draining seton as the first stage of fistula repair (advancement flap or ligation of the internal fistula tract [LIFT] procedure) for more than 1 cm of muscle. An advancement flap or LIFT procedure is more successful than a fistula plug or fibrin glue in achieving healing.

Superficial Trans-sphincteric Fistula

The track passes through the lower one-fourth of the internal sphincter and often through some of the external sphincter. The external opening is close to the anus but away from the anal verge. This sort of fistula can be treated by fistulotomy, delayed fistulotomy using a cutting seton, or a staged repair procedure, depending on the state of the sphincter and the position of the fistula. In patients with a short anal canal, or women with an anterior fistula, no muscle should be cut.

Deep Trans-sphincteric Fistula

The track passes through the body of both sphincter muscles, so fistulotomy would have a significant chance of creating anal seepage or incontinence. The external opening can be anywhere on the perineum. These fistulas must be repaired, using either advancement flap or LIFT techniques (see Suggested Readings).

Suprasphincteric Fistula

The track leaves the infected duct opening at the dentate line and passes up in the intersphincteric plane, arching over and through the levator muscle before descending through the ischiorectal space to the external opening. An advancement flap repair can cure these fistulas if they are cryptoglandular in origin. The challenge is to get a probe around the track to the internal opening for insertion of a seton. This is best done by a dual approach, probing through both the infected crypt and the external opening.

Extrasphincteric Fistulas

The track leaves the external opening and passes straight into the rectum above the level of the levator muscle. These are usually iatrogenic fistulas. Direct repair of the rectal opening by one of many transrectal surgical techniques is usually effective as long as the track is counterdrained. Be cautious: there may be a missed real internal opening at the dentate line with a suprasphincteric track. Look carefully for this and treat as determined by the correct anatomy of the real fistula.

PRINCIPLES OF THE TREATMENT OF ANAL FISTULAS

1. Control of the internal opening is the key, and identification of the correct opening is crucial. As the source of the sepsis it must be closed or obliterated.
2. Simplify the primary track before definitive management using a seton drain (Fig. 33.5); drain associated abscesses or cavities, and associated tracks using setons and mushroom catheters.
3. Allow the sepsis to resolve and fibrosis to occur before doing a repair. Inflamed, edematous tracks are fragile and do not heal well with sutures. Use preliminary seton drainage for at least 6 weeks.
4. Assess the strength and length of the anal canal before treatment. In patients with short, weak sphincters, division of any muscle should be avoided.
5. Operate according to the foundations of perianal surgery: a. no dead space; b. no tension; c. big bites; d. good hemostasis; e. manage the track (the most common cause of failed fistula repair is a track abscess.) In short fistulas, debride the external opening widely; in long fistulas, use a mushroom drain for 120 days.

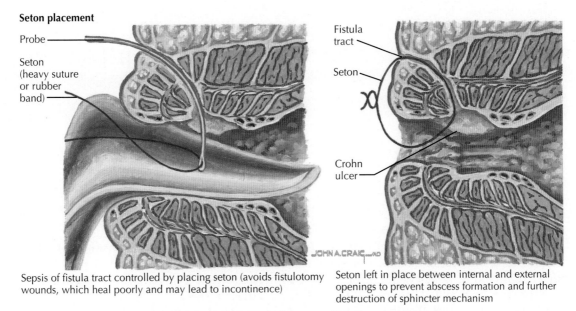

Seton placement

Probe

Seton (heavy suture or rubber band)

Fistula tract

Seton

Crohn ulcer

JOHN A.CRAIG—AD

Sepsis of fistula tract controlled by placing seton (avoids fistulotomy wounds, which heal poorly and may lead to incontinence)

Seton left in place between internal and external openings to prevent abscess formation and further destruction of sphincter mechanism

FIGURE 33.5 Insertion of a seton drain in an anal fistula.

COMPLICATED PERIANAL SEPSIS

Crohn's Disease

Perianal sepsis occurs in patients with Crohn's disease under two circumstances: with normal perianal tissues and with perianal/perineal tissues affected by Crohn's disease (see Suggested Readings). Clinical suspicion of perineal Crohn's disease is confirmed if granulomas are found in the tissue. "Normal" perianal sepsis can be treated in the same way as any patient with an abscess or fistula. Patients with perineal Crohn's disease tend to have edematous, shiny perineal skin that does not heal when incised. The sepsis is drained but with minimal incisions, and fecal diversion may be necessary. The disease is controlled by biologic therapy, and then surgical repair can be considered.

Vaginal Fistulas

The vagina is a favorite site for anterior perianal sepsis to drain because the distance between the two organs is short, and there may be septal scarring from obstetric misadventures. Setons are not needed because sepsis is rare. Repair requires a flap. Simple flaps can work if the perineum is of normal thickness, but with a thin perineum, augment the distance between anus and vagina by episioproctotomy, sphincteroplasty, Martius flap, or gracilis flap.

Pouch Fistulas

Anal fistulas may arise from the ileal pouch-anal anastomosis (IPAA) itself, or from the dentate line below a stapled IPAA. Fistulas to perianal skin are drained with a seton and then repaired. Vaginal fistulas are drained if there is sepsis. Fistulas associated with Crohn's disease are drained and treated with biologics, and repair is considered. Anastomotic pouch fistulas can be treated locally by excision of the defect in the anastomosis and resuture, transanal pouch advancement, or a redone transabdominal pouch. The same options exist for cryptoglandular fistulas in pouch patients, although an advancement flap can be considered if there is enough anoderm between the anastomosis and the dentate line. Repair of pouch vaginal fistulas is most difficult of all because of the lack of tissue between the pouch and the vagina. Sphincteroplasty and Martius and gracilis flaps are options.

SUGGESTED READINGS

Abbas MA, Lemus-Rangel R, Hamadani A. Long-term outcome of endorectal advancement flap for complex anorectal fistulae. Am Surg 2008;74:921–4.

Bleier JI, Moloo H, Goldberg SM. Ligation of the intersphincteric fistula tract: an effective new technique for complex fistulas. Dis Colon Rectum 2010;53:43–6.

Bolshinsky V, Church J. How to insert a draining seton correctly. Dis Colon Rectum 2018;61:1121–3.

Christoforidis D, Pieh MC, Madoff RD, Mellgren AF. Treatment of transsphincteric anal fistulas by endorectal advancement flap or collagen fistula plug: a comparative study. Dis Colon Rectum 2009;52:18–22.

Figg RE, Church JM. Perineal Crohn's disease: an indicator of poor prognosis and potential proctectomy. Dis Colon Rectum 2009;52:646–50.

Garcia-Aguilar J, Belmonte C, Wong WD, Goldberg SM, Madoff RD. Anal fistula surgery: factors associated with recurrence and incontinence. Dis Colon Rectum 1996;39:723–9.

Ghahramani L, Minaie MR, Arasteh P, Hosseini SV, Izadpanah A, Bananzadeh AM, et al. Antibiotic therapy for prevention of fistula in-ano after incision and drainage of simple perianal abscess: a randomized single blind clinical trial. Surgery 2017;162:1017–25.

Hanley PH. Conservative surgical correction of horseshoe abscess and fistula. Dis Colon Rectum 1965;8:364–8.

Jarrar A, Church J. Advancement flap repair: a good option for complex anorectal fistulas. Dis Colon Rectum 2011;54:1537–41.

Lin H, Jin Z, Zhu Y, Diao M, Hu W. Anal fistula plug vs rectal advancement flap for the treatment of complex cryptoglandular anal fistulas: a system review and meta-analysis of studies with long-term follow-up. Colorectal Dis 2018. https://doi.org/10.1111/codi.14504. [Epub ahead of print].

Malik AI, Nelson RL, Tou S. Incision and drainage of perianal abscess with or without treatment of anal fistula. Cochrane Database Syst Rev 2010;7(7):CD006827.

Pearce L, Newton K, Smith SR, Barrow P, Smith J, Hancock L, North West Research Collaborative, et al. Multicentre observational study of outcomes after drainage of acute perianal abscess. Br J Surg 2016;103:1063–8.

Rojanasakul A, Pattanaarun J, Sahakitrungruang C, Tantiphlachiva K. Total anal sphincter saving technique for fistula-in-ano: the ligation of intersphincteric fistula tract. J Med Assoc Thai 2007;90:581–6.

Sahnan K, Adegbola SO, Tozer PJ, Watfah J, Phillips RK. Perianal abscess. BMJ 2017;356:j475. https://doi.org/10.1136/bmj.j475.

Suture Rectopexy and Ventral Mesh Rectopexy

Sherief Shawki

INTRODUCTION

Full-thickness external rectal prolapse is herniation of the rectum through the anal orifice. More commonly seen in older women, rectal prolapse can occur in both genders and even at a young age. The underlying mechanism of rectal prolapse is poorly understood. However, a mid-to-low rectal intussusception is thought to be the initiating step. Chronic straining is also thought to be a precipitating factor.

The goals of surgical repair are to fix the prolapsed rectum with a durable repair to minimize recurrence while maintaining or improving continence and bowel function. More than 100 surgical procedures have been proposed for the surgical management of rectal prolapse, indicating that an optimal operation has not been defined. The majority of these encompass several concepts that can be undertaken via a transabdominal or transperineal approach. The choice depends on the surgeon's experience and training, as well as his or her understanding of the anatomic defect, patient condition, and fitness for the operation. These options include the following:

- Narrowing the patulous anus
- Restoration of the pelvic floor
- Obliteration of the peritoneal pouch of Douglas
- Bowel resection by an abdominal or perineal approach
- Fixation and/or suspension of the rectum to the sacrum
- A combination of these modalities

This chapter focuses on suture and ventral mesh rectopexy, because they are two of the more commonly used procedures in management of full-thickness prolapse.

ANATOMY FOR RECTOPEXY AND PELVIC DISSECTION

During surgery there are some alterations in the pelvic anatomy associated with rectal prolapse that are typically observed and are worth mentioning. These include increased tissue laxity, a deepened rectovaginal or rectovesical pouch of Douglas (Fig. 34.1A through C), and increased mobility of the rectum, which is more extensively covered with thickened peritoneum when compared with the normal findings. A weak pelvic floor musculature and diastasis of the levator ani muscle complex are often encountered as well. Whether these are causative factors or merely associated anatomic variations remains debatable.

It is important to recognize that tissue laxity and thickened peritoneum render traction and countertraction challenging and may result in drifting or deviation from the correct trajectory during dissection.

For suspension procedures, the anterior sacral longitudinal ligament overlying the sacral promontory must be used to anchor the mobilized rectum or mesh/graft. During this portion of the procedure, awareness of the surrounding structures ensures proper technique and avoids injury to nearby structures. Fig. 34.1D and E and Fig. 34.2A through C show the surrounding anatomic structures.

The median sacral artery lies in the midline, which will be to the left of the cleared area (Fig. 34.1D). On the same side but running obliquely from left to right is the left iliac vein. Distally and traveling from left to right is the right hypogastric nerve. The right iliac artery is proximal, heading caudad from left to right and the right ureter runs on the right lateral side (Fig. 34.1D). The area in between these structures overlying the sacral promontory is a suitable landing zone for the anchoring stitches (Fig. 34.1E). All of these are extrafascial and retroperitoneal structures and therefore can be easily encountered when suturing to the underlying anterior sacral longitudinal ligament, which is posterior to these structures.

When placing the anchoring stitches, the surgeon must take care to avoid suturing distally and further to the right of the promontory, because this may risk injuring the right first sacral nerve (Fig. 34.1D and E).

Occasionally, especially with visceral obesity, the sacral promontory is covered by fatty tissues, which makes this dissection very challenging.

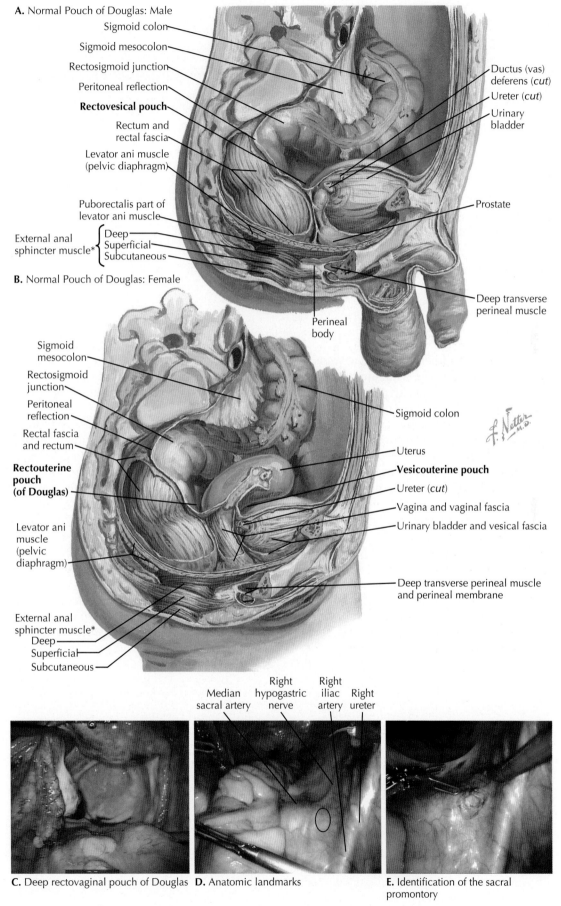

A. Normal Pouch of Douglas: Male
- Sigmoid colon
- Sigmoid mesocolon
- Rectosigmoid junction
- Peritoneal reflection
- **Rectovesical pouch**
- Rectum and rectal fascia
- Levator ani muscle (pelvic diaphragm)
- Puborectalis part of levator ani muscle
- External anal sphincter muscle*
  - Deep
  - Superficial
  - Subcutaneous

- Ductus (vas) deferens (*cut*)
- Ureter (*cut*)
- Urinary bladder
- Prostate
- Deep transverse perineal muscle
- Perineal body

B. Normal Pouch of Douglas: Female
- Sigmoid mesocolon
- Rectosigmoid junction
- Peritoneal reflection
- Rectal fascia and rectum
- **Rectouterine pouch (of Douglas)**
- Levator ani muscle (pelvic diaphragm)
- External anal sphincter muscle*
  - Deep
  - Superficial
  - Subcutaneous

- Sigmoid colon
- Uterus
- **Vesicouterine pouch**
- Ureter (*cut*)
- Vagina and vaginal fascia
- Urinary bladder and vesical fascia
- Deep transverse perineal muscle and perineal membrane

- Median sacral artery
- Right hypogastric nerve
- Right iliac artery
- Right ureter

C. Deep rectovaginal pouch of Douglas **D.** Anatomic landmarks **E.** Identification of the sacral promontory

FIGURE 34.1 Anatomy for rectopexy and pelvic dissection.

SUTURE RECTOPEXY

The anatomic landmarks for pelvic dissection in rectopexy are the same as in rectal cancer. These are shown in Fig. 34.2. Similar to the promontory area, a knowledge of structures surrounding the rectum in the pelvis (including the great vessels, nerves, and ureters) is crucial before performing any type of rectal surgery.

In this procedure, a posterior rectal dissection is undertaken in a very similar fashion to when dissecting in rectal cancer. The peritoneum overlying the rectosigmoid junction is incised (Fig. 34.2A through C). The goal is to enter the plane between the mesentery and Toldt's fascia, keeping the ureters and the autonomic nerves away from harm as they pass from the abdomen toward the pelvis lying underneath this fascia. Once in the correct plane, the rectum is mobilized posteriorly and caudally until the levator ani muscle is encountered (Fig. 34.2A through C). After pulling up the rectum, its mesentery is secured to the sacral promontory with two nonabsorbable sutures (Fig. 34.2D and E). It is often helpful to use a mattress-type technique to avoid pulling the suture through the mesentery. In addition, some surgeons prefer to place sutures on one side the mesentery, whereas others prefer bilateral sutures; this appears to be at the discretion of the surgeon, and no good data support either approach.

It is important that the posterior mobilization is adequate to completely reduce the prolapse, and this is confirmed by digital rectal examination at the completion of dissection to ensure that the prolapse is adequately reduced. In some patients, some proximal lateral dissection may be necessary to get adequate reduction.

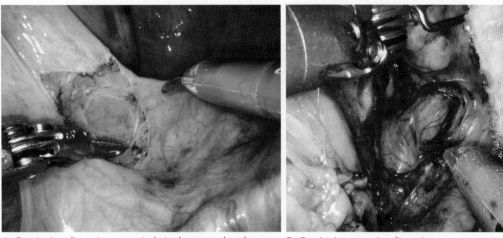

A. Continuing dissection posteriorly in the avascular plane   **B.** Continuing posterior dissection

Levator ani   Distal rectum   Levator ani

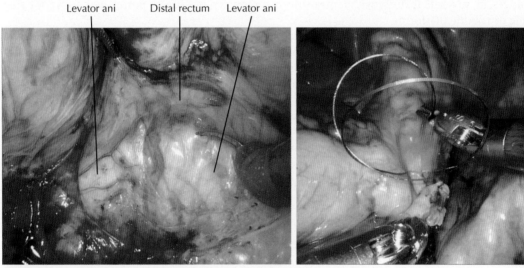

C. Dissection is carried down to the pelvic floor   **D.** Placing the sutures

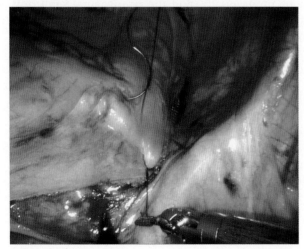

E. Securing the rectopexy

FIGURE 34.2 Suture rectopexy.

MINIMALLY INVASIVE VENTRAL MESH RECTOPEXY

In some series, patients who have abdominal repair of rectal prolapse may have increased constipation rates, and the posterior dissection may have caused denervation of the rectum with resultant emptying difficulties. A ventral dissection avoids denervation by limiting the dissection anterior to the rectum in the rectovaginal septum. It has been shown to be associated with resolution of constipation in more than 80% of patients. With minimally invasive surgery and advances in surgical techniques, ventral mesh rectopexy is usually performed using laparoscopic or robotic platforms.

The peritoneum on the right side of the rectosigmoid junction is incised. The anterior sacral longitudinal ligament is identified. Care should be exercised to protect the surrounding structures as discussed earlier. A peritoneal flap is subsequently created by incising the peritoneum along the right pararectal gutter. Only the peritoneum overlying the anterior right side of the mesorectum is incised (Fig. 34.3A and B). The mesorectum should remain in place and is not mobilized. The incision is then extended caudally until the right side of pouch of Douglas is reached.

Caution should be exercised to resist drifting laterally while dissecting. This can happen easily because of the laxity of tissues, again making traction and countertraction challenging. Outlining the peritoneal flap with electrocautery may help. In female patients, identifying the right uterosacral ligament and keeping it on the right side avoids injury of the right ureter, which typically runs lateral to the ligament.

Entering and dissecting in the rectovaginal septum occurs in a way similar to dissection in rectal cancer, during which the apex of the vagina is retracted anterocaudally. An EEA sizer may be inserted in the vagina to facilitate this part of the procedure. Countertraction is applied on the rectum, and the peritoneum is incised transversely (Fig. 34.3C and D). The fine avascular areolar tissue starts to appear and opens up gradually, and the rectovaginal septum is entered. In this areolar tissue plan, dissection is carried out caudally, exposing the anterior wall of the rectum until the level of the pelvic floor (Fig. 34.3C and D).

A synthetic mesh or a biologic collagen graft can be used. Some sort of tailoring may be needed to enable fitting in the pocket. The mesh/graft is introduced into the abdomen through one of the trocars and placed distally in the pelvis overlying the rectum. It is then anchored to the anterior rectal wall with three rows of absorbable interrupted sutures (Fig. 34.3E and F).

Subsequently, the other end of the mesh/graft is fixed to the initially cleared area in the sacral promontory (Fig. 34.3G and H). This can be done with a tacking instrument such as the ProTack Fixation Device (Medtronic, St. Paul, MN), or in the conventional fashion using nonabsorbable suture. The excess length is trimmed before reperitonealization of the pelvis.

The cul-de-sac is closed, creating a neo-pouch of Douglas. Finally, the initially created peritoneal flap on the right pararectal side is closed over the mesh/graft (Fig. 34.3I).

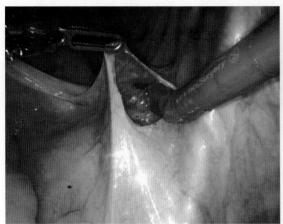

A. Opening the right side of the peritoneum

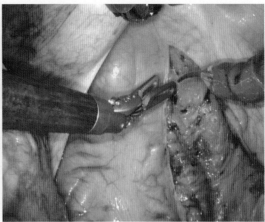

B. Mobilizing along the right anteriorly

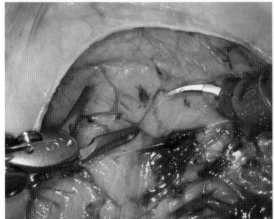

C. Note the avascular plane

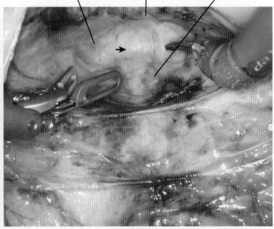

Perineal body   Distal posterior   Distal anterior
                 vaginal wall   rectal wall

D. Shows incising the peritoneum in pouch of Douglas, entering rectovaginal septum, dissecting in the rectovaginal septum, and end of distal dissection to the perineal body if needed.

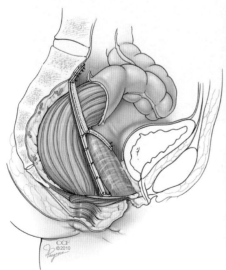

E. Cross-section demonstrating mesh fixation for the sacrocolpopexy

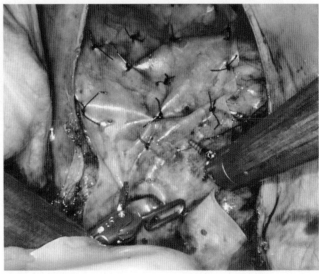

F. The graft anchored to the anterior rectal wall.

FIGURE 34.3 **Laparoscopic/robotic ventral mesh rectopexy—cont'd** *(Part E reprinted with permission, Cleveland Clinic Center for Medical Art & Photography © 1994-2019. All Rights Reserved.)*

Continued

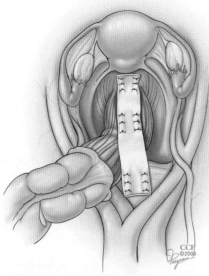

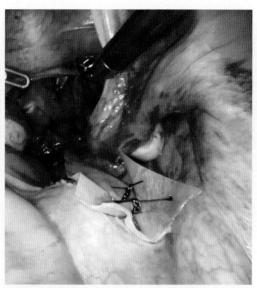

G. Mesh secured to the anterior rectal wall

H. Shows securing the graft to the sacral promontory with a permanent suture

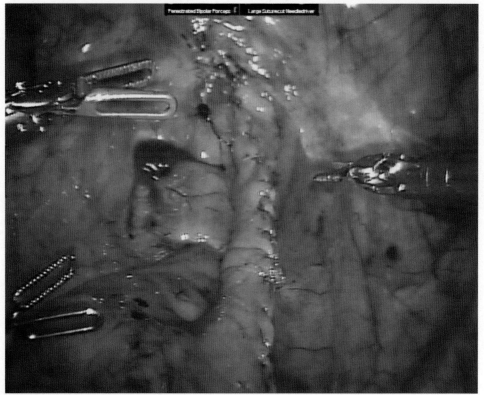

I. Demonstrating pelvic re-peritonealization.

FIGURE 34.3 Laparoscopic/robotic ventral mesh rectopexy—(cont'd)

(Part G reprinted with permission, Cleveland Clinic Center for Medical Art & Photography © 1994-2019. All Rights Reserved.)

SUGGESTED READINGS

Gurland B, Zutschi M. Rectal prolapse. In: Steele SR, Hull TL, Read TE, Saclarides TJ, Senagore AJ, Whitlow CB, editors. The ASCRS Textbook of Colon and Rectal Surgery. 3rd ed. New York: Springer; 2016.

Lindsey I, Nicholls RJ. Rectal prolapse (internal and external). Solitary rectal ulcer, descending perineum syndrome, and rectocele. In: Corman ML, Bergamaschi RCM, Nicholls RJ, Fazio VW, editors. Corman's Colon and Rectal Surgery. 6th ed. Philadelphia: Lippincott Williams & Wilkins; 2013.

Russ AJ, Delaney CP. Rectal prolapse. In: Fazio VW, Church JM, Delaney CP, Kiran RP, editors. Current Therapy in Colon and Rectal Surgery. 3rd ed. Philadelphia: Elsevier; 2017.

Ileal Pouch Anal Anastomosis

Emre Gorgun

VIDEOS

35.1 Single Incision Total Abdominal Colectomy (First Stage Restorative Proctectomy/Ileal Pouch Anal Anastomosis)
35.2 Completion Proctectomy/J-Pouch Construction

INTRODUCTION

An ileal pouch anal anastomosis (IPAA) is performed to reconstruct intestinal continuity after proctocolectomy to treat a number of pathologies. Common indications include mucosal ulcerative colitis (MUC), familial adenomatous polyposis (FAP), and Lynch syndrome. The technique restores gastrointestinal continuity, re-establishes transanal defecation, and avoids a permanent stoma. It is technically demanding and associated with low mortality rates. To avoid early and late complications, it is crucial to be familiar with the anatomy and key steps of the procedure.

SURGICAL PRINCIPLES

The current standard of care for patients with medically refractory ulcerative colitis is a restorative proctocolectomy with IPAA. A J-shaped ileal pouch with a stapled anastomosis has been the preferred technique because it is fast, safe, and has good functional outcomes. Complete removal of the colon and rectum and surrounding mesorectum can be performed in stages. Generally, leaving a short anal canal cuff of 2 to 3 cm before the anastomosis is important to preclude future inflammation of the retained mucosa. In general, this procedure is performed in conjunction with ligation of the ileocolic, middle colic, and superior mesenteric artery and vein, and mobilization of the hepatic and splenic flexures (see Chapters 27, 28, 29; Fig. 35.1A). In addition, as the dissection proceeds into the pelvis, it is important that the autonomic nerves are carefully protected.

In patients with severe fulminant colitis or toxic megacolon, restorative proctocolectomy with ileal pouch-anal anastomosis is most commonly performed in three stages. At the time of the first stage, a total or subtotal colectomy with end ileostomy is performed. This can be completed by single-incision laparoscopic surgery (SILS) (Video 35.1), multiport laparoscopic approach, or through an open incision. If the specimen is opened, the amount of mucosal disease can easily be appreciated in a patient with medically refractory ulcerative colitis (Fig. 35.1B).

A. Arteries of the colon.

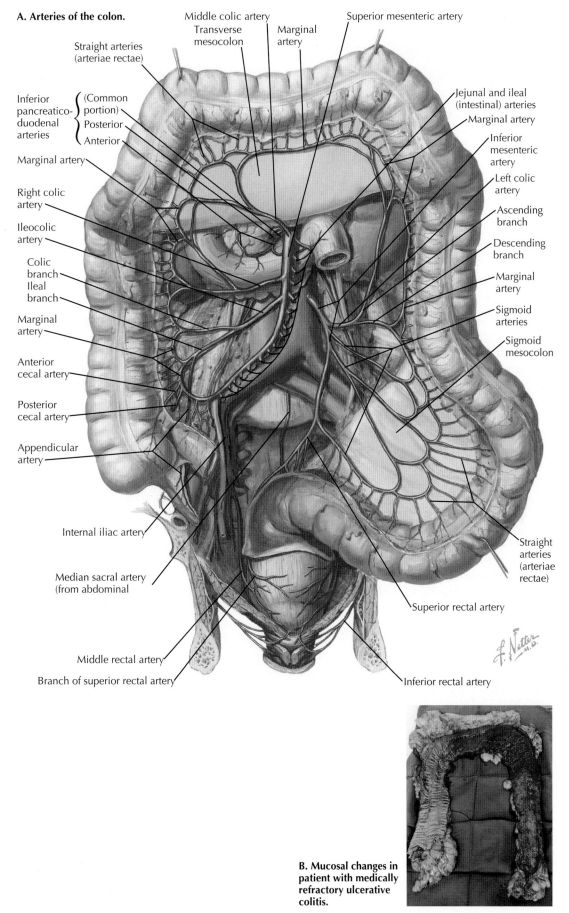

Middle colic artery

Transverse mesocolon

Marginal artery

Superior mesenteric artery

Straight arteries (arteriae rectae)

Inferior pancreatico- duodenal arteries { (Common portion) Posterior Anterior

Marginal artery

Right colic artery

Ileocolic artery

Colic branch

Ileal branch

Marginal artery

Anterior cecal artery

Posterior cecal artery

Appendicular artery

Internal iliac artery

Median sacral artery (from abdominal

Middle rectal artery

Branch of superior rectal artery

Jejunal and ileal (intestinal) arteries

Marginal artery

Inferior mesenteric artery

Left colic artery

Ascending branch

Descending branch

Marginal artery

Sigmoid arteries

Sigmoid mesocolon

Straight arteries (arteriae rectae)

Superior rectal artery

Inferior rectal artery

B. Mucosal changes in patient with medically refractory ulcerative colitis.

FIGURE 35.1 (A) Arteries of the colon. (B) Mucosal changes in patient with medically refractory ulcerative colitis.

SURGICAL PRINCIPLES (Continued)

At the second stage, which is typically performed 6 months later, a completion proctectomy with ileal pouch anal anastomosis (CP/IPAA) and diverting loop ileostomy is created. The final stage constitutes reversal of the diverting loop ileostomy.

Laparoscopically assisted total proctocolectomy and IPAA has evolved over the years.

Although some surgeons prefer the hand-assisted device, a single-incision or multiport laparoscopic approach is preferred (Video 35.2). In the presence of dysplasia or cancer, a complete total mesorectal excision (TME) is performed. In benign conditions similar to rectal cancer operations, a complete posterior TME dissection is performed, in which the pelvis is entered between the layers of fascia propria of the mesorectum and presacral fascia. During the second stage of completion proctectomy with IPAA in benign cases, to maximally protect the presacral autonomic nerves, the dissection to enter the avascular plane posterior to the mesorectum (i.e., "holy plane") is slightly anterior to that of typical rectal cancer "oncologic" operations (Fig. 35.2A). Thus the hypogastric nerve plexus at the pelvic rim is preserved (Fig. 35.2B). Inferiorly, the pelvic dissection is continued in the midline between Waldeyer's fascia and the rectum to the level of the levator muscle (Fig. 35.2C). Anteriorly and laterally it is crucial to stay close to the rectum to avoid any nerve injury (Fig. 35.3A).

Subsequently, bilateral incisions on the pelvic peritoneum are made and joined on the anterior rectal wall at the peritoneal reflection.

Anteriorly, dissection is performed on the lower border of the prostate gland or lower one-third of the vagina (Fig. 35.3B).

Denonvilliers' fascia is preserved in patients without a carcinoma to minimize the risk of damage to the plexus near the prostate. At this stage, the rectum is fully mobilized. A transanal digital assessment with the index finger is performed to determine the level of transection by a linear stapler, which should be approximately 1.5 to 2 cm above the dentate line (Figs. 35.3C and D and 35.4).

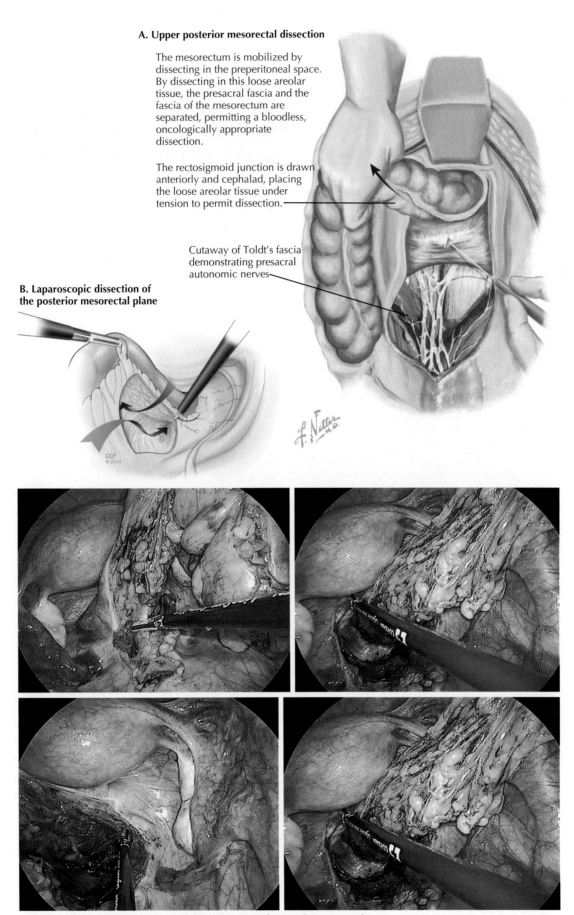

A. Upper posterior mesorectal dissection

The mesorectum is mobilized by dissecting in the preperitoneal space. By dissecting in this loose areolar tissue, the presacral fascia and the fascia of the mesorectum are separated, permitting a bloodless, oncologically appropriate dissection.

The rectosigmoid junction is drawn anteriorly and cephalad, placing the loose areolar tissue under tension to permit dissection.

Cutaway of Toldt's fascia demonstrating presacral autonomic nerves

B. Laparoscopic dissection of the posterior mesorectal plane

C. Laparoscopic posterior mesorectal dissection/TME down to levator muscles

FIGURE 35.2 Dissection of posterior mesorectal space.

TME, Total mesorectal excision. *(B, Reprinted with permission, Cleveland Clinic Center for Medical Art & Photography © 2014-2019. All Rights Reserved.)*

A. Laparoscopic lateral and anterior dissection of the rectum

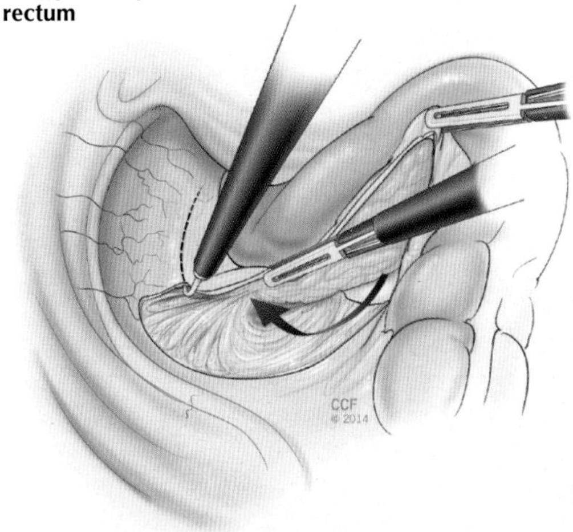

B. Laparoscopic anterior rectal dissection

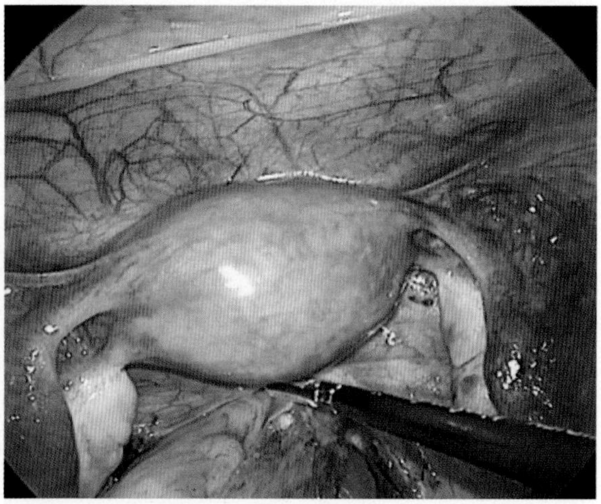

C. The anatomy of the pelvic floor

Superior view

Pubic symphysis

Inguinal ligament (Poupart's)

Inferior (arcuate) pubic ligament
Deep dorsal vein of clitoris
Transverse perineal ligament
Fascia of deep perineal muscles
Urethra
Vagina
Obturator canal
Obturator fascia (over obturator internus muscle)
Pubococcygeus muscle (part of levator ani muscle)
Tendinous arch of levator ani muscle
Rectum
Iliococcygeus muscle (part of levator ani muscle)
Ischial spine
Levator plate (median raphe) of levator ani muscle
Coccygeus (ischiococcygeus) muscle
Piriformis muscle

Coccyx

Anterior sacro-coccygeal ligament

Sacral promontory

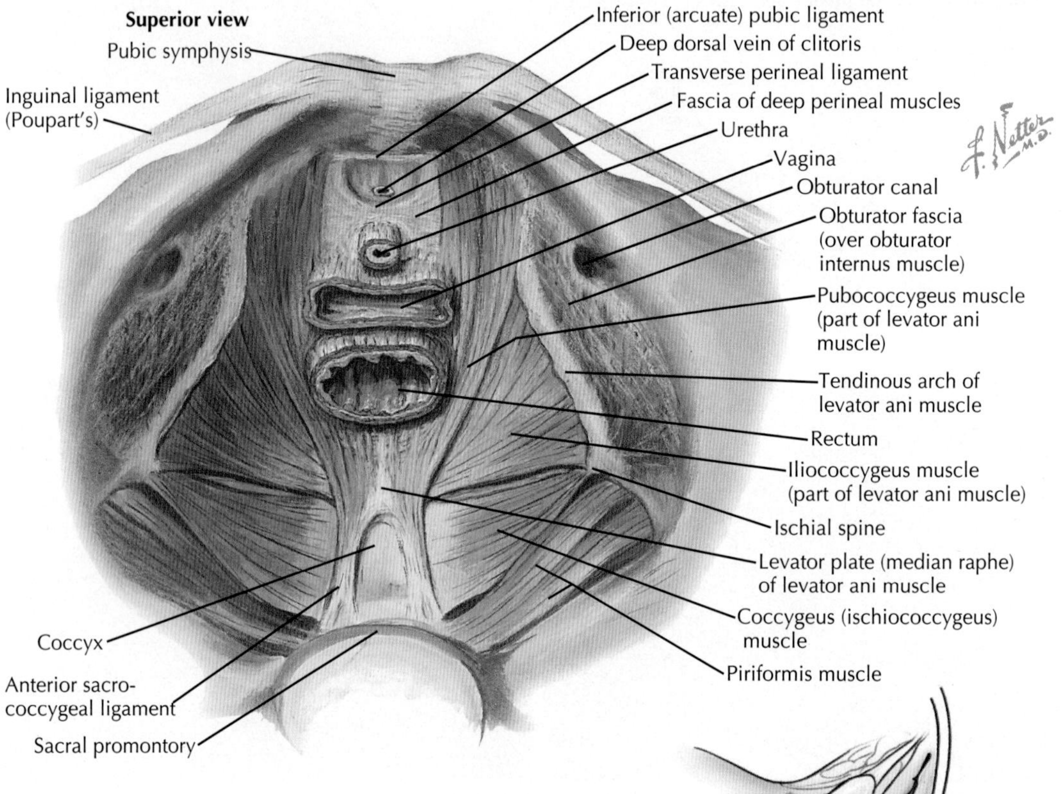

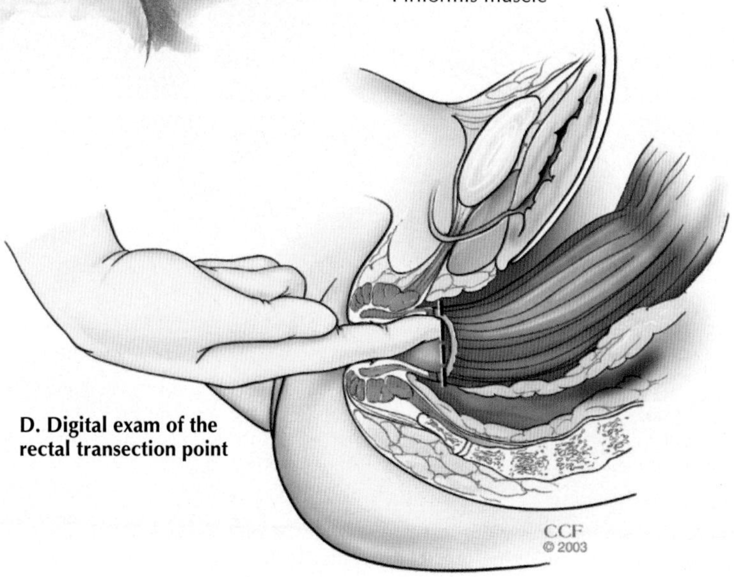

D. Digital exam of the rectal transection point

FIGURE 35.3 **Dissection of the rectum, anatomy of the pelvic floor, and digital rectal examination.** *(A and D, Reprinted with permission, Cleveland Clinic Center for Medical Art & Photography © 2014-2019. All Rights Reserved.)*

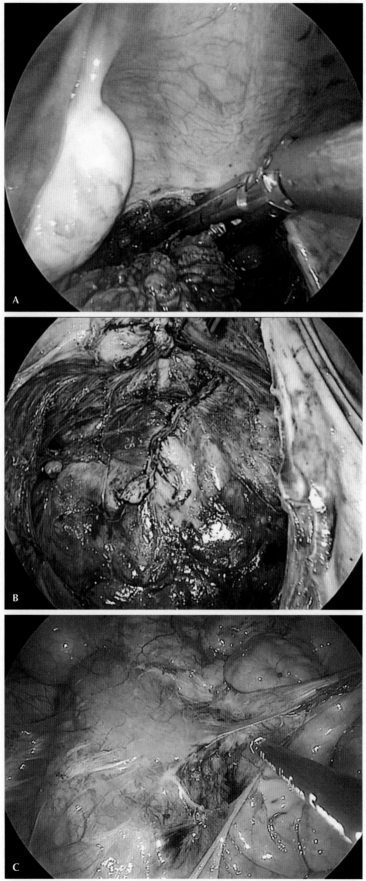

Transection of the rectum at the anorectal junction (**A** and **B**). Mobilization of SMA up to 3rd part of the duodenum and pancreas (**C**).

FIGURE 35.4 Transection of the rectum at the anorectal junction and mobilization of superior mesenteric artery (SMA).

ILEOANAL POUCH AND ANASTOMOSIS

The key to success in an IPAA is to maximize "reach" and ensure there is a tension-free anastomosis. For this purpose, the small bowel mesentery (Fig. 35.4C) should be fully mobilized, freeing the posterior attachments of the mesentery and superior mesenteric vessels as far as the upper border of the third part of the duodenum (Video 35.2). This is especially important if there is limited reach, such as in overweight patients or in patients with shortened mesentery. If there is still tension, additional maneuvers, such as incising the mesenteric surface on the anterior and posterior of the superior mesenteric vessels, are performed (i.e., relaxing incisions) (Fig. 35.5A).

The J-pouch is constructed from the terminal small bowel segment by folding this portion of the bowel into two 15-cm segments. An approximately 2-cm enterotomy is made longitudinally at the pouch apex to construct the side-to-side anastomosis. This is performed by using two cartridges of a 100-mm linear stapler introduced through the enterotomy at the apex (Fig. 35.5B).

The blind tip of the J-pouch is closed using a TA stapler and is generally oversewn by a continuous suture (Fig. 35.5C). After a 2-0 polypropylene purse-string suture is applied to the apical enterotomy, insufflation using normal saline is performed to confirm the integrity of the pouch (Fig. 35.6A), before inserting the anvil to complete the stapled ileal pouch-anal anastomosis.

After the IPAA anastomosis (Fig. 35.6B), an intraoperative pouchoscopy (Fig. 35.6C) with a leak test is performed (Video 35.2).

A diverting loop ileostomy is usually created at the completion of the ileal pouch-anal anastomosis.

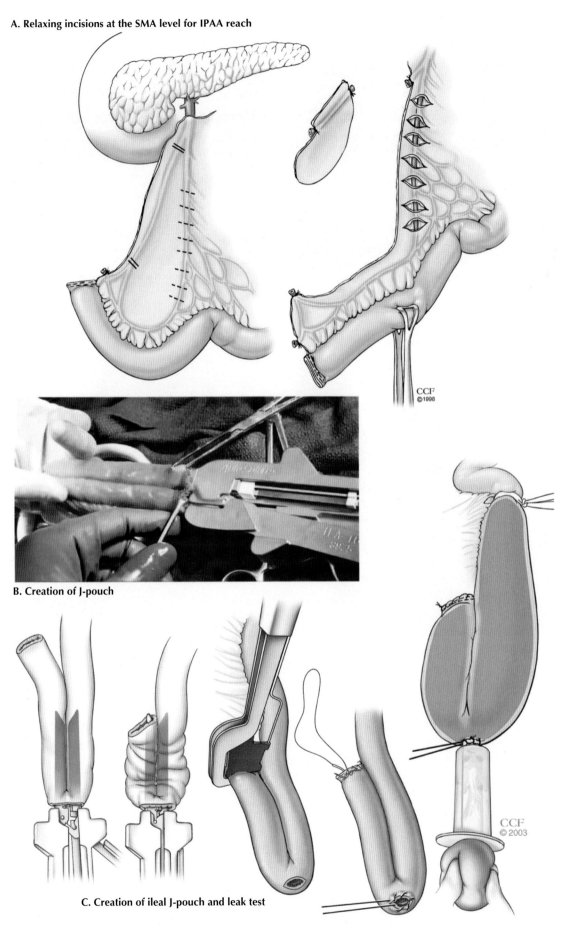

A. Relaxing incisions at the SMA level for IPAA reach

B. Creation of J-pouch

C. Creation of ileal J-pouch and leak test

FIGURE 35.5 Creation of ileal anal pouch.

IPAA; Ileal pouch anal anastomosis; *SMA,* superior mesenteric artery. *(A and C, Reprinted with permission, Cleveland Clinic Center for Medical Art & Photography © 2014-2019. All Rights Reserved.)*

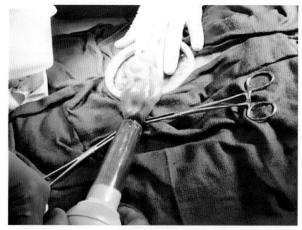

A. Leak test

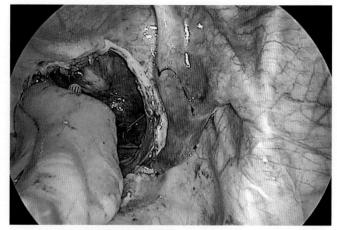

B. Creation of pouch anal anastomosis under laparoscopic view

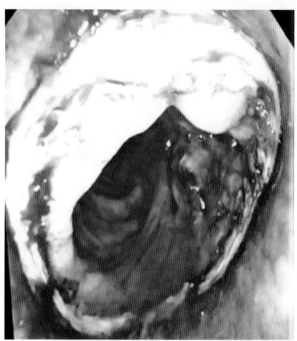

C. Pouchoscopy and intraoperative leak test

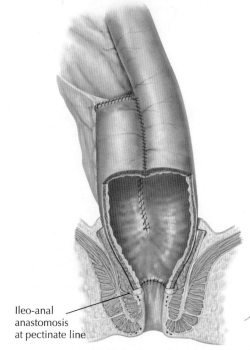

Ileo-anal anastomosis at pectinate line

D. Ileal "J" pouch-anal anastomosis

FIGURE 35.6 Anastomosis and leak test.

SUGGESTED READINGS

Fazio VW, Ziv Y, Church JM, et al. Ileal pouch-anal anastomoses complications and function in 1005 patients. Ann Surg 1995;222(2):120–7.

Remzi FH, Fazio VW, Gorgun E, et al. The outcome after restorative proctocolectomy with or without defunctioning ileostomy. Dis Colon Rectum 2006;49(4):470–7.

CHAPTER

36

Sphincter Repair and Sacral Neuromodulation

Massarat Zutshi

INTRODUCTION

Fecal incontinence is a devastating problem. The incidence has been cited between 1% and 18% based on several studies. However, even at this rate, this symptom seems to be under-reported, with true incontinence (that excludes incontinence of flatus) thought to be around 7% to 8%.

The initial treatment of fecal incontinence is usually by conservative means involving diet and bowel management. This is done by eliminating foods that may contribute to diarrhea and exploring food allergies. Inclusion of fiber may also help decrease symptoms in some patients. Kegel exercises, by patient alone or using a physical therapist to direct sphincter contractions, are a mainstay of initial approaches. Antidiarrheals and probiotics may be other medications that are often necessary to control symptoms. Finally, rectal irrigation is an option for patients who have fairly normal bowel movements but continue to leak after a bowel movement. However, despite this multimodality approach, many patients still experience symptoms affecting quality of life.

When conservative management fails, future options are based on an assessment of patient symptoms and expectations. Nonoperative management involves the use of anal plugs such as the Renew insert or the Procon 2 device. Other nonoperative managements include the Eclipse device and the Secca procedure. Surgical options also still exist. Sphincteroplasty is an option for patients who have a sphincter defect of less than 180 degrees, and sacral neuromodulation with an implantable device has more recently had significant success at improving incontinence. In this chapter, we explore the latter two procedures in the treatment of fecal incontinence.

SPHINCTEROPLASTY (OVERLAPPING SPHINCTER REPAIR)

An incision usually about 1 to 1.5 cm is made over the perineum between the rectum and the vagina beyond the anal verge for obstetric injuries. To avoid nerve injury, the arc of the incision should not extend to the extreme posterolateral position. The anterior and posterior flaps are then dissected away using sharp dissection. Hemostasis is secured using electrocautery. It is important to keep the operative field "dry" to have precise view of the planes. Often there is scar tissue between the two edges of the muscle that may be visible in the floor of the incision. If this is seen, it is incised in the middle and the muscle is dissected laterally. If it is not seen, then the edges of the muscle are identified and dissected laterally, taking care not to go too lateral to avoid injury to the nerves. It is necessary to avoid buttonhole defects into the anal mucosa or vagina. The dissection is carried laterally to the ischiorectal fat. Any tears in the anal mucosa are repaired with a 4-0 chromic suture.

If the internal anal sphincter was not injured (Fig. 36.1), and therefore not divided, for the overlapping repair, a plication can be done using 2-0 Vicryl suture before the sphincteroplasty. The sphincter ends that have been sufficiently mobilized to allow overlapping of the muscle are grasped. These ends can be approximated end-to-end if the length is not sufficient to perform an overlapping repair. However, if possible, the preferred technique is an overlapping sphincter repair. The repair is performed by using 2-0 polyglactin sutures, which are placed as a mattress sutures starting at the lateral end of one muscle that is overlapped and proceeding to the cut end. This is done so that about three sutures are taken: one at the cut end, one in the middle, and one at the lateral end, each in a vest-over-pants repair. The sutures are tied loosely so as not to cause necrosis of the muscle. Throughout the procedure, irrigation with an antibiotic solution is carried out and hemostasis is secured. The wound is then closed in layers, and any dead space can be drained using a fine drain (e.g., ½-inch Penrose), which can be inserted and then removed on approximately day 5. Although often not necessary, a diverting stoma may be used at the discretion of the surgeon.

SACRAL NEUROMODULATION

This is a procedure currently done more commonly because it can treat patients with anatomic defects as well as neurologic issues.

The procedure is performed in two stages. In the first stage, which is the test phase, the electrode is inserted into the S3 foramina under fluoroscopy control and connected to an external stimulator. During the next 2 weeks the patient assesses his or her symptoms and returns to decide whether the generator can be attached to the device or the devices removed and the absence of any improvement. Alternatively, occasionally a PNE test is done in the office, where a thin electrode is placed blindly in the region of S3, and the patients symptoms are assessed over a week. If symptoms are improved more than 50% compared with the preoperative state, then both stage 1 and 2 may be done at the same sitting.

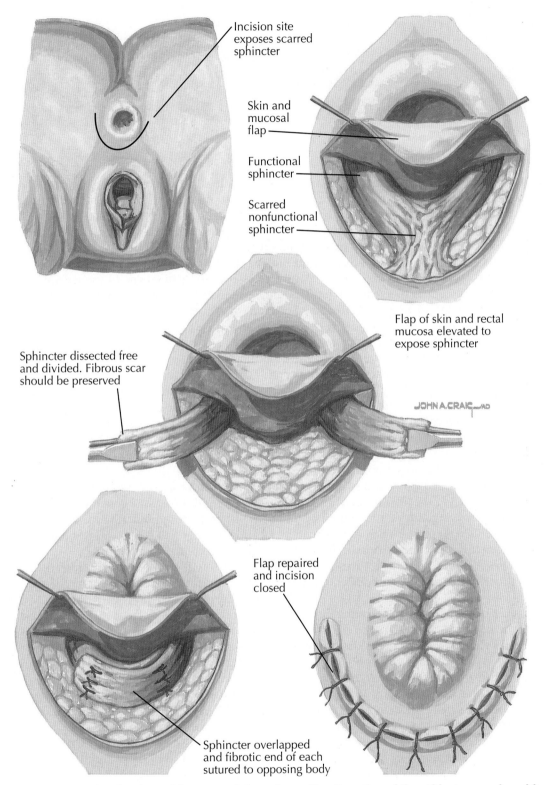

FIGURE 36.1 **Overlapping sphincter repair is performed by dissection of the sphincter muscles with overlapping sutured repair.**

STAGE 1: IMPLANTATION OF THE ELECTRODE

This procedure is done under sedation and local anesthesia. The patient is placed in a prone position, and the bony points and the chest are well supported on pillows. The patient's feet are left hanging off a pillow so that they can be accessed during the procedure. The area of the implantation of the electrode and the creation of the pocket is then cleaned and draped. The anatomic location of S3 is judged based on landmarks such as the tip of the coccyx. A distance of 9 cm is marked toward the sacrum, and radiopaque guidewires or needles are placed horizontally to assess the level of S3 and vertically to assess the medial edge of the foramina (Fig. 36.2A). Fluoroscopy is then carried out, and the needles and guidewire may be moved according to the location of S3 on fluoroscopy. Local anesthesia is used to infiltrate the site of the intended needle placement on both sides. The needle is then advanced and guided into S3 (Fig. 36.2B). Fluoroscopy will assess the depth of the needle, and it is advanced so that the tip is just outside the foramen on the dorsal side of the sacrum.

The needle is then stimulated, and reflex contractions of the anus called "bellows" and flexion of the big toe are assessed. Stimulation of nerve root S2 results in contraction of the calf muscle, whereas S4 stimulation does not cause any flexion of the toe.

Once the correct site is identified for stimulation, the incision area is enlarged using a No. 11 blade, and the obturator within the needle is removed. A guidewire is then passed within the needle groove and the needle is removed. The trocar is advanced over the guidewire so that it sits just inside the dorsal portion of the S3 foramina (Fig. 36.2C). The curved stylet is then assembled. The needle is removed and the stylet is passed into the trocar so that the curve goes from the medial to the lateral side. This is performed under fluoroscopic guidance so that three electrodes are lying outside the foramina and one is just at the foramina. All four electrodes are then tested for the motor responses. The ideal location is where all electrodes respond to both the anal bellows and the flexion of the big toe at a low-frequency stimulation.

A pocket is then created on the right or the left side below the posterior iliac crest in an area that is below the beltline and does not interfere with sitting. The side is picked by the patient, often based on sleeping habits. An incision is made and deepened below Scarpa's fascia, where a pocket is then created. The tunneling tool is used to tunnel the electrode from its insertion into the pocket (Fig. 36.2D). The electrode is cleaned of body fluids and a plastic boot is passed over the electrodes. The electrodes are then inserted into the external stimulator and held in position with 4 screws, which are tightened (Fig. 36.2E). The external stimulating electrode is tunneled from the pocket to the opposite side to prevent any infection of the pocket. The pocket is closed in layers (Fig. 36.2F). The incision is closed over the electrode in the S3 region using a single stitch. The device is finally connected to the external stimulator, and a dressing is applied to include the external stimulator and an incision over the pocket.

At stage 2 surgery, the pocket is opened and the electrode is delivered and inserted into the head of the generator (Fig. 36.2G). The pocket is then enlarged so that it will fit the generator. The pocket is irrigated with an antibiotic solution and hemostasis is secured. The generator is then inserted into the pocket with the markings on the stimulator facing toward the skin. The impedance is checked via a device that is inserted into a sterile pocket and placed over the incision. Once impedance checking is completed, the wound is closed in layers and a dressing is applied.

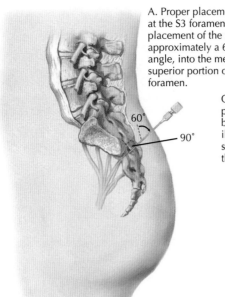

A. Proper placement of needle at the S3 foramen. Optimal placement of the needle is at approximately a 60-degree angle, into the medial and superior portion of the S3 foramen.

B. A guidewire is inserted, and the needle is removed after testing the motor response from S3. A trocar is inserted over a guidewire, and its depth is checked radiologically and the curved stylet is advanced under fluoroscopic guidance.

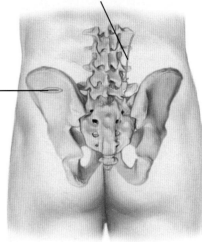

C. A subcutaneous pocket is created below the posterior iliac crest on the side picked by the patient.

D. The electrode is tunneled into the pocket using the tunneling device.

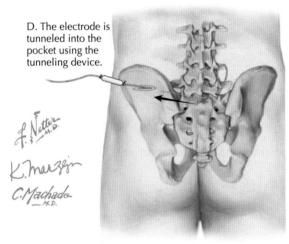

E. The electrode is tunneled to the opposite side to exit away from the pocket. The sutures over the boot are to protect the electrode from body fluids.

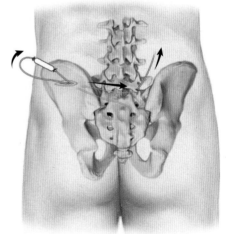

F. The electrode is connected the external stimulator. Stage 1.

G. Stage 2: The pocket is opened and the electrode is disconnected from the external stimulator and inserted into the generator for permanent stimulation.

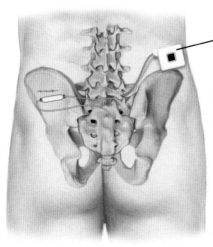

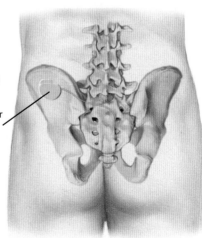

FIGURE 36.2 Stage 1 implantation of the electrode.

SUGGESTED READINGS

Johanson JF, Lafferty J. Epidemiology of fecal incontinence: the silent affliction. Am J Gastroenterol 1996;91:33.

Jorge JM, Wexner SD. Etiology and management of fecal incontinence. Dis Colon Rectum 1993;36:77.

Oliveira L, Pfeifer J, Wexner SD. Physiological and clinical outcome of anterior sphincteroplasty. Br J Surg 1996;83:502.

Vaizey CJ, Norton C, Thornton MJ, et al. Long-term results of repeat anterior anal sphincter repair. Dis Colon Rectum 2004;47:858.

Hernia

SECTION EDITOR: Michael J. Rosen

Laparoscopic Inguinal Hernia Repair

Aldo Fafaj and Steven Rosenblatt

INTRODUCTION

Since the first laparoscopic cholecystectomy was successfully performed in 1987, there has been a remarkable adoption of minimally invasive techniques, which has dramatically changed the field of general surgery. The surgical management of inguinal hernias, traditionally one of the most commonly performed procedures by the general surgeon, has paralleled the natural evolution of such surgical innovation. Compared with the open tension-free technique, laparoscopic inguinal hernia repair has been found to be associated with less postoperative pain, as well as a more rapid return to normal activities. In addition, the laparoscopic approaches are advantageous for patients with bilateral hernias because the same incisions can be used to access and repair both sides. Similarly, by avoiding the anterior scarring and previously placed mesh, these minimally invasive surgical (MIS) techniques are optimal in repairing recurrences associated with a prior open repair. A thorough understanding of the anatomy of the groin is crucial for both techniques to achieve a durable repair and minimize the risk of complications.

LAPAROSCOPIC APPROACHES

The transabdominal preperitoneal (TAPP) and the totally extraperitoneal (TEP) are the most commonly performed of the available MIS techniques. Broadly speaking, the major difference between the two approaches is in the access and development of the preperitoneal space. Otherwise, the tenets associated with each operation are essentially the same.

The TAPP approach first requires entry into the abdomen and then the creation of the preperitoneal space. An incision of the peritoneum just lateral to the medial umbilical ligament is extended laterally to the level of the anterior superior iliac spine (ASIS). The peritoneal flap is developed by bluntly dissecting the peritoneum from the transversalis fascia. The hernias are exposed and reduced. Ultimately the pocket for placing the mesh into the preperitoneal space is created. Upon completion of mesh placement, the peritoneal flap is then closed so that the mesh is excluded from the abdominal viscera.

In contrast, the TEP approach does not require entry into the peritoneal cavity. Rather, a balloon dissector or blunt telescopic dissection can be used to develop the preperitoneal space directly. Mesh is then placed and secured in a similar manner to the TAPP technique. Closure of the peritoneum is therefore not necessary.

KEY ANATOMIC CONCEPTS FOR LAPAROSCOPIC REPAIR

Myopectineal Orifice

Initially named by Dr. Henri Fruchaud, the myopectineal orifice is a critically important feature of groin anatomy (Fig. 37.1, *dashed ovals*). All groin hernias originate from within this area of weakness, which is covered only by the transversalis fascia and the peritoneum. Superiorly and medially, this aperture is bordered by the rectus muscle and the conjoined tendon, inferiorly by the superior pubic ramus and the pectineal (Cooper's) ligament, and laterally by the iliopsoas muscle and the lateral border of the femoral sheath. The myopectineal orifice is divided into two by the inguinal ligament. The suprainguinal region contains the spermatic cord in males or the round ligament in females, and the infrainguinal region contains the femoral nerve, femoral artery, and femoral vein. The goal of mesh placement in either inguinal hernia repair is coverage of the entire region.

A. Anterior view

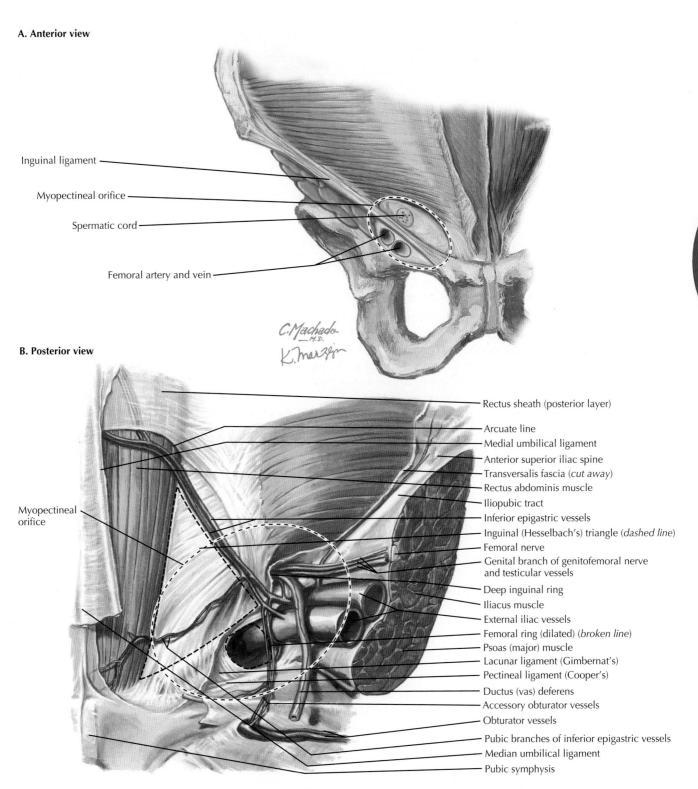

Inguinal ligament

Myopectineal orifice

Spermatic cord

Femoral artery and vein

B. Posterior view

Myopectineal orifice

Rectus sheath (posterior layer)

Arcuate line

Medial umbilical ligament

Anterior superior iliac spine

Transversalis fascia (*cut away*)

Rectus abdominis muscle

Iliopubic tract

Inferior epigastric vessels

Inguinal (Hesselbach's) triangle (*dashed line*)

Femoral nerve

Genital branch of genitofemoral nerve
and testicular vessels

Deep inguinal ring

Iliacus muscle

External iliac vessels

Femoral ring (dilated) (*broken line*)

Psoas (major) muscle

Lacunar ligament (Gimbernat's)

Pectineal ligament (Cooper's)

Ductus (vas) deferens

Accessory obturator vessels

Obturator vessels

Pubic branches of inferior epigastric vessels

Median umbilical ligament

Pubic symphysis

FIGURE 37.1 Anterior and posterior views of the myopectineal orifice.

Inguinal Ligament Versus Ileopubic Tract

The inguinal (Poupart's) ligament is a fibrous band that extends from the ASIS to the pubic tubercle. The inferior edge of the external oblique aponeurosis folds upon itself posteriorly to form the "shelving edge," which is used to secure the inferior border of mesh in an open inguinal hernia repair. The iliopubic tract is a thickening of the transversalis fascia that runs posterior and parallel to the inguinal ligament extending from the pubic tubercle medially and passing over the femoral vessels to insert to the ASIS laterally. Because the inguinal ligament is not visualized during a laparoscopic inguinal hernia repair, the iliopubic tract becomes an important landmark as its position is verified by palpation of instruments across the abdominal wall (Fig. 37.2A). Lateral to the internal ring, no fixation devices should be fired below the palpated iliopubic tract because of the risk of injury to the lateral femoral cutaneous, genitofemoral, and femoral nerves.

Pectineal Ligament

The pectineal (Cooper's) ligament refers to the periosteum found along the superior ramus of the pubic bone, posterior to the iliopubic tract (Fig. 37.2B). This ligament is an extension of the lacunar (Gimbernat's) ligament, which connects the inguinal ligament to Cooper's ligament near their insertion site at the pubic tubercle. Cooper's ligament is an important landmark during laparoscopic hernia repair, because it is frequently used for medial fixation of the mesh because of the ability to hold tacks.

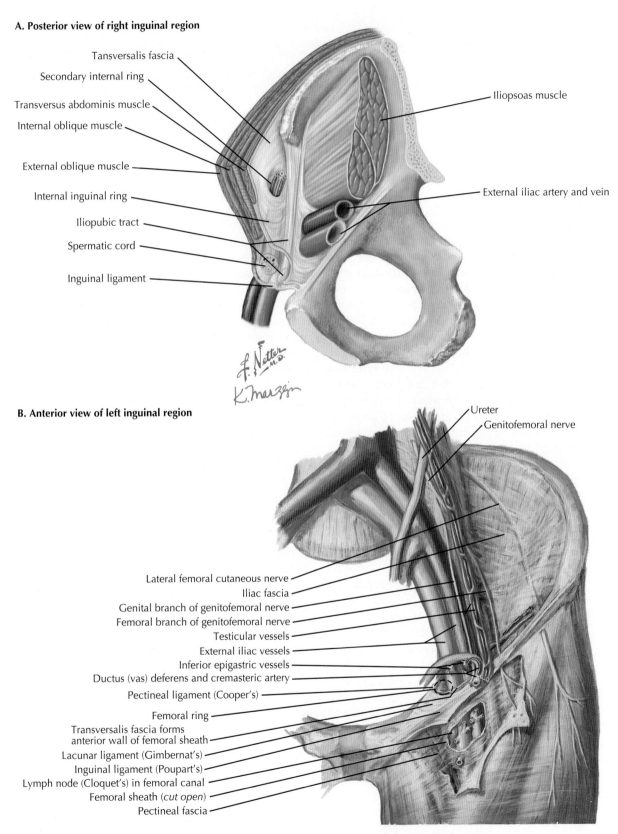

A. Posterior view of right inguinal region

Tansversalis fascia

Secondary internal ring

Transversus abdominis muscle

Internal oblique muscle

External oblique muscle

Internal inguinal ring

Iliopubic tract

Spermatic cord

Inguinal ligament

Iliopsoas muscle

External iliac artery and vein

B. Anterior view of left inguinal region

Ureter

Genitofemoral nerve

Lateral femoral cutaneous nerve

Iliac fascia

Genital branch of genitofemoral nerve

Femoral branch of genitofemoral nerve

Testicular vessels

External iliac vessels

Inferior epigastric vessels

Ductus (vas) deferens and cremasteric artery

Pectineal ligament (Cooper's)

Femoral ring

Transversalis fascia forms
anterior wall of femoral sheath

Lacunar ligament (Gimbernat's)

Inguinal ligament (Poupart's)

Lymph node (Cloquet's) in femoral canal

Femoral sheath (*cut open*)

Pectineal fascia

FIGURE 37.2 Posterior and anterior views of the inguinal region.

Inguinal Geometry

Hesselbach's triangle is bordered by the inferior epigastric vessels laterally, the rectus abdominis muscle medially, and the inguinal ligament inferiorly (see Fig. 37.1B). A direct hernia occurs medial to the inferior epigastric vessels and directly through the triangle, whereas indirect hernias are found lateral to the inguinal triangle and, similarly, the inferior epigastric vessels.

The "triangle of doom" is marked by the ductus deferens or round ligament medially, the gonadal vessels laterally, and the cut edge of the peritoneum inferiorly. Within these boundaries, the external iliac artery and vein (Fig. 37.3A) are found. Dissection here must be undertaken with extreme caution because of the potential for severe bleeding.

The "triangle of pain" is bound by the gonadal vessels medially, the iliopubic tract laterally, and the cut edge of the peritoneum inferiorly. The lateral femoral cutaneous nerve, the femoral branch of the genitofemoral nerve, and the femoral nerve (see Fig. 37.3A) are within this perimeter. Extreme care must be taken when dissecting these areas, and no fixation devices should be placed in these regions to avoid neurovascular injuries.

The "circle of death," also known as corona mortis, is an anatomic variant in which a vascular ring forms from an anastomosis between the obturator and the external iliac or epigastric arteries or veins (Fig. 37.3B). It is located about 5 cm from the pubic symphysis arching over the pectineal ligament. Significant bleeding that can be difficult to control can occur if this ring is injured, so no fixation should be placed in this region.

PRINCIPLES OF LAPAROSCOPIC REPAIR

General anesthesia is indicated for TEP and TAPP repairs. Intraoperative Foley catheterization for bladder decompression is routinely used. However, it is also acceptable to ask the patient to void before entering the operating room instead. Identification and exposure of the anatomic landmarks of Cooper's ligament medially, the psoas muscle inferiorly, as well as the peritoneal sac, gonadal vessels, round ligament or vas deferens, iliac vessels, and the iliopubic tract are key to operative safety and efficacy. Separation of the hernia sac from the cord structures before reduction of the sac helps avoid injury to the gonadal vessels and vas deferens.

Identification and complete reduction of the hernia sac are critical to preventing recurrent hernias, as is the dissection of a wide pocket for placement of the mesh and ample coverage of the direct, indirect, and femoral spaces. If tacks are to be used to secure the mesh, they should be used sparingly. Similarly, as previously mentioned, fixation should be avoided within the triangle of pain to avoid chronic postoperative pain.

A. Triangle of doom and pain

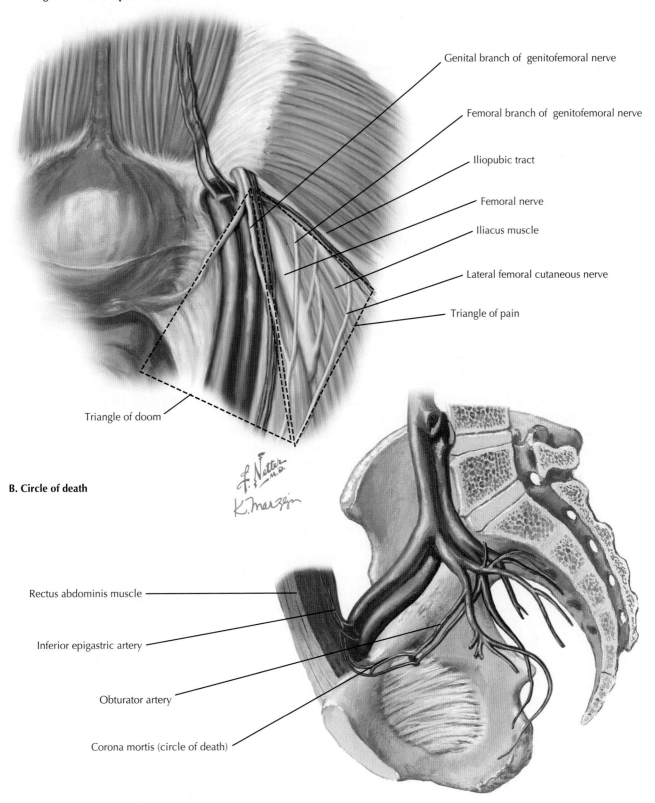

Genital branch of genitofemoral nerve

Femoral branch of genitofemoral nerve

Iliopubic tract

Femoral nerve

Iliacus muscle

Lateral femoral cutaneous nerve

Triangle of pain

Triangle of doom

B. Circle of death

Rectus abdominis muscle

Inferior epigastric artery

Obturator artery

Corona mortis (circle of death)

FIGURE 37.3 Inguinal landmarks in hernia repair: warning triangles and corona mortis.

TRANSABDOMINAL PREPERITONEAL APPROACH

The patient is placed supine on the operating room table with both arms tucked at the side. To gain access into the abdomen via the open cut-down (Hasson) technique at the umbilicus and placement of a 10-mm trocar is preferred. Another option is to use a 5-mm optical trocar and the 0-degree scope to enter the abdomen in a more superior location. A thorough diagnostic laparoscopy is performed, followed by careful inspection of the inguinal areas to evaluate for hernias. Two additional 5-mm ports are placed just lateral to the inferior epigastric vessels on either side and cephalad to the umbilicus. A 5-mm, 30-degree laparoscope is placed into the port that is ipsilateral to the hernia. The working ports are the umbilical and the contralateral 5-mm port. Identification of the following landmarks is critical to begin dissection: medial umbilical ligament (containing obliterated umbilical artery), testicular vessels, inferior epigastric vessels (lateral umbilical ligament), and external iliac vessels (Fig. 37.4A).

The peritoneum is incised using the scissors with electrocautery just lateral to the medial umbilical fold. To maximize the working space required to place an adequately sized piece of mesh, this incision should start as high and close to the umbilicus as possible. The edge of the cut peritoneum is then grasped, and the peritoneum is bluntly dissected away from the transversalis fascia, which should remain on the anterior abdominal wall. This dissection is ideal because it allows for the development of a single plane, which will eventually allow for placement of the mesh. If the surgeon is in this correct plane, he or she should not see the muscle belly of the rectus muscle but rather the transversalis fascia. In some patients, the peritoneum can be thin and prone to tearing, so alternatively the pretransversalis plane can be entered. This plane can be confirmed by seeing the muscle belly of the rectus muscle. Although following this plane out laterally makes the development of the flap easier, the surgeon must eventually enter the preperitoneal plane because the trasversalis fascia inserts onto the iliopubic tract. This can be safely done just lateral to the inferior epigastric vessels. Once the correct plane is identified, the peritoneal incision is continued laterally in a straight line, ending just short of the ASIS.

The peritoneal flap is then created by blunt sweeping motions medial to the inferior epigastric vessels until Cooper's is identified as a white, glistening structure along the superior pubic ramus. This ligament marks the medial extent of the dissection. When creating this peritoneal flap, the surgeon must take great care to avoid injury to the epigastric vessels and to sweep all layers toward the anterior abdominal wall, except the thin peritoneum (Fig. 37.4B). If the dissection is performed superficial to this layer, then fatty tissue will be encountered, which often leads to bleeding. The dissection is carried down to the peritoneum until the cord structures are identified. At this point, the triangles of "doom" and "pain" can be exposed, and the lateral dissection is complete. Inferiorly, the dissection should continue until the edge of the psoas muscle is visible.

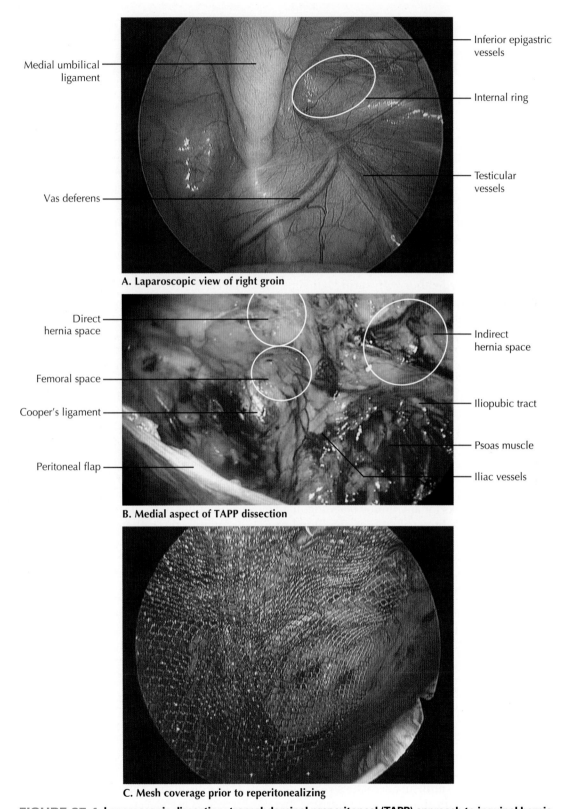

Medial umbilical ligament

Inferior epigastric vessels

Internal ring

Vas deferens

Testicular vessels

A. Laparoscopic view of right groin

Direct hernia space

Indirect hernia space

Femoral space

Cooper's ligament

Iliopubic tract

Psoas muscle

Peritoneal flap

Iliac vessels

B. Medial aspect of TAPP dissection

C. Mesh coverage prior to reperitonealizing

FIGURE 37.4 Laparoscopic dissection: transabdominal preperitoneal (TAPP) approach to inguinal hernia.

TRANSABDOMINAL PREPERITONEAL APPROACH (Continued)

Obviously, it is then crucial to evaluate both potential hernia spaces and rule out an unexpected pantaloon hernia. For direct hernias, the contents should be dissected carefully from the transversalis fascia using small, rather than large, bites, with appropriate countertension. Exposure of the pectineal ligament from the pubis to the iliac vessels confirms the completed dissection. Visualization of the iliac vein is necessary to avoid missing an occult femoral hernia. In the case of indirect hernias, dissection is started laterally with appropriate traction. Such dissection lateral to the spermatic cord is mandatory to identify and reduce the cord lipoma, if present. The indirect hernia sac is often deeply invested within the spermatic cord, so it is important to separate the cord structures from the sac before reducing it. This will minimize bleeding and inadvertent injury to the cord vessels and the vas deferens.

Once the hernia sac is completely reduced, and the entire myopectineal orifice has been exposed, the pocket is ready for mesh placement. Depending on their size, any peritoneal defects are repaired either with sutures or clips. A flat piece of 15-cm by 10-cm heavyweight polypropylene mesh is used, which is introduced into the abdomen and placed into the space through the umbilical port. The mesh should cover the entire myopectineal orifice (and thereby the three potential hernia sites) with significant overlap, especially inferiorly because this is the location of most recurrences (Fig. 37.4C). A laparoscopic tacker with permanent tacks to fixate the mesh is used. Typically, two tacks are placed on the pectineal ligament, and one tack high on each side of the inferior epigastric vessels. For the superior and lateral tacks, it is important to palpate the tip of the device before placing the tack to confirm that it will be placed above the iliopubic tract, the superior border of the "triangle of pain" (see Fig. 37.3A).

The peritoneal flap is then reapproximated over the mesh with the tacker, again palpating the tip before firing. Naturally, this defect can also be closed using intracorporeal suturing, depending on the preference of the surgeon. No large gaps should remain in the peritoneal closure, which would both expose the mesh to the bowel and potentially allow for it to herniate through the peritoneal flap. At the conclusion of the procedure, the surgeon carefully inspects the repair and looks for any undue bleeding. If a Foley catheter has been placed, then the anesthesiologist is asked to evaluate for any blood or CO_2 gas within the catheter. The trocars are then removed, and the insufflation is released. The fascia and then the skin are closed, and the wounds are dressed. The Foley is removed.

TOTALLY EXTRAPERITONEAL APPROACH

As the preperitoneal space is directly accessed in the TEP repair, the initial port is positioned off of the midline. It is our preference to place this incision on the opposite side of the hernia or, in the case of bilateral defects, on the contralateral location from the largest hernia. Just inferior to the umbilicus, a transverse incision is created lateral to the linea alba, overlying the rectus muscle. It is crucial to attain optimal exposure to create the extraperitoneal space; for this reason, it is important that the incision is large enough, which is dependent on the patient's body habitus. The subcutaneous dissection is then carried down to the level of the anterior fascia using electrocautery. The anterior rectus sheath is cleared off and grasped between two Kocher clamps and sharply incised vertically. The rectus abdominis muscle is exposed and retracted laterally so that the posterior sheath is visualized. Along this plane, the dissecting balloon is inserted until the tip reaches the pubic symphysis (Fig. 37.5). The balloon should be inflated under direct visualization until an adequate space is developed. The dissecting balloon is deflated and replaced with a blunt-tipped structural trocar. Two 5-mm trocars are placed in the midline after needle localization and under direct visualization.

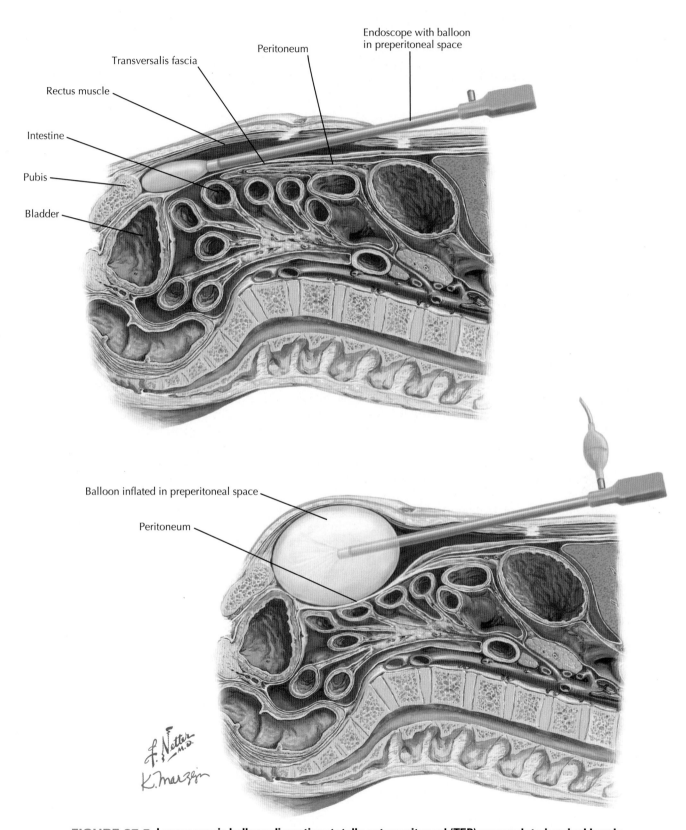

FIGURE 37.5 Laparoscopic balloon dissection: totally extraperitoneal (TEP) approach to inguinal hernia.

TOTALLY EXTRAPERITONEAL APPROACH (Continued)

Using laparoscopic Kittner dissectors, Cooper's ligament is exposed in a medial to lateral fashion. Moving out laterally to the inferior epigastric vessels, upward retraction is maintained on the abdominal wall with one hand while the other Kittner exposes the edge of the peritoneum. The peritoneum must be gently dissected from the transversalis fascia from the level of the ASIS medially to below the iliopubic tract. A window is gently created around the spermatic cord. Unlike the TAPP technique, the indirect space must always be more carefully inspected because a hernia here may not be readily apparent. Dissection between the vas and the vessels to reduce any adherent peritoneum that could act as a lead point for a future recurrence is traditionally done. At this point, the steps of the TAPP (as described earlier) are performed. If the peritoneal cavity is violated during dissection, insufflation of the abdomen may obscure the working space. Although not usually necessary, such a peritoneal defect may be closed with clips.

When the hernia sac or sacs have been reduced, the mesh is ready for implantation, as in a TAPP approach. The choice of whether to use tacks depends on surgeon preference. To secure the mesh by placing two tacks in the pectineal ligament, one in the superolateral corner of the mesh, two tacks on each side of the inferior epigastric on the superior edge of the mesh, and a last tack superiomedially is preferred. Once the mesh is positioned in a satisfactory manner, the insufflation is released as graspers hold the lower edge of the mesh in place. This maneuver verifies that the mesh remains below the peritoneum. All trocars are removed, and the anterior rectus fascia at the 10-mm port site is closed. The skin is closed, and the Foley catheter is removed.

In comparison of TAPP and TEP outcomes, there are similar rates of recurrence, seromas, nerve injuries, and chronic pain. Although rare, there are some complication differences related to each technique. TAPP is associated with more visceral injuries, whereas there are more vascular injuries associated with TEP. Ultimately, the approach to any inguinal hernia is dependent on the surgeon and the patient and may entail a TAPP, a TEP, or an open repair.

SUGGESTED READINGS

Cameron JL, Cameron AM. Current surgical therapy. 12th ed. Elsevier Inc.; 2018.

Köckerling F, Simons MP. Current concepts of inguinal hernia repair. Visc Med. 2018;34(2): 145–50.

Rosen MJ. Chapter 22—transabdominal preperitoneal inguinal hernia repair. 2nd ed. Elsevier Inc.; 2016.

Scott-Conner CEH. Essential operative techniques and anatomy, 4th ed. Philadelphia: Lippincott, Williams & Wilkins; 2014.

Wake BL, McCormack K, Fraser C, Vale L, Perez J, Grant A. "Transabdominal pre–peritoneal (TAPP) vs totally extraperitoneal (TEP) laparoscopic techniques for inguinal hernia repair. Cochrane Database Syst. Rev., no. 1, 2005.

Surgical Approach to Chronic Groin Pain Following Inguinal Hernia Repairs

David M. Krpata

INTRODUCTION

Chronic postoperative inguinal pain (CPIP) has become an increasingly appreciated complication of one of the most common operations performed in surgery, the inguinal hernia repair. The rate of CPIP after inguinal hernia repair is greater than the risk of developing an inguinal hernia recurrence. Chronic groin pain is defined as having pain that persists for more than 3 months after an inguinal hernia repair; 15% of patients undergoing an inguinal hernia repair have pain that affects their ability to concentrate on a daily basis 1 year after surgery; 1% to 3% have severe pain that requires medical or surgical intervention.

There are multiple risk factors for developing CPIP after an inguinal hernia repair, including a younger age, preoperative pain, prior groin surgery within the past 3 years, severe postoperative pain, postoperative complications, and female gender. To reduce the incidence and treat chronic groin pain, surgeons must have a thorough understanding of the inguinal neuroanatomy, as surgical technique also plays a role in CPIP.

INGUINAL NEUROANATOMY

All approaches to inguinal hernia repair have the potential for development of CPIP. This includes anterior approaches with mesh, primary tissue repairs, and minimally invasive totally extraperitoneal and transabdominal preperitoneal repairs. An anterior approach, or open inguinal hernia repair, is typically considered a greater risk of developing chronic groin pain because of the potential direct contact to the inguinal nerves. The three most important nerves are the iliohypogastric, ilioinguinal, and genitofemoral nerves (Fig. 38.1A). These nerves originate from the lumbar plexus with the iliohypogastric nerve from T12-L1, ilioinguinal nerve from L1, and the genitofemoral nerve from L2 (Fig. 38.1B).

Importantly for anterior repairs, the iliohypogastric and ilioinguinal nerves pierce through the transversus abdominis muscle in the lateral abdominal wall and run between the transversus abdominis muscle and internal oblique, eventually piercing through the internal oblique muscle. The iliohypogastric can most commonly be found 2 to 3 cm above the level of the internal ring, whereas the ilioinguinal will run more inferiorly and travel along the anterior portion of the spermatic cord in the inguinal canal for males and the round ligament for females. The genital branch of the genitofemoral nerve also has the potential for direct injury or contact during an anterior inguinal hernia repair. The genital branch of the genitofemoral nerves runs along the anterior surface of the psoas muscle and through the internal ring along the inferior portion of the spermatic cord adjacent to the spermatic vein in males.

A. Anterior view of the inguinal neuroanatomy

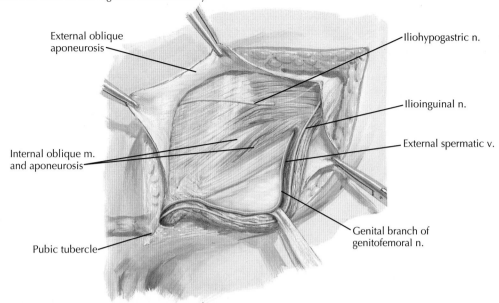

External oblique aponeurosis

Iliohypogastric n.

Ilioinguinal n.

External spermatic v.

Internal oblique m. and aponeurosis

Genital branch of genitofemoral n.

Pubic tubercle

B. Iliohypogastric, Ilioinguinal, Genitofemoral, and Obturator Nerves

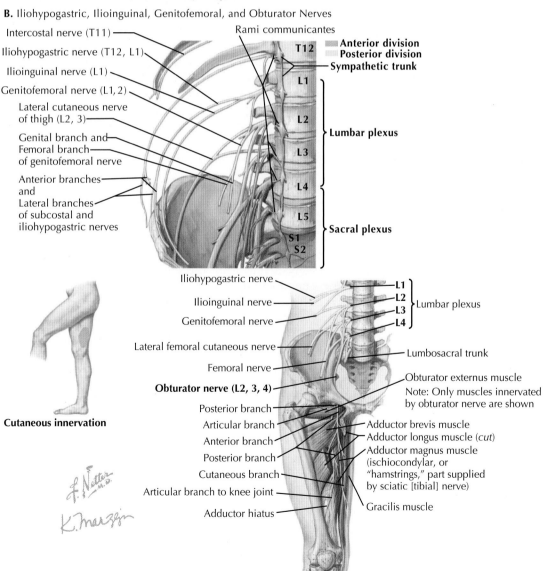

Intercostal nerve (T11)

Iliohypogastric nerve (T12, L1)

Ilioinguinal nerve (L1)

Genitofemoral nerve (L1, 2)

Lateral cutaneous nerve of thigh (L2, 3)

Genital branch and Femoral branch of genitofemoral nerve

Anterior branches and Lateral branches of subcostal and iliohypogastric nerves

Rami communicantes

T12

L1

L2

L3

L4

L5

S1

S2

Anterior division
Posterior division
Sympathetic trunk

Lumbar plexus

Sacral plexus

Iliohypogastric nerve

Ilioinguinal nerve

Genitofemoral nerve

Lateral femoral cutaneous nerve

Femoral nerve

Obturator nerve (L2, 3, 4)

Posterior branch

Articular branch

Anterior branch

Posterior branch

Cutaneous branch

Articular branch to knee joint

Adductor hiatus

L1
L2
L3
L4

Lumbar plexus

Lumbosacral trunk

Obturator externus muscle

Note: Only muscles innervated by obturator nerve are shown

Adductor brevis muscle

Adductor longus muscle (*cut*)

Adductor magnus muscle (ischiocondylar, or "hamstrings," part supplied by sciatic [tibial] nerve)

Gracilis muscle

Cutaneous innervation

FIGURE 38.1 Inguinal neuroanatomy.

SURGICAL INTERVENTIONS FOR CHRONIC POSTOPERATIVE INGUINAL PAIN

Patients with CPIP after inguinal hernia repair should be assessed in a stepwise approach that is beyond the scope of this chapter. Before considering surgery, patients should undergo examination, review of prior operative reports, and imaging. Nonsurgical interventions such as nerve blocks, nerve ablation, medical pain management, and physical therapy should also be considered. If all else fails and surgery is deemed the most appropriate next step, two main questions must be addressed. First, would the patient benefit from inguinal mesh removal, neurectomy, or both? Second, which approach is better, an open (anterior) approach or laparoscopically with a posterior approach? For mesh removal, prior anterior approaches are best addressed through an anterior approach, and prior laparoscopic mesh is best removed through a minimally invasive approach. One exception is for patients who have had a mesh plug without a patch. These plugs can be completely removed from a posterior approach while providing the surgeon the main benefit of direct visualization of the inferior epigastric vessels, which typically approximate the mesh (Fig. 38.2A).

When the need for a neurectomy is determined, it is useful to perform dermatomal mapping during the physical exam. Patients are mapped with a skin marker from the umbilicus to the mid-thigh marking every 3 to 4 cm for pain, numbness, or normal sensation. When patients have patterns of pain that fall within a specific dermatome (Fig. 38.2B) and neuropathic pain complaints, they should be considered for neurectomy. The iliohypogastric nerve provides cutaneous innervation to the abdominal wall skin from the anterior superior iliac spine to the pubis above the inguinal ligament. The ilioinguinal nerve provides cutaneous innervation to the upper and medial portion of the thigh as well as the base of the penis and part of the scrotum for men and mons pubis and labia majora for women. The genital branch of the genitofemoral nerve provides sensation to the scrotum in men and mons pubis and labia majora in women. The femoral branch of the genitofemoral nerve runs under the inguinal ligament and provides cutaneous innervation to the upper, anterior thigh (Fig. 38.3). It is important to map down the thigh for patients who have had a prior laparoscopic repair, because dermatomal mapping can also identify lateral femoral cutaneous nerve injury with pain down the lateral thigh (Fig. 38.4).

A. Posterior view of the inguinal anatomy

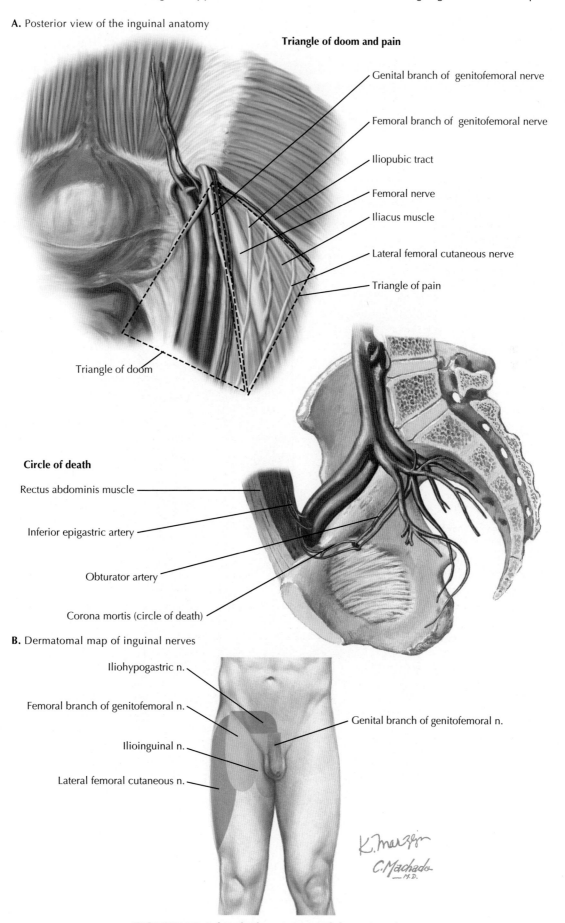

Triangle of doom and pain

Genital branch of genitofemoral nerve

Femoral branch of genitofemoral nerve

Iliopubic tract

Femoral nerve

Iliacus muscle

Lateral femoral cutaneous nerve

Triangle of pain

Triangle of doom

Circle of death

Rectus abdominis muscle

Inferior epigastric artery

Obturator artery

Corona mortis (circle of death)

B. Dermatomal map of inguinal nerves

Iliohypogastric n.

Femoral branch of genitofemoral n.

Ilioinguinal n.

Lateral femoral cutaneous n.

Genital branch of genitofemoral n.

FIGURE 38.2 Inguinal anatomy and dermatomal map.

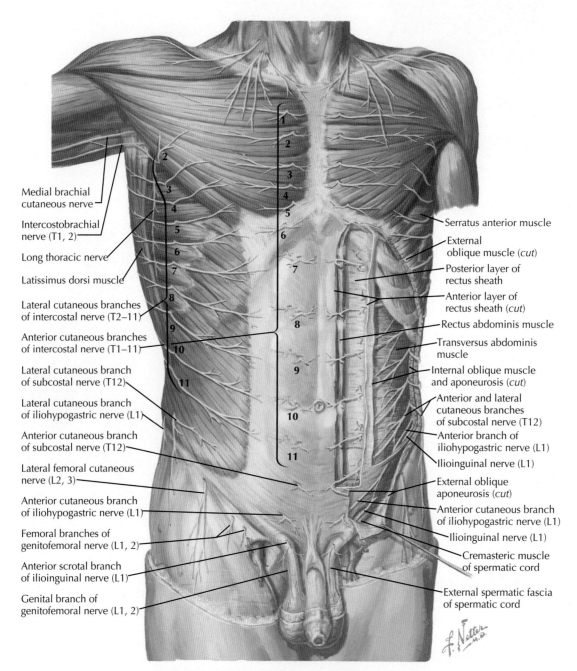

Medial brachial
cutaneous nerve

Intercostobrachial
nerve (T1, 2)

Long thoracic nerve

Latissimus dorsi muscle

Lateral cutaneous branches
of intercostal nerve (T2–11)

Anterior cutaneous branches
of intercostal nerve (T1–11)

Lateral cutaneous branch
of subcostal nerve (T12)

Lateral cutaneous branch
of iliohypogastric nerve (L1)

Anterior cutaneous branch
of subcostal nerve (T12)

Lateral femoral cutaneous
nerve (L2, 3)

Anterior cutaneous branch
of iliohypogastric nerve (L1)

Femoral branches of
genitofemoral nerve (L1, 2)

Anterior scrotal branch
of ilioinguinal nerve (L1)

Genital branch of
genitofemoral nerve (L1, 2)

Serratus anterior muscle

External
oblique muscle (*cut*)

Posterior layer of
rectus sheath

Anterior layer of
rectus sheath (*cut*)

Rectus abdominis muscle

Transversus abdominis
muscle

Internal oblique muscle
and aponeurosis (*cut*)

Anterior and lateral
cutaneous branches
of subcostal nerve (T12)

Anterior branch of
iliohypogastric nerve (L1)

Ilioinguinal nerve (L1)

External oblique
aponeurosis (*cut*)

Anterior cutaneous branch
of iliohypogastric nerve (L1)

Ilioinguinal nerve (L1)

Cremasteric muscle
of spermatic cord

External spermatic fascia
of spermatic cord

FIGURE 38.3 Innervation of the abdominal wall.

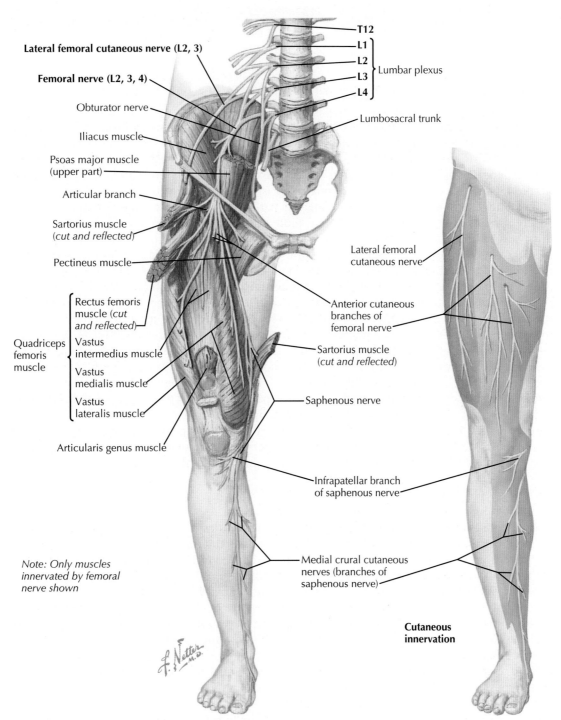

Lateral femoral cutaneous nerve (L2, 3)

Femoral nerve (L2, 3, 4)

Obturator nerve

Iliacus muscle

Psoas major muscle
(upper part)

Articular branch

Sartorius muscle
(*cut and reflected*)

Pectineus muscle

Rectus femoris
muscle (*cut
and reflected*)

Quadriceps
femoris
muscle

Vastus
intermedius muscle

Vastus
medialis muscle

Vastus
lateralis muscle

Articularis genus muscle

*Note: Only muscles
innervated by femoral
nerve shown*

T12

L1

L2

L3

L4

Lumbar plexus

Lumbosacral trunk

Lateral femoral
cutaneous nerve

Anterior cutaneous
branches of
femoral nerve

Sartorius muscle
(*cut and reflected*)

Saphenous nerve

Infrapatellar branch
of saphenous nerve

Medial crural cutaneous
nerves (branches of
saphenous nerve)

**Cutaneous
innervation**

FIGURE 38.4 Lateral femoral cutaneous nerve.

Open Inguinal Mesh Removal and Triple Neurectomy

Mesh removal presents particular challenges: previously placed mesh is encased in scar tissue and is in proximity to major structures such as the spermatic cord for anterior repairs or iliac vessels for posterior repairs. For open mesh removal, male patients should be aware of the potential to compromise the testicular blood supply. Open mesh removal should begin with a generous inguinal incision that typically extends medially and laterally to the initial hernia repair. The external oblique aponeurosis is opened toward the external inguinal ring and extended laterally along the tissue fibers as with a traditional open inguinal hernia repair. Before mesh removal, the ilioinguinal and iliohypogastric nerves are identified lateral to the prior surgical field, and the spermatic cord is encircled with a Penrose drain over the pubis medial to hernia mesh (Fig. 38.5A). With control of the spermatic cord, the mesh can be separated from the cord in an attempt to preserve all its contents. The lateral edge of the mesh is then freed form the underlying internal oblique muscle until the lateral edge of the internal ring is identified. The mesh is then divided from the lateral edge to the internal ring recreating the two lateral tails of a Lichtenstein repair. The superior edge of the mesh is then elevated off the conjoint tendon toward the pubis. The medial portion of the mesh is freed from the pubis, which should then leave mesh only attached to the shelving edge of the inguinal ligament. The superior flap of mesh is passed under the cord and the inferior edge of the mesh is freed form the shelving edge of the inguinal ligament (Fig. 38.5B). Any hernia that is present after mesh removal can be addressed with a primary tissue repair. A Bassini repair approximating the conjoint tendon to the shelving edge of the inguinal ligament can be used as long as there is no femoral defect. For patients with a femoral defect, a McVay or Cooper's ligament repair would be required. Mesh replacement is avoided whenever possible; however, in instances of significant abdominal wall defects resulting from mesh removal, a mesh repair may be necessary.

Laparoscopic Inguinal Mesh Removal

Removing inguinal hernia mesh that has been placed in the plane posterior to the abdominal musculature is more challenging than removing anterior mesh. The proximity to major vascular structures such as the iliac artery and vein as well as the inferior epigastric vessels, which originate from the iliac vessels, presents risks that are not typical with anterior mesh. Removal of this mesh should begin at the most superior edge of the mesh, completely freeing up the edge of the mesh. Dissection is carried out laterally using electrocautery to dissect the mesh of the abdominal wall. Dissecting lateral and inferior to the edge of the mesh allows for identification of the gonadal vessels in the retroperitoneum, as preservation is typically possible. The main goal during dissection of the mesh should be to obtain a medial plane toward the pubis and Cooper's ligament and freeing up of the mesh laterally so that the epigastric vessels are well defined as they travel to the iliac vessels (Fig. 38.6). Careful dissection of the epigastric vessels off the mesh is not always possible and either the vessels need to be ligated or a small amount of mesh is left behind to prevent injury to the iliac vessels. Any hernia that is present after mesh removal can be repaired through an open primary tissue repair, open mesh repair, or laparoscopically if a peritoneal flap has been preserved.

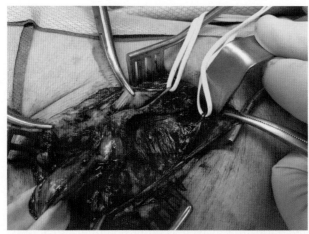

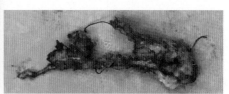

A. Open inguinal mesh removal (Penrose drain encircles the spermatic cord medially, ilioinguinal and iliohypogastric nerves identified laterally).

B. Excised inguinal mesh with the ilioinguinal nerve scarred to the edge laterally.

FIGURE 38.5 **Open inguinal mesh removal and triple neurectomy.**

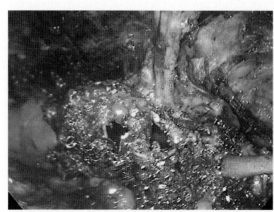

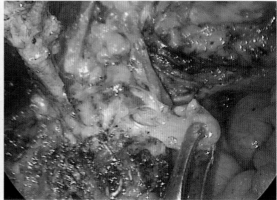

A. Laparoscopic inguinal mesh excision

B. Laparoscopic inguinal mesh excision

FIGURE 38.6 **Laparoscopic inguinal mesh removal.**

Laparoscopic Triple Neurectomy

Patients who are refractory to mesh removal or inguinal neurectomy may be candidates for retroperitoneal triple neurectomy. In a retroperitoneal triple neurectomy the iliohypogastric, ilioinguinal, and genitofemoral nerves are transected within the retroperitoneum, where there is no prior surgical scar, making it easier to identify the neuroanatomy (Fig. 38.7). The retroperitoneal triple neurectomy results in a much greater area of numbness than an inguinal neurectomy, and patients should be educated about this as well as other potential side effects, including hyperesthesia and possible bulging of the lower quadrant on the neurectomized side.

To perform this operation, patients are placed in the lateral decubitus position with the affected side up. The bed is flexed to separate the costal margin and the iliac crest to improve the working space (Fig. 38.8A). A 10-mm incision is made two fingerbreadths superior to the iliac crest in the midaxillary line with a 5-mm port placed medial and inferior to the 10-mm port. Dissection is carried through the external oblique muscle, internal oblique muscle, and transversus abdominis muscle until the retroperitoneum is entered. A balloon dissector is placed in the retroperitoneum and blown up under direct visualization. Once the balloon is removed and the retroperitoneum is insufflated, several key anatomic structures must be identified before any nerves are divided. Superiorly, the 12th rib is identified with the psoas muscle medially and the quadratus lumborum muscle lateral to the psoas muscle and inferior to the 12th rib. The iliohypogastric and ilioinguinal nerve can be identified as they come from beneath the psoas muscle and run on top of the quadratus lumborum muscle (Fig. 38.8B). Inferiorly, the psoas muscle is completely cleared to its medial boarder. This will help to identify the ureter, iliac artery, and gonadal vessels (Fig. 38.8C). The genitofemoral nerve can be identified on the superior aspect of the psoas muscle running down the muscle and splitting into the femoral branch, which runs under the inguinal ligament, and the genital branch, which will run into the internal ring (Fig. 38.8D). Once all anatomy has been defined, all three nerves are transected proximally and distally and a long segment is removed.

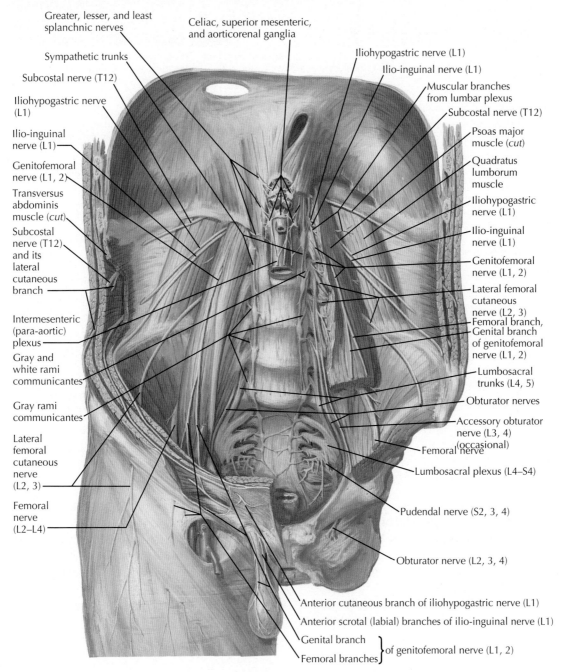

Greater, lesser, and least splanchnic nerves

Sympathetic trunks

Subcostal nerve (T12)

Iliohypogastric nerve (L1)

Ilio-inguinal nerve (L1)

Genitofemoral nerve (L1, 2)

Transversus abdominis muscle (*cut*)

Subcostal nerve (T12) and its lateral cutaneous branch

Intermesenteric (para-aortic) plexus

Gray and white rami communicantes

Gray rami communicantes

Lateral femoral cutaneous nerve (L2, 3)

Femoral nerve (L2–L4)

Celiac, superior mesenteric, and aorticorenal ganglia

Iliohypogastric nerve (L1)

Ilio-inguinal nerve (L1)

Muscular branches from lumbar plexus

Subcostal nerve (T12)

Psoas major muscle (*cut*)

Quadratus lumborum muscle

Iliohypogastric nerve (L1)

Ilio-inguinal nerve (L1)

Genitofemoral nerve (L1, 2)

Lateral femoral cutaneous nerve (L2, 3)

Femoral branch, Genital branch of genitofemoral nerve (L1, 2)

Lumbosacral trunks (L4, 5)

Obturator nerves

Accessory obturator nerve (L3, 4) (occasional)

Femoral nerve

Lumbosacral plexus (L4–S4)

Pudendal nerve (S2, 3, 4)

Obturator nerve (L2, 3, 4)

Anterior cutaneous branch of iliohypogastric nerve (L1)

Anterior scrotal (labial) branches of ilio-inguinal nerve (L1)

Genital branch
Femoral branches } of genitofemoral nerve (L1, 2)

FIGURE 38.7 Inguinal nerve anatomy in the retroperitoneum.

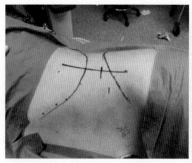

A. Positioning for a laparoscopic retroperitoneal triple neurectomy

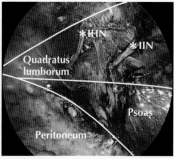

B. Laparoscopic retroperitoneal triple neurectomy- Iliohypogastric and ilioinguinal nerves

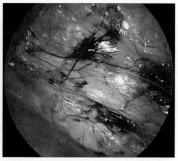

C. Laparoscopic retroperitoneal triple neurectomy-Identification of the iliac artery, ureter and gonadal vessels

D. Genitofemoral nerve with genital and femoral branches

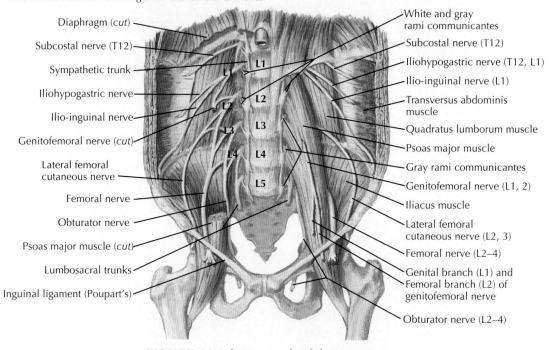

Diaphragm (*cut*)
Subcostal nerve (T12)
Sympathetic trunk
Iliohypogastric nerve
Ilio-inguinal nerve
Genitofemoral nerve (*cut*)
Lateral femoral cutaneous nerve
Femoral nerve
Obturator nerve
Psoas major muscle (*cut*)
Lumbosacral trunks
Inguinal ligament (Poupart's)

White and gray rami communicantes
Subcostal nerve (T12)
Iliohypogastric nerve (T12, L1)
Ilio-inguinal nerve (L1)
Transversus abdominis muscle
Quadratus lumborum muscle
Psoas major muscle
Gray rami communicantes
Genitofemoral nerve (L1, 2)
Iliacus muscle
Lateral femoral cutaneous nerve (L2, 3)
Femoral nerve (L2–4)
Genital branch (L1) and Femoral branch (L2) of genitofemoral nerve
Obturator nerve (L2–4)

FIGURE 38.8 Laparoscopic triple neurectomy.

SUGGESTED READINGS

Chen DC, Hiatt JR, Amik PK. Operative management of refractory neuropathic inguinodynia by a laparoscopic retroperitoneal approach. JAMA Surg 2013;148(10):962–7.

Hu QL, Chen DC. Approach to the patient with chronic groin pain. Surg Clin North Am 2018;98(3):651–65.

Lange JF, Kaufmann R, Wijsmuller AR, et al. An international consensus algorithm for management of chronic postoperative inguinal pain. Hernia 2015;19(1):33–43.

Open Flank and Lumbar Hernia Repair

Luciano Tastaldi and Ajita Prabhu

INTRODUCTION

Lumbar and flank hernias are caused by defects originating in the lateral abdominal wall. Such defects can be congenital or acquired as a consequence of surgery, trauma, or progressive weakening of native tissues. There are some specific challenges associated with these hernias that require surgeons who repair them to have a profound knowledge of the abdominal wall and anatomy. First, their anatomic location is bordered by bony prominences and neurovascular structures, thus calling for the identification of important anatomic landmarks to perform a safe and efficient dissection. Second, the close location to the costal margin and iliac crest limits mesh overlap, which is a key tenet for an adequate hernia repair. Similarly, proximity to bony structures and retroperitoneal vessels, nerves, and ureter poses a challenge to obtain adequate mesh fixation along all the edges of the mesh. Consequently, understanding the unique anatomic challenges imposed by a flank/lumbar hernia is necessary to provide the patient with a durable hernia repair.

ANATOMY AND CLASSIFICATION

Differentiation between lumbar and flank hernias and overlapping nomenclature and classifications is confusing and can be overwhelming for the surgeon. Nevertheless, the surgical management of lumbar and flank hernias does not differ significantly. A suggested nomenclature and classification was developed by the European Hernia Society and has been endorsed by hernia societies worldwide, standardizing reporting and facilitating the communication between surgeons. Lateral hernias are those occurring lateral to the rectus sheath and linea semilunaris and involving the posterolateral abdominal wall. They occur within the limits of the costal margin (cranially), inguinal ligament (caudally), the lateral border of the rectus sheath or the linea semilunaris (medially), and the lumbar region (laterally). These are further divided into four different zones, each with its own anatomic boundaries: subcostal (L1), occurring between the costal margin and an imaginary horizontal line 3 cm above the umbilicus; flank (L2), occurring lateral to the rectus sheath and within 3 cm above and below the umbilicus; iliac (L3), between an imaginary horizontal line 3 cm below the umbilicus and the inguinal region; and lumbar hernias (L4), those located posteriorly to the anterior axillary line (Fig. 39.1A).

Acquired hernias, particularly after surgery or trauma, tend to be larger and often extend into more than one of the aforementioned zones (Fig. 39.1B). Congenital hernias are the true lumbar hernias and are usually limited to the lumbar area (posteriorly to the anterior axillary line): 12th rib superiorly, erector spinae muscle laterally, the iliac crest inferiorly, and the external oblique muscle medially. The Petit hernia occurs within the inferior lumbar triangle, which is defined by the iliac crest inferiorly, the latissimus dorsi muscle posteriorly, and the external oblique muscle anteriorly. A Grynfeltt hernia occurs below the latissimus dorsi muscle, where the superior lumbar triangle is located. Anatomic limits are the 12th rib superiorly, the erector spinae muscle posteriorly, the internal oblique muscle inferiorly, and the external oblique muscle anteriorly (Fig. 39.1C). Fig. 39.1D illustrates a Petit hernia.

CLINICAL PRESENTATION

Bulging is the most common symptom associated with flank/lumbar hernias, which are also often accompanied by discomfort and pain. Symptomatic patients should benefit from elective repair if medically fit for surgery. The risk for bowel incarceration and strangulation in flank/lumbar hernias is disputed. Therefore, the repair of asymptomatic hernias remains debatable.

IMAGING

An abdominopelvic computed tomography (CT) scan is an important adjunct for the diagnosis and management of flank/lumbar hernias. It provides valuable information on the abdominal wall anatomy and condition of the musculature of the abdominal wall, hernia limits, and hernia sac contents. More importantly, it assists the surgeon in planning the approach, anticipated mesh overlap, and strategy for mesh fixation. For example, for a true flank hernia (as opposed to lumbar hernia), the surgeon may choose a midline approach for favorable defects in patients with a smaller body habitus, where a transversus abdominus release will allow plenty of lateral and posterior coverage. A midline approach to transversus abdominus release is outside of the scope of this chapter and is described elsewhere. In contrast, a true lumbar hernia or a very large flank hernia may necessitate a lateral approach through a flank incision, which is described in the following section.

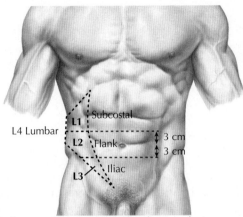

A. European Hernia Society classification of primary and incisional abdominal wall hernias

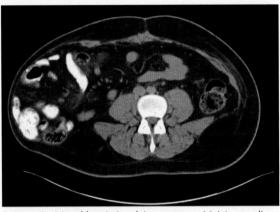

B. Large incisional hernia involving segments L1-L4 according to the classification suggested by the European Hernia Society.

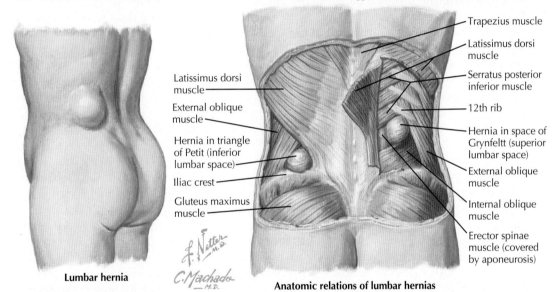

Lumbar hernia

Anatomic relations of lumbar hernias

C. Lumbar and obturator hernias

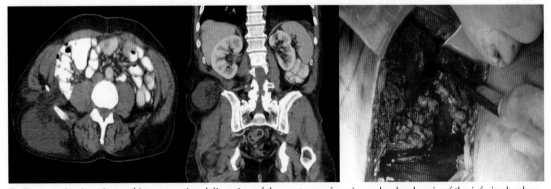

D. Preoperative imaging and intraoperative delineation of the anatomy of a primary lumbar hernia of the inferior lumbar triangle (Petit hernia).

FIGURE 39.1 Anatomy and classifications of flank and lumbar hernias.

SURGICAL ANATOMY AND OPERATIVE STEPS

For an open approach, a Foley catheter is placed routinely. The patient is positioned in a lateral decubitus position, and a bean bag is used to stabilize the torso. A double arm board may be used to support the arms, or alternatively a single arm board with a pillow placed between the arms may be used. The patient is secured to the surgical table, and all surfaces are appropriately padded. It is important to ensure that the umbilicus is lined up with the area where the table flexes to maximize the distance between the costal margin and the iliac spine, because this directly affects operative space. The table is then flexed to increase the distance between the costal margin and the iliac spine and therefore maximize exposure.

The costal margin, the iliac crest, and the palpable hernia are marked for reference. A transverse incision is performed two to three fingerbreadths above the iliac crest (Fig. 39.2A). Upon dividing the subcutaneous tissue, the surgeon can identify the external oblique muscle. The muscles of the lateral abdominal wall (external oblique, internal oblique, and transversus abdominis) are divided, exposing the underlying preperitoneal space (Fig. 39.2B).

A blunt dissection of the preperitoneal space is performed in all directions to create a large pocket to accommodate the mesh. The extent of this dissection will be dictated by the size of the defect and the amount of mesh overlap for the particular case. For larger hernias, a cranial dissection in the preperitoneal plane permits the peritoneum to be separated off the diaphragm, extending mesh overlap above the costal margin. Similarly, in a caudal direction, dissection can be extended into the pelvic preperitoneal space, exposing the ipsilateral Cooper's ligament. In some instances, especially in large hernias, mesh coverage up to the midline may be necessary to have sufficient mesh overlap. In such instances, the retrorectus space can be accessed by incising the posterior rectus sheath medially to the linea semilunaris. This has been called informally a "reverse TAR," or reverse transversus abdominus release, because it is performing a similar operation to the standard transversus abdominus release but from an opposite approach (lateral to medial as opposed to medial to lateral).

If performing this procedure, the surgeon identifies the linea semilunaris in the medial aspect of the field. The posterior rectus sheath is incised in a vertical orientation, and the rectus abdominus muscle is visible on the "ceiling" of the dissection. The surgeon must take care to avoid injury to the deep inferior epigastric vessels, which must be mobilized and preserved. Dissection can then be continued in the retrorectus space all the way to the midline, affording a wide ventral coverage to the midline.

Posteriorly, the psoas muscle is the main anatomic landmark during this dissection and should be identified below and above the hernia sac before any attempts to encircle and reduce the hernia sac are performed. Neurovascular structures are lying along the medial border of the psoas, and care should be taken to avoid injuries to the gonadal vessels, ureter, and innervation of the abdominal wall (Fig. 39.2C). The hernia sac is gently dissected off the fascia and bony structures and reduced. Any holes made in the peritoneum should be repaired with simple absorbable sutures. Upon reducing the hernia sac and completing dissection of the preperitoneal/retroperitoneal spaces, the peritoneal surface can be retracted medially, exposing the pocket that was created for mesh placement (Fig. 39.2D).

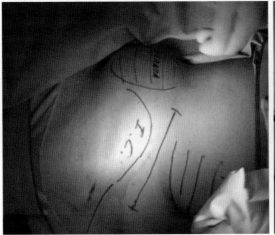

A. Surface anatomy with demarcation of the iliac crest, costal margin, hernia, and transverse incision location.

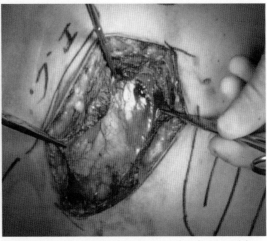

B. Exposure of the preperitoneal space after division of the skin, subcutaneous tissue and musculature of the lateral abdominal wall (external oblique, internal oblique, and transversus abdominis muscles).

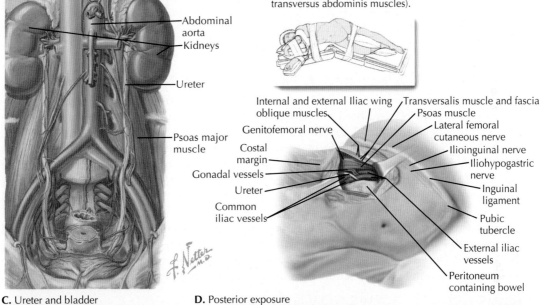

Abdominal aorta

Kidneys

Ureter

Psoas major muscle

Internal and external oblique muscles

Iliac wing

Transversalis muscle and fascia

Psoas muscle

Genitofemoral nerve

Lateral femoral cutaneous nerve

Costal margin

Ilioinguinal nerve

Gonadal vessels

Iliohypogastric nerve

Ureter

Inguinal ligament

Common iliac vessels

Pubic tubercle

External iliac vessels

Peritoneum containing bowel

C. Ureter and bladder

D. Posterior exposure

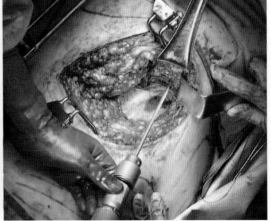

E. A piece of mesh is trimmed to size and inserted to cover the entire pocket, lying in the retroperitoneum over the lateral border of the psoas posteriorly, and gently folded to cover the preperitoneal space of the lateral abdominal wall, in the direction of the midline.

F. Mesh also should extend underneath the costal margin and below the iliac crest. The mesh is typically fixated over the lateral border of the psoas muscle with a limited number of simple stitches of a 2-0 absorbable suture. When necessary, the mesh is secured to the iliac bone using bone anchors with permanent sutures.

FIGURE 39.2 Surgical anatomy and operative steps.

(D, Reused with permission from LaPinska MP, Rosen MJ. Open flank hernia repair. In Rosen MJ, ed. Atlas of Abdominal Wall Reconstruction, 2nd ed. Philadelphia: Elsevier; 2016:110-123, Fig. 6-4.)

SURGICAL ANATOMY AND OPERATIVE STEPS (Continued)

A piece of mesh is trimmed to size and inserted to cover the entire pocket, lying in the retroperitoneum over the lateral border of the psoas posteriorly, and gently folded to cover the preperitoneal space of the lateral abdominal wall, in the direction of the midline (Fig. 39.2E). Mesh also should extend underneath the costal margin and below the iliac crest. The mesh is typically fixated over the lateral border of the psoas muscle with a limited number of simple stitches of a 2-0 absorbable suture. When necessary, the mesh is secured to the iliac bone using bone anchors with permanent sutures (Fig. 39.2F). Similarly, the mesh is fixated to the costal margin with slowly absorbable monofilament sutures. The most medial edges of the mesh that extend into the lateral abdominal wall are fixated using full-thickness transfascial sutures of slowly absorbable monofilament material, with the aid of a suture passer. Upon completion of mesh fixation, a closed suction drain is placed above the mesh and underneath the musculature of the lateral abdominal wall. Subcutaneous tissue and skin are closed in layers.

SUGGESTED READINGS

Beffa LR, Margiotta AL, Carbonell AM. Flank and lumbar hernia repair. Surg Clin North Am 2018;98(3):593–605. https://doi.org/10.1016/j.suc.2018.01.009.

Campanelli G, Bruni PG, Morlacchi A, Lombardo F, Cavalli M. Flank hernia. In: Campanelli G, editor. The Art of Hernia Surgery. Springer; 2018. p. 527–32. https://doi.org/10.1007/978-3-319-72626-7_53.

La Pinska MP, Rosen MJ. Open flank hernia repair. In: Rosen MJ, editor. Atlas of Abdominal Wall Reconstruction. 2nd ed. Elsevier; 2017. p. 110–23.

Muysoms FE, Miserez M, Berrevoet F, et al. Classification of primary and incisional abdominal wall hernias. Hernia 2009;13:407–14.

Open Retromuscular Hernia Repair

Clayton C. Petro

 VIDEO

40.1 Open Transversus Abdominis Release (TAR)

INTRODUCTION

Approximately 300,000 to 400,000 ventral hernias are fixed yearly in the United States, encompassing primary defects as well as the 20% to 25% of incisional hernias that occur after midline laparotomy and 24% to 43% of recurrences even after mesh repair. Even for the smallest primary defects, long-term follow-up of randomized controlled data has found that mesh reinforcement demonstrates superiority to suture repair. Still, the frequency of hernias only seems to be increasing despite the ubiquity of this disease and high-level evidence supporting the use of mesh.

There are three considerations relevant to decision making for management of hernias:
- *The patient:* including demographics, medical comorbidities (e.g., smoking status, body mass index, diabetes control) and impact of the hernia on the patient's quality of life
- *The hernia:* including width, length, location (midline vs. proximity to bony prominences), level of contamination, and context of presentation (elective vs. emergent)
- *The repair:* variables include choice of mesh (synthetic vs. biologic vs. biosynthetic), location of mesh relative to the abdominal wall, technique (open vs. laparoscopic vs. robotic), and use of adjuncts such as component separation techniques or skin flaps

These considerations are all intimately related, making comparisons of techniques or the identification of high-risk patient/hernia characteristics challenging. Although a detailed discussion of each component is beyond the scope of this chapter, one should always have a skeptical approach to the review of hernia literature, as claims of superiority regarding a type of mesh or technique may not have controlled for the other variables relevant to the outcome of interest.

Despite the growing complexity of this field and seemingly innumerable permutations of treatment options, open retromuscular hernia repair (ORHR) has recently gained tremendous popularity, decades after its initial depiction. French surgeon Jean Rives first described retrorectus mesh reinforcement for large ventral eventrations in 1973, but it was not until 1989 that his colleague Rene Stoppa published the technique in English. Although laparoscopic ventral hernia repair was popularized in the 1990s, several modifications to the Rives-Stoppa retrorectus dissection were described from 2006 to 2012, culminating in the description of the transversus abdominis release (TAR). These modifications extended the benefits of the Rives-Stoppa repair to even larger hernias, and as such the TAR has enjoyed wide dissemination among surgeons in the past decade. Here we review the benefits of all open retromuscular repair techniques and the steps to these operations that are guided by a comprehensive understanding of abdominal wall anatomy.

SURGICAL PRINCIPLES

Retromuscular mesh placement with concomitant reconstruction of the linea alba offers several key advantages over other techniques:

- Retromuscular mesh placement (Fig. 40.1A) allows for mesh reinforcement of the hernia defect without exposure of the prosthetic to the viscera as in an underlay (i.e., intraperitoneal onlay mesh [IPOM] placement).
- Because the prosthetic is not exposed to the viscera in the retromuscular space, uncoated meshes are used, which are more resilient to infection and substantially less expensive than coated or barrier meshes.
- Mesh in the retromuscular space also has direct face-to-face apposition of posterior fascia and muscle anteriorly to allow for prosthetic ingrowth and separates the mesh from superficial wound morbidity. Alternatively, mesh placed in the "onlay" position—above fascia—is subjected to potentially devascularized subcutaneous tissue when flaps are raised to accommodate the reinforcement material.
- In contrast to open and laparoscopic bridged repairs, ORHR also allows for re-creation of the linea alba, which has been shown to provide benefits in regard to core abdominal strength—both by returning the rectus muscles to the midline and by re-establishing a firm re-insertion point for the lateral oblique muscles.

RETROMUSCULAR REPAIRS AND ADJUNCTS

The Rives-Stoppa retrorectus dissection allows for all the aforementioned benefits with mesh placement in the retrorectus space (Fig. 40.1B and C).

A. Consensus on mesh position

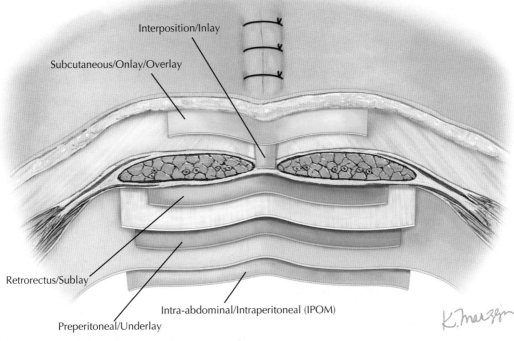

Interposition/Inlay

Subcutaneous/Onlay/Overlay

Retrorectus/Sublay

Intra-abdominal/Intraperitoneal (IPOM)

Preperitoneal/Underlay

B. Rives-Stoppa cephalad to the arcuate line

Aponeurosis of
external oblique muscle

Aponeurosis of
internal oblique muscle

Aponeurosis of transversus
abdominis muscle

Anterior layer of rectus sheath

Rectus abdominis muscle

Linea alba

External
oblique muscle

Internal
oblique muscle

Transversus
abdominis muscle

Peritoneum

Posterior layer
of rectus sheath

Transversalis fascia

C. Rives-Stoppa caudad to the arcuate line

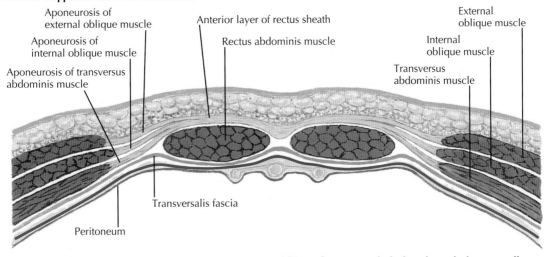

Aponeurosis of
external oblique muscle

Aponeurosis of
internal oblique muscle

Aponeurosis of transversus
abdominis muscle

Anterior layer of rectus sheath

Rectus abdominis muscle

External
oblique muscle

Internal
oblique muscle

Transversus
abdominis muscle

Transversalis fascia

Peritoneum

FIGURE 40.1 Retromuscular mesh placement and Rives-Stoppa cephalad and caudad arcuate lines.

Rives-Stoppa Retrorectus Dissection

- The dissection is achieved by incising the posterior rectus sheath just lateral to its insertion point on the linea alba. Visualization of the rectus muscle confirms the retrorectus space is entered.
- Below the arcuate line, the posterior rectus sheath is contiguous with peritoneum and transversalis fascia, which encase the rectus muscle. Again, these layers are dissected away from the rectus muscle (Fig. 40.2A).
- Separation of the posterior rectus sheath (above the arcuate line) and peritoneum/transversalis fascia (below the arcuate line) allows for a retrorectus dissection lateral as far as the linea semilunaris (Fig. 40.2B).
- The inferior and superior epigastric vessels are visible at the most cephalad and caudad portions of the dissection before coursing within the rectus abdominis muscle.
- Laterally perforating neurovascular bundles traveling between the internal oblique and transversus abdominis muscle pierce the posterior lamella of the internal oblique to enter the retrorectus space just medial to the linea semilunaris. These are visualized as the retrorectus dissection approaches the linea semilunaris and should be salvaged to preserve innervation of the rectus abdominis muscle.
- The medial course of the intercostal nerves just anterior to the transversus abdominis can be observed in Fig. 40.2C through F. Similarly, intercostal vessels and tributaries of the deep circumflex arteries follow an analogous course medially toward the rectus muscles.

The most notable limitation to the Rives-Stoppa retrorectus dissection is that the lateral dissection ends at the linea semilunaris creating challenges for larger defects. First, the posterior sheath closure can be under considerable tension. Second, the lateral mesh overlap is limited by the width of each rectus muscle. Third, there is no release of a lateral oblique muscle to aid in the closure of the anterior fascia. Several modifications were subsequently described to address these limitations.

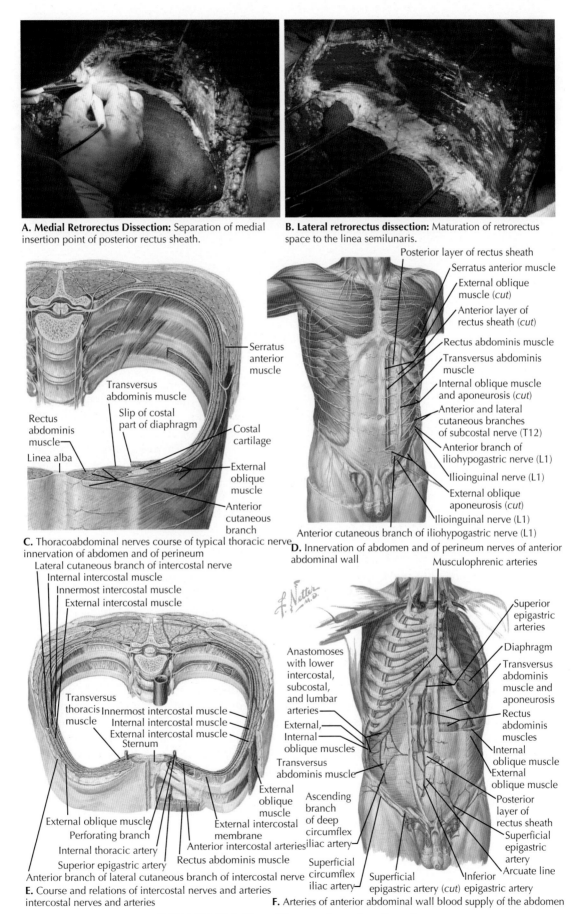

A. Medial Retrorectus Dissection: Separation of medial insertion point of posterior rectus sheath.

B. Lateral retrorectus dissection: Maturation of retrorectus space to the linea semilunaris.

Serratus anterior muscle

Transversus abdominis muscle

Rectus abdominis muscle

Linea alba

Slip of costal part of diaphragm

Costal cartilage

External oblique muscle

Anterior cutaneous branch

C. Thoracoabdominal nerves course of typical thoracic nerve innervation of abdomen and of perineum

Posterior layer of rectus sheath

Serratus anterior muscle

External oblique muscle (*cut*)

Anterior layer of rectus sheath (*cut*)

Rectus abdominis muscle

Transversus abdominis muscle

Internal oblique muscle and aponeurosis (*cut*)

Anterior and lateral cutaneous branches of subcostal nerve (T12)

Anterior branch of iliohypogastric nerve (L1)

Ilioinguinal nerve (L1)

External oblique aponeurosis (*cut*)

Ilioinguinal nerve (L1)

Anterior cutaneous branch of iliohypogastric nerve (L1)

D. Innervation of abdomen and of perineum nerves of anterior abdominal wall

Lateral cutaneous branch of intercostal nerve
Internal intercostal muscle
Innermost intercostal muscle
External intercostal muscle

Transversus thoracis muscle
Innermost intercostal muscle
Internal intercostal muscle
External intercostal muscle
Sternum

External oblique muscle
Perforating branch
Internal thoracic artery
Superior epigastric artery
Anterior branch of lateral cutaneous branch of intercostal nerve

External oblique muscle
External intercostal membrane
Anterior intercostal arteries
Rectus abdominis muscle

E. Course and relations of intercostal nerves and arteries intercostal nerves and arteries

Musculophrenic arteries

Superior epigastric arteries

Diaphragm

Transversus abdominis muscle and aponeurosis

Rectus abdominis muscles

Internal oblique muscle

External oblique muscle

Posterior layer of rectus sheath

Superficial epigastric artery

Arcuate line

Inferior epigastric artery

Anastomoses with lower intercostal, subcostal, and lumbar arteries

External, Internal oblique muscles

Transversus abdominis muscle

Ascending branch of deep circumflex iliac artery

Superficial circumflex iliac artery

Superficial epigastric artery (*cut*)

F. Arteries of anterior abdominal wall blood supply of the abdomen

FIGURE 40.2 Rives-Stoppa retrorectus dissection.

Preperitoneal Approach

Described by Novitsky et al in 2006, the preperitoneal dissection addresses the limitation of the aforementioned lateral dissection.

- Once the lateral extent of the retrorectus dissection is achieved, the lateral posterior rectus sheath is divided to re-enter the preperitoneal plane, which can be continued laterally toward the retroperitoneum.
- Alternatively, the preperitoneal plane can be developed from the midline, working medial to lateral without entering the posterior rectus space, although this can be challenging as the peritoneum and posterior rectus sheath are commonly fused in the mid-abdomen, particularly in cases who have had prior abdominal surgery (Fig. 40.3A and B).

The preperitoneal approach creates a large retromuscular pocket for wide mesh overlap, and separation of the peritoneum from the anterior muscles allows for significant advancement of the posterior rectus sheaths. A major limitation is that staying in the preperitoneal plane without tearing the thin peritoneum—particularly as it fuses with the posterior rectus sheath—can be technically challenging to reproduce. Finally, the technique does not divide any lateral oblique to aid with anterior fascial advancement.

Intramuscular Dissection

Described by Carbonell in 2008, the intramuscular dissection is an alternative way to address the lateral limitation of the linea semilunaris above the arcuate line.

- After maturing the retrorectus space to the linea semilunaris, the posterior lamella of the internal oblique can be divided to enter the space between the internal oblique and transversus abdominis muscles.
- Lateral development of this plane creates a large pocket for mesh placement between these muscles (Fig. 40.3C and D).

A major limitation of this approach is that it requires division of all the laterally perforating neurovascular bundles that supply the rectus abdominis muscle, although admittedly, the clinical significance of this is unknown. Although dividing the posterior lamella of the internal oblique separates the anterior muscle bellies—internal and external obliques—from the posterior transversus abdominis (i.e., a "posterior component separation"), this likely provides little myofascial advancement of the anterior segments. Likewise, the posterior rectus sheath is not liberated from the transversus abdominis muscle and therefore does not benefit from additional medialization.

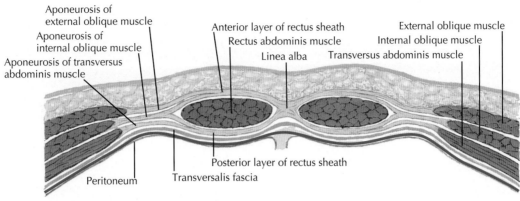

A. Pure preperitoneal - Cephalad to the arcuate line

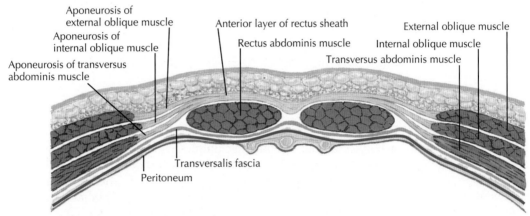

B. Pure preperitoneal - Caudad to the arcuate line

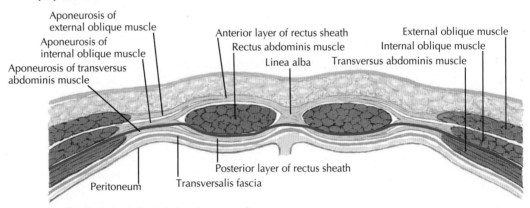

C. Intramuscular dissection - Cephalad to the arcuate line

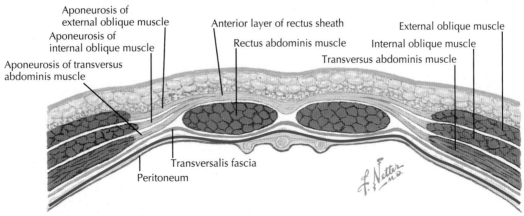

D. Intramuscular dissection - Caudad to the arcuate line

FIGURE 40.3 Preperitoneal and intramuscular dissections.

Transversus Abdominis Release

The TAR borrows from each of the aforementioned techniques. The described advantages have led to its growing popularity and as such will be described in greater detail.

- At the lateral extent of the retrorectus dissection, the posterior rectus sheath—consisting of fibers of the posterior lamella of the internal oblique—are divided just medial to the lateral perforating neurovascular bundles to preserve them (Fig. 40.4A through C).
- Above the arcuate line, this exposes the transversus abdominis muscle. In the upper one-third of the abdomen, the transversus abdominis muscle belly is exposed (Fig. 40.4D), and in the middle one-third of the abdomen, the aponeurosis of the transversus abdominis is exposed.
- It is then possible to divide the transversus abdominis muscle or associated aponeurosis while preserving the underlying peritoneum (Fig. 40.4E).
- Next, the preperitoneal plane can be matured laterally to the retroperitoneum as far back as the psoas muscle (Fig. 40.4F through H).
- Below the arcuate line, care should be taken to preserve the inferior epigastric vessels. Often, transversalis fascia must be divided to separate the peritoneum from these vessels.
- Lateral to the inferior epigastric vessels, the spermatic cord structures or round ligament can be dissected free from the peritoneum as the preperitoneal plane is matured toward the psoas.

The ability of this lateral dissection to create a wide space for mesh placement, allow for significant advancement of the posterior rectus sheath, and release the transversus abdominis muscle for anterior fascial advancement all without sacrificing lateral neurovascular bundles is what makes this technique appear to be the ideal adjunct to the Rives-Stoppa dissection.

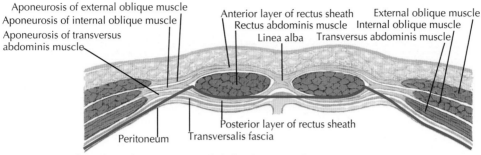

Aponeurosis of external oblique muscle
Aponeurosis of internal oblique muscle
Aponeurosis of transversus abdominis muscle
Anterior layer of rectus sheath
Rectus abdominis muscle
Linea alba
External oblique muscle
Internal oblique muscle
Transversus abdominis muscle
Posterior layer of rectus sheath
Transversalis fascia
Peritoneum

A. Transversus Abdominis Release (TAR) - Cephalad to the arcuate line

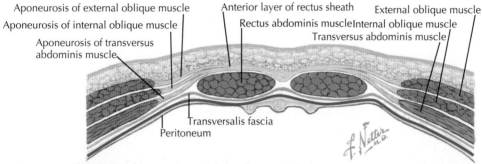

Aponeurosis of external oblique muscle
Aponeurosis of internal oblique muscle
Aponeurosis of transversus abdominis muscle
Anterior layer of rectus sheath
Rectus abdominis muscle
External oblique muscle
Internal oblique muscle
Transversus abdominis muscle
Transversalis fascia
Peritoneum

B. Transversus Abdominis Release (TAR) - Caudad to the arcuate line

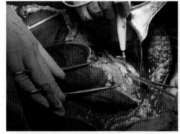

C. Inferior Tar Dissection. Division of the posterior lamina of the internal oblique and underlying aponeurosis of the transversus abdominis muscle

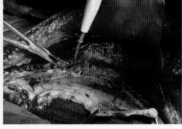

D. Superior TAR Dissection. Superiorly, division of the posterior lamellae of the internal oblique exposes the muscle of the transversus abdominis muscle which is divided.

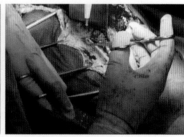

E. Middle TAR Dissection. The inferior 2/3 of the TAR dissection is of the aponeurotic portion of the transversus abdominis muscle.

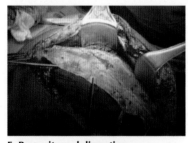

F. Preperitoneal dissection

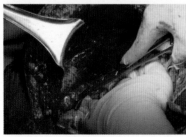

G. Exposure of the psoas muscle. Note that some of the retroperitoneal fat is pushed laterally to expose the psoas during this preperitoneal dissection.

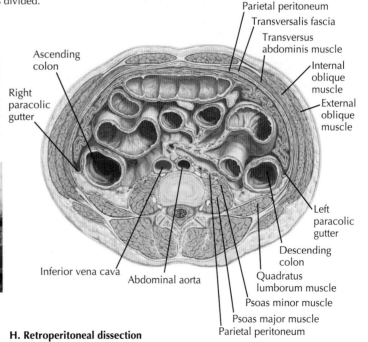

Ascending colon
Right paracolic gutter
Parietal peritoneum
Transversalis fascia
Transversus abdominis muscle
Internal oblique muscle
External oblique muscle
Left paracolic gutter
Descending colon
Quadratus lumborum muscle
Psoas minor muscle
Psoas major muscle
Parietal peritoneum
Inferior vena cava
Abdominal aorta

H. Retroperitoneal dissection

FIGURE 40.4 Transversus abdominis release (TAR).

Exposure of Cooper's Ligament and Space of Retzius

- Medial to the epigastric vessels, the retrorectus space is matured to expose Cooper's ligament on either side of the pubis. If this space has not been previously violated, the preperitoneal plane can be bluntly matured to expose the space of Retzius inferior to the pubis (Fig. 40.5A).
- In a reoperative pelvis, care should be taken during this medial preperitoneal dissection so as not to injure the bladder. Rather than blunt dissection, this should be done sharply and under direct visualization.

Exposure of the Subxiphoid Space and Central Tendon of the Diaphragm

- Cephalad, the medial insertion of the posterior rectus sheath is divided as it approaches the xiphoid process. This makes the preperitoneal subxiphoid fat plane contiguous with the retrorectus space.
- At its apex, the posterior rectus sheath is ultimately transected from lateral to medial at the costal margin. Cephalad to the costal margin the lateral and medial preperitoneal planes are married and subsequently matured to the central tendon of the diaphragm (Fig. 40.5B).

Once the lateral, superior, and inferior dissections are complete, the posterior rectus sheaths can be closed along the midline, generally using a 2-0 absorbable suture. All holes in the posterior sheath and contiguous peritoneal layer, which may have occurred from scarring from prior surgery, should be closed to completely isolate the underlying viscera (Fig. 40.5C). If needed, holes can be patched with underlying omentum or if absolutely necessary a piece of Vicryl mesh can be used as a bridge.

Mesh Placement

- The mesh is placed in the retromuscular pocket with wide overlap of the fascial repair (Fig. 40.5D).
- Although there are no data to support transfascial suture fixation of mesh, this is preferred to keep the mesh flat and off-load the midline fascial closure. A superior, inferior, and three lateral transfascial fixation sutures are used on each side.
- Bilateral suction drains are placed on the mesh in the retromuscular space.

Reconstruction of the Linea Alba

- The fascia is apposed in the midline, using a number 1 slowly absorbable suture either in a running fashion or with interrupted figure-of-8 sutures if there is much tension on the closure.

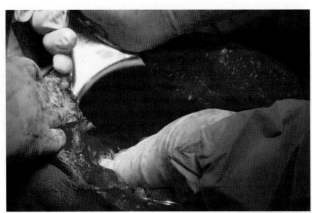

A. Development of the space of Retzius. Cooper's ligament exposed bilaterally

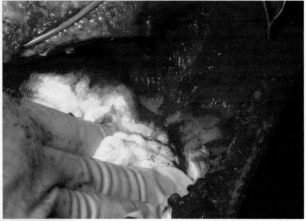

B. Retroxyphoid dissection. Central tendon of the diaphragm exposed

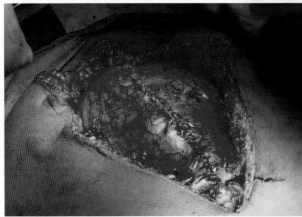

C. Posterior rectus sheath closed

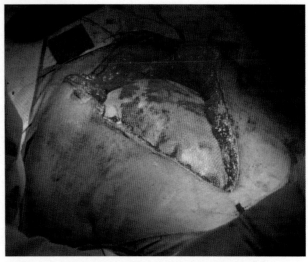

D. Mesh placed in retromuscular space

FIGURE 40.5 Exposure of Cooper's ligament, subxiphoid space, and mesh placement.

SUGGESTED READINGS

Blatnik JA, et al. In vivo analysis of the morphologic characteristics of synthetic mesh to resist MRSA adherence. J Gastrointest Surg 2012;16(11):2139–44.

Burger JW, et al. Long-term follow-up of a randomized controlled trial of suture versus mesh repair of incisional hernia. Ann Surg 2004;240(4):578–83; discussion 583–5.

Carbonell AM, Cobb WS, Chen SM. Posterior components separation during retromuscular hernia repair. Hernia 2008;12(4):359–62.

Criss CN, et al. Functional abdominal wall reconstruction improves core physiology and quality-of-life. Surgery 2014;156(1):176–82.

Haskins IN, et al. Effect of transversus abdominis release on core stability: short-term results from a single institution. Surgery 2019;165(2):412–6.

Kaufmann R, et al. Mesh versus suture repair of umbilical hernia in adults: a randomised, double-blind, controlled, multicentre trial. Lancet 2018;391(10123):860–9.

Luijendijk RW, et al. A comparison of suture repair with mesh repair for incisional hernia. N Engl J Med 2000;343(6):392–8.

Muysoms F, Jacob B. International hernia collaboration consensus on nomenclature of abdominal wall hernia repair. World J Surg 2018;42(1):302–4.

Muysoms F, et al. EuraHS: the development of an international online platform for registration and outcome measurement of ventral abdominal wall hernia repair. Hernia 2012;16(3):239–50.

Novitsky YW, et al. Open preperitoneal retrofascial mesh repair for multiply recurrent ventral incisional hernias. J Am Coll Surg 2006;203(3):283–9.

Novitsky YW, et al. Transversus abdominis muscle release: a novel approach to posterior component separation during complex abdominal wall reconstruction. Am J Surg 2012;204(5):709–16.

Poulose BK, et al. Epidemiology and cost of ventral hernia repair: making the case for hernia research. Hernia 2012;16(2):179–83.

Stoppa RE. The treatment of complicated groin and incisional hernias. World J Surg 1989;13(5):545–54.

Vascular

Carotid Endarterectomy

David M. Hardy and Will Perry

INTRODUCTION

Carotid endarterectomy (CEA) is one of the most commonly performed vascular operations, with the majority of these procedures being performed for carotid bifurcation atherosclerotic disease (Fig. 41.1A). Two landmark multicenter randomized trials, North American Symptomatic Carotid Endarterectomy Trial (NASCET) and the European Carotid Surgery Trial, have demonstrated the reduction of stroke risk with CEA in patients with ipsilateral symptomatic carotid stenosis. Reduction of stroke risk for asymptomatic disease has also been demonstrated for moderate to severe stenosis in three randomized clinical trials.

There are many potential complications from CEA, which include stroke, cranial nerve injury, hematoma, and restenosis. For all patient subgroups, the perioperative stroke risk for CEA ranges from 1% to 4%. Persistent cranial nerve injury at the time of discharge is around 4%, with the majority of these deficits resolving on subsequent follow-ups. The execution of a technically sound operation is paramount in reducing these pitfalls.

SURGICAL EXPOSURE

Patient positioning and incision: The patient is placed in the supine position with the affected side at the edge of the table to facilitate surgeon access. To provide adequate exposure, the neck is extended and the head turned to the opposite side and placed upon a gel ring. A shoulder roll can be placed to provide elevation of the shoulders, enhancing further neck extension. Depending on surgeon preference, the table may be placed in a neutral, slight reverse Trendelenburg or beach-chair position. The upper chest, neck, lower face along the mandible, and lower ear are prepped and draped into the field. The key anatomic boundaries are the sternocleidomastoid muscle (SCM), the midline, and the mandible (Fig. 41.1B). Incision is made along the anterior border of the SCM, extending from clavicular head to the retromandibular area, curving the distal portion of the incision so that it extends inferior to the lobe of the ear (see Fig. 41.1B). Curving the distal aspect of the incision in a posterior fashion one fingerbreadth below the angle of the mandible avoids injury to the marginal mandibular branch of the facial nerve. Paralleling the incision to the SCM will allow exposure of the cervical course of the carotid artery. The bifurcation can also be marked and mapped before incision with use of a duplex ultrasound. Marking the bifurcation with ultrasound before incision may limit the size of the incision.

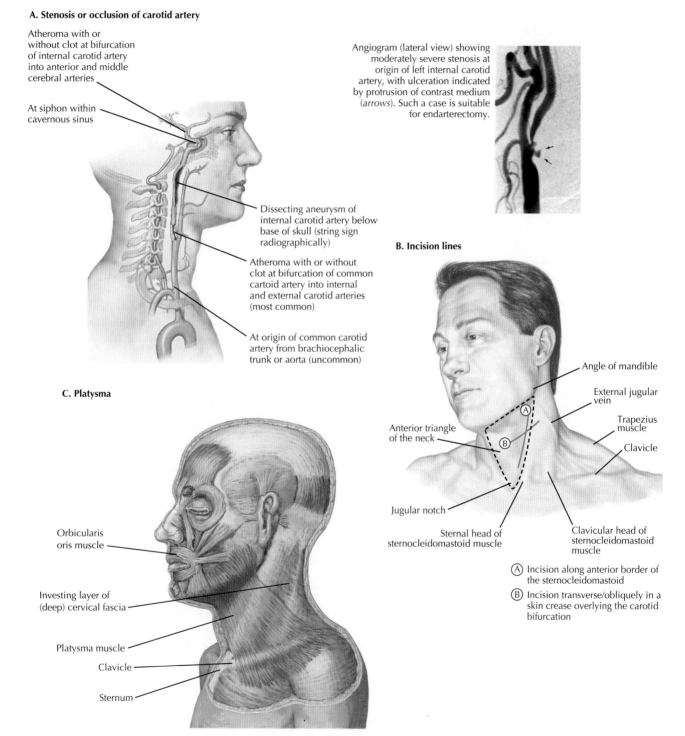

A. Stenosis or occlusion of carotid artery

Atheroma with or without clot at bifurcation of internal carotid artery into anterior and middle cerebral arteries

At siphon within cavernous sinus

Angiogram (lateral view) showing moderately severe stenosis at origin of left internal carotid artery, with ulceration indicated by protrusion of contrast medium (*arrows*). Such a case is suitable for endarterectomy.

Dissecting aneurysm of internal carotid artery below base of skull (string sign radiographically)

Atheroma with or without clot at bifurcation of common cartoid artery into internal and external carotid arteries (most common)

At origin of common carotid artery from brachiocephalic trunk or aorta (uncommon)

B. Incision lines

Angle of mandible

External jugular vein

Trapezius muscle

Clavicle

Anterior triangle of the neck

Jugular notch

Sternal head of sternocleidomastoid muscle

Clavicular head of sternocleidomastoid muscle

Ⓐ Incision along anterior border of the sternocleidomastoid

Ⓑ Incision transverse/obliquely in a skin crease overlying the carotid bifurcation

C. Platysma

Orbicularis oris muscle

Investing layer of (deep) cervical fascia

Platysma muscle

Clavicle

Sternum

FIGURE 41.1 Carotid stenosis, incision lines for endarterectomy, and platysma.

CAROTID BIFURCATION EXPOSURE

The incision is carried through the platysma muscle (Fig. 41.1C), and the investing layer of the deep cervical fascia is opened on the anterior border of the SCM. The SCM is mobilized along the medial border and separated from the underlying vascular sheath with sharp dissection. There should be minimal bleeding if you are in the correct plane at this step of the procedure. Small branches and perforating vessels can be ligated to allow for further mobilization of the SCM. The SCM is retracted posterolaterally, identifying the carotid sheath. The sheath is opened superior to the omohyoid muscle, which can be divided if more proximal exposure is necessary (Fig. 41.2). The internal jugular vein, which lies lateral and anterior to the common carotid artery (CCA), is dissected along the medial border and retracted in similar fashion with the SCM. This retraction and maneuver require ligation and division of the common facial vein, an important landmark that typically overlays the carotid bifurcation. Mobilization and retraction of the internal jugular vein exposes the CCA as well as the vagus nerve, which usually lies posterior to the artery but may occasionally be anterior.

Dissection of the CCA and its branches is performed next with delicate and exact movements. The vagus nerve should be identified and protected. The Ansa cervicalis nerve often runs along the anterior surface of the CCA and can be divided without any clinical consequence (see Fig. 41.2). The patient is heparinized once the CCA is exposed but before manipulating and placing silastic vessel (or umbilical tape) loops around the CCA. 80 to 100 units/kg intravenous heparin are given and activated clotting time (ACT) is checked; it should be 1.5 to 2 times the preoperative value. The initial ACT is checked at 3 to 5 minutes after initial heparin administration and repeated every 30 minutes to ensure adequate anticoagulation. Isolation and dissection of the CCA and its distal branches should be performed before the carotid bifurcation. A "no-touch" technique should be implemented during arterial mobilization, especially along the carotid bulb and bifurcation, to prevent dislodgement of plaque or thrombus. The CCA is isolated first using sharp dissection, freeing the surrounding tissue from the artery as far proximally as the omohyoid muscle, after which can be encircled with an elastic vessel loop. The external carotid artery (ECA) is dissected next, which is typically located anterior and lateral to the internal carotid artery (ICA). ECA mobilization should be performed at the bifurcation with sharp dissection and encircled with an elastic vessel loop. Encircling the artery more proximally will avoid injuring the superior laryngeal nerve as it courses behind the ECA. The superior thyroid artery is encountered near the bifurcation medially and may require isolation, arising as a branch from the CCA or ECA. The ICA is isolated next and is found deep to the internal jugular vein. Dissection of the medial border of the vein in the superior wound will expose the ICA away from the bifurcation. Lymphatic tissue and small venous or arterial branches above the level of the facial vein can be identified and ligated with careful dissection. The hypoglossal nerve crosses the ICA in a medial course at variable positions away from the bifurcation and should be identified (Fig. 41.3A and B). Following the ansa cervicalis to its junction with the hypoglossal can facilitate identification. Mobilization and careful retraction of the hypoglossal nerve anteriorly enable more distal exposure of the ICA to the level of the digastric muscle. Mobilization of the hypoglossal nerve requires ligation of the "sling vessels," consisting of small veins and lymphatics. Once the ICA is freed, it can be encircled with an elastic vascular loop, distal to the visible extent of atheromatous disease.

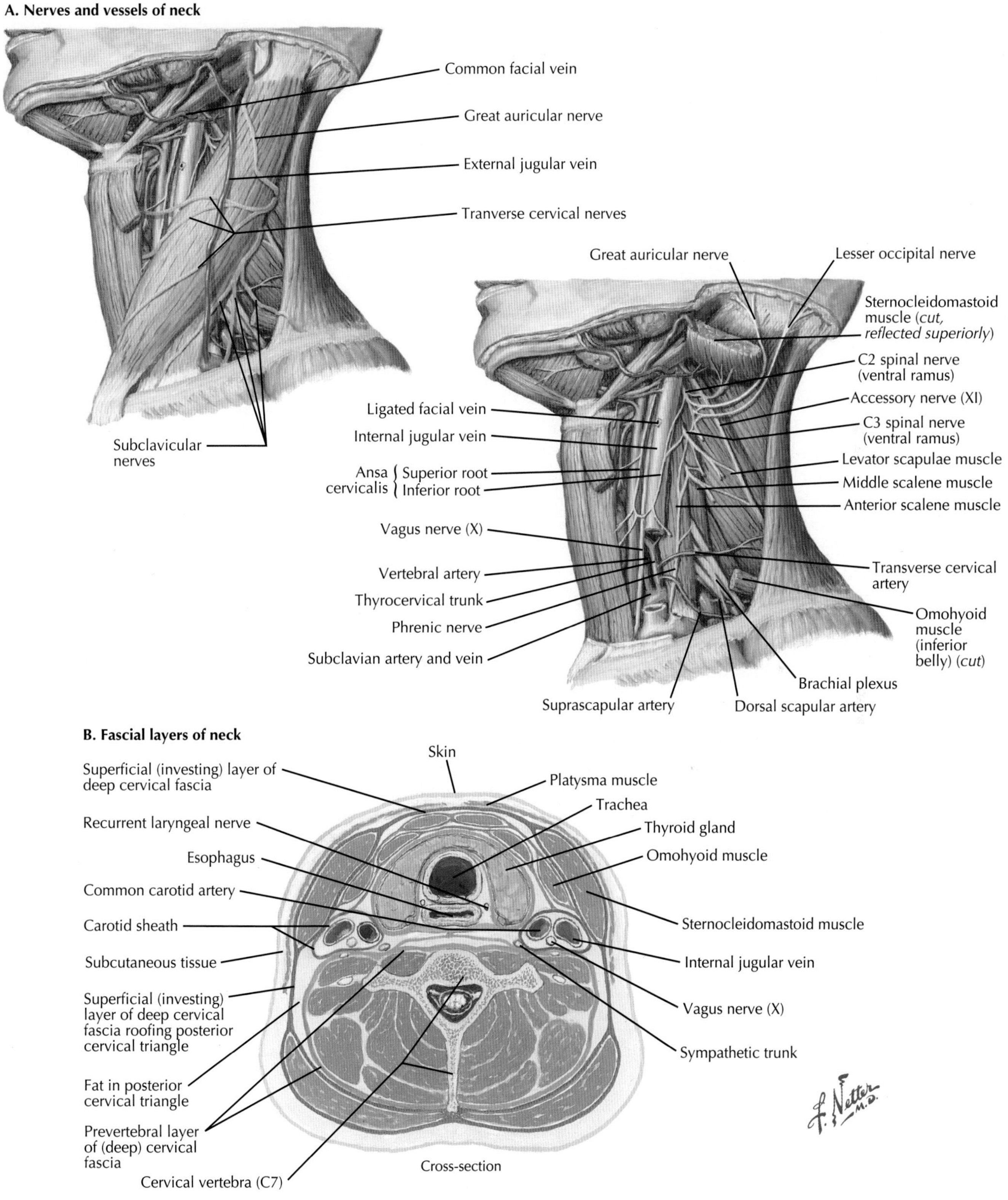

A. Nerves and vessels of neck

Common facial vein

Great auricular nerve

External jugular vein

Tranverse cervical nerves

Subclavicular nerves

Great auricular nerve

Lesser occipital nerve

Sternocleidomastoid muscle (*cut, reflected superiorly*)

C2 spinal nerve (ventral ramus)

Accessory nerve (XI)

C3 spinal nerve (ventral ramus)

Levator scapulae muscle

Middle scalene muscle

Anterior scalene muscle

Transverse cervical artery

Omohyoid muscle (inferior belly) (*cut*)

Brachial plexus

Dorsal scapular artery

Suprascapular artery

Ligated facial vein

Internal jugular vein

Ansa cervicalis { Superior root / Inferior root

Vagus nerve (X)

Vertebral artery

Thyrocervical trunk

Phrenic nerve

Subclavian artery and vein

B. Fascial layers of neck

Skin

Superficial (investing) layer of deep cervical fascia

Recurrent laryngeal nerve

Esophagus

Common carotid artery

Carotid sheath

Subcutaneous tissue

Superficial (investing) layer of deep cervical fascia roofing posterior cervical triangle

Fat in posterior cervical triangle

Prevertebral layer of (deep) cervical fascia

Cervical vertebra (C7)

Platysma muscle

Trachea

Thyroid gland

Omohyoid muscle

Sternocleidomastoid muscle

Internal jugular vein

Vagus nerve (X)

Sympathetic trunk

Cross-section

FIGURE 41.2 Nerves and fascial layers of neck.

CAROTID BIFURCATION EXPOSURE (Continued)

In circumstances of a high carotid bifurcation or extensive disease in the ICA, exposure of the upper cervical segment of the ICA can be achieved by several different maneuvers. Division of the posterior belly of the digastric muscle allows further exposure of the ICA within 2 cm of the skull base. Gentle cephalad retraction must be taken to avoid compression of the marginal mandibular branch of the facial nerve. General anesthesia with nasotracheal intubation and mandibular subluxation can expose the distal cervical segment of the ICA, but this must be planned for preoperatively. Higher exposure can be obtained with removal of the styloid process after division of the stylohyoid ligament and stylopharyngeus and styloglossus muscles.

The carotid bifurcation should be dissected last in a precise manner and is most safely done after the artery is clamped. The surrounding tissue should be dissected free with care to prevent distal embolization from atherosclerotic plaque. The tissues within the carotid bifurcation contain the ascending pharyngeal artery and the baroreceptor nerve of Hering, a branch of the glossopharyngeal nerve to the carotid sinus, which communicates with the vagus nerve and sympathetic trunk. Excessive manipulation and dissection around these tissues may cause reflexive vagal nerve function, resulting in hypotension and bradycardia. Some surgeons advocate inactivating this reflex by injecting local sodium-chloride channel blocker (1% lidocaine) at the carotid bifurcation in the subadventitial plane. Rarely and almost exclusively on the right side, a nonrecurrent laryngeal nerve anomaly leaves the vagus nerve at the level of the bifurcation and is at risk for injury during this dissection. When completed, this dissection should permit gentle lifting of the vessels toward the surface of the wound. After completion of exposure, mobilization and control of the CCA and its branches, the arteriotomy and endarterectomy can be performed.

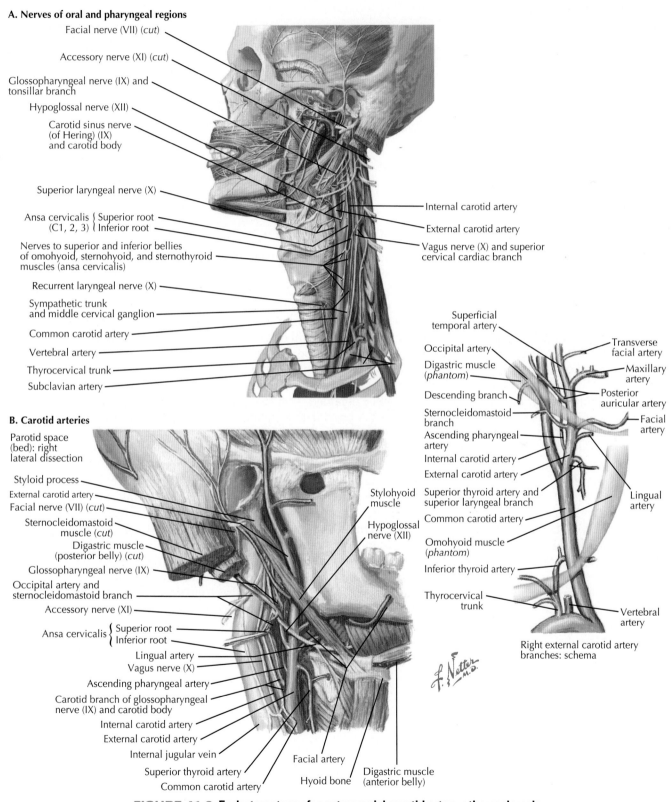

A. Nerves of oral and pharyngeal regions

Facial nerve (VII) (*cut*)

Accessory nerve (XI) (*cut*)

Glossopharyngeal nerve (IX) and tonsillar branch

Hypoglossal nerve (XII)

Carotid sinus nerve (of Hering) (IX) and carotid body

Superior laryngeal nerve (X)

Ansa cervicalis { Superior root (C1, 2, 3) { Inferior root

Nerves to superior and inferior bellies of omohyoid, sternohyoid, and sternothyroid muscles (ansa cervicalis)

Recurrent laryngeal nerve (X)

Sympathetic trunk and middle cervical ganglion

Common carotid artery

Vertebral artery

Thyrocervical trunk

Subclavian artery

Internal carotid artery

External carotid artery

Vagus nerve (X) and superior cervical cardiac branch

B. Carotid arteries

Parotid space (bed): right lateral dissection

Styloid process

External carotid artery

Facial nerve (VII) (*cut*)

Sternocleidomastoid muscle (*cut*)

Digastric muscle (posterior belly) (*cut*)

Glossopharyngeal nerve (IX)

Occipital artery and sternocleidomastoid branch

Accessory nerve (XI)

Ansa cervicalis { Superior root { Inferior root

Lingual artery

Vagus nerve (X)

Ascending pharyngeal artery

Carotid branch of glossopharyngeal nerve (IX) and carotid body

Internal carotid artery

External carotid artery

Internal jugular vein

Superior thyroid artery

Common carotid artery

Stylohyoid muscle

Hypoglossal nerve (XII)

Facial artery

Hyoid bone

Digastric muscle (anterior belly)

Superficial temporal artery

Occipital artery

Digastric muscle (*phantom*)

Descending branch

Sternocleidomastoid branch

Ascending pharyngeal artery

Internal carotid artery

External carotid artery

Superior thyroid artery and superior laryngeal branch

Common carotid artery

Omohyoid muscle (*phantom*)

Inferior thyroid artery

Thyrocervical trunk

Transverse facial artery

Maxillary artery

Posterior auricular artery

Facial artery

Lingual artery

Vertebral artery

Right external carotid artery branches: schema

FIGURE 41.3 Endarterectomy for extracranial carotid artery atherosclerosis.

CAROTID ENDARTERECTOMY TECHNIQUE

Before the arteriotomy and clamping, heparin (80–100 units/kg) is administered intravenously. As stated previously, heparin is administered once the carotid has been exposed. The ICA is clamped first on a soft portion of the artery distal to the plaque. Clamping of the ICA first prevents distal embolization that can occur with clamping of the CCA or ECA. Depending on surgeon preference, cerebral monitoring or carotid stump pressure can be obtained after ICA clamping to be used for selective shunting. A test clamp on the distal ICA should be applied for several minutes, and the cerebral monitoring method can be observed to assess for any neurologic changes. In the circumstance of observed changes, the artery should be unclamped to allow cerebral reperfusion, and a shunt may be used for cerebral perfusion during the endarterectomy. If carotid stump pressures are to be obtained, after ICA clamping a needle connected to a pressure line is placed into the distal CCA proximal to the bifurcation. This confirms arterial flow and can confirm lack of proximal significant stenosis. The common carotid and external carotid are then clamped to confirm isolation of this segment from flow; then the internal carotid is unclamped and the stump pressure is obtained. Shunting is generally used when stump pressures are lower than 40 mm Hg systolic.

Once the stump pressures are recorded, arteriotomy is made in the anterolateral aspect of the CCA, extending on to the ICA beyond the atheromatous plaque using Potts scissors (Fig. 41.4A). If a shunt is to be used, it is placed into the distal ICA, and retrograde flow is confirmed. During placement, if retrograde flow is suddenly stopped, there may be an iatrogenic dissection of the distal ICA or the shunt lumen may be up against the side wall in a tortuous segment of artery; thus, the shunt is never to be forced. It is then temporarily occluded with a finger and the proximal end is placed into the lumen of the CCA under direct visualization to prevent inadvertent embolization. The angled vascular clamp on the CCA is removed, the shunt is advanced into the CCA, and silastic or Rummel tourniquets are tightened around the shunt. Flow through the shunt must be evaluated by Doppler flow probe to ensure there is unimpeded flow without an obstructive "waterhammer" signal.

A. Internal carotid artery shunting

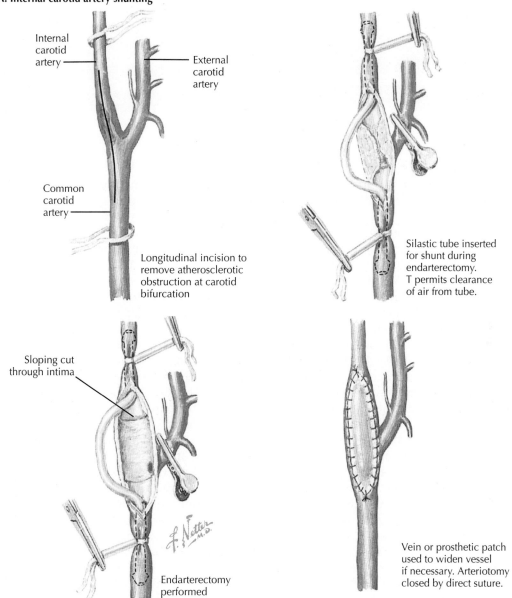

Internal carotid artery

External carotid artery

Common carotid artery

Longitudinal incision to remove atherosclerotic obstruction at carotid bifurcation

Silastic tube inserted for shunt during endarterectomy. T permits clearance of air from tube.

Sloping cut through intima

Endarterectomy performed

Vein or prosthetic patch used to widen vessel if necessary. Arteriotomy closed by direct suture.

B. Endarterectmoized plaque from carotid bifurcation

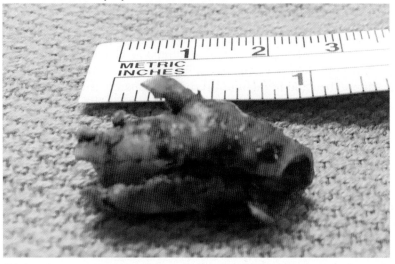

FIGURE 41.4 (A) Arteriotomy, shunt placement, endarterectomy, and patch angioplasty of carotid artery. (B) Endarterectomized plaque from carotid bifurcation.

CAROTID ENDARTERECTOMY TECHNIQUE (Continued)

After shunt placement, or if a shunt is not used, the endarterectomy portion is begun in the CCA by dissecting the layer between the media and adventitia using a Freer elevator. Forceps are used to retract the vessel wall as the wall is pushed away from the plaque. The dissection should be started in the CCA, and the proximal endpoint is established in the distal CCA by trimming the plaque in that location in a beveled fashion. The endarterectomy is then continued into the ECA orifice and separated by eversion technique. The plaque and dissection can be carried into the ICA. Achieving a smooth endpoint in the ICA is critical to prevent postoperative stroke and recurrent stenosis. The endpoint and endarterectomy should be terminated in normal ICA with gradual tapering transition to normal intima. Be careful to avoid pulling down or out on the plaque, which could result in an abrupt step off, or worse, distal dissection of the plaque. A tacking suture can be placed in the distal endpoint, if the endpoint is loose or not adherent. Fig. 41.4B demonstrates endarterectomized plaque from the bifurcation. Heparinized-saline irrigation is used to wash the wall of the artery, exposing any loose fragments that can be removed with forceps. It is believed that repairing the arteriotomy with patch angioplasty represents the standard of care in practice, with routine use of prosthetic (Dacron, bovine pericardium, or polytetrafluoroethylene) or vein patch. A double-armed 6-0 polypropylene suture is started at the distal end of the arteriotomy in the apex of the ICA. The patch is sewn to one side of the artery with constant gentle tension on the artery. The contralateral side of the patch is then sewn to the artery progressing toward the CCA using constant gentle traction until the suture line is met in the middle on one side of the artery and nearly completed, but allowed enough opening to remove the shunt. If a shunt is used, the CCA and ICA are reclamped and the shunt is removed. Both clamps are briefly released to flush debris and air out of the arteries. The clamps are then replaced proximal and distal to the endarterectomized and patched site. The carotid bifurcation is then flushed with heparinized saline and inspected again for intimal flap or debris before the arteriotomy is closed. Again, the ICA clamp is released to fill the bifurcation with blood and reclamped, while the clamps on the CCA and ECA are released to flush remaining debris to the ECA. Now, the ICA clamp is removed. Any bleeding from the suture is addressed at this time.

CLOSURE

Hemostasis should be evaluated, including the patch angioplasty, jugular vein, ligated facial vein, SCM, and surrounding tissues. Protamine should be given to reverse heparinization, and this has been shown not to increase the risk of thrombosis or stroke. A closed suction drain can be left in the surgical bed and brought out through a separate incision. Absorbable 3-0 suture is used to close the platysma, and the skin is approximated with absorbable 4-0 subcuticular suture. The patient should remain in the operating room until neurologic status is established and there are no findings that warrant re-exploration.

SUGGESTED READINGS

Counsell CE, Salinas R, Naylor R, Warlow CP. A systematic review of the randomised trials of carotid patch angioplasty in carotid endarterectomy. Eur J Vasc Endovasc Surg 1997;13:345.

Hertzer NR, Beven EG, Greenstreet RL, Humphries AW. Internal carotid back pressure, intraoperative shunting, ulcerated atheromata, and the incidence of stroke during carotid endarterectomy. Surgery 1978;83:306.

Ricotta JJ, et al. Updated Society for Vascular Surgery guidelines for management of extracranial carotid disease. J Vasc Surg 2011;54:e1-e31.

Carotid Subclavian Bypass/ Transposition and Vertebral Transposition

Jocelyn M. Beach and Behzad S. Farivar

SUBCLAVIAN ARTERY RECONSTRUCTION

Introduction

Cervical reconstruction of arch branch vessels requires detailed understanding of neck and thoracic outlet anatomy. Revascularization of the subclavian arteries using a carotid subclavian bypass or transposition can be used to improve or preserve blood flow to the left subclavian and its branch vessels. Proximal occlusive lesions of the subclavian can be treated using these procedures avoiding open chest reconstruction and as an alternative if endovascular stenting has failed. Coronary and subclavian steal syndromes secondary to a proximal subclavian stenosis can be similarly treated. With increased use of thoracic endovascular aortic repair (TEVAR), the left subclavian artery may have to be intentionally covered to achieve an adequate proximal sealing zone in the treatment of thoracic aneurysms and dissections. This vessel can be revascularized with one of these techniques to preserve arterial perfusion to the vertebral artery and upper extremity and decrease the risk of spinal cord ischemia. A right-sided operation can also be performed to revascularize an aberrant right subclavian artery.

Surgical Planning

Decision making regarding the use of a carotid subclavian bypass versus transposition is based on clinical situation, anatomy, and surgeon experience/comfort. An absolute contraindication for a subclavian-to-carotid transposition is a patent left internal thoracic artery (ITA) to left anterior descending coronary artery bypass graft. In this situation, a carotid subclavian bypass is performed to maintain perfusion to the coronary artery bypass graft while the subclavian artery is clamped distal to the ITA. A very proximal vertebral artery may prohibit transposition of the subclavian. Other relative reasons to consider a bypass over a transposition are large arch aneurysms that displace the left subclavian artery and may make the dissection and mobilization challenging as well as presence of dominant vertebral artery.

In the setting of TEVAR, a benefit of a transposition as opposed to a bypass is that an additional procedure to embolize or occlude the origin of the subclavian is not necessary as the proximal subclavian artery is ligated during a transposition. For an elective TEVAR, current guidelines recommend routine preoperative revascularization; however, these recommendations are based on very low–quality evidence.

Preparation

To perform these procedures the patient is placed in the supine position with the head at the top of the operating table and with the neck extended and rotated toward the contralateral side. This can be facilitated with the use of a shoulder roll and positioning the bed in semi-Fowler, or "beach-chair," position.

CAROTID SUBCLAVIAN BYPASS

Dissection

A transverse incision is made approximately one fingerbreadth above the clavicle and starting lateral to the clavicular head of the sternocleidomastoid muscle (Fig. 42.1A). Subplatysmal flaps are created superior and inferior to the incision. Dissection between the sternal and clavicular head of the sternocleidomastoid muscle is begun with blunt separation of the heads. For carotid subclavian bypass the clavicular head of the sternocleidomastoid can be transected to facilitate medial exposure. The dissection is carried out lateral to the internal jugular vein, mobilizing the scalene fat pad along its medial and inferior borders. Careful attention to the ligation of lymphatics within the fat pad, including the thoracic duct if visualized, is imperative to avoid lymphatic leaks. Deep to the fat pad lies the anterior scalene with overlying phrenic nerve. The phrenic nerve should be dissected off of the anterior scalene and protected. The anterior scalene is then sharply transected as close as possible to its inferior attachments to the first rib. The sub-clavian artery is found deep to the anterior scalene. At this level, the thyrocervical trunk will be visible, and proximal clamping can be achieved distal to the internal thoracic and vertebral arteries, preserving flow to these vessels during the anastomosis (see Fig. 42.1A).

The common carotid is then found medial and deep to the internal jugular vein. The internal jugular should be retracted medially and the common carotid dissected circumferentially and controlled with vessel loops. The vagus nerve is found within the carotid sheath and usually found posterior; however, an anterior vagus is possible.

Bypass and Anastomosis

For a carotid subclavian bypass, 6- to 8-mm Dacron or ringed polytetrafluoroethylene (PTFE) is typically used as conduit. Vein provides no additional patency benefit, is at risk of compression within the neck, and should be reserved for use only in an infected field. The objective is to create a short bypass from the common carotid to the subclavian artery distal to the vertebral and internal thoracic arteries (Fig. 42.1B).

After systemically heparinizing the patient, the subclavian anastomosis is typically performed first. An aortic punch can be used to remove an ellipse of the artery to facilitate the creation of the anastomosis. The subclavian artery is typically soft and can be easily torn. Minimal manipulation of the vessel with forceps is recommended. A running anastomosis with 6-0 Prolene is performed. Flow is restored in the subclavian artery and the graft can be clamped. The graft is then placed posterior to the internal jugular vein before completion of the common carotid anastomosis. The carotid is clamped proximally and distally, and an arteriotomy on the posterior lateral wall is facilitated by gently rotating the vessel with the clamps. A running anastomosis is performed with 6-0 Prolene. The graft and artery is flushed and de-aired before restoring flow. The graft is unclamped first, followed by the proximal common carotid, then the distal common carotid artery. Doppler insonation should be done to confirm low-resistance flow pattern.

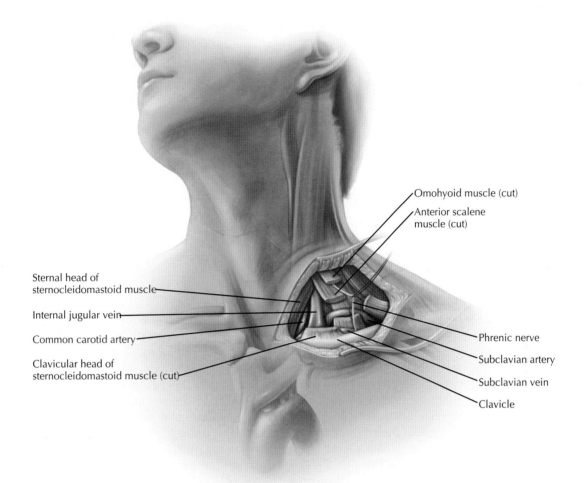

Omohyoid muscle (cut)

Anterior scalene
muscle (cut)

Sternal head of
sternocleidomastoid muscle

Internal jugular vein

Common carotid artery

Clavicular head of
sternocleidomastoid muscle (cut)

Phrenic nerve

Subclavian artery

Subclavian vein

Clavicle

A. Exposure for left carotid subclavian bypass

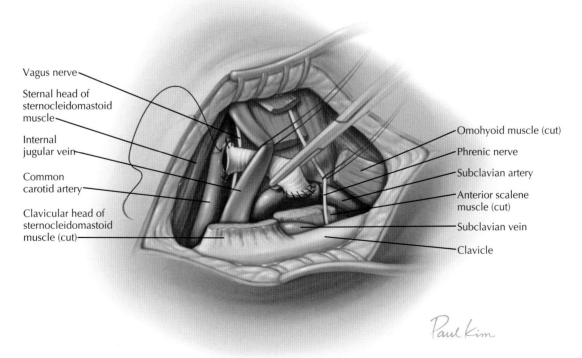

Vagus nerve

Sternal head of
sternocleidomastoid
muscle

Internal
jugular vein

Common
carotid artery

Clavicular head of
sternocleidomastoid
muscle (cut)

Omohyoid muscle (cut)

Phrenic nerve

Subclavian artery

Anterior scalene
muscle (cut)

Subclavian vein

Clavicle

Paul Kim

B. Graft anastomosis for carotid subclavian bypass

FIGURE 42.1 Carotid subclavian bypass.

SUBCLAVIAN-TO-CAROTID TRANSPOSITION
Dissection

In contrast to a carotid subclavian bypass, the incision for a subclavian-to-carotid transposition is a transverse incision made 1 cm above the clavicle and extending from the sternal notch over both the sternal and clavicular heads of the sternocleidomastoid muscle. The incision is carried through the subcutaneous tissues and platysma. Again, superior and inferior subplatysmal flaps are created to assist with the dissection. Care is taken to preserve the external jugular. The dissection is carried down to the internal jugular and dissected along the medial edge and reflected laterally. The common carotid is then dissected and mobilized deep toward the mediastinum and controlled with vessel loops. The omohyoid will be visualized and can be mobilized superiorly or transected. Careful attention should be paid to the thoracic duct, which is typically located near the junction of the left subclavian vein and internal jugular confluence and should be securely ligated (Fig. 42.2A through C). Even if the procedure is performed on the right, lymphatics are still present and should be ligated. Unlike a carotid subclavian bypass dissection, this dissection is performed medially to the fat pad and therefore medial to the anterior scalene and phrenic nerve. One of the key landmarks of this dissection is the vertebral vein, which is found deep and just lateral to the carotid. The vertebral vein is ligated, revealing the subclavian and vertebral arteries. The subclavian artery as well as the proximal branches—vertebral and internal thoracic arteries—and the thyrocervical trunk should all be identified and controlled. Medially the subclavian should be dissected and controlled deep into the mediastinum, proximally to the vertebral artery.

After adequate heparization, the distal subclavian can be clamped followed by the proximal subclavian with a right-angle clamp proximal to the vertebral. The subclavian artery is then transected, and the proximal stump is expeditiously ligated and oversewn. Loss of control of the proximal stump has clear devastating consequences.

Arteriotomy and Anastomosis

The common carotid is then clamped in preparation for the arteriotomy. The arteriotomy should be made slightly posterolaterally on the proximal common carotid. An end-to-side anastomosis between the transected subclavian artery and the common carotid artery is then performed (Fig. 42.2D).

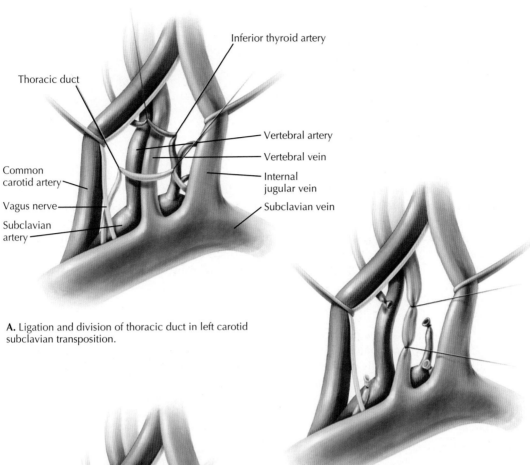

Inferior thyroid artery

Thoracic duct

Vertebral artery

Vertebral vein

Common
carotid artery

Internal
jugular vein

Vagus nerve

Subclavian vein

Subclavian
artery

A. Ligation and division of thoracic duct in left carotid subclavian transposition.

B. Ligation and division of left vertebral vein in left carotid subclavian transposition.

C. Vessel loops around LCCA, LSCA, and left vertebral artery in left carotid subclavian transposition.

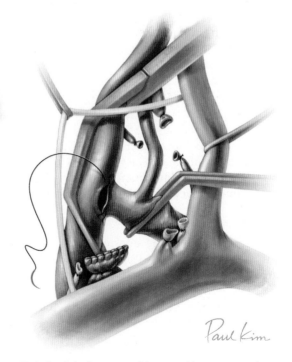

D. Left subclavian-to-carotid transposition anastomosis.

FIGURE 42.2 Subclavian-to-carotid transposition.

VERTEBRAL TRANSPOSITION

Surgical Anatomy

The extracranial vertebral artery is described as having four segments, V1-V4, from proximal to distal. The vertebral artery originates from the proximal subclavian artery. The V1 segment is surgically accessible from its origin to its entrance into the bony transverse foramina canal at the C5-C6 vertebrae. The V2 segment is within the C2-C6 bony canal of the transverse foramina and is difficult to access surgically. The V3 segment is also surgically accessible, where it exits the foramina at C2 before penetration of the dura through the foramen magnum. V4 segment is intracranial from the foramen magnum to the confluence of the two vertebral arteries into the basilar artery.

Indications

A vertebral transposition can be performed to treat ostial occlusive lesions of the V1 segment of the vertebral artery. Approximately 15% of people have a vertebral artery with an origin off of the aortic arch, most commonly between the left common carotid and left subclavian arteries. In the setting of TEVAR, similar to the subclavian, a vertebral transposition may be necessary to extend a proximal landing zone to the origin of the left common carotid artery.

Dissection

The incision and dissection for a vertebral transposition is the same as the subclavian-to-carotid transposition. The vertebral vein overlies proximal V1 segment of the vertebral artery and is similarly ligated proximally. The vertebral artery is dissected from its proximal origin off of the subclavian artery to the longus colli tendon distally. On the anterior surface lies the sympathetic chain often with ganglia overlying the vessel (Fig. 42.3). Care should be taken when dissecting the chain to avoid injury and Horner syndrome. After the vertebral artery is dissected, the common carotid can be located medially and posterior to the internal jugular vein. After systemic heparinization, the vertebral artery is clamped distally just proximally to the longus colli tendon, and the proximal vertebral artery is clamped and transected distal to disease. The stump is then ligated and oversewn.

Arteriotomy and Anastomosis

The vertebral artery is mobilized to identify anastomotic site on the common carotid. The carotid is clamped, and a 5- to 7-mm arteriotomy is created. An aortic punch can facilitate creation of an elliptical arteriotomy. The transected vertebral artery is brought posterior to the sympathetic chain and is anastomosed in a parachute fashion to the common carotid (see Fig. 42.3). Standard flushing maneuvers are performed before complete closure of the anastomosis, clamps are removed, and hemostasis is confirmed.

Closure

After completion of the anastomoses and achieving hemostasis, closure is performed in a similar fashion for all of the earlier-mentioned operations. Unique to the carotid subclavian bypass, the fat pad is replaced; however, after all procedures, careful examination ensures no visible lymphatic vessels are draining. The platysma is then re-approximated and skin is closed. Placement of a drain under the platysma closure is recommended. This drain is kept in place until the patient resumes and tolerates a diet to ensure there are no lymphatic leaks.

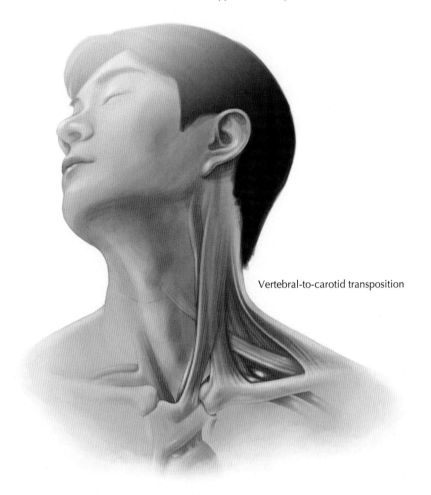

Vertebral-to-carotid transposition

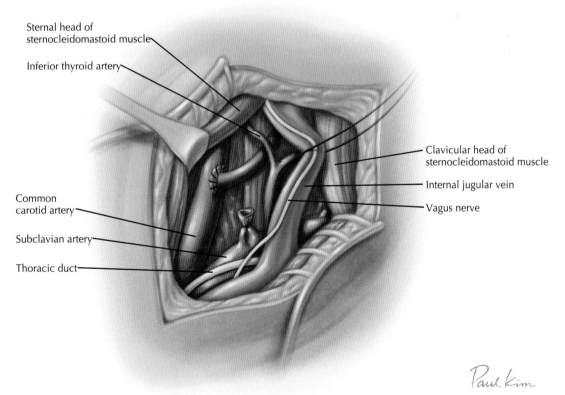

Sternal head of
sternocleidomastoid muscle

Inferior thyroid artery

Clavicular head of
sternocleidomastoid muscle

Internal jugular vein

Vagus nerve

Common
carotid artery

Subclavian artery

Thoracic duct

FIGURE 42.3 Vertebral transposition.

SUGGESTED READINGS

Lee CJ, Morasch MD. Treatment of vertebral disease: appropriate use of open and endovascular techniques. Semin Vasc Surg 2011 1;24(1):24–30.

Matsumura JS, Lee WA, Mitchell RS, Farber MA, Murad MH, Lumsden AB, Society for Vascular Surgery, et al. The Society for Vascular Surgery Practice Guidelines: management of the left subclavian artery with thoracic endovascular aortic repair. J Vasc Surg 2009;50(5):1155–8.

Morasch MD. Technique for subclavian to carotid transposition, tips, and tricks. J Vasc Surg 2009;49(1):251–4.

Aortic Aneurysm Repair and Thoracoabdominal Aneurysm Repair

Sungho Lim and Francis J. Caputo

 VIDEO

43.1 Abdominal Aortic Aneurysm

INTRODUCTION

Aneurysms and dissections are the most common disease processes of the aorta. Several factors contribute to their formation and growth. Although most aneurysms are now treated through endovascular techniques, open surgical reconstruction of the aorta is still necessary in certain anatomic and physiologic constraints. Open aortic reconstruction was first described by Dubost et al in 1951 and has undergone continuous improvement and refinement. Infrarenal or juxtarenal aortic aneurysm may be treated with a midline transperitoneal approach, although the retroperitoneal or thoracoabdominal approach may be used if higher-level proximal aortic control is required.

SURGICAL PLANNING

A preoperative computed tomographic angiogram (CTA) is mandatory to investigate the extent of the disease and determine the level of aortic control. The ideal criteria for the proximal aortic cross-clamping are lack of atherosclerotic plaque or mural thrombus without aneurysmal degeneration. There are two widely accepted surgical approaches to expose the aorta: transperitoneal and retroperitoneal. The transperitoneal approach requires the supine position and midline incision. This approach is familiar to many surgeons and offers rapid access to the abdominal cavity and infrarenal aorta. This is a relatively easy way to gain access to the right renal artery and to the right iliac segment when concomitant reconstruction is necessary. As compared with a transperitoneal approach, a retroperitoneal approach, usually via a left 10th intercostal space, requires right lateral decubitus position and oblique left flank incision. The retroperitoneal approach allows superior exposure of the paravisceral or supraceliac abdominal aorta as well as thoracoabdominal aortic aneurysm (TAAA). The retroperitoneal approach is also preferred in patients with previous peritonitis or multiple abdominal surgeries to avoid intra-abdominal adhesions.

TRANSPERITONEAL APPROACH

The patient is placed on the operating room table in supine position. The abdomen is prepped and draped from the nipples to the knees. A midline abdominal incision is made from the xiphoid process to below the umbilicus for an appropriate distance (Fig. 43.1A). An abdominal aortic aneurysm (AAA) not involving the common iliac arteries, and for which a predetermined tube graft reconstruction will be performed, is sufficiently exposed with a shorter abdominal incision to just below the umbilicus.

Then the greater omentum and the transverse colon are retracted cephalad. The small bowel is moved to the right hemi-abdomen, and the sigmoid colon is gently retracted to the left. When possible, small bowel is not eviscerated to prevent unnecessary bowel edema and insensible fluid loss. A self-retraining retractor can facilitate the exposure at this point. The main dissection of the aorta then proceeds (Fig. 43.1B). The ligament of Treitz is incised, and the fourth portion of duodenum is mobilized. The peritoneum between the duodenum and the inferior mesenteric vein is divided. This incision starts to the left of the aorta at the ligament of Treitz but should course to the right of the aortic midline to prevent injury to the inferior mesenteric artery (IMA), sigmoid mesentery, and autonomic nervous plexus at the aortic bifurcation. Leaving some peritoneal cuff at the inferior border of the duodenum helps, providing adequate tissue to close the retroperitoneum at the end of the aortic repair (Fig. 43.1C).

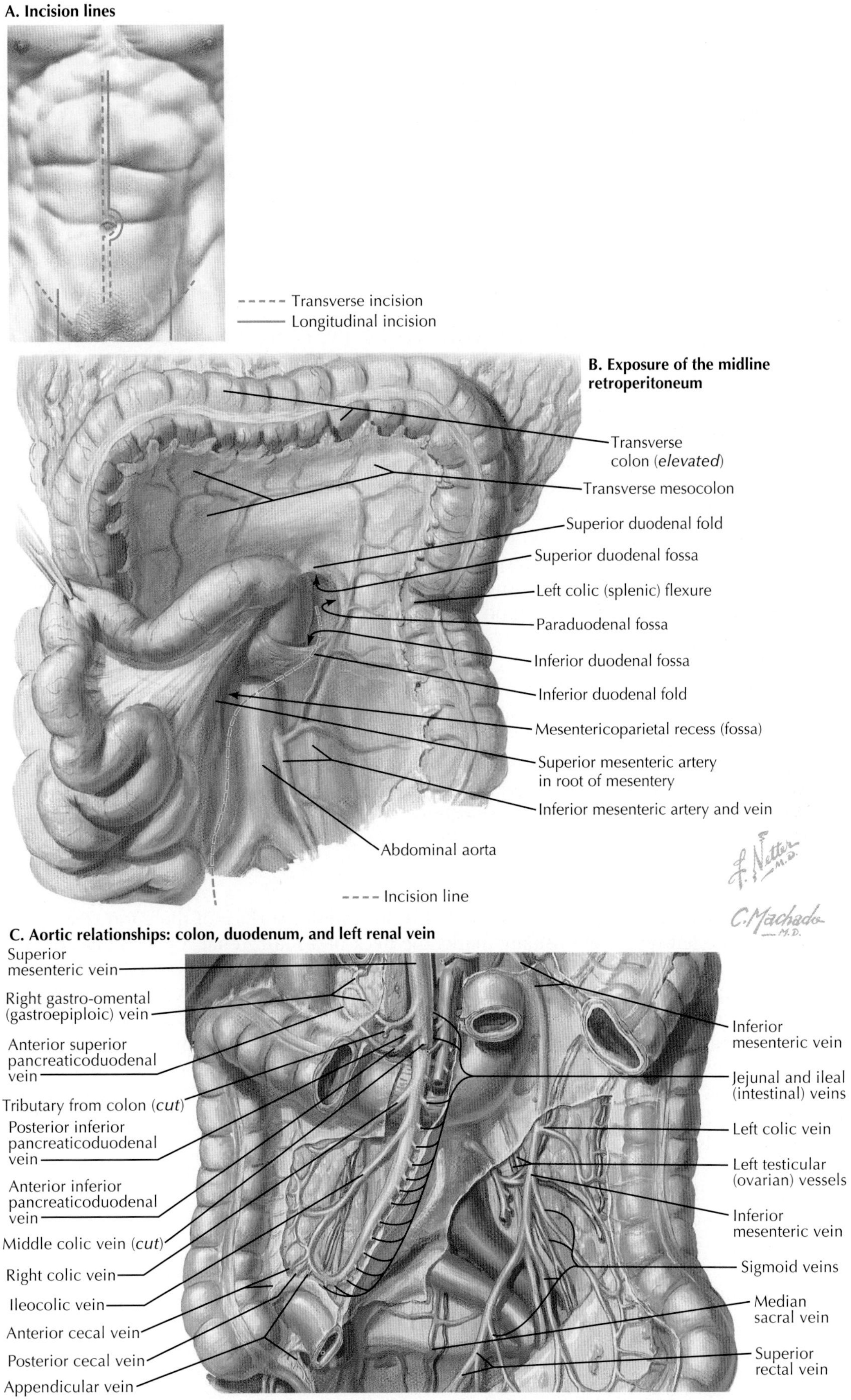

A. Incision lines

----- Transverse incision
——— Longitudinal incision

B. Exposure of the midline retroperitoneum

Transverse colon (*elevated*)

Transverse mesocolon

Superior duodenal fold

Superior duodenal fossa

Left colic (splenic) flexure

Paraduodenal fossa

Inferior duodenal fossa

Inferior duodenal fold

Mesentericoparietal recess (fossa)

Superior mesenteric artery in root of mesentery

Inferior mesenteric artery and vein

Abdominal aorta

----- Incision line

C. Aortic relationships: colon, duodenum, and left renal vein

Superior mesenteric vein

Right gastro-omental (gastroepiploic) vein

Anterior superior pancreaticoduodenal vein

Tributary from colon (*cut*)

Posterior inferior pancreaticoduodenal vein

Anterior inferior pancreaticoduodenal vein

Middle colic vein (*cut*)

Right colic vein

Ileocolic vein

Anterior cecal vein

Posterior cecal vein

Appendicular vein

Inferior mesenteric vein

Jejunal and ileal (intestinal) veins

Left colic vein

Left testicular (ovarian) vessels

Inferior mesenteric vein

Sigmoid veins

Median sacral vein

Superior rectal vein

FIGURE 43.1 Abdominal incision lines and exposure of midline transperitoneal approach.

Iliac Exposure

Palpation of the aortic bifurcation identifies the midline, and the pelvic retroperitoneum is incised. The ureter crosses the iliac vessels anteriorly and at the level of the common iliac bifurcation bilaterally (Fig. 43.2A). Depending on the level of anastomosis, vessel loops can be placed around the right external and internal iliac arteries or around the distal common iliac artery, respecting the intimate relationship between the iliac arteries and veins. The most common atherosclerotic pattern demonstrates disease at the distal common iliac artery, so vessel loops around the external and internal iliac arteries are preferred. The vessels are usually soft at this location and will provide the most flexibility in constructing the anastomosis.

The left common iliac bifurcation reveals the same anatomic pattern of ureter anteriorly and a close relationship between the arteries and the fragile veins. Accessing the left common iliac bifurcation is more difficult because of the colonic mesentery. Traction is applied to the mesentery to visualize the desired plane. A layer of tissue that usually contains sympathetic nerves is left over the left common iliac artery, and the left iliac bifurcation is palpated. The ureter is then found, and the entire mass of tissue containing the ureter and sigmoid colon mesentery is gently retracted to dissect the bifurcation and carefully place vessel loops.

Lateral Iliac Exposure

An alternate approach to the left iliac bifurcation is a lateral approach, reflecting the sigmoid colon's mesentery to the right and incising the peritoneum over the left external iliac artery (Fig. 43.2B). This approach is helpful in patients with a large, left common iliac artery aneurysm, or if the retractors used to access the left iliac bifurcation from the medial side place too much tension on the ureter or sigmoid colon mesentery. With a larger common iliac artery aneurysm, if there is known internal iliac artery occlusion, the lateral approach could allow an end-to-end anastomosis to the left external iliac artery and thus exclude the entire aneurysm.

Renal Vasculature

The left renal vein has intimate relationship with the anterior surface of the aorta (Fig. 43.2C through E). The left renal vein usually marks the neck of an infrarenal AAA and lies slightly caudal to the renal arteries. Often, it can be dissected free and retracted cephalad to achieve exposure of the aorta and renal arteries (Fig. 43.3). However, if the AAA is juxtarenal, thus suprarenal control of the aorta is necessary; the surgeon should decide whether the renal vein should be retracted or divided. If the left renal vein must be cut, its adrenal, gonadal, and lumbar branches should remain intact (see Fig. 43.3). Alternatively, the gonadal and lumbar branches can be ligated to maximize mobility of the renal vein if to avoid ligation of the left renal vein. Dissection of a small amount of inferior vena cava (IVC) at its confluence with the left renal vein also facilitates exposure of the suprarenal aorta.

Care should also be taken not to damage lumbar vessels. These vessels originate from the posterior half of the aorta between lumbar vertebrae. Therefore, instrument or finger dissection must be performed posterior to the aorta to have a clear clamp site between the aorta and the vertebrae (Fig. 43.4A). With a large AAA, there is anterior deviation or angulation of the neck, allowing less dissection and still sufficient purchase for safe, complete clamping of the aorta (Fig. 43.4B and C).

A. Arteries of ureters and urinary bladder

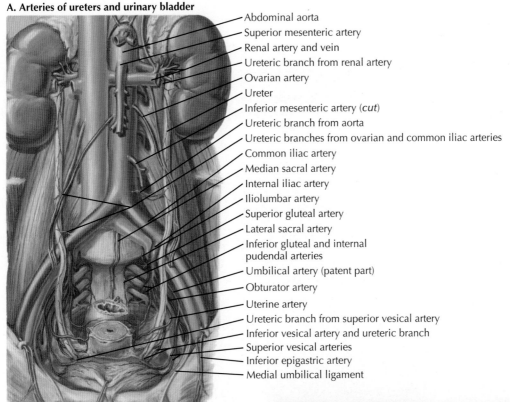

- Abdominal aorta
- Superior mesenteric artery
- Renal artery and vein
- Ureteric branch from renal artery
- Ovarian artery
- Ureter
- Inferior mesenteric artery (*cut*)
- Ureteric branch from aorta
- Ureteric branches from ovarian and common iliac arteries
- Common iliac artery
- Median sacral artery
- Internal iliac artery
- Iliolumbar artery
- Superior gluteal artery
- Lateral sacral artery
- Inferior gluteal and internal pudendal arteries
- Umbilical artery (patent part)
- Obturator artery
- Uterine artery
- Ureteric branch from superior vesical artery
- Inferior vesical artery and ureteric branch
- Superior vesical arteries
- Inferior epigastric artery
- Medial umbilical ligament

B. Mesenteric relations of intestines (reflected)

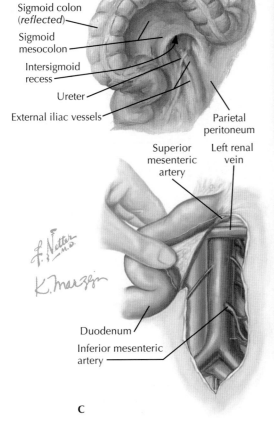

- Sigmoid colon (*reflected*)
- Sigmoid mesocolon
- Intersigmoid recess
- Ureter
- External iliac vessels
- Parietal peritoneum
- Superior mesenteric artery
- Left renal vein
- Duodenum
- Inferior mesenteric artery

C

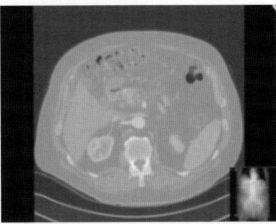

D. CT angiogram showing the usual relationship between the aorta, superior mesenteric artery, and left-to-right crossing left renal vein.

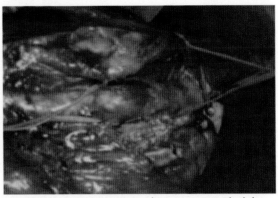

E. Infrarenal aorta in preparation for aortic repair. The left renal vein is seen to the right, the vena cava superiorly, and the suction device pointing to the right renal artery.

FIGURE 43.2 Aortic and iliac arterial relationships with retroperitoneal structures.

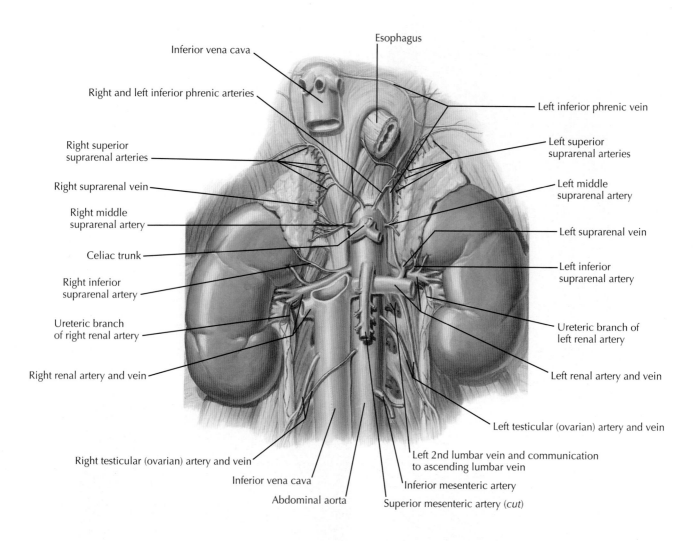

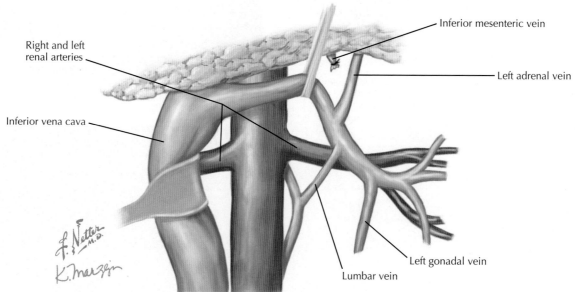

FIGURE 43.3 Aortic relationships with retroperitoneum and left renal vein.

A. Abdominal wall

Lesser omentum

Hepatic portal vein and proper hepatic artery in right margin of lesser omentum

Omental bursa (lesser sac)

Stomach

Middle colic artery

Transverse mesocolon

Transverse colon

Greater omentum

Small intestine

T12

L1

L2

L3

L4

L5

S1

S2

Omental (epiploic) foramen (of Winslow)

Celiac trunk

Splenic vessels

Renal vessels

Pancreas

Superior mesenteric artery

Lumbar vessels

Inferior (horizontal, or 3rd) part of duodenum

Abdominal aorta

Parietal peritoneum (of posterior abdominal wall)

Mesentery of small intestine

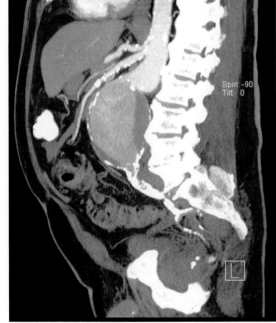

B. Sagittal CT angiogram showing the angulation of the neck of a large 8-cm AAA. Also seen is an accentuated concavity in the lumbar vertebrae.

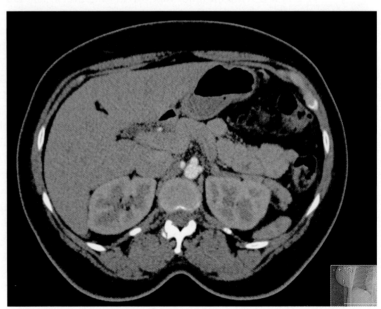

C. CT angiogram showing contrast in the aorta, renal arteries, and origin of the superior mesenteric artery. Note the proximity of these vessels.

FIGURE 43.4 Aortic relationships with lumbar spine and visceral vessels. *AAA,* Abdominal aortic aneurysm.

Medial Visceral Rotation

Suprarenal aneurysm is best approached using a retroperitoneal approach, but the paravisceral aorta still can be accessed transperitoneally using a left medial visceral rotation. The left white line of Toldt is incised, and the left colon and the sigmoid colon mesentery are mobilized medially. The incision is carried cephalad, dividing the phrenicocolic ligament. The plane between the posterior aspect of Gerota's fascia and posterior abdominal wall is developed. The spleen, colon, tail of the pancreas, and the left kidney are reflected medially. Alternatively, the plane anterior to Gerota's fascia can be developed and the left kidney left in the renal fossa (Fig. 43.5A). When visceral vessels require transaortic endarterectomy or in the setting of retroaortic left renal vein, the left kidney is usually left in situ. The rest of exposure is the same as retroperitoneal aortic exposure.

RETROPERITONEAL EXPOSURE

The patient is placed in the lazy right lateral decubitus position, and the break in the operating table should be just above the iliac crest. An axillary roll is placed below the right axilla, and the hip is tilted approximately 60 degrees so that both femoral arteries can be accessible if needed. The left knee can be flexed, and a pillow is placed between the legs. The left arm is secured to an arm board with shoulder flexion at 90 degrees. The elbow and shoulder should be well padded and secured with adhesive tape. The table is now to be flexed, and the bean bag is vacuumed into a supportive shape (Fig. 43.5B).

The proximal portion of the incision is made along the superior border of the 11th rib (10th intercostal space), starting at the posterior axillary line and subsequently curved down toward the lateral edge of the rectus sheath. The distal end of the incision can be between the level of the umbilicus and pubis as dictated by the distal extent of the aneurysm. The skin and subcutaneous tissue are divided, and the external, internal, and transversus abdominis muscles are sequentially opened. Care should be taken not to violate the peritoneum, which should be bluntly dissected free from the abdominal wall. Fibroadipose retroperitoneal tissue is opened and psoas muscle is identified. Peritoneal contents, the left kidney, renal artery, and ureter are reflected medially (Fig. 43.5C). In some cases, a limited incision in the diaphragm is required to separate the 10th and the 11th ribs. The diaphragm can be primarily repaired using nonabsorbable monofilament sutures during closure with a small chest tube left in the pleural space. The left renolumbar vein, which runs from the vertebrae to the left renal vein, must be ligated to prevent avulsion. The left renal artery is usually palpable, identified and isolated at its aortic origin. Proceeding cephalad, the SMA and celiac axis can be identified and dissected. These are usually surrounded by fibrous tissue and a nerve plexus. The median arcuate ligament and left crus of the diaphragm may be divided to facilitate the exposure (Fig. 43.5D and E).

A. Transperitoneal medial visceral rotation leaving kidney in situ

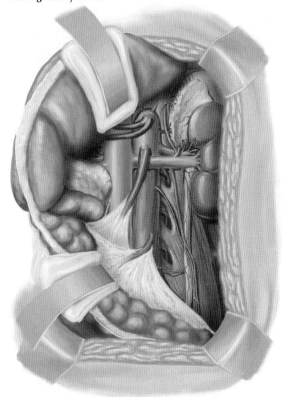

B. Patient positioning for retroperitoneal approach

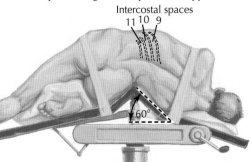

Intercostal spaces
11 10 9

60°

C. Planes of dissection from medial visceral rotation approach illustrating planes in front and behind left kidney

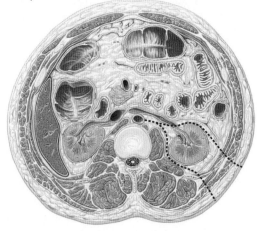

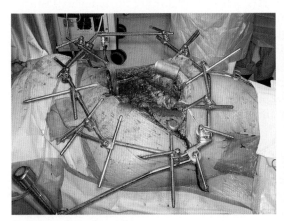

D. Retroperitoneal exposure.
Retractors and patient position.

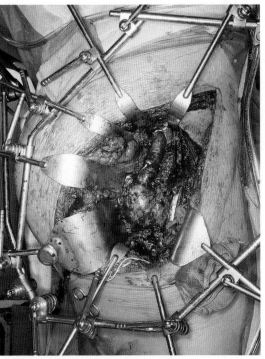

E. Thoracoretroperitoneal aortic exposure via 10th intercostal space.

FIGURE 43.5 Retroperitoneal exposures. Position and dissection plane.

Iliac Exposure

The left common iliac artery is exposed following the same plane that developed for aortic exposure. Care is taken not to injure the ureter under the retractor or by accidentally placing the clamp directly on the ureter. The retroperitoneal tissue can be mobilized to the right side of the aorta to identify the origin of the right common iliac artery for clamping. It can be difficult to dissect distal to the iliac bifurcation. In some instances, the right iliac artery can be controlled intraluminally using Fogarty balloons. When the inferior mesenteric artery is chronically occluded, it can be divided at its origin to facilitate retraction of the intestines off the aorta, allowing better access to the right common and external and internal iliac vessels.

THORACOABDOMINAL AORTIC ANEURYSM

Patient position for TAAA repair is identical to retroperitoneal aortic exposure. However, the precise location and extent of the incision does vary and is mainly dictated by the specific area of aorta to be exposed. The modified Crawford classification is the most widely used, which divides this disease into five different anatomic types: type I extends from the left subclavian artery to just above the renal arteries; type II, the most extensive, descends from the left subclavian artery to the infrarenal aorta; type III from the mid–descending thoracic aorta to the aortic bifurcations; type IV from the diaphragmatic aorta to the iliac bifurcations; and type V from the mid–descending thoracic aorta to just above the renal arteries (Fig. 43.6A). The proximal incision is typically made at the 5th intercostal space for type I and II TAAA and at the 6th intercostal space for type III and V TAAA, whereas type IV TAAA requires incision at 8th or 9th intercostal space. Higher-level ribs can be accessed posteriorly if more proximal exposure is required in the thoracic cavity. When exposing the thoracic aorta, it is important to avoid injury to the phrenic nerve, the vagus, and its recurrent branch because these nerves increase the risk of pulmonary and other complications. The left vagus nerve enters the chest cavity between the left common carotid artery and left subclavian artery and lies in front of the transverse aortic arch near the left subclavian artery. It gives rise to the left recurrent laryngeal nerve, which hooks around the aortic arch and ascends between the trachea and cervical esophagus. The remainder of the vagus nerve descends parallel to the descending thoracic aorta and the thoracic esophagus (Fig. 43.6B).

Avoiding Visceral, Renal, and Spinal Cord Ischemia

Spinal cord protection may be achieved through spinal fluid drainage. Lumbar drains should be placed preoperatively, and the CSF pressure should be maintained less than 10 mm Hg for 3 days postoperatively. Lowering the CSF pressure will maximize perfusion pressure of the spinal cord and is protective against ischemia. Patent intercostal arteries, especially T8-T12, are recommended to be reattached immediately to increase spinal cord perfusion. This can be done by a side-biting aortic graft and by using either a separate graft or a direct anastomosis as an island patch. In addition to CSF drainage and intercostal artery reimplantation, distal aortic perfusion by partial bypass from the left atrium to the distal aorta or to the left femoral artery has proven efficacy to prevent visceral and renal ischemia. The bypass allows retrograde perfusion to the visceral and renal artery while the proximal aorta undergoing reconstruction using sequential clamping (Fig. 43.6C).

A. Modified Crawford TAAA classification

Extent I   Extent II   Extent III   Extent IV   Extent V

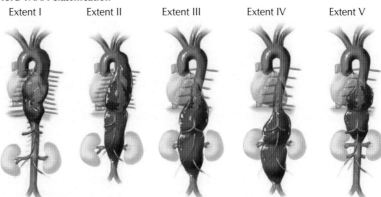

B. Aortic relationships with supra-aortic trunks, esophagus, and vagus nerve

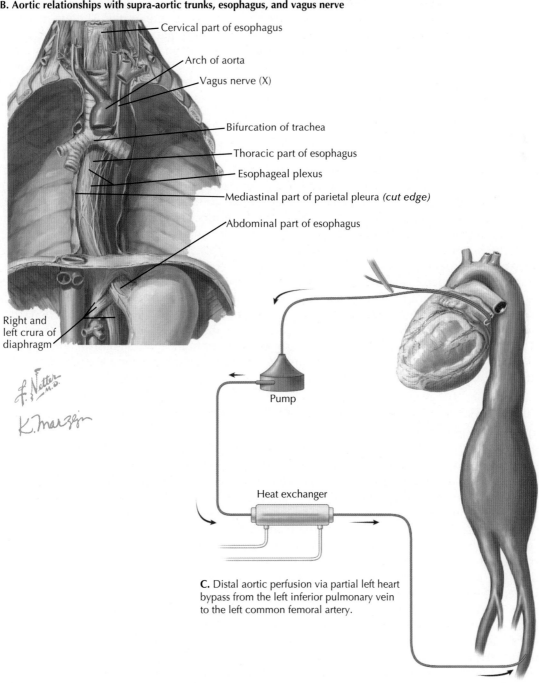

Cervical part of esophagus

Arch of aorta

Vagus nerve (X)

Bifurcation of trachea

Thoracic part of esophagus

Esophageal plexus

Mediastinal part of parietal pleura *(cut edge)*

Abdominal part of esophagus

Right and left crura of diaphragm

Pump

Heat exchanger

C. Distal aortic perfusion via partial left heart bypass from the left inferior pulmonary vein to the left common femoral artery.

FIGURE 43.6 Thoracoabdominal aortic aneurysm (TAAA).

(A, reused with permission from Frederick JR, Woo YJ. Mycotic thoracoabdominal aneurysms. Ann Cardiothorac Surg 2012;1[3]:277-285. https://doi.org/10.3978/j.issn.2225-319X.2012.09.01, Fig. 1.)

SPECIAL CONCERNS

Dissection of the suprarenal aorta can then be done with finger and instrument dissection, but usually not circumferentially. The surgeon must always be cognizant of the superior mesenteric artery (SMA) and avoiding injury to the middle colic branch during SMA retraction. A space usually exists between the lateral takeoff of the renal arteries and the midline anterior origin of the SMA. The space for suprarenal clamping can vary but can be anticipated from careful inspection of the preoperative CT scan (see Fig. 43.4BC). In presence of atherosclerotic and thrombus burden or aneurysmal degeneration in the suprarenal aorta, supraceliac clamping is warranted.

Another potential area of concern or danger is variable venous anatomy. The main venous variations or anomalies are (1) transposition (left-sided) or duplication (bilateral) of the IVC and (2) the retroaortic left renal vein, which usually travels from lower left posterior to upper right, where it connects to the vena cava. The retroaortic left renal vein is usually not perpendicular to the aorta, as is the normal left renal vein. When preoperative CT scans demonstrate these variations, the clamp should be carefully placed to avoid potentially fatal venous injury.

AORTOBIFEMORAL BYPASS

If an aortobifemoral bypass is indicated for aortoiliac occlusive disease, a shorter incision is usually made from the xiphoid to just below the umbilicus. The groin incisions are made transversely or vertically depending on the complexity of the femoral reconstruction (see Fig. 43.1). Vertical incisions can be easily extended proximally and distally if the external iliac, superficial, and/or deep femoral arteries need reconstruction. Exposure of the infrarenal aorta down to its bifurcation usually provides enough space to create a proximal anastomosis (see Fig. 43.2E).

Both end-to-end and end-to-side proximal anastomosis are viable options. An end-to-end anastomosis provides improved hemodynamics and decreased perianastomotic turbulent flow, and recurrent atheroma formation. It is easy to cover with retroperitoneal tissue and poses less chance of graft-enteric fistula. An end-to-side anastomosis is preferred when preservation of a large accessory renal artery or patent inferior mesenteric artery (IMA) is required. Then, tunnels are created along the iliac vessels with gentle blunt dissection from the groins to the aorta. A retroureteral tunnel is created to prevent hydroureter from mechanical obstruction from the iliac graft limb. The tunnels are usually marked with an umbilical tape or a Penrose drain, and the limbs are pulled through the tunnels at the appropriate time (Fig. 43.7A).

RUPTURED ABDOMINAL AORTIC ANEURYSM

The open approach to the ruptured AAA is usually the same as previously described, with a midline incision and dissection into the retroperitoneum to the right of midline, then along the duodenum, pushing it to the right. Care is taken not to injure the duodenum or incise the retroperitoneum too far to the left, where collaterals to the sigmoid colon or the IMA may travel. The renal vein can be difficult to identify because of the hematoma and the tissue staining, making the entire retroperitoneum the same deep-maroon, purple color.

Occasionally, clamping the aorta at the diaphragmatic hiatus is necessary to gain proximal control. This technique can be an especially helpful maneuver in the trauma victim with a central hematoma (Fig. 43.7B). The falciform ligament is divided and taken down off the dome of the liver; the surgeon follows it to the insertion on the diaphragm. The anterior and posterior leaflets of the left triangular ligament are divided and followed medially to the level of the vena cava. This allows mobilization and retraction of the left lobe of the liver. The gastrohepatic ligament is divided and the lesser sac entered. Then, bluntly dissect the distal esophagus to retract the stomach and esophagus to the patient's left. This dissection is greatly facilitated by placing a nasogastric tube to assist identification of the esophagus to avoid injury during the dissection. A small portion of patients will have a replaced right hepatic artery, which must be identified and avoided. The anterior portion of the crus of the diaphragm is incised with cautery overlying the aorta. With exposure of the supraceliac segment of the aorta, it allows pressure with a sponge stick or occlusion with a straight aortic clamp.

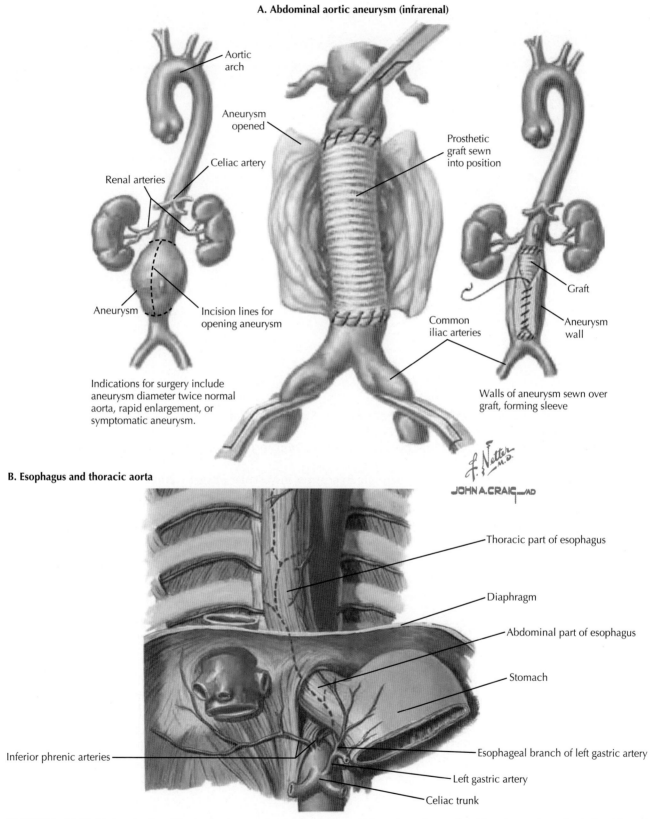

A. Abdominal aortic aneurysm (infrarenal)

Aortic arch

Aneurysm opened

Celiac artery

Renal arteries

Prosthetic graft sewn into position

Aneurysm

Incision lines for opening aneurysm

Graft

Common iliac arteries

Aneurysm wall

Indications for surgery include aneurysm diameter twice normal aorta, rapid enlargement, or symptomatic aneurysm.

Walls of aneurysm sewn over graft, forming sleeve

B. Esophagus and thoracic aorta

Thoracic part of esophagus

Diaphragm

Abdominal part of esophagus

Stomach

Inferior phrenic arteries

Esophageal branch of left gastric artery

Left gastric artery

Celiac trunk

FIGURE 43.7 Abdominal aortic aneurysm and anatomy. Completion of aortic repair with tube graft and relationships of supraceliac aorta, stomach, and crus of stomach.

SUGGESTED READINGS

Moore W, editor. Vascular and Endovascular Surgery: a Comprehensive Review. 9th ed. Philadelphia: Saunders-Elsevier; 2018.

Turnipseed WD, Carr SC, Tefera G, et al. Minimal incision aortic surgery. J Vasc Surg 2001;34:47–53.

Valentine RJ, Wind GG, editors. Anatomic Exposures in Vascular Surgery. 2nd ed. Philadelphia: Lippincott, Williams & Wilkins; 2003.

Wahlberg E, Olofsson P, Goldstone J. Emergency Vascular Surgery: a Practical Guide. Berlin: Springer; 2007. (See Chapter 7 on AAA for illustrations of supraceliac cross-clamp technique.)

Visceral Bypass

Nathan Droz and F. Ezequiel Parodi

INTRODUCTION

Mesenteric ischemia can be an acute or chronic process. Acute mesenteric ischemia is caused by embolism or thrombosis of one or more mesenteric blood vessels. Embolism is generally a result of a recent cardiac event or arrhythmia. Acute mesenteric ischemia patients have elevated lactic acid and often "pain out of proportion" to the physical exam. Urgent angiographic imaging should reveal filling defects in one or more mesenteric vessels. Additional findings on axial imaging may reveal stigmata of bowel ischemia (e.g., bowel wall thickening, mesenteric edema, or pneumatosis). Patients with thrombotic or occlusive disease tend to have prodromal symptoms such as postprandial abdominal pain before their acute presentation.

Chronic mesenteric ischemia is a result of advanced mesenteric vessel atherosclerosis. Patients have comorbidities consistent with peripheral arterial disease. Classic symptoms include postprandial abdominal pain, weight loss, and food fear. In most cases, two of the three mesenteric vessels must be involved for symptoms to occur. Duplex ultrasound and arteriographic findings of severe ostial stenosis confirm the diagnosis. Symptomatic patients with occlusive disease of at least two of the three mesenteric vessels (celiac axis, superior, and inferior mesenteric arteries) are often considered for revascularization.

SURGICAL ANATOMY

The mesenteric vessels of the visceral aorta include the celiac axis, superior, and inferior mesenteric arteries. The celiac axis is a short common arterial trunk that originates on the anterior surface of the abdominal aorta as it passes through the diaphragmatic crura at the 12th thoracic vertebra (T12). Most commonly within 2 cm of its origin the celiac divides into the left gastric, splenic, and common hepatic arteries (Fig. 44.1). These arterial branches and their tributaries supply the stomach, proximal duodenum, liver, spleen, and portions of the pancreas. Important for mesenteric revascularization is the common hepatic artery. The common hepatic artery traverses the gastrohepatic ligament toward the portal triad and may be used as a target vessel in revascularization procedures.

The superior mesenteric artery (SMA) arises approximately 1 cm distal to the celiac axis on the anterior surface of the aorta at the first lumbar vertebra (L1) (see Fig. 44.1). The SMA is the dominant blood supply to the distal duodenum, small bowel, and ascending and transverse colon. The SMA has a robust collateral network to both the celiac axis and the inferior mesenteric artery (IMA). The celiac communicates with the SMA via the pancreaticoduodenal arcades and with the IMA via the marginal artery of Drummond. The SMA's intimate relationship with the pancreas also deserves mention. The SMA travels behind the neck of the pancreas, medial to the superior mesenteric vein, but then traverses the uncinate process and third portion of the duodenum in an anterior position. Finally, an important landmark for identification of the SMA during surgical exposure is the middle colic artery, which is the first major branch of the infrapancreatic SMA and may be traced to its origin to identify the SMA.

SURGICAL PLANNING AND REVASCULARIZATION

There are two main transperitoneal revascularization options for chronic mesenteric ischemia: antegrade mesenteric bypass and retrograde mesenteric bypass. Antegrade allows for a more anatomic orientation of the bypass graft and provides access to the often minimally diseased supraceliac aorta. It does require exposure of the supraceliac aorta, supraceliac clamping, and creation of a retropancreatic tunnel. Although a retrograde bypass can often be accomplished without aortic clamping, patients with patent, minimally diseased iliac arteries and chronic mesenteric ischemia are uncommon.

The mesenteric arteries may also be approached through a retroperitoneal incision, which provides unparalleled access to the proximal portions of the mesenteric vessels. In patients with ostomies or a hostile abdomen, the retroperitoneal approach offers a useful approach. In brief, patients are placed left side up, and the operating room table is flexed. A left thoraco-retroperitoneal or thoracoabdominal incision is made. The peritoneum is identified and reflected medially. The left kidney is kept down in its normal anatomic location and the space between the left colon mesentery and Gerota's fascia is developed. The left renal vein will cross the aorta and the left renal artery can be found underneath the renal vein. The advantage of leaving the kidney in situ is that it allows exposure of the entire lateral wall of the superior mesenteric artery. The superior mesenteric artery can be dissected out from the aorta to past the middle colic artery in the same area where a bypass is done when exposed from the anterior approach.

A. Celiac axis and its branches

Left hepatic artery

Common hepatic artery

Left gastric artery

Splenic branches of splenic artery

Right hepatic artery

Proper hepatic artery

Right gastric artery

Splenic artery

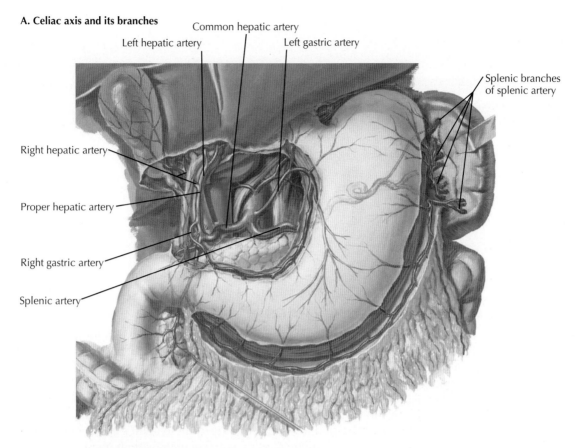

B. Superior mesenteric artery and its relationship to the pancreas

Left gastric artery

Common hepatic artery

Middle colic artery (*cut*)

Inferior pancreaticoduodenal artery

Superior mesenteric artery

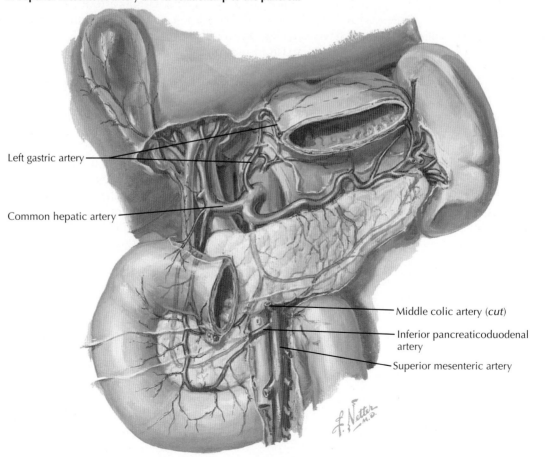

FIGURE 44.1 Celiac axis and superior mesenteric artery (SMA).

ANTEGRADE MESENTERIC BYPASS

Patients are placed supine on a standard operating table. Entrance to the abdomen is gained through a generous midline incision. In an antegrade bypass, the supraceliac aorta is the first structure to be exposed. The falciform ligament is taken down almost to the vena cava. From this point, the left triangular ligament of the liver is then incised to mobilize the left lobe of the liver (Fig. 44.2A). Careful attention must be paid to the left hepatic vein during this maneuver. The liver is then retracted to the patient's right. The gastrohepatic ligament is then opened. The esophagus and lesser curve of the stomach are retracted to the patient's left to expose the right crus of the diaphragm (Fig. 44.2B). The median arcuate ligament is then incised for a few centimeters to reveal the supraceliac aorta. If present, any crossing phrenic arteries at this level should be controlled. Dissecting caudally along the anterior surface of the aorta will expose the celiac origin. The celiac plexus will have to be ligated to fully reveal the underlying celiac axis (Fig. 44.2C). Depending on the intended anastomotic configuration, control of the common trunk or the celiac branches may be necessary.

The SMA is then exposed at the inferior border of the pancreas. The transverse colon is retracted cranially and the small bowel reflected to the patient's right. The middle colic artery is identified and traced to the base of the mesentery. Palpation should help to identify the SMA, but if the SMA cannot be identified, the superior mesenteric vein can act as a landmark because the artery is medial to the vein. The anterior peritoneum is opened overlying the artery (Fig. 44.2D). There are no anterior branches of the SMA at this level, although multiple jejunal branches are present and should be preserved if possible. The SMA is then encircled with vessel loops. At this point, a retropancreatic tunnel is formed by blunt finger dissection from the distal SMA anastomoses location toward the supraceliac aorta. The tunnel is then preserved with a vessel loop or umbilical tape. A bifurcated graft is then introduced to the field and tunneled.

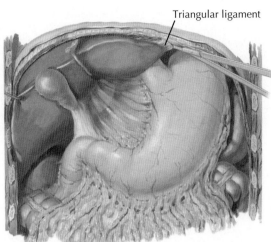

Triangular ligament

A. Incision of the left triangular ligament to facilitate exposure of the supraceliac aorta

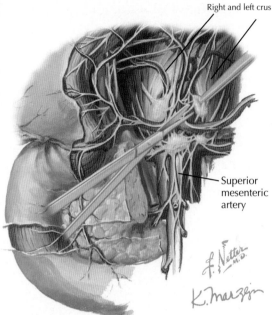

Right and left crus

Superior mesenteric artery

B. Incision of celiac plexus to expose the celiac axis and SMA origins

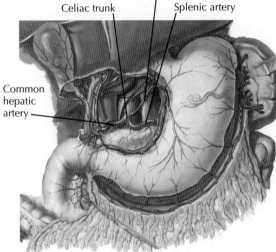

Left gastric artery

Celiac trunk

Splenic artery

Common hepatic artery

C. Exposure of the celiac branches

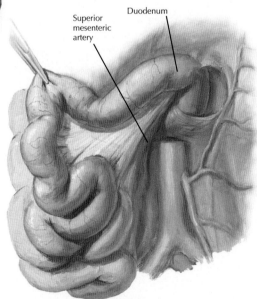

Superior mesenteric artery

Duodenum

D. Incision at base of small bowel mesentery to expose SMA distal to location occlusion

FIGURE 44.2 Surgical exposure of supraceliac aorta, superior mesenteric artery (SMA), and reconstruction.

ANTEGRADE MESENTERIC BYPASS (Continued)

The patient is then systemically heparinized and monitored by activated clotting times. The aorta is clamped, and an end-to-side anastomosis is performed with a bifurcated graft. The anastomosis is then tested. If the celiac artery is to be used as outflow, an end to side anastamosis may be performed. The common hepatic artery is typically soft and an ideal target to sew to in an end-to-side fashion. A limb of the bifurcated graft is tunneled retropancreatically to the SMA. Finally, the SMA anastomosis is performed in an end to side fashion (Fig. 44.3). Doppler ultrasound confirms distal flow, and the peritoneum over the SMA is closed to protect the graft from the overlying intestine. The intestine is then returned to its anatomic position, and the abdominal incision is closed.

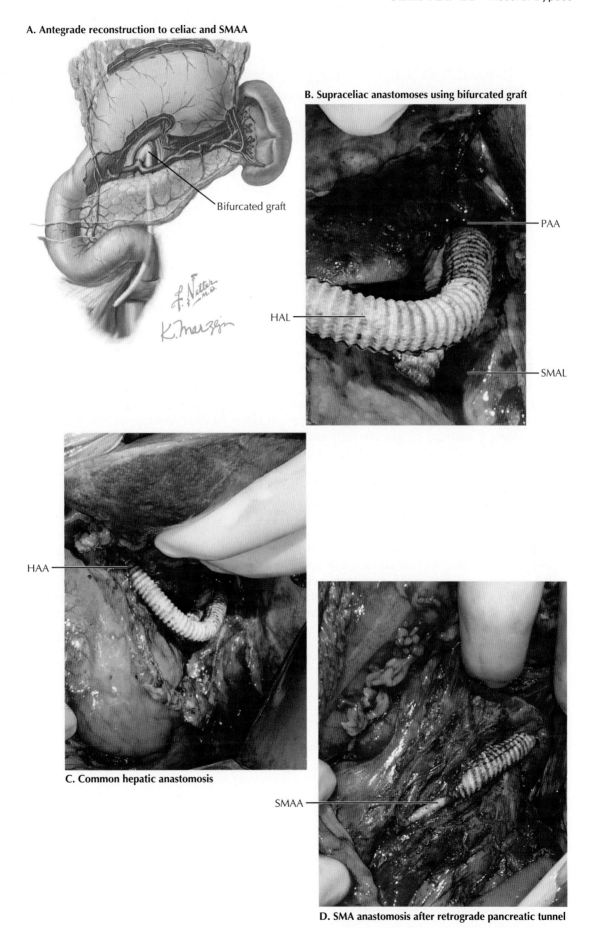

A. Antegrade reconstruction to celiac and SMAA

Bifurcated graft

B. Supraceliac anastomoses using bifurcated graft

PAA

HAL

SMAL

HAA

C. Common hepatic anastomosis

SMAA

D. SMA anastomosis after retrograde pancreatic tunnel

FIGURE 44.3 Tunneling and reconstruction of antegrade mesenteric bypass. *HAA,* Hepatic artery anastomosis; *HAL,* hepatic artery limb; *PAA,* proximal aortic anastomosis; *SMAA,* SMA anastomosis; *SMAL,* SMA limb.

RETROGRADE MESENTERIC BYPASS

The abdomen is entered in a standard fashion, and the colon and small bowel are retracted to expose the retroperitoneum overlying the infrarenal aorta. Classically, the right iliac is used as inflow for a retrograde mesenteric bypass, although the least diseased iliac may be preferred. Alternatively, if anatomy allows, the infrarenal aorta may be used as inflow for a short aorta to SMA bypass. The retroperitoneum over the selected iliac artery is opened with careful attention to the underlying iliac vein. The ligament of Treitz is mobilized to facilitate SMA dissection. With the duodenum mobilized, the root of the small bowel mesentery may be grasped and the SMA palpated (Fig. 44.4). The anterior peritoneum over the SMA is opened and the SMA exposed and dissected. The celiac or common hepatic artery are then exposed in the fashion described earlier.

The most critical aspect of the retrograde bypass is tunneling. The grafts must lay in a gentle C-loop configuration to avoid kinking and undue tension on the anastomosis. The graft is tunneled along the left crus of the diaphragm behind the pancreas and spleen toward the celiac in gentle curve (Fig. 44.4). The tunnel is preserved with a vessel loop or umbilical tape, and the graft is passed through the tunnel. The patient is then heparinized, and the anastomosis to the iliac is then performed with a bifurcated graft. The SMA and celiac anastomoses are performed with attention to the orientation to avoid kinking of the graft. Doppler is used to confirm patency, before the retroperitoneum is then closed to cover the grafts.

A. Opening of the retroperitoneum to expose the infrarenal aorta and iliac arteries

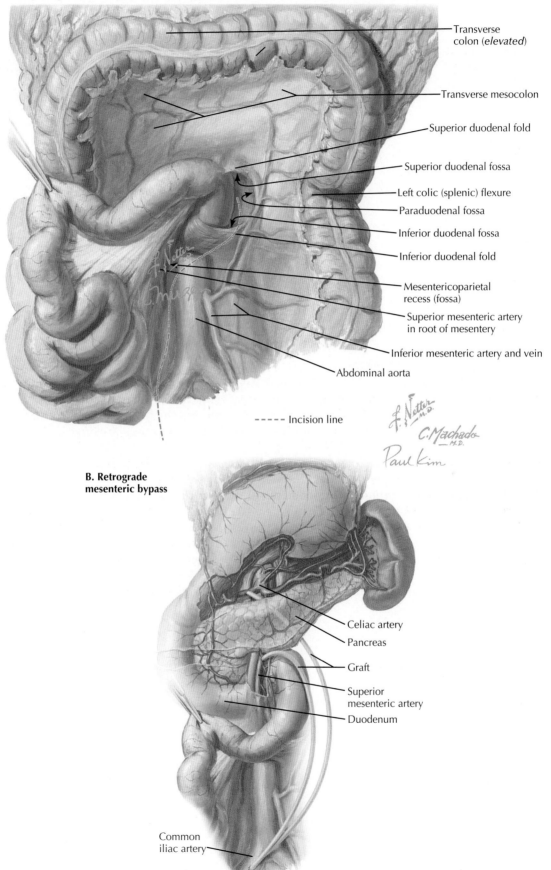

Transverse colon (*elevated*)

Transverse mesocolon

Superior duodenal fold

Superior duodenal fossa

Left colic (splenic) flexure

Paraduodenal fossa

Inferior duodenal fossa

Inferior duodenal fold

Mesentericoparietal recess (fossa)

Superior mesenteric artery in root of mesentery

Inferior mesenteric artery and vein

Abdominal aorta

- - - - - Incision line

B. Retrograde mesenteric bypass

Celiac artery

Pancreas

Graft

Superior mesenteric artery

Duodenum

Common iliac artery

FIGURE 44.4 Retrograde mesenteric bypass.

SUGGESTED READINGS

Celiac and mesenteric arteries. In Wind GG and Valentine RJ editors. Anatomic Exposure in Vascular Surgery, 3rd ed. Philadelphia: Lippincott Williams and Wilkins; 2013.

Coleman DM, Criado E. Arterial bypass for chronic mesenteric ischemic. In Stanley JC, Veith F, Wakefield TW editors. Current Therapy in Vascular and Endovascular Surgery, 5th ed. Saunders; 2014.

McPhee JT, Carruthers TN. Retrograde ilio-SMA and celiac bypass. In: Darling RC and Ozaki CK, editors. Vascular Surgery Arterial Procedures. Philadelphia: Wolters Kluwer; 2016.

Oderich GS, Ribeiro M. Chronic mesenteric arterial disease: clinical evaluation, open surgical and endovascular treatment. In: Sidawy AP and Perler BA, editors. Rutherford's Vascular and Endovascular Therapy. 9th ed. Philadelphia: Elsevier; 2019.

Quinones-Bladrich WJ. Antegrade aorto-SMA and Celiac artery bypass. In: Darling RC and Ozaki CK, editors. Vascular Surgery Arterial Procedures. Philadelphia: Wolters Kluwer; 2016.

Wyers MC, Martin MC. Acute Mesenteric Arterial Disease. In: Sidawy AP and Perler BA, editors. Rutherford's Vascular and Endovascular Therapy. 9th ed. Philadelphia: Elsevier; 2019.

Radiocephalic, Brachiocephalic, and Brachiobasilic Fistula

Abdul Q. Alarhayem and Lee Kirksey

INTRODUCTION

Hemodialysis continues to be the predominant form of renal replacement. Arteriovenous fistulas (AVFs) are the preferred hemodialysis (HD) vascular access. Compared with arteriovenous grafts (AVGs) and tunneled central venous catheters (CVCs), they have lower complication and infection rates, reduced rates of vascular access thrombosis and access-related hospitalizations, and reduced overall health care costs.

Both the 2006 Kidney Disease Outcomes Quality Initiative (KDOQI) and the 2008 Society of Vascular Surgery (SVS) guidelines suggest upper-extremity autogenous access be considered first. Although the "Fistula First" initiative has resulted in a significant increase in the number of autogenous dialysis access created, an unintended consequence has been failure of maturation of up to 50% of AVFs, which in turn has resulted in an increase in concomitant CVC use. This prompted the amendment of the original initiative to "fistula first and catheter last."

PREOPERATIVE EVALUATION

Preoperative evaluation of patients for dialysis access requires a multidisciplinary approach including the patient, the nephrologist, surgeon, and dialysis provider and is best performed with a patient-centered approach to planning.

Timely referral is essential to allow for adequate maturation as well as potential revisions if the access fails to mature. Patients with a glomerular filtration rate (GFR) less than 25 mL/min who opt for HD should be referred for surgical planning and instructed to avoid blood-pressure checks, venipuncture, or peripheral intravenous (IV) placement to preserve vein integrity in the nondominant arm. The preservation of the arm with the most ideal venous anatomy is preferred, hand dominance notwithstanding.

Thorough preoperative planning is essential to creation of a functional dialysis access.

This begins with a detailed history and physical examination. Hand dominance, prior central catheters or pacemakers, history of congestive heart failure, prior chest or arm trauma, and a history of thrombotic episodes should be noted. Diabetes mellitus is more frequently associated with nonmaturation and steal syndrome because of fixed, calcified macrovascular and microvascular disease. Heart failure, particularly diastolic dysfunction, increases the risk of high output failure after access creation. The presence of transvenous pacemakers can create central stenosis, even in the absence of radiographic evidence of such.

The physical exam should assess functionality of the upper extremities, prior failed access, overlying skin conditions, and the strength and symmetry of the brachial, radial, and ulnar pulses. Blood pressure should be measured in both upper extremities. A significant discrepancy may indicate inadequate inflow. Dilated chest wall veins and arm edema should raise suspicion for central venous stenosis or occlusion.

Vein mapping, usually via Doppler ultrasound, is useful in directing the surgical approach and should be performed in all patients before access creation. The diameter of the artery and veins should be more than 2.0 and 2.5 mm, respectively. A comprehensive assessment should note vein diameter, patency, depth, tributaries, and areas of stenosis or thrombosis.

Vein wall fibrosis increases nonmaturation, notwithstanding absolute vein size.

TECHNICAL CONSIDERATIONS

Both SVS and KDOQI recommend that the first access should be placed as far distally as possible to preserve proximal sites for future accesses. In order of preference, the radiocephalic AVF is preferred, followed by the brachiocephalic AVF, and then the transposed brachial-basilic vein fistula. Our practice is to choose the basilic over the cephalic vein in patients who will require superficialization, having found this approach to be associated with a lower rate of nonmaturation.

An AVF is created by anastomosing a vein to the artery. In the end stage kidney disease (ESKD) patient population, this may prove challenging. Tissues are often fragile, arteries may be calcified or diseased, and surgical wounds may heal slowly or poorly. Therefore, meticulous technique, use of fine instruments, and gentle tissue handling are essential to avoid complications. Care must be taken to avoid cautery or retraction trauma to nearby sensorimotor nerves. Minimizing vessel manipulation can reduce vasospasm of artery or vein.

End-to-side or side-to-side AV anastomosis may be performed, although it is thought that the former is associated with a lower incidence of venous hypertension and arterial steal. End-to-side anastomosis to facilitate single-vessel maturation is preferred. Anastomosis diameter must be gauged relative to the size of the inflow artery and outflow vein to allow for adequate inflow for fistula maturation while minimizing the chances of arterial steal from the hand circulation.

Surface venous anatomy varies considerably, particularly near the antecubital fossa; adjustment in placement of the skin incision or use of draining venous side branches may be necessary. To this end, the use of intraoperative ultrasound facilitates incision site selection, enabling adjustment based on vessel size and quality, such that the anastomosis does not incorporate disease vascular structures.

RADIOCEPHALIC FISTULA

The approach for radiocephalic AVF is through a longitudinal skin incision along the anterolateral distal forearm that allows exposure of both the cephalic vein and the radial artery proximal to the flexor retinaculum. If anatomy permits, the anatomic "snuff box" may be used. The cephalic vein should be adequately mobilized and dissected, and small tributaries should be ligated. Once the distal cephalic vein is transected, the vein should be able to lie adjacent to the artery without tension or kinking. An attempt to orient the vein in a directly parallel path to the artery is made. The artery is then controlled proximally and distally. An arteriotomy is then made using a #11 blade scalpel, and extended using Potts' scissors. The vein is then spatulated, and the arteriovenous anastomosis is constructed using 7-0 running polypropylene suture. Upon completion, there should be a thrill at the fistula and a strong radial artery pulse (Fig. 45.1).

The superficial branch of the radial nerve, a small sensory branch, is often identified in the surgical field; excessive traction or transection may cause annoying numbness along the posterior thumb or lateral dorsum of the hand.

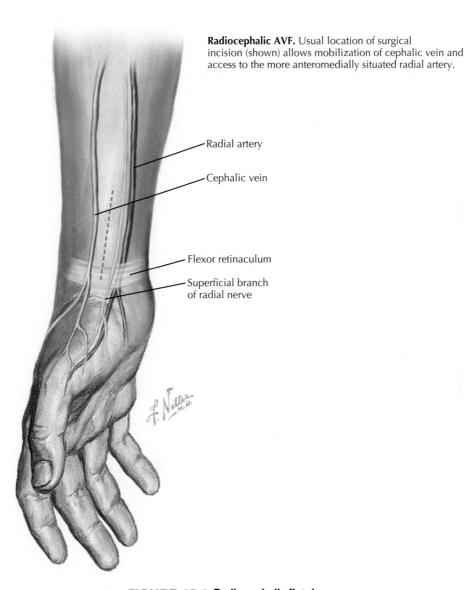

Radiocephalic AVF. Usual location of surgical incision (shown) allows mobilization of cephalic vein and access to the more anteromedially situated radial artery.

Radial artery

Cephalic vein

Flexor retinaculum

Superficial branch of radial nerve

FIGURE 45.1 Radiocephalic fistula.
AVF, Arteriovenous fistula.

BRACHIOCEPHALIC FISTULA

The approach for brachiocephalic AVF is through a transverse or curvilinear skin incision at or just distal to the antecubital crease. In standard anatomy, the cephalic vein is most proximate to the brachial artery below the cutaneous antecubital crease. The cephalic vein must be mobilized sufficiently to deliver it medially and into the deeper plane, where the brachial artery resides. The median antecubital vein represents the distal continuation of the cephalic vein in the antecubital fossa; its branches can be incorporated to create a larger hood for the anastomosis. Attention is then directed to exposure of the brachial artery, which requires incision of the biceps tendinous aponeurosis. Care must be taken to not confuse a high radial artery takeoff for the brachial artery. A smaller-caliber artery encountered in a more superficial location should alert the surgeon to this variation.

Once the brachial artery is dissected, systemic heparin is administered, and the artery is clamped proximally and distally. The anastomosis is constructed using running 6-0 running polypropylene suture. The brachial artery is back-bled and forward-flushed before completion of the anastomosis. There should be a palpable thrill at the fistula and a strong brachial and radial artery pulse (Fig. 45.2A).

The large median nerve is frequently encountered close to the brachial artery, and care should be taken to avoid inadvertent injury. Interruption of sensory nerves such as branches of the lateral or medial antebrachial cutaneous nerves may result in numbness over lateral or medial forearm, respectively (Fig. 45.2B).

BRACHIOBASILIC FISTULA

The basilic vein, often inaccessible with venipuncture, can be a good choice in patients with failed radiocephalic or brachiocephalic AVFs, or in those without suitable cephalic or median cubital veins. Its medial and deep location protects it from venipuncture but requires its transposition to a more superficial and anterior location for comfortable arm position during cannulation and to mitigate inadvertent brachial artery puncture in thin patients.

One may choose to construct a basilic vein transposition in one or two stages. There is evidence to suggest that the two-stage procedure achieves higher maturation rates, especially if the basilic vein is small.

The first stage involves creating a brachiobasilic fistula at the elbow. Once the vein matures sufficiently, usually at around 6 weeks, the vein is then transposed or superficialized. The site of the skin incision is based on arterial and basilic/antecubital surface venous anatomy.

Whether done in one or two stages, the basilic vein is harvested from the antecubital fossa up to its entry into the axillary vein via continuous or split incisions along the medial arm. Side branches are divided between ligatures. The medial antebrachial cutaneous nerve and its branches are often entwined around the basilic vein. Avoiding injury to this nerve often requires dividing the basilic vein and delivering it from under the nerve branch.

A tunnel is then created along the anterolateral aspect of the upper arm from the antecubital area to the axillary fossa using a curved tunneler. The vein is passed into the tunnel with great care taken to avoid kinking it. After systemic heparinization, the anastomosis is constructed between the spatulated end of the vein and the brachial artery (Fig. 45.2C).

Alternatively, the basilic vein may be superficialized by approximating the subcutaneous tissue below the vein without tunneling it. The advantages to this approach compared with transposition include avoidance of vein kinking (at the swing-point) and tunnel bleeding.

The vein, however, may lie immediately beneath the skin incision and thus may be vulnerable if the wound were to break down. This can be avoided by elevating skin flaps and creating a subcutaneous pocket.

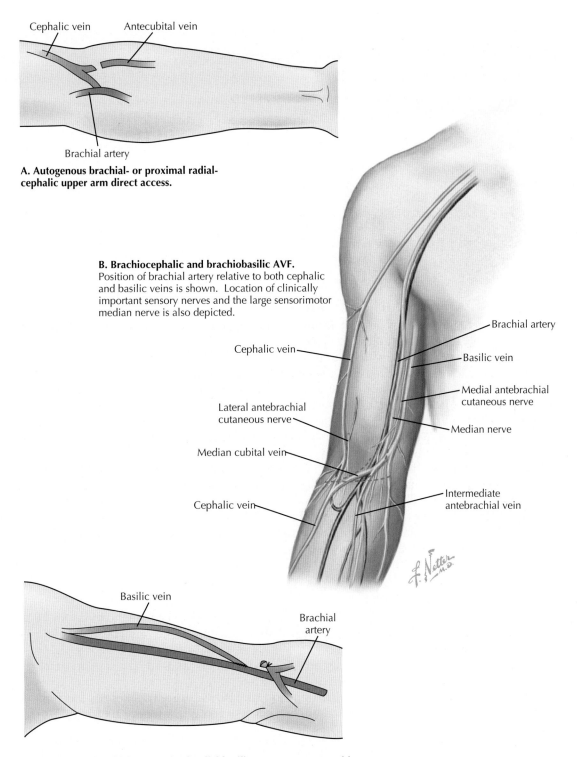

Cephalic vein   Antecubital vein

Brachial artery

A. Autogenous brachial- or proximal radial-cephalic upper arm direct access.

B. Brachiocephalic and brachiobasilic AVF.
Position of brachial artery relative to both cephalic and basilic veins is shown. Location of clinically important sensory nerves and the large sensorimotor median nerve is also depicted.

Brachial artery

Cephalic vein

Basilic vein

Medial antebrachial cutaneous nerve

Lateral antebrachial cutaneous nerve

Median nerve

Median cubital vein

Cephalic vein

Intermediate antebrachial vein

Basilic vein

Brachial artery

C. Autogenous brachial- or proximal radial-basilic upper arm transposition.

FIGURE 45.2 **Brachiocephalic fistula, vascular and nerve anatomy of the upper extremity, and basilica vein transposition.**

AVF, Arteriovenous fistula.

(A and C reused with permission from Macsata RA, Sidawy AN. Hemodialysis Access: General Considerations and Strategies to Optimize Access Placement. In Sidaway AN, Perler BA, eds. Rutherford's Vascular Surgery and Endovascular Therapy. Elsevier; 2018; Chapter 175, pp 2288-2299, Figures 175-9 and 175-10.)

POSTOPERATIVE MONITORING

A mature, functional fistula is defined as one that has adequate blood flow to support dialysis and is large and superficial enough for successful repetitive cannulation. The "Rule of 6s" is often cited; at 6 weeks postcreation, the fistula should be at least 6 mm in diameter, 6 cm in length, no more than 0.6 cm deep, and the blood flow rate should be at least 600 mL/min. The reasons for failure of an AVF to mature include stenosis at the arterial anastomosis, outflow vein narrowing, or large side branches. Aggressive management of these conditions may assist with successful maturation.

The KDOQI and SVS Clinical Practice Guidelines recommend regular monitoring (i.e., via physical exam) and surveillance (flow or venous pressure) to detect access dysfunction. Timely detection of dysfunction is crucial to preventing complications and loss of access. Arm edema and dilated veins suggest a central venous stenosis. A strong thrill/bruit throughout the access during both systole and diastole indicates good flow, whereas a weak thrill, or one felt only during systole, indicates poor flow. Failure of the fistula to collapse when the arm is elevated and lack of pulse augmentation are also suggestive of underlying stenosis. Difficulty with cannulation, inability to achieve target dialysis blood flow or delivered dialysis dose, and prolonged bleeding from needle puncture sites should prompt further investigation.

SUGGESTED READINGS

Found NK. KDOQI clinical practice guidelines and clinical practice recommendations for 2006 updates: hemodialysis adequacy, peritoneal dialysis adequacy and vascular access. Am J Kidney Dis 2006;48(Suppl. 1):S1–322.

Rodriguez A, Shalhub S. Hemodialysis access: fundamentals and advanced management. Hemodialysis Access. Cham: Springer; 2017. p. 281–8.

Sidawy AN, et al. The Society for Vascular Surgery: clinical practice guidelines for the surgical placement and maintenance of arteriovenous hemodialysis access. J Vasc Surg 2008;48(5):S2–25.

Femoral Endarterectomy and Femoral Popliteal Bypass

Christopher J. Smolock and Keith Glover

INTRODUCTION

Lower-extremity peripheral arterial disease (PAD) symptoms range from asymptomatic to claudication, which may be lifestyle limiting, to chronic limb-threatening ischemia consisting of rest pain and/or tissue loss. The usual minimum threshold for treatment is lifestyle-limiting claudication. However, this is considered on a case-by-case basis because this stage of PAD is not limb threatening. Chronic limb-threatening ischemia, as the name suggests, mandates treatment. Although the use of endovascular treatment for PAD has been consistently increasing, there remain some patients and situations that are best treated with open surgery. This chapter describes three common, open infrainguinal procedures to treat PAD. These procedures are commonly termed *femoral endarterectomy, femoral to above-knee popliteal artery bypass,* and *femoral to below-knee popliteal artery bypass.* In these cases, "femoral" often refers to the common femoral artery (CFA), which is typically the focus of the endarterectomy and the origin of the bypasses. Femoral endarterectomy is sometimes performed concomitantly with a bypass to the popliteal artery.

ANATOMY AND TOPOGRAPHIC LANDMARKS

The CFA, contiguous with the external iliac artery, begins at the inguinal ligament and continues in the upper anterior thigh until it branches into the superficial femoral artery (SFA) and profunda femoris artery (PFA) (Fig. 46.1). The CFA resides in the femoral canal, which has lateral, medial, and superior borders of the sartorius, adductor longus, and the inguinal ligament, respectively. The mnemonic NAVEL refers to these structures deep to the inguinal ligament, from lateral to medial: femoral Nerve, common femoral Artery (CFA), common femoral Vein (CFV), Empty space in femoral canal containing lymph vessels and lymph nodes, and lacunar Ligament (see Fig. 46.1).

The popliteal artery begins at the adductor hiatus, where the passage of the femoral vessels from anterior to posterior thigh occurs between the adductor magnus muscle and the femur. This is the termination of the adductor, or Hunter's canal. The popliteal artery continues behind the knee, coursing through the popliteal fossa (defined by four borders: semimembranosus, biceps femoris, medial head of the gastrocnemius, and lateral head of the gastrocnemius), ending at the lower border of the popliteus muscle, where it branches into the anterior tibial artery and the tibioperoneal trunk (see Fig. 46.1).

COMMON FEMORAL ARTERY EXPOSURE

With the patient in the supine position, the femoral artery is located at the medial one-third of the span of the inguinal ligament, which runs from the anterior superior iliac spine (ASIS) to the pubic tubercle (see Fig. 46.1). A vertical or oblique incision is made overlying this area, starting just caudad to the inguinal ligament. The incision is deepened through the Camper's and Scarpa's fascia to reveal the superficial inguinal lymphatics. Once the lymphatic tissue is carefully divided and ligated, to decrease the risk of future lymphocele formation, the fascia lata is encountered. The fascia lata is opened vertically on the medial border of the sartorius muscle and the sartorius muscle is retracted laterally. The proximal aspect of the incision is extended cephalad to the inguinal ligament, which is freed up from the surrounding tissue. At this point, the femoral sheath is identified at the bottom of the incision and opened vertically on top of the CFA. Once the femoral sheath is open, the CFA should be dissected out from the surrounding tissue. The proximal extent of the CFA dissection is above the inferior epigastric and lateral circumflex vessels, which are located under the inguinal ligament. When exposing the proximal CFA, the surgeon must take care to identify and ligate the deep circumflex iliac vein, colloquially termed the "vein of sorrow" or "vein of pain." Once the CFA is exposed, it can be controlled with a vessel loop. The distal extent of the exposure should be beyond the distal extent of disease, which may be at the proximal SFA or PFA or 10 cm down the SFA or to second- or third-order PFA branches. The origins of the SFA and PFA are identified at the distal CFA by a caliber decrease. The PFA is usually found posterior and lateral to the distal CFA. During the PFA dissection, care is taken to identify and ligate the lateral femoral circumflex vein that crosses over the proximal portion of this artery. When exposing the second- and third-order PDA branches, the surgeon encounters small profunda veins and ligates them, but the main profunda vein should be spared. When the SFA and PFA are exposed beyond the distal extent of disease, they are controlled with vessel loops.

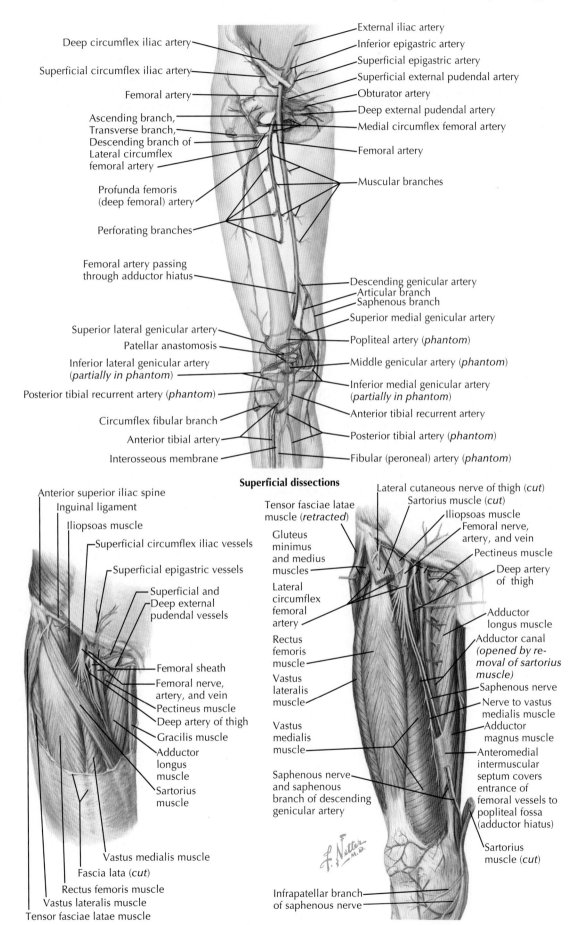

Deep circumflex iliac artery

Superficial circumflex iliac artery

Femoral artery

Ascending branch,
Transverse branch,
Descending branch of
Lateral circumflex
femoral artery

Profunda femoris
(deep femoral) artery

Perforating branches

Femoral artery passing
through adductor hiatus

Superior lateral genicular artery

Patellar anastomosis

Inferior lateral genicular artery
(partially in phantom)

Posterior tibial recurrent artery (phantom)

Circumflex fibular branch

Anterior tibial artery

Interosseous membrane

External iliac artery

Inferior epigastric artery

Superficial epigastric artery

Superficial external pudendal artery

Obturator artery

Deep external pudendal artery

Medial circumflex femoral artery

Femoral artery

Muscular branches

Descending genicular artery
Articular branch
Saphenous branch

Superior medial genicular artery

Popliteal artery (phantom)

Middle genicular artery (phantom)

Inferior medial genicular artery
(partially in phantom)

Anterior tibial recurrent artery

Posterior tibial artery (phantom)

Fibular (peroneal) artery (phantom)

Superficial dissections

Anterior superior iliac spine

Inguinal ligament

Iliopsoas muscle

Superficial circumflex iliac vessels

Superficial epigastric vessels

Superficial and
Deep external
pudendal vessels

Femoral sheath

Femoral nerve,
artery, and vein

Pectineus muscle

Deep artery of thigh

Gracilis muscle

Adductor
longus
muscle

Sartorius
muscle

Vastus medialis muscle

Fascia lata (cut)

Rectus femoris muscle

Vastus lateralis muscle

Tensor fasciae latae muscle

Tensor fasciae latae
muscle (retracted)

Gluteus
minimus
and medius
muscles

Lateral
circumflex
femoral
artery

Rectus
femoris
muscle

Vastus
lateralis
muscle

Vastus
medialis
muscle

Saphenous nerve
and saphenous
branch of descending
genicular artery

Lateral cutaneous nerve of thigh (cut)

Sartorius muscle (cut)

Iliopsoas muscle

Femoral nerve,
artery, and vein

Pectineus muscle

Deep artery
of thigh

Adductor
longus muscle

Adductor canal
(opened by re-
moval of sartorius
muscle)

Saphenous nerve

Nerve to vastus
medialis muscle

Adductor
magnus muscle

Anteromedial
intermuscular
septum covers
entrance of
femoral vessels to
popliteal fossa
(adductor hiatus)

Sartorius
muscle (cut)

Infrapatellar branch
of saphenous nerve

FIGURE 46.1 Arteries and nerves of thigh and knee.

ENDARTERECTOMY AND PATCH ANGIOPLASTY

Control of the CFA is obtained proximally at the external iliac artery just under the inguinal ligament and distally at the SFA and PFA past the level of disease, which may be 10 cm down the SFA or to second- or third-order PFA branches or both. A longitudinal arteriotomy is made on the anterior aspect of the CFA and carried down to the SFA or PFA, and in some cases both, past the distal extent of disease. The atherosclerotic plaque is removed in a layer between the intima and media. Any remaining intimal flaps are tacked with monofilament suture. The arteriotomy is then closed with patch angioplasty (Fig. 46.2A). Common patches include autologous vein, such as greater saphenous vein (GSV), or prosthetic materials such as Dacron, PTFE (polytetrafluoroethylene), or bovine pericardium.

SUPRAGENICULATE POPLITEAL ARTERY EXPOSURE

The patient is placed in the supine position with the hip externally rotated and the knee slightly bent. A rolled-up towel or "bump" may be placed below the knee to aid in exposure. An incision is made on the distal medial thigh and anterior to the sartorius muscle (Fig. 46.2B). The sartorius is then retracted posteriorly and the vastus medialis anteriorly, revealing the fascial bridge connecting the abductor magnus and semimembranosus. Opening this fascial bridge gains access to the popliteal fossa above the knee (Fig. 46.2C). The artery is then carefully dissected out and controlled with vessel loops. The popliteal vein is often duplicated in this location, but venous anatomy can be variable.

A. Femoral endartectomy with greater saphenous vein (GSV) patch angioplasty

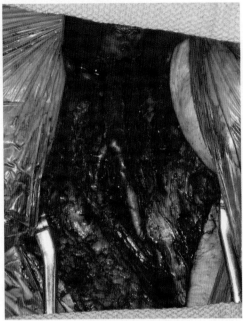

B. Knee: medial view

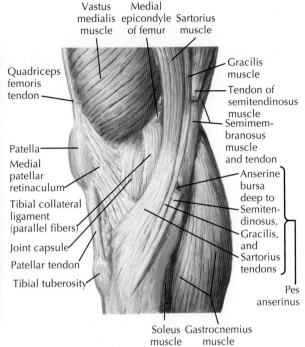

Vastus medialis muscle
Medial epicondyle of femur
Sartorius muscle
Quadriceps femoris tendon
Gracilis muscle
Tendon of semitendinosus muscle
Semimembranosus muscle and tendon
Patella
Medial patellar retinaculum
Anserine bursa deep to Semitendinosus, Gracilis, and Sartorius tendons
Tibial collateral ligament (parallel fibers)
Joint capsule
Patellar tendon
Tibial tuberosity
Pes anserinus
Soleus muscle
Gastrocnemius muscle

C. Cross-sectional anatomy of thigh

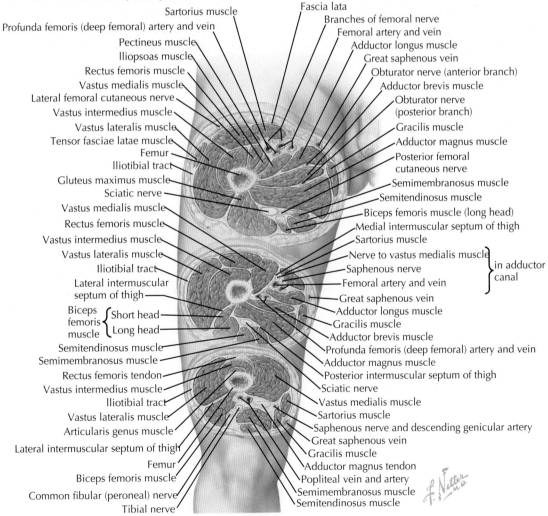

Sartorius muscle
Profunda femoris (deep femoral) artery and vein
Pectineus muscle
Iliopsoas muscle
Rectus femoris muscle
Vastus medialis muscle
Lateral femoral cutaneous nerve
Vastus intermedius muscle
Vastus lateralis muscle
Tensor fasciae latae muscle
Femur
Iliotibial tract
Gluteus maximus muscle
Sciatic nerve
Vastus medialis muscle
Rectus femoris muscle
Vastus intermedius muscle
Vastus lateralis muscle
Iliotibial tract
Lateral intermuscular septum of thigh
Biceps femoris muscle { Short head / Long head }
Semitendinosus muscle
Semimembranosus muscle
Rectus femoris tendon
Vastus intermedius muscle
Iliotibial tract
Vastus lateralis muscle
Articularis genus muscle
Lateral intermuscular septum of thigh
Femur
Biceps femoris muscle
Common fibular (peroneal) nerve
Tibial nerve

Fascia lata
Branches of femoral nerve
Femoral artery and vein
Adductor longus muscle
Great saphenous vein
Obturator nerve (anterior branch)
Adductor brevis muscle
Obturator nerve (posterior branch)
Gracilis muscle
Adductor magnus muscle
Posterior femoral cutaneous nerve
Semimembranosus muscle
Semitendinosus muscle
Biceps femoris muscle (long head)
Medial intermuscular septum of thigh
Sartorius muscle
Nerve to vastus medialis muscle
Saphenous nerve
Femoral artery and vein
Great saphenous vein
Adductor longus muscle
Gracilis muscle
Adductor brevis muscle
Profunda femoris (deep femoral) artery and vein
Adductor magnus muscle
Posterior intermuscular septum of thigh
Sciatic nerve
Vastus medialis muscle
Sartorius muscle
Saphenous nerve and descending genicular artery
Great saphenous vein
Gracilis muscle
Adductor magnus tendon
Popliteal vein and artery
Semimembranosus muscle
Semitendinosus muscle

} in adductor canal

FIGURE 46.2 Anatomy of the knee and thigh.

INFRAGENICULATE POPLITEAL ARTERY EXPOSURE

The patient is placed in the supine position with the hip externally rotated and the knee slightly bent. A rolled-up towel or "bump" may be placed above the knee to aid in exposure. An incision is made on the medial lower leg, one fingerbreadth posterior to the tibia extending from the tibial plateau to approximately one-third down the length of the leg (Fig. 46.3A). The GSV lies in this approximate location, and care should be taken to preserve it during this dissection. Incising the crural fascia overlying the gastrocnemius and retracting the muscle posteriorly gains access to the popliteal fossa. Keep in mind that this dissection starts cranial to the soleus muscle. Exposure can be extended proximally by dividing the pes anserinus (sartorius, gracilis, and semitendinosus) (see Fig. 46.2B) and distally by releasing the soleus muscle from the tibia. The artery is then dissected away from the vein, which is commonly encountered first during this exposure, and controlled with vessel loops.

BYPASS CONDUITS

Common bypass conduits are autologous, GSV as well as arm vein, homografts such as cadaveric vein, and prosthetic materials such as PTFE and Dacron. Each conduit has its benefits and drawbacks. In general, ipsilateral GSV is preferred followed by contralateral GSV.

TUNNELING

Once the proximal and distal arterial targets are identified and prepared, the bypass conduit must be tunneled between the above incisions. Tunneling can be done in an anatomic or subcutaneous plane. In most cases, anatomic tunneling is preferred because it requires a shorter conduit and has muscle coverage. During the anatomic femoral to above-knee popliteal bypass, the bypass conduit is passed from the femoral incision through the femoral canal, which is located under the sartorius muscle to the suprageniculate popliteal artery incision (see Figs. 46.1 and 46.3B). The anatomic femoral to below-knee popliteal bypass can be done in either one or two steps. During the one-step tunneling, the bypass graft is tunneled from the femoral incision to the infrageniculate popliteal artery incision, through the femoral canal and in between the two heads of the gastrocnemius muscle (see Fig. 46.3B). In the two-step tunneling, the bypass graft is first tunneled from the femoral incision to the suprageniculate popliteal and subsequently tunneled to the infrageniculate popliteal artery incision.

A. Cross-Section of the Leg: Axial View

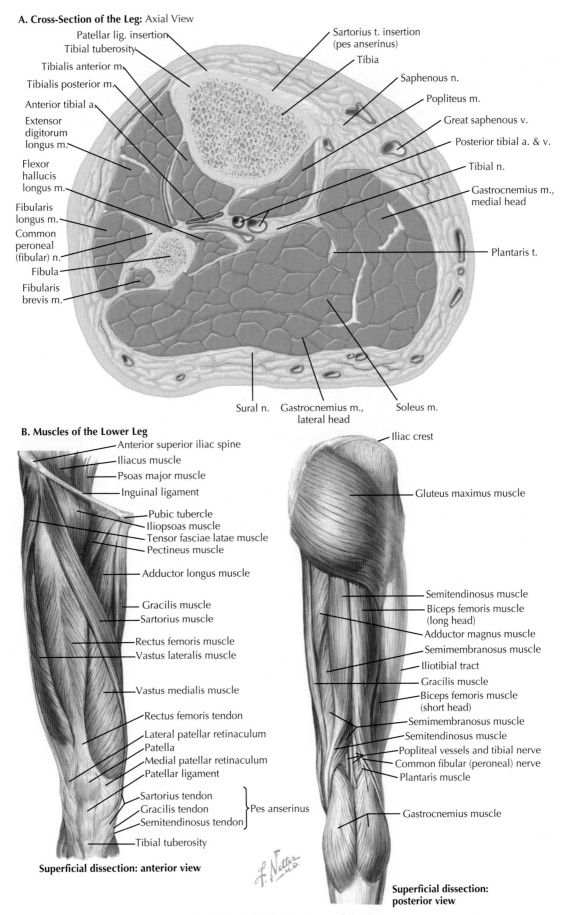

Patellar lig. insertion
Tibial tuberosity
Tibialis anterior m.
Tibialis posterior m.
Anterior tibial a.
Extensor digitorum longus m.
Flexor hallucis longus m.
Fibularis longus m.
Common peroneal (fibular) n.
Fibula
Fibularis brevis m.

Sartorius t. insertion (pes anserinus)
Tibia
Saphenous n.
Popliteus m.
Great saphenous v.
Posterior tibial a. & v.
Tibial n.
Gastrocnemius m., medial head
Plantaris t.

Sural n.   Gastrocnemius m., lateral head   Soleus m.

B. Muscles of the Lower Leg

Anterior superior iliac spine
Iliacus muscle
Psoas major muscle
Inguinal ligament
Pubic tubercle
Iliopsoas muscle
Tensor fasciae latae muscle
Pectineus muscle
Adductor longus muscle
Gracilis muscle
Sartorius muscle
Rectus femoris muscle
Vastus lateralis muscle
Vastus medialis muscle
Rectus femoris tendon
Lateral patellar retinaculum
Patella
Medial patellar retinaculum
Patellar ligament
Sartorius tendon
Gracilis tendon   } Pes anserinus
Semitendinosus tendon
Tibial tuberosity

Superficial dissection: anterior view

Iliac crest
Gluteus maximus muscle
Semitendinosus muscle
Biceps femoris muscle (long head)
Adductor magnus muscle
Semimembranosus muscle
Iliotibial tract
Gracilis muscle
Biceps femoris muscle (short head)
Semimembranosus muscle
Semitendinosus muscle
Popliteal vessels and tibial nerve
Common fibular (peroneal) nerve
Plantaris muscle
Gastrocnemius muscle

Superficial dissection: posterior view

FIGURE 46.3 Anatomy of the leg.

SUGGESTED READINGS

Adam DJ, Beard JD, Cleveland T, Bell J, Bradbury AW, Forbes JF, Storkey H. Bypass versus angioplasty in severe ischaemia of the leg (BASIL): multicentre, randomised controlled trial. Lancet 2005;366(9501):1925–34. https://doi.org/10.1016/s0140-6736(05)67704-5.

Ambler GK, Twine CP. Graft type for femoro-popliteal bypass surgery. Cochrane Database Syst Rev 2018;2:Cd001487. https://doi.org/10.1002/14651858.CD001487.pub3.

Anton S, Perler B. Rutherford's Vascular Surgery and Endovascular Therapy. 9th ed. Philadelphia, PA: Elsevier; 2018. pp.1438–1462 [Chapter 109].

Conte MS. Bypass versus Angioplasty in Severe Ischaemia of the Leg (BASIL) and the (hoped for) dawn of evidence-based treatment for advanced limb ischemia. J Vasc Surg 2010;51(5 Suppl):69s–75s. https://doi.org/10.1016/j.jvs.2010.02.001.

Norgren L, Hiatt WR, Dormandy JA, Nehler MR, Harris KA, Fowkes FG. Inter-Society Consensus for the Management of Peripheral Arterial Disease (TASC II). J Vasc Surg 2007;45(Suppl. S):S5–67. https://doi.org/10.1016/j.jvs.2006.12.037.

Femoral Tibial Bypass

Sean P. Steenberge and Francis J. Caputo

INTRODUCTION

Infrainguinal arterial bypasses are major arterial reconstructions with the proximal anastomotic site below the inguinal ligament that are commonly used in the setting of chronic limb-threatening ischemia manifested by rest pain and/or tissue loss. The goal of these reconstructions is to provide inline arterial flow below the level(s) of the significant arterial stenosis or arterial occlusion. When a bypass is considered, it is imperative to evaluate the arterial inflow, bypass conduit, and arterial outflow to determine an operative plan that will optimize distal arterial perfusion and bypass graft patency. These bypasses can be created using autogenous, prosthetic, or cadaveric conduits, which have varying long-term patencies depending on the arterial inflow, site of distal bypass insertion, and arterial outflow. In this chapter, we focus on the anatomic exposure and techniques used for femoral artery to tibial arterial bypasses.

FEMORAL–POSTERIOR TIBIAL

Adequate exposure of the proximal anastomotic site is imperative to ensuring a successful infrainguinal arterial bypass. This typically involves exposure of the common femoral artery, but the profunda femoris artery may also be used when trying to avoid the common femoral artery because of infection or to avoid a reoperative field. The superficial femoral artery is often too diseased to allow it to be a suitable candidate for the proximal anastomotic site of a femoral-tibial bypass, but it may be used in some settings, if necessary. For this chapter, we focus on exposure of the common femoral artery and profunda femoris arteries.

FEMORAL–POSTERIOR TIBIAL (Continued)

First, the patient is placed in the supine position. After the patient is shaved and prepped from the level of the umbilicus through the foot, the common femoral artery exposure is typically achieved through a vertical incision directly over the femoral pulse with two-thirds of the incision below the inguinal ligament and one-third of the incision above the inguinal ligament. The inguinal ligament is identified via a straight line from the anterior superior iliac spine to the pubic tubercle. The common femoral artery is usually approximately two fingerbreadths from the pubic tubercle. When there is no palpable pulse, a continuous-wave Doppler can be used to assist with identification of the femoral artery location. If there is no Doppler signal, the vertical incision should be made just medial to the middle of the inguinal ligament. Typically the diseased vessel can be palpated by rolling fingers over the location to feel the hardened longitudinal tube structure through the skin. Oblique incisions may be used because they may decrease wound complications, but these typically limit the exposure needed for bypass creation. If any oblique incision is to be made, it is parallel and just above the groin crease. Once the incision has been made, the incision is deepened through the Camper's and Scarpa's fascia. At this point, the superficial inguinal lymph node lymphatics as well as the superficial epigastric and superficial circumflex iliac vessels are encountered. Lymphatic tissue should be carefully divided and ligated to decrease the risk of future lymphocele formation. One may also divide the superficial epigastric and circumflex iliac vessels when deepening the incision toward the common femoral artery. Once the lymphatic tissue has been divided, the fascia lata is encountered.

The fascia lata is opened vertically on the medial border of the sartorius muscle. The sartorius muscle is retracted laterally, and the proximal aspect of the incision is extended cephalad until the inguinal ligament is identified. Once identified, the inguinal ligament is freed up from the surrounding tissue. At this point, the femoral sheath is identified at the bottom of the incision and opened vertically on top of the common femoral artery. Once the femoral sheath is open, the common femoral artery should be dissected out from the surrounding areolar tissue to allow for arterial control to be obtained. When attempting to obtain proximal common femoral artery control, the surgeon must try to identify the deep circumflex iliac vein, commonly referred to as the "vein of sorrow" or "vein of pain," which usually crosses the very proximal common femoral artery or distal external iliac artery. Identification and ligation of this vein allow for more proximal arterial control, but its ligation can also help avoid significant venous bleeding that can be difficult to control during the initial or a subsequent common femoral artery exposure. A right angle can be used to pass a silicone vessel loop twice around the proximal aspect of the vessel to ensure adequate proximal arterial control has been achieved. The common femoral vein is immediately medial to the common femoral artery, and conscientious care should be taken to avoid inadvertent injury to the vessel during dissection and while obtaining control of the common femoral artery (Fig. 47.1). After obtaining proximal common femoral artery control, the surgeon uses dissection along the anterior surface of the common femoral artery until a caliber change is noted in the artery. This approach helps to avoid injury to the profunda femoris artery and branches off the common femoral artery. The caliber change in the common femoral artery identifies where the common femoral artery bifurcates into the profunda femoris artery and superficial femoral artery.

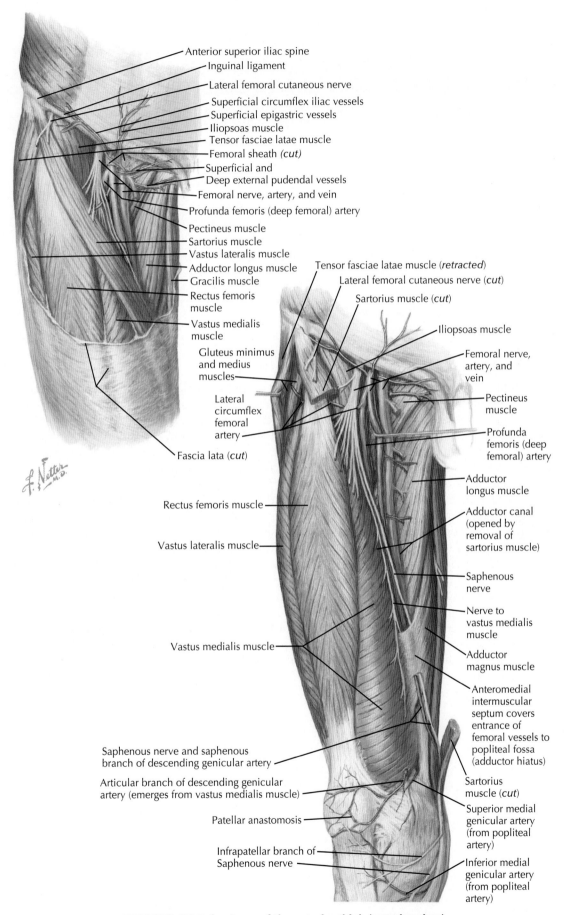

Anterior superior iliac spine

Inguinal ligament

Lateral femoral cutaneous nerve

Superficial circumflex iliac vessels

Superficial epigastric vessels

Iliopsoas muscle

Tensor fasciae latae muscle

Femoral sheath *(cut)*

Superficial and

Deep external pudendal vessels

Femoral nerve, artery, and vein

Profunda femoris (deep femoral) artery

Pectineus muscle

Sartorius muscle

Vastus lateralis muscle

Adductor longus muscle

Gracilis muscle

Rectus femoris muscle

Vastus medialis muscle

Tensor fasciae latae muscle *(retracted)*

Lateral femoral cutaneous nerve *(cut)*

Sartorius muscle *(cut)*

Iliopsoas muscle

Femoral nerve, artery, and vein

Gluteus minimus and medius muscles

Lateral circumflex femoral artery

Pectineus muscle

Profunda femoris (deep femoral) artery

Fascia lata *(cut)*

Rectus femoris muscle

Vastus lateralis muscle

Adductor longus muscle

Adductor canal (opened by removal of sartorius muscle)

Saphenous nerve

Nerve to vastus medialis muscle

Vastus medialis muscle

Adductor magnus muscle

Anteromedial intermuscular septum covers entrance of femoral vessels to popliteal fossa (adductor hiatus)

Saphenous nerve and saphenous branch of descending genicular artery

Articular branch of descending genicular artery (emerges from vastus medialis muscle)

Patellar anastomosis

Sartorius muscle *(cut)*

Superior medial genicular artery (from popliteal artery)

Infrapatellar branch of Saphenous nerve

Inferior medial genicular artery (from popliteal artery)

FIGURE 47.1 Anatomy of the anterior thigh (anterior view).

FEMORAL–POSTERIOR TIBIAL (Continued)

The profunda femoris artery typically is identified posterior and lateral to the common femoral artery. During the isolation of the profunda femoris artery, it is imperative to avoid injuring the lateral femoral circumflex vein, which often crosses anterior to the proximal aspect of the profunda femoris artery and can be easily injured during dissection. Dissection of the profunda femoris artery should be extended distal to the extent of arterial disease to allow for potential endarterectomy of the artery, if needed. This may require dissection of the profunda femoris artery to its second or third order, but it is crucial to ensure that the surgeon performs the anastomosis to a disease-free vessel. For dissections that require extension to the second or third order of the profunda femoris artery, it is imperative to identify the main profunda femoris vein and avoid its ligation because there will be many small crossing veins at this level that will likely require ligation for adequate exposure of distal profunda femoris artery. For details on femoral endarterectomy, see Chapter 46, Femoral Endarterectomy and Femoral Popliteal Bypass. After the profunda femoris is controlled with a silicone vessel loop, the superficial femoral artery can be dissected out to control the proximal portion of the artery with a silicone vessel loop (Fig. 47.2A). Care should be taken to obtain control of all branches off the common femoral artery before opening the common femoral artery because there can be significant back bleeding from uncontrolled branches (Fig. 47.2B). Once adequate control of the common femoral artery has been obtained, a moistened sponge can be placed into the incision, and attention can be turned to the posterior tibial artery dissection.

A. Profunda femoris artery control

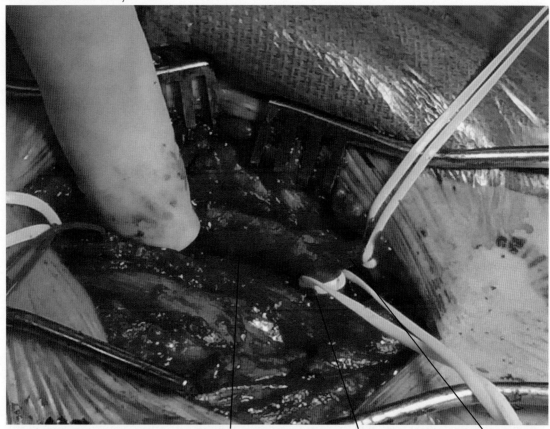

Common femoral artery   Profunda femoris artery   Superficial femoris artery

B. Common femoral artery control

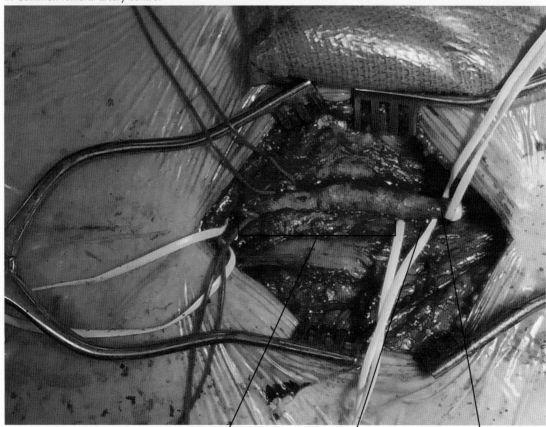

Common femoral artery   Profunda femoris artery   Superficial femoris artery

FIGURE 47.2 Profunda femoris artery control and common femoral artery control.

FEMORAL–POSTERIOR TIBIAL (Continued)

The posterior tibial artery is located in the deep posterior compartment and can often be exposed in the mid-lower leg via a medial approach (Fig. 47.3A). A rolled-up towel should be used as a lateral support ("bump") behind a partially flexed (45 to 60 degrees) and externally rotated knee to assist with visualization. After identifying the posterior aspect of the tibia, an approximately 10-cm incision is made 1 fingerbreadth (~2 cm) below the tibia. This incision is deepened until the crural fascia is reached. At this point the crural fascia is incised in the same direction as the incision. Next, the soleal attachments to the tibia are encountered and subsequently freed up with a combination of blunt and sharp dissection. The soleus is then retracted posteriorly, and blunt dissection is used to create a plane between the soleus and flexor digitorum longus muscles. Within this created plane, the posterior tibial artery can be identified with surrounding areolar tissue and venous branches crossing the artery. These veins can be ligated and divided, as needed, to create an adequate length of exposure for the bypass. At this point, the posterior tibial artery can be encircled proximally and distally with silicone vessel loops to obtain adequate control of the vessel (Fig. 47.3B). Another technique for distal tibial artery control is through the use of a tourniquet that should be applied to the thigh. One advantage of using a tourniquet is that it avoids the need for extensive dissection of the tibial artery to obtain adequate control of the vessel. Decreasing the extent of the dissection results in a lower risk of vein injury and bleeding while dissecting the numerous venous branches that cross over the artery.

Sometimes the conduit length for the bypass requires that a femoral artery to posterior tibial artery be performed to the proximal posterior tibial artery. Although the dissection to the mid-posterior tibial artery is easier, the proximal posterior tibial artery can be exposed in a similar fashion to the mid-posterior tibial artery. With the patient's leg partially flexed (45 to 60 degrees) and externally rotated with the support of a "bump," a 10-cm vertical incision that starts just below the knee is made one fingerbreadth (~2 cm) below the tibia. The incision is deepened until the crural fascia is reached and then incised in the same manner as the incision. During the dissection, one must be mindful to avoid injuring the great saphenous vein that runs through this region. With the crural fascia incised, the medial of the gastrocnemius muscle is identified and retracted posteriorly, exposing the distal popliteal artery and soleus muscle. At this point, the soleal attachments to the tibia are divided carefully, exposing the proximal anterior tibial artery and tibioperoneal artery trunk. As more of the soleal attachments are freed, the proximal posterior tibial artery is identified usually 2 to 3 cm from the takeoff of the anterior tibial artery, and a disease-free area is dissected free. At this point, the posterior tibial artery can be encircled proximally and distally with silicone vessel loops, or a tourniquet can be used for arterial control, as described above. Again, the surgeon must be careful during the dissection to avoid injury to the numerous crossing veins that overly the artery with its usually paired veins.

A. Cross section just above middle of leg

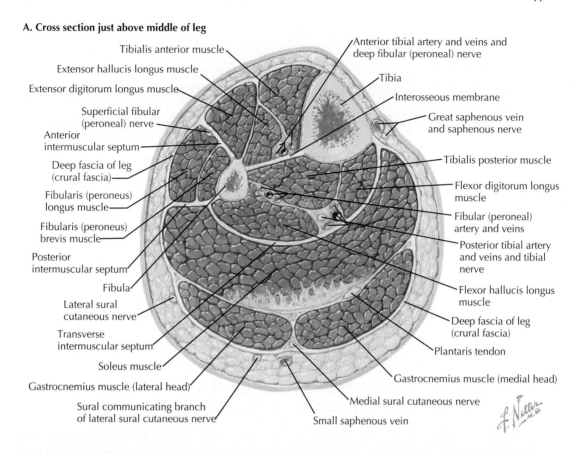

Tibialis anterior muscle

Extensor hallucis longus muscle

Extensor digitorum longus muscle

Superficial fibular (peroneal) nerve

Anterior intermuscular septum

Deep fascia of leg (crural fascia)

Fibularis (peroneus) longus muscle

Fibularis (peroneus) brevis muscle

Posterior intermuscular septum

Fibula

Lateral sural cutaneous nerve

Transverse intermuscular septum

Soleus muscle

Gastrocnemius muscle (lateral head)

Sural communicating branch of lateral sural cutaneous nerve

Anterior tibial artery and veins and deep fibular (peroneal) nerve

Tibia

Interosseous membrane

Great saphenous vein and saphenous nerve

Tibialis posterior muscle

Flexor digitorum longus muscle

Fibular (peroneal) artery and veins

Posterior tibial artery and veins and tibial nerve

Flexor hallucis longus muscle

Deep fascia of leg (crural fascia)

Plantaris tendon

Gastrocnemius muscle (medial head)

Medial sural cutaneous nerve

Small saphenous vein

B. Posterior tibial artery control

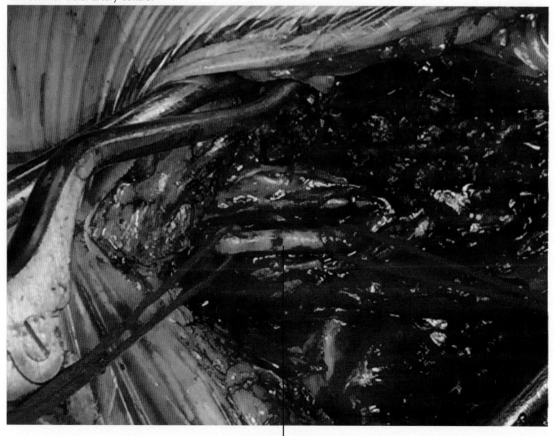

Posterior tibial

FIGURE 47.3 **Anatomy of lower leg and posterior tibial artery control.**

FEMORAL–POSTERIOR TIBIAL (Continued)

Once the proximal and distal bypass targets are controlled, the bypass conduit can be tunneled either anatomically or subcutaneously using a rigid tunneling device. It is imperative to ensure that the conduit does not have any kinking or twisting within it while being tunneled because this can cause the bypass to fail in the early postoperative period. With the conduit in place, vascular clamps can be used to clamp the common femoral artery, and the artery can be checked to ensure cessation of a pulse. If no pulse is palpated after the clamps have been placed, a longitudinal arteriotomy is made and the proximal portion of the bypass conduit can be sewn to the artery, typically using a 6-0 nonabsorbable, monofilament suture with a "heel," "heel and toe," or "parachute" technique. The proximal anastomosis should be flushed with heparinized saline, adequately de-aired, and then tested for hemostasis. Repair sutures can be applied as needed. Similarly, vascular clamps can be applied to the posterior tibial artery before making a longitudinal arteriotomy. However, sometimes it is possible to tighten the silicone vessel loops or to use a tourniquet to create cessation of flow while avoiding potentially damaging clamps. Once the longitudinal arteriotomy is performed, the distal anastomosis can be performed using a 6-0 or 7-0 nonabsorbable, monofilament suture with a "heel," "heel and toe," or "parachute" technique. Before releasing the vascular clamps, the surgeon should flush the graft and distal anastomosis with heparinized saline. The graft and anastomosis should then be de-aired and tested for hemostasis. Once hemostasis has been achieved, the groin and lower leg incisions should be closed in multiple layers.

FEMORAL–ANTERIOR TIBIAL

The patient is placed in the supine position and subsequently shaved and prepped from the umbilicus through the foot. The common femoral artery is exposed and controlled as described in the Femoral–Posterior Tibial bypass section. The anterior tibial artery located in the anterior compartment of the leg is typically exposed using an anterolateral lower-leg incision (see Fig. 47.3A). Given the position of the anterior tibial artery in the anterior compartment of the leg, the leg must be internally rotated with the knee flexed at 30 degrees and supported with a "bump." The tibia and fibula are identified on the anterolateral aspect of the leg, and then an approximately 10-cm vertical incision is made between these two structures. The incision is deepened to the crural fascia, which is opened along the lateral border of the tibialis anterior muscle. At this point, a plane can be created using blunt dissection between the extensor digitorum longus and tibialis anterior muscle to identify the anterior tibial artery against the interosseus membrane. The first structure to be encountered in the neurovascular bundle containing the anterior tibial artery should be the anterior tibial vein. This can be carefully isolated using silicone vessel loops to retract it out of the way. There are also numerous venous branches that may require ligation around the anterior tibial artery. The deep peroneal nerve is typically posterior to the anterior tibial artery, but this should be identified to ensure no injury to the nerve occurs while obtaining control of the anterior tibial artery. Proximal and distal control of the anterior tibial artery should be obtained with silicone vessel loops.

Once control of the anterior tibial artery has been obtained, the graft can be tunneled subcutaneously along the lateral aspect of the thigh or anatomically. When tunneling subcutaneously, the tunneler should pass posterior to the lateral femoral condyle. The bypass can be tunneled anatomically in a subsartorial plane, but a separate incision on the medial leg must be made similar to the incision used to expose the posterior tibial artery to protect those vessels as well as to bring the tunneler out in that region. Once the bypass conduit is in the leg, the interosseous membrane can be incised and then traversed at a 45-degree angle using the tunneler to cross from the medial to lateral lower leg. It is important to ensure that the interosseous membrane defect is large enough so that two fingers can fit through the membrane. This prevents potential kinking of the conduit as it comes through the interosseous membrane. At this point, the vessels can be clamped or controlled with vessel loops, and the anastomoses can be performed as described in the Femoral–Posterior Tibial bypass section.

FEMORAL–PERONEAL

The patient is placed in the supine position and subsequently shaved and prepped from the umbilicus through the foot. The common femoral artery is exposed and controlled as described in the Femoral–Posterior Tibial bypass section. The peroneal artery located in the deep posterior compartment is usually exposed through a vertical incision along the medial aspect of mid-lower leg (Fig. 47.3A). Therefore the leg is externally rotated with the knee flexed at 30 degrees and supported with a "bump." The tibia is identified in the middle third of the lower leg, and an approximately 10-cm incision is made through a vertical incision that is 2 cm below the posterior border of the tibia. The incision is deepened through the subcutaneous tissue until the crural fascia is encountered. At this point, the crural fascia is incised in the direction of the incision. Next, the soleal attachments to the tibia are freed up with a combination of blunt and sharp dissection. The soleus is then retracted posteriorly, and blunt dissection is used to create a plane between the soleus and flexor digitorum longus muscles. The posterior tibial vessels should be identified and protected while further dissection deeper into the wound occurs. At this point, the peroneal vessels are identified along the anterior surface of the flexor hallucis longus muscle and dissected free to obtain an adequate length for the bypass with adequate proximal and distal control using silicone vessel loops. Next, the bypass conduit can be tunneled either anatomically or subcutaneously using a rigid tunneling device. It is imperative to ensure that the conduit does not have any kinking or twisting within it while being tunneled, because this can cause the bypass to fail in the early postoperative period. At this point, the vessels can be clamped or controlled with vessel loops, and the anastomoses can be performed as described in the Femoral–Posterior Tibial bypass section.

The peroneal artery may also be exposed using a lateral approach. When a lateral approach is performed, the patient is prepped and draped in the same manner as the medial approach, but the supine patient has the leg flexed to a 45- to 60-degree angle and then internally rotated with the support of a "bump." The region of eventual anastomosis is identified, and a 10-cm vertical incision is made directly over the fibula with the incision centered over that region. The incision is deepened through the subcutaneous tissue until the crural fascia is encountered, which is incised in the direction of the incision. At this point, the muscular attachments to the fibula are dissected off the fibula, while careful attention is paid to identify and protect the common peroneal nerve from injury as it courses around the proximal aspect of the fibula. As the muscular attachments are freed of the fibula from lateral to medial, care must be taken to avoid inadvertent injury to the peroneal vessels lying on the medial aspect of the fibula. Once the fibula within the incision is freed of all muscular attachments, that portion of the fibula is resected with a saw or bone cutter, exposing the peroneal vessels deep within the incision. With the partial fibulectomy completed, the peroneal vessels are dissected free to obtain adequate length for the bypass. The artery is encircled proximally and distally with silicone vessel loops, unless a tourniquet is going to be used for arterial control. Next, the bypass conduit is tunneled subcutaneously using a rigid tunneling device, ensuring there are no kinks or twisting of the conduit during the tunneling process. At this point, the peroneal artery can be clamped, controlled with vessel loops, or the tourniquet can be inflated. Finally, the anastomoses can be performed as described in the Femoral–Posterior Tibial bypass section.

FEMORAL–FOOT OR ANKLE ARTERIES

Femoral–Dorsalis Pedis

The patient is positioned in the supine position and subsequently shaved and prepped from the umbilicus through the foot. The common femoral artery is exposed and controlled as described in the Femoral–Posterior Tibial bypass section. The dorsalis pedis artery is found on the dorsal aspect of the foot and is exposed using a vertical incision. The vertical incision is made between the first and second metatarsals in the middle third of the foot. The incision is deepened through the subcutaneous tissue, and the dorsal branch of the superficial peroneal nerve is identified and retracted laterally to protect it during further dissection. The incision is deepened to the deep fascia, which is incised in the direction of the incision. At this point, the extensor hallucis longus and brevis muscles are identified and separated, exposing the dorsalis pedis artery lying lateral to the deep peroneal nerve. At this point, the dorsalis pedis artery is carefully dissected free and controlled with vessel loops. Next, the bypass conduit can be tunneled anatomically or subcutaneously using a rigid tunneling device. It is imperative to ensure that the conduit does not have any kinking or twisting within it while being tunneled, because this can cause the bypass to fail in the early postoperative period. At this point, the vessels can be clamped or controlled with vessel loops, and the anastomoses can be performed as described in the Femoral–Posterior Tibial bypass section.

Femoral–Distal Posterior Tibial

The patient is positioned in the supine position and subsequently shaved and prepped from the umbilicus through the foot. The common femoral artery is exposed and controlled as described in the Femoral–Posterior Tibial bypass section. A rolled-up towel should be used as a lateral support ("bump") behind a partially flexed (45 to 60 degrees) and externally rotated knee to assist with visualization. After identifying the posterior aspect of the distal tibia, the surgeon makes an approximately 5-cm curvilinear incision 1 fingerbreadth (~2 cm) below the tibia around the medial malleolus. The incision is deepened through the crural fascia, and the flexor retinaculum is subsequently incised, revealing the distal posterior tibial neurovascular bundle. At this point, the posterior tibial artery can be encircled proximally and distally with silicone vessel loops or a tourniquet can be used for arterial control. When encircling the artery, the surgeon must pay careful attention not to injure the tibial nerve, which is posterior to the artery. If more exposure is needed to safely control the artery, the flexor digitorum longus can be mobilized and retracted toward the medial malleolus. Next, the bypass conduit can be tunneled anatomically or subcutaneously using a rigid tunneling device. It is imperative to ensure that the conduit does not have any kinking or twisting within it while being tunneled, because this can cause the bypass to fail in the early postoperative period. At this point, the vessels can be clamped or controlled with vessel loops, and the anastomoses can be performed as described in the Femoral–Posterior Tibial bypass section.

ADJUNCTS FOR BYPASS SUCCESS

Autogenous vein is the best conduit for infrainguinal bypasses, but it is not uncommon for there to be a lack of autogenous vein available because of prior harvesting for a previous operation. In the instances in which autogenous vein is not available, a prosthetic graft or cadaveric graft can be used as the bypass conduit. When a nonautogenous conduit is used, there are a couple of considerations that improve the likelihood of bypass success. The first is the use of vein cuffs at the distal bypass site. Although no randomized control trials have evaluated the efficacy of vein cuffs with respect to bypass patency, several studies have demonstrated improved patency with the use of a vein cuff. There are several types of vein cuffs that may be used based on surgeon preference, which include the Miller cuff, Taylor patch, St. Mary's boot, and Linton patch. In addition, the "Achilles heel" of any nonautogenous graft is infection. Therefore routine use of an iodine-impregnated adhesive drapes and avoiding contact of the conduit with the skin are recommended to decrease the risk of infection. Similarly, when a bypass that does not extend to the foot is performed, the foot can be placed in an impermeable isolation bag and then wrapped with sterile wrap if needed to prevent contamination of the surgical field from the foot.

SUGGESTED READINGS

Davis FM, Henke PK. Infrainguinal bypass graft for lower extremity arterial occlusive disease. In: Hans SS, Shepard AD, Weaver MR, Bove PG, Long GW, editors. Endovascular and Open Vascular Reconstruction: a Practical Approach. Boca Raton: CRC Press; 2018.

Mills JL. Infrainguinal disease: surgical treatment. In: Sidawy AN, Perler BA, editors. Rutherford's Vascular Surgery and Endovascular Therapy. 9th ed. Philadelphia: Elsevier; 2019.

Minjarez RC, Moneta GL. Direct surgical repair of tibial-peroneal arterial occlusive disease. In: Chaikof EL, Cambria RP, editors. Atlas of Vascular Surgery and Endovascular Therapy: Anatomy and Technique. Philadelphia: Saunders; 2014.

Wind GG, Valentine RJ. Common femoral artery. Anatomic Exposures in Vascular Surgery. 3rd ed. Philadelphia: Lippincott, Williams & Wilkins; 2013.

Wind GG, Valentine RJ. Vessels of the leg. Anatomic Exposures in Vascular Surgery. 3rd ed. Philadelphia: Lippincott, Williams & Wilkins; 2013.

Above-Knee and Below-Knee Amputation

David M. Hardy and David J. Laczynski

INTRODUCTION

Amputations above and below the knee are common surgical procedures performed by vascular, orthopedic, and general surgeons. The indications for these procedures include infection, irreversible acute ischemia, chronic progressive ischemia, trauma, intractable pain, neuropathy, and non-healing wounds. In developed countries, the primary indications for lower-extremity amputation are complications of peripheral vascular disease and diabetes mellitus.

PREOPERATIVE EVALUATION

Recognition of the importance of amputation as the first step of the patient's rehabilitation to recovery of functional status should be emphasized to the patient and health care team. Successful rehabilitation depends on aggressive postoperative physical and occupational therapy. Group amputee therapy can be helpful in patients with psychological issues surrounding the actual amputation.

Preoperative evaluation and optimization prepare the patient for surgery and minimize perioperative complications. Glucose control, nutrition, and cardiopulmonary status should be evaluated and optimized before operating. Occasionally, initial guillotine amputation is indicated to provide source control of deep space infection, with a secondary procedure for definitive closure planned when clinical and infection status have improved.

The level of amputation is predicated on surgical site healing capacity and ambulatory potential of the patient. The below-knee amputation (BKA) requires significantly less energy expenditure for postoperative mobilization, affording patients a higher likelihood of successful rehabilitation with their prosthesis. The above-knee amputation (AKA), although decreasing ambulatory potential, improves the chance of wound healing, reduces need for amputation revision, and eliminates complications from contractures. Physical examination and noninvasive vascular laboratory testing are helpful in determining the appropriate level of amputation for successful healing.

SURGICAL PRINCIPLES

Surgical technique emphasizes minimal handling of the skin edges, appropriate flap size to minimize tension on stump closure, strict hemostasis, use of viable tissue for closure, and ligation of nerves under tension to allow retraction out of the area of surgical incision. Retraction and atrophy of tissues associated with normal healing and scarring should be considered when transection of bone is performed to avoid the complication of pressure-induced necrosis. The identification of the fascial layers for closure and meticulous handling of the tissues are critical (Fig. 48.1). Understanding the bony landmarks, arterial supply, nerves, and compartments of the lower extremity is essential to perform an appropriate procedure (Figs. 48.2 and 48.3).

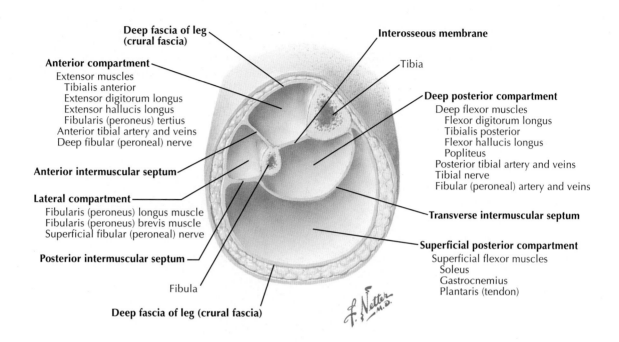

Cross section just above middle of leg

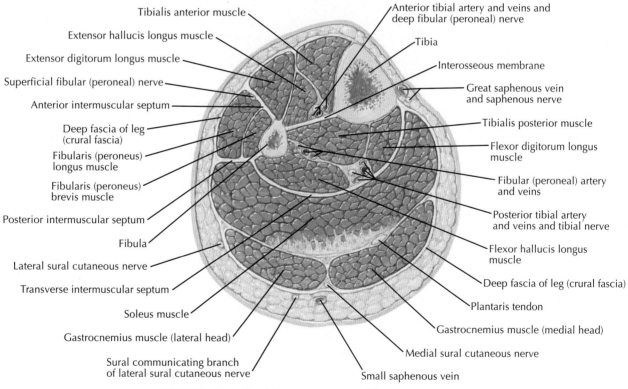

FIGURE 48.1 Fascial compartments of leg.

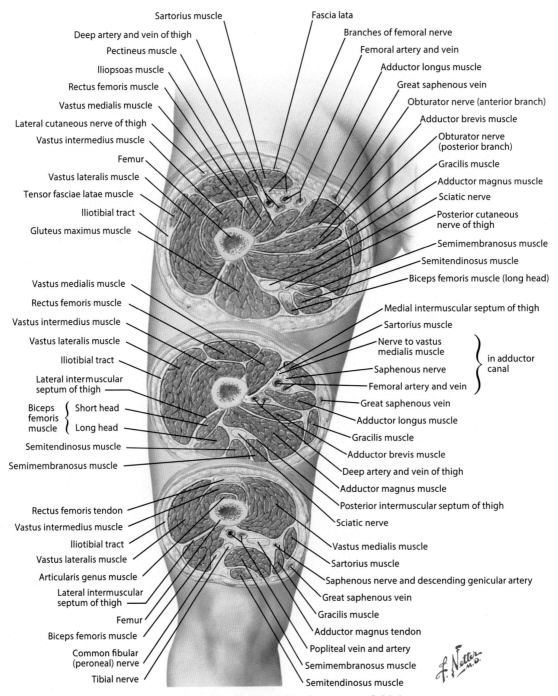

Sartorius muscle
Deep artery and vein of thigh
Pectineus muscle
Iliopsoas muscle
Rectus femoris muscle
Vastus medialis muscle
Lateral cutaneous nerve of thigh
Vastus intermedius muscle
Femur
Vastus lateralis muscle
Tensor fasciae latae muscle
Iliotibial tract
Gluteus maximus muscle

Vastus medialis muscle
Rectus femoris muscle
Vastus intermedius muscle
Vastus lateralis muscle
Iliotibial tract
Lateral intermuscular septum of thigh
Biceps femoris muscle { Short head / Long head }
Semitendinosus muscle
Semimembranosus muscle

Rectus femoris tendon
Vastus intermedius muscle
Iliotibial tract
Vastus lateralis muscle
Articularis genus muscle
Lateral intermuscular septum of thigh
Femur
Biceps femoris muscle
Common fibular (peroneal) nerve
Tibial nerve

Fascia lata
Branches of femoral nerve
Femoral artery and vein
Adductor longus muscle
Great saphenous vein
Obturator nerve (anterior branch)
Adductor brevis muscle
Obturator nerve (posterior branch)
Gracilis muscle
Adductor magnus muscle
Sciatic nerve
Posterior cutaneous nerve of thigh
Semimembranosus muscle
Semitendinosus muscle
Biceps femoris muscle (long head)

Medial intermuscular septum of thigh
Sartorius muscle
Nerve to vastus medialis muscle
Saphenous nerve
Femoral artery and vein
} in adductor canal
Great saphenous vein
Adductor longus muscle
Gracilis muscle
Adductor brevis muscle
Deep artery and vein of thigh
Adductor magnus muscle
Posterior intermuscular septum of thigh
Sciatic nerve

Vastus medialis muscle
Sartorius muscle
Saphenous nerve and descending genicular artery
Great saphenous vein
Gracilis muscle
Adductor magnus tendon
Popliteal vein and artery
Semimembranosus muscle
Semitendinosus muscle

FIGURE 48.2 Cross-sectional anatomy of thigh.

Superficial nerves and veins (anterior view)

Arteries of leg

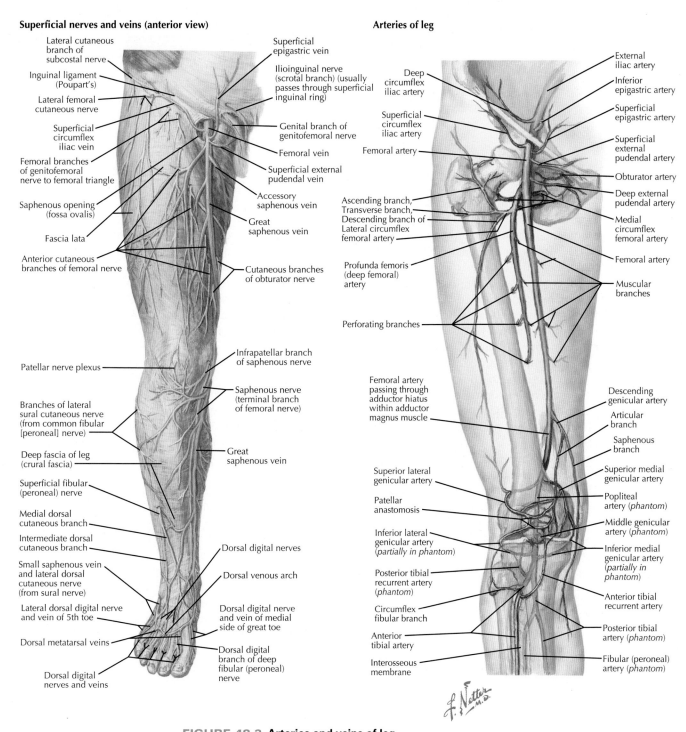

Lateral cutaneous branch of subcostal nerve

Inguinal ligament (Poupart's)

Lateral femoral cutaneous nerve

Superficial circumflex iliac vein

Femoral branches of genitofemoral nerve to femoral triangle

Saphenous opening (fossa ovalis)

Fascia lata

Anterior cutaneous branches of femoral nerve

Patellar nerve plexus

Branches of lateral sural cutaneous nerve (from common fibular [peroneal] nerve)

Deep fascia of leg (crural fascia)

Superficial fibular (peroneal) nerve

Medial dorsal cutaneous branch

Intermediate dorsal cutaneous branch

Small saphenous vein and lateral dorsal cutaneous nerve (from sural nerve)

Lateral dorsal digital nerve and vein of 5th toe

Dorsal metatarsal veins

Dorsal digital nerves and veins

Superficial epigastric vein

Ilioinguinal nerve (scrotal branch) (usually passes through superficial inguinal ring)

Genital branch of genitofemoral nerve

Femoral vein

Superficial external pudendal vein

Accessory saphenous vein

Great saphenous vein

Cutaneous branches of obturator nerve

Infrapatellar branch of saphenous nerve

Saphenous nerve (terminal branch of femoral nerve)

Great saphenous vein

Dorsal digital nerves

Dorsal venous arch

Dorsal digital nerve and vein of medial side of great toe

Dorsal digital branch of deep fibular (peroneal) nerve

Deep circumflex iliac artery

Superficial circumflex iliac artery

Femoral artery

Ascending branch, Transverse branch, Descending branch of Lateral circumflex femoral artery

Profunda femoris (deep femoral) artery

Perforating branches

Femoral artery passing through adductor hiatus within adductor magnus muscle

Superior lateral genicular artery

Patellar anastomosis

Inferior lateral genicular artery (*partially in phantom*)

Posterior tibial recurrent artery (*phantom*)

Circumflex fibular branch

Anterior tibial artery

Interosseous membrane

External iliac artery

Inferior epigastric artery

Superficial epigastric artery

Superficial external pudendal artery

Obturator artery

Deep external pudendal artery

Medial circumflex femoral artery

Femoral artery

Muscular branches

Descending genicular artery

Articular branch

Saphenous branch

Superior medial genicular artery

Popliteal artery (*phantom*)

Middle genicular artery (*phantom*)

Inferior medial genicular artery (*partially in phantom*)

Anterior tibial recurrent artery

Posterior tibial artery (*phantom*)

Fibular (peroneal) artery (*phantom*)

FIGURE 48.3 Arteries and veins of leg.

BELOW-KNEE (TRANSTIBIAL) AMPUTATION

The myocutaneous skin flap can be measured using the "two-thirds/one-third leg circumference rule" or created freehand but should be marked before the incision is made. For a typical posterior flap, the transverse anterior skin incision is made approximately 10 to 12 cm below the tibial tuberosity, extending two-thirds of the circumference of the leg. The flap length should be approximately one-third of the circumference; however, the tendency is to be slightly more generous, knowing this tissue can always be shortened later. In some patients, typically with thin lower legs, a two-thirds circumference may leave the posterior flap too thin, so the anterior incision may be shortened.

The skin and fascia are transected with care in the same vertical plane to the level of the fascia. The posterior skin and muscle flap are transected to fascia, ensuring adequate hemostasis, and then attention is turned back to the anterior portion. The anterior compartment musculature is transected. The anterior tibial artery and vein are identified beneath these muscles, lying on the interosseous membrane with the peroneal nerve, and are individually ligated. Medially, the musculature is transected. The tibia is dissected clear of surrounding tissues, and then the periosteum is separated proximally 2 to 3 cm with periosteal elevator. The fibula is also dissected circumferentially.

The tibia is then transected proximal to the level of the skin incision by using a power sagittal or Gigli saw (Fig. 48.4A and B). The anterior tibia is beveled 60 degrees, and the edges are smoothed with a rasp. The fibula is then transected 1 to 2 cm proximal to the tibia. This technique permits exposure of the posterior tibial and peroneal neurovascular bundles, which are individually ligated.

The posterior flap is fashioned with an amputation knife by separating the posterior compartments in a plane just deep to the tibia and fibula. Strict hemostasis is achieved; placement of a drain is optional. Closure is performed first by deep fascial approximation with absorbable sutures. 0 or 2-0 polyglactin is typically chosen for fascial closure. Special care is taken with the skin closure, using subcuticular skin approximation, staples, or nonabsorbable vertical mattress sutures, minimizing tension along the suture line (Fig. 48.4C and D). A well-padded sterile dressing is applied. The knee should be immobilized with a splint or cast to minimize contracture.

A. Below-knee amputation

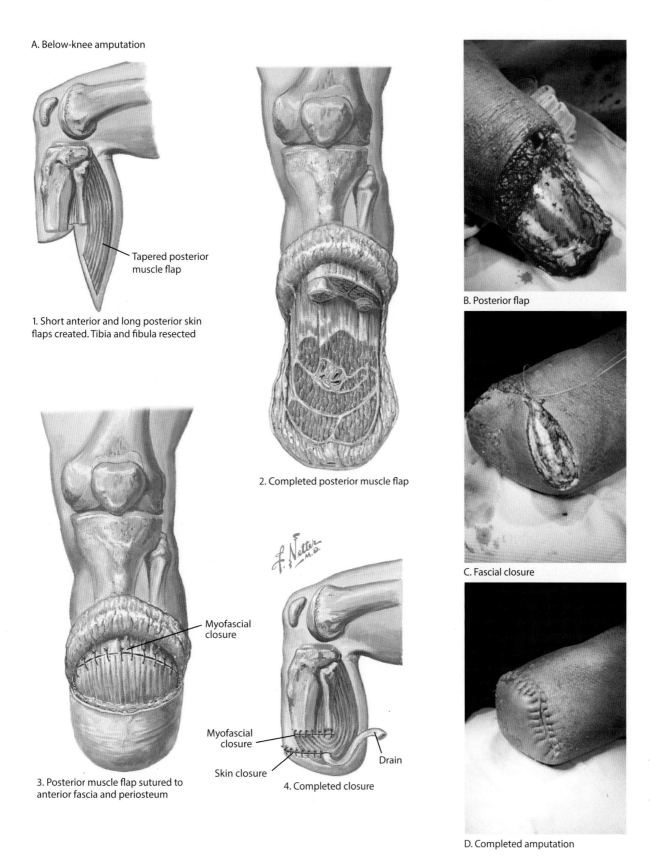

Tapered posterior muscle flap

1. Short anterior and long posterior skin flaps created. Tibia and fibula resected

2. Completed posterior muscle flap

Myofascial closure

3. Posterior muscle flap sutured to anterior fascia and periosteum

Myofascial closure

Skin closure

Drain

4. Completed closure

B. Posterior flap

C. Fascial closure

D. Completed amputation

FIGURE 48.4 Below-knee amputation and closure.

ABOVE-KNEE (TRANSFEMORAL) AMPUTATION

The most common closure in AKA is an anteroposterior fish-mouth incision, but as in BKA, this can be modified to obtain adequate tissue coverage, provided there is adequate soft tissue coverage of the femur (Fig. 48.5A). The stump is traditionally created between the middle and distal third of the femur; however, a shorter stump may be necessary. A short fish-mouth incision, with equal-size anterior and posterior myocutaneous flaps, minimizes the length of incision in AKA. The incision is carried down to the level of the fascia, which is transected. The quadriceps muscles are transected with cautery. Medial division of the sartorius muscle allows entry into the popliteal fossa, where the femoral artery and vein are ligated and transected. Laterally, the iliotibial band and intermuscular septum are divided, along with the large lateral muscles.

The femur is dissected clear of surrounding tissues. The periosteum is raised to at least 2 cm above the skin incision (Fig. 48.5B). The femur is transected with a power sagittal or Gigli saw. The bone should be transected generously proximal to the skin incision, allowing for skin retraction during healing and avoiding tension on the distal incision by the remaining femur. The posterior flap is then fashioned with an amputation knife or cautery. The sciatic nerve is encountered posterior to femur, which is ligated as far proximal as possible, then allowed to retract with transection. This maneuver will help prevent neuroma formation.

Strict hemostasis is achieved with cautery and silk ligatures. The fascia is approximated with absorbable sutures, generally using 0 or 2-0 polyglactin with interrupted "figure-of-8" sutures to approximate the fascia. The skin is closed with subcuticular absorbable suture, staples, or nonabsorbable suture (Fig. 48.5C and D). A padded sterile dressing is applied with a final application of an impervious dressing.

POSTOPERATIVE CARE

The use of barrier occlusive dressing is recommended to avoid postoperative soiling, especially in the elderly, incontinent patient. Mild compression in the surgical dressing also helps control edema, which can lead to ischemia and necrosis of the wound edges. Early indications to evaluate the amputation site include significant pain, hematoma, and unexplained fever. Otherwise, the initial operative dressing is maintained for 3 days. Proper positioning of the stump and use of knee immobilizers to prevent contracture are imperative. Compression of stump with a "shrinker" stocking after the dressings are removed on day 3 is also important to reduce edema. Early transfer to rehabilitation minimizes deconditioning and optimizes functional outcome in the patient with lower-extremity amputation.

A. Above-knee amputation

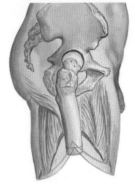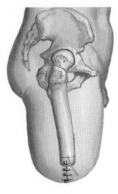

Skin and myofascial flaps
tailored for closure

Myofascial and skin flaps
closed over drain

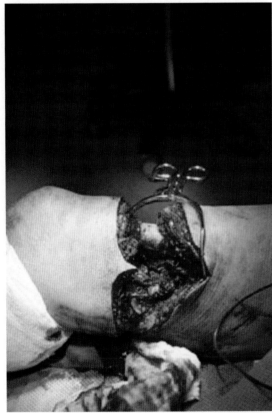

B. Anterior posterior fish-mouth incision

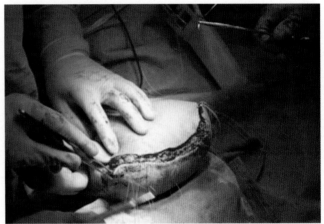

C. Fascial closure

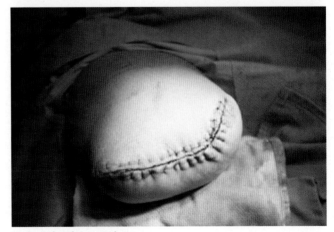

D. Completed amputation

FIGURE 48.5 Above-knee amputation and closure.

SUGGESTED READING

Rios AL, Eidt JF. Lower extremity amputations: operative techniques and results. In: Sidawy AN, Perler BA, editors. Rutherford's Vascular Surgery. 9th ed. Philadelphia: Elsevier; 2019.

Vascular Access, Emergency and Trauma Procedures

SECTION EDITOR: Tony R. Capizzani

Tracheal Intubation and Endoscopic Anatomy

Kristen Holler and Tony R. Capizzani

INTRODUCTION

The well-trained airway expert has a key understanding of the anatomy and challenges that may cause possible complications during airway placement. There are several essential steps when considering an airway placement. The provider must understand the indications for intubation and have a standardized method of assessing the patient's anatomy. With more complex airway placement encounters, the provider should be familiar with numerous difficult airway adjuncts and be familiar with the anatomy, innervation, and pitfalls of various equipment choices. Even under those extreme conditions of a challenging airway, familiarity with basic anatomy serves as a cornerstone for definitive airway placement.

AIRWAY ANATOMY

The pulmonary system consists of the lungs and a series of airways that are subdivided into upper and lower segments.

Upper Airway

The airway passage is divided into three anatomic areas of the pharyngeal cavity. The nasopharynx is defined by superiorly and anteriorly by the nasal septum and inferiorly by the soft palate; it communicates with the oropharynx via the pharyngeal isthmus. The oropharynx borders extend inferiorly from the soft palate to the superior margin of the epiglottis. The most inferior cavity, the laryngopharynx, is bounded by the landmarks of the epiglottis superiorly and the lower border of the cricoid cartilage inferiorly (Fig. 49.1). Inspiratory patency of the pharynx is maintained primarily by contraction of the tensor palatine, genioglossus, and hyoid bone muscles. Loss of muscle tone, as occurs during general anesthesia and sedation, leads to pharyngeal collapse because of a decrease in the anteroposterior diameter of the pharynx at the level of the soft palate and epiglottis.

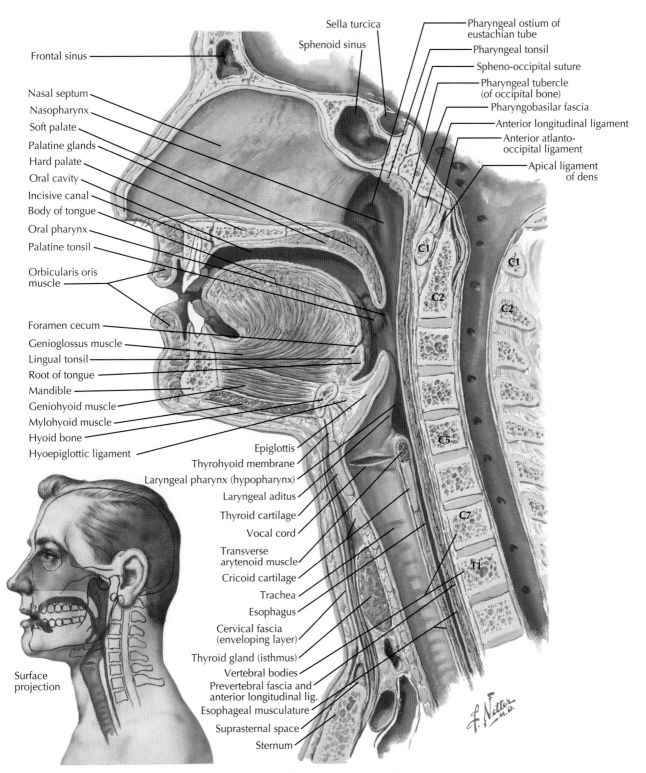

Frontal sinus

Nasal septum
Nasopharynx
Soft palate
Palatine glands
Hard palate
Oral cavity
Incisive canal
Body of tongue
Oral pharynx
Palatine tonsil
Orbicularis oris muscle

Foramen cecum
Genioglossus muscle
Lingual tonsil
Root of tongue
Mandible
Geniohyoid muscle
Mylohyoid muscle
Hyoid bone
Hyoepiglottic ligament

Sella turcica
Sphenoid sinus

Pharyngeal ostium of eustachian tube
Pharyngeal tonsil
Spheno-occipital suture
Pharyngeal tubercle (of occipital bone)
Pharyngobasilar fascia
Anterior longitudinal ligament
Anterior atlanto-occipital ligament
Apical ligament of dens

C1
C2
C5
C7
T1

C1
C2

Epiglottis
Thyrohyoid membrane
Laryngeal pharynx (hypopharynx)
Laryngeal aditus
Thyroid cartilage
Vocal cord
Transverse arytenoid muscle
Cricoid cartilage
Trachea
Esophagus
Cervical fascia (enveloping layer)
Thyroid gland (isthmus)
Vertebral bodies
Prevertebral fascia and anterior longitudinal lig.
Esophageal musculature
Suprasternal space
Sternum

Surface projection

FIGURE 49.1 Sagittal section of pharynx.

Larynx

The larynx serves as the connecting structure between the upper and lower airways. The adult larynx extends from the fourth to the sixth cervical vertebra, and it is composed of nine cartilages, with six paired and three single components. The three single cartilages include the thyroid, cricoid, and epiglottic. The paired cartilages include the arytenoid, corniculate, and cuneiform. The vocal folds extend in an anterior-posterior plane from the thyroid cartilage to the arytenoid cartilages, and the former acts as a protective housing anteriorly for the vocal mechanism (Fig. 49.2). Laryngeal movement is controlled by two muscle groups: the extrinsic muscles, which move the larynx as a whole, and the intrinsic muscles, which move the various cartilages. The larynx is innervated by two branches of the vagus nerve on each side, the superior laryngeal and recurrent laryngeal nerves. The recurrent laryngeal nerve innervates all intrinsic laryngeal muscles except for the cricothyroid muscle, and injury can lead to vocal cord dysfunction. Airway patency is typically preserved in unilateral nerve injury; however, this isolated defect may still impair the ability of the larynx to protect against aspiration. The superior laryngeal nerve also supplies sensory innervation to the airway extending from the epiglottis to above the vocal folds and is an important target for anesthetizing the airway for awake intubation.

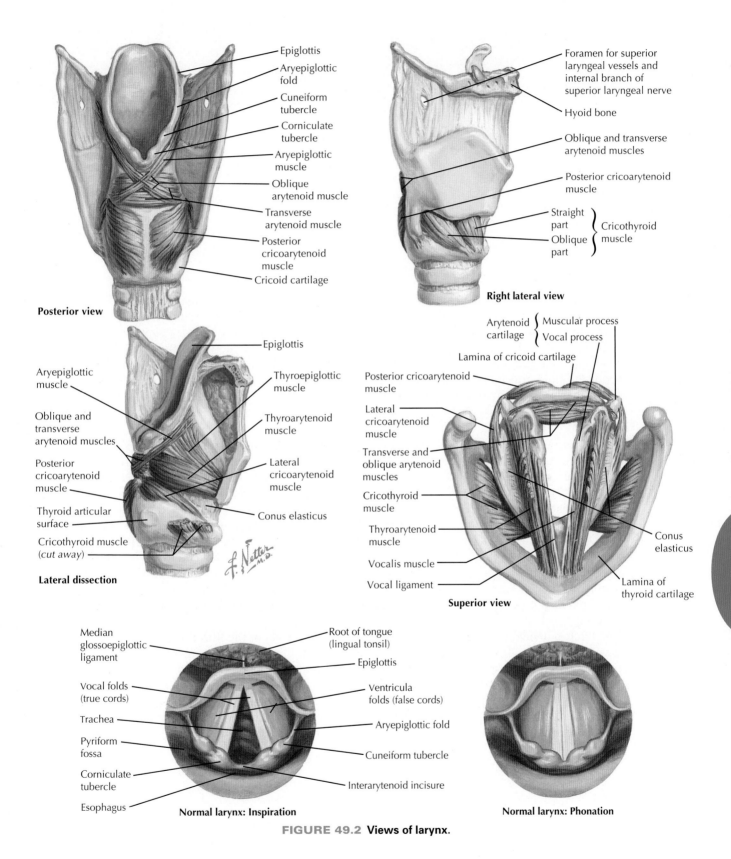

Epiglottis
Aryepiglottic fold
Cuneiform tubercle
Corniculate tubercle
Aryepiglottic muscle
Oblique arytenoid muscle
Transverse arytenoid muscle
Posterior cricoarytenoid muscle
Cricoid cartilage

Posterior view

Foramen for superior laryngeal vessels and internal branch of superior laryngeal nerve
Hyoid bone
Oblique and transverse arytenoid muscles
Posterior cricoarytenoid muscle
Straight part
Oblique part
Cricothyroid muscle

Right lateral view

Aryepiglottic muscle
Oblique and transverse arytenoid muscles
Posterior cricoarytenoid muscle
Thyroid articular surface
Cricothyroid muscle (cut away)

Epiglottis
Thyroepiglottic muscle
Thyroarytenoid muscle
Lateral cricoarytenoid muscle
Conus elasticus

Lateral dissection

Arytenoid cartilage {Muscular process / Vocal process}
Lamina of cricoid cartilage
Posterior cricoarytenoid muscle
Lateral cricoarytenoid muscle
Transverse and oblique arytenoid muscles
Cricothyroid muscle
Thyroarytenoid muscle
Vocalis muscle
Vocal ligament
Conus elasticus
Lamina of thyroid cartilage

Superior view

Median glossoepiglottic ligament
Vocal folds (true cords)
Trachea
Pyriform fossa
Corniculate tubercle
Esophagus

Root of tongue (lingual tonsil)
Epiglottis
Ventricula folds (false cords)
Aryepiglottic fold
Cuneiform tubercle
Interarytenoid incisure

Normal larynx: Inspiration

Normal larynx: Phonation

FIGURE 49.2 Views of larynx.

Nose and Nasopharynx

Nasotracheal intubation (NTI) is an alternative approach to orotracheal intubation and is discussed later in this chapter. The two nasal fossae extend from the nostrils to the nasopharynx through the choana. The nasal fossae are divided by the midline cartilaginous septum and medial portions of the lateral cartilages (Fig. 49.3) and inferiorly by the turbinate bones. The mucosa covering the middle turbinate is highly vascular, receiving its blood supply from the anterior ethmoid artery and also containing a large plexus of veins. The middle turbinate is susceptible to avulsion by trauma, causing massive epistaxis.

Lower Airway

The lower airway consists of the trachea, bronchus, bronchioles, respiratory bronchioles, and alveoli. The adult trachea begins at the cricoid cartilage at the level of the sixth cervical vertebra and contains 16 to 20 incomplete cartilaginous rings. The posterior trachea is devoid of cartilage (Fig. 49.3B). The cricothyroid membrane is an externally identified structure between the thyroid cartilage and the cricoid cartilage. This landmark is important when evaluating patients with a known or suspected difficult airway, because it is the preferred puncture or incision site for emergent surgical airway placement. The cricoid cartilage, unlike the tracheal rings, is a complete cartilaginous ring. Pressure over the cricoid cartilage (Sellick maneuver) is often applied during rapid-sequence induction and intubation (RSI) to minimize the risk of aspiration in patients with known or suspected full stomachs. However, cricoid pressure may distort airway anatomy, making intubation more difficult and has not been shown to decrease risk of aspiration.

The trachea divides into two bronchi at the carina, at the level of the fifth thoracic vertebra. The right main bronchus is larger in diameter and bifurcates at a less acute angle than the left main bronchus, causing aspirated materials as well as a malpositioned endotracheal tube (ETT) to be more likely to enter the right mainstem bronchus.

Bronchial divisions continue down the respiratory tree into increasingly smaller airways. The alveoli are the terminus of the airways and are the areas of primary gas exchange, where oxygen enters the bloodstream and carbon dioxide is removed.

A. Lateral view of the nose

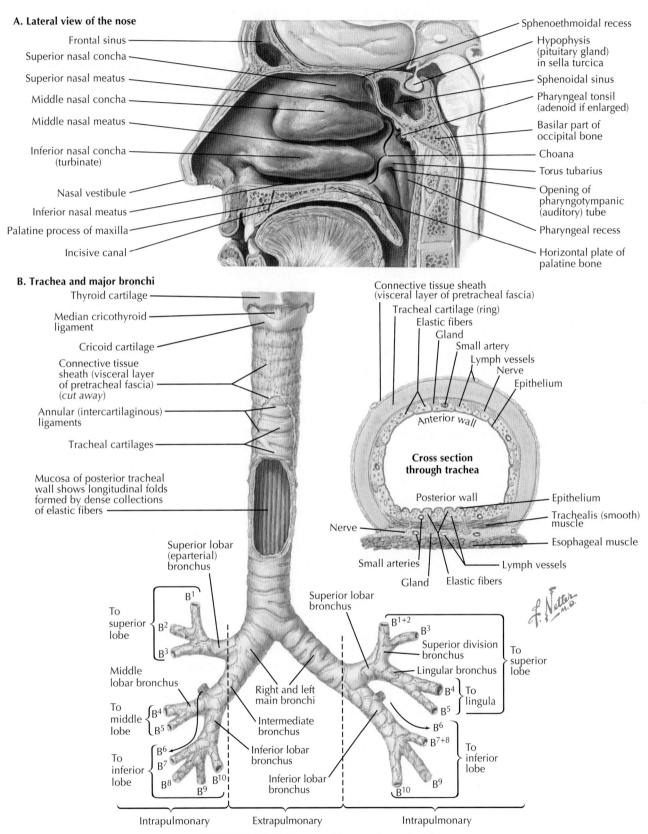

Frontal sinus
Superior nasal concha
Superior nasal meatus
Middle nasal concha
Middle nasal meatus
Inferior nasal concha (turbinate)
Nasal vestibule
Inferior nasal meatus
Palatine process of maxilla
Incisive canal

Sphenoethmoidal recess
Hypophysis (pituitary gland) in sella turcica
Sphenoidal sinus
Pharyngeal tonsil (adenoid if enlarged)
Basilar part of occipital bone
Choana
Torus tubarius
Opening of pharyngotympanic (auditory) tube
Pharyngeal recess
Horizontal plate of palatine bone

B. Trachea and major bronchi

Thyroid cartilage
Median cricothyroid ligament
Cricoid cartilage
Connective tissue sheath (visceral layer of pretracheal fascia) (cut away)
Annular (intercartilaginous) ligaments
Tracheal cartilages
Mucosa of posterior tracheal wall shows longitudinal folds formed by dense collections of elastic fibers

Connective tissue sheath (visceral layer of pretracheal fascia)
Tracheal cartilage (ring)
Elastic fibers
Gland
Small artery
Lymph vessels
Nerve
Epithelium
Anterior wall

Cross section through trachea

Posterior wall
Epithelium
Trachealis (smooth) muscle
Esophageal muscle
Nerve
Small arteries
Gland
Elastic fibers
Lymph vessels

Superior lobar (eparterial) bronchus

B^1
To superior lobe
B^2
B^3

Middle lobar bronchus

To middle lobe
B^4
B^5

To inferior lobe
B^6
B^7
B^8
B^{10}
B^9

Right and left main bronchi
Intermediate bronchus
Inferior lobar bronchus
Inferior lobar bronchus

Superior lobar bronchus
B^{1+2}
B^3
Superior division bronchus
Lingular bronchus
B^4 To lingula
B^5
To superior lobe
B^6
B^{7+8}
B^{10} B^9
To inferior lobe

Intrapulmonary   Extrapulmonary   Intrapulmonary

FIGURE 49.3 Nose and lower airway/trachea.

INDICATIONS FOR INTUBATION

When ventilation or oxygenation is compromised, definitive airway placement may be required to prevent hypoxia and brain injury. Indications for endotracheal intubation include respiratory failure, airway protection or compromise resulting from aspiration risk or decreased level of consciousness, high inspired oxygen requirements, cardiac arrest, and inadequate bag mask or noninvasive ventilation strategies.

Initial respiratory support is usually focused on relieving upper airway obstruction via suctioning, jaw thrust, and oral or nasal airway placement. As the patient progresses to require bag mask ventilation (BMV), a systematic approach should include assessing the airway, anticipated medications, and equipment to support a successful airway rescue.

PREINTUBATION AIRWAY EVALUATION

Airway examination should focus on identifying risk factors for both difficult BMV as well as difficult intubation. Presence of a beard, obesity, lack of teeth, and history of snoring are predictive of potential difficulty with BMV, whereas small mouth opening (<3 cm), short thyromental distance (<6 cm), and Mallampati score (>3) are predictive of difficult intubation. No single risk factor alone has been shown to be highly sensitive in predicting difficulty, although when used in combination, the incidence of difficult intubation increases with an increasing number of risk factors. The Mallampati assessment of the oral cavity hinges on the provider's ability to inspect the varying degrees of visibility of the patient's uvula, faucial pillars, and soft palate, resulting in a score of 1 to 4. Although it has long been the mainstay of airway evaluation, this score assessment requires an awake and cooperative patient.

Anatomic factors must also be considered. Congenital syndromes affecting the airway, infections or tumors of the airway, and trauma can contribute to increased difficulty in airway placement.

For initial evaluation of the patient, the LEMON system is a simple way to assess for airway challenges: Look externally, Evaluate, Mallampati score, Obstruction, and Neck mobility.

ANESTHESIA AND AIRWAY INNERVATION

Once airway placement is deemed imminent, appropriate anesthesia is necessary for ETT placement. Anesthetic choices include general anesthesia with or without neuromuscular blockade or topical anesthesia. When topical anesthesia is used, sedation is typically provided.

Knowledge of airway innervation is critical when ETT placement is planned without general anesthesia. The three main cranial nerves innervating the airway include the trigeminal nerve (V), the glossopharyngeal nerve (IX), and the vagus nerve (X). The trigeminal nerve includes branches for ophthalmic, maxillary, and mandibular distribution (Fig. 49.4). The maxillary branch (V2) can be anesthetized successfully with inhaled aerosolized lidocaine or topical viscous lidocaine applied to the surface of a nasopharyngeal airway if a nasotracheal airway is anticipated (see Fig. 49.4). Mucosal vasoconstriction is used before airway insertion to reduce the risk of bleeding. The glossopharyngeal (IX) nerve provides sensory innervation to the posterior one-third of the tongue and the pharynx above the epiglottis. The superior laryngeal nerve and recurrent laryngeal nerve, both branches of the vagus nerve (X), supply mucosa from the epiglottis to the level of the vocal cords and mucosa below the cords, respectively. The recurrent laryngeal nerve innervates all of the intrinsic laryngeal muscles except for the cricothyroid muscle, which is innervated by the external branch of the superior laryngeal nerve.

Complete anesthesia of the glossopharyngeal, superior laryngeal, and recurrent laryngeal nerves can be achieved via a variety of methods to facilitate awake intubation. Aerosolized lidocaine, and viscous lidocaine oral rinse after pretreatment with an anti-sialagogue are most frequently used. A number of airway nerve blocks such as transtracheal lidocaine injection can be used to decrease the total amount of local anesthetic needed.

Key anatomic relationships of the airway as well as the reflexes they affect should be understood before anesthetizing the cranial nerves of the airway because nerve blocks and local anesthetic injections will abolish these reflexes. This can be detrimental when patients are unable to protect their airway because of neurologic or physiologic impairment: lack of airway reflexes may lead to aspiration.

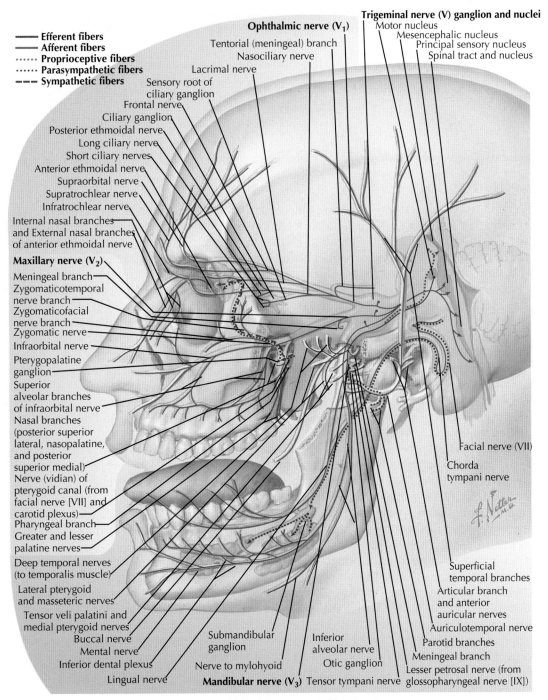

Efferent fibers
Afferent fibers
Proprioceptive fibers
Parasympathetic fibers
Sympathetic fibers

Ophthalmic nerve (V₁)
Tentorial (meningeal) branch
Nasociliary nerve
Lacrimal nerve
Sensory root of ciliary ganglion
Frontal nerve
Ciliary ganglion
Posterior ethmoidal nerve
Long ciliary nerve
Short ciliary nerves
Anterior ethmoidal nerve
Supraorbital nerve
Supratrochlear nerve
Infratrochlear nerve
Internal nasal branches and External nasal branches of anterior ethmoidal nerve

Maxillary nerve (V₂)
Meningeal branch
Zygomaticotemporal nerve branch
Zygomaticofacial nerve branch
Zygomatic nerve
Infraorbital nerve
Pterygopalatine ganglion
Superior alveolar branches of infraorbital nerve
Nasal branches (posterior superior lateral, nasopalatine, and posterior superior medial)
Nerve (vidian) of pterygoid canal (from facial nerve [VII] and carotid plexus)
Pharyngeal branch
Greater and lesser palatine nerves
Deep temporal nerves (to temporalis muscle)
Lateral pterygoid and masseteric nerves
Tensor veli palatini and medial pterygoid nerves
Buccal nerve
Mental nerve
Inferior dental plexus
Lingual nerve

Trigeminal nerve (V) ganglion and nuclei
Motor nucleus
Mesencephalic nucleus
Principal sensory nucleus
Spinal tract and nucleus

Facial nerve (VII)
Chorda tympani nerve

Superficial temporal branches
Articular branch and anterior auricular nerves
Auriculotemporal nerve
Parotid branches
Meningeal branch
Lesser petrosal nerve (from glossopharyngeal nerve [IX])

Submandibular ganglion
Inferior alveolar nerve
Otic ganglion
Nerve to mylohyoid
Mandibular nerve (V₃) Tensor tympani nerve

FIGURE 49.4 Trigeminal nerve (CN V): schema.

LARYNGOSCOPY

Before induction of anesthesia for airway placement the patient should be preoxygenated via a nonrebreather oxygen mask or bag mask. A sniffing position, external auditory meatus aligned at the height of the sternal notch, and jaw thrust or chin lift allow for easier BMV and alignment of the oral and pharyngeal axis needed for direct laryngoscopy. Establishing adequate BMV allows for careful evaluation of the airway via laryngoscopy without jeopardizing that patient's oxygenation status. With the neck slightly extended, the laryngoscope handle is held in the left hand and the blade gently placed into the hypopharynx to the right of the patient's tongue. A confident anterior lift with the blade correctly positioned in the posterior aspect of the hypopharynx, blade tip in close position to the hyoid bone, allows visualization of the glottic region and vocal cords (Fig. 49.5).

During intubation, varying views of the vocal cords are achieved, depending on patient anatomy and operator skills. Using the Cormack-Lehane classification, these views are graded 1 to 4 similar to Mallampati and are based on how much of the glottic aperture and epiglottis is visible. Application of cricoid pressure in a BURP (back upward rightward and posterior) fashion often improves the visualization grade.

The endotracheal tube is placed into the right lateral aspect of the oral cavity and advanced into the posterior cavity and through the vocal cords under direct vision until the cuff is completely past the cords. The endotracheal tube balloon is insufflated at a level above the carina to ensure bilateral bronchial ventilation. In adults this is typically achieved at a depth of 20 to 24 cm measured at the patient's lip. Confirmation of airway placement should include visual inspection, bilateral breath sounds, and an end-tidal CO_2 detection by waveform or pH-sensitive colorimetric capnography.

With video laryngoscopes, a camera is embedded at the distal tip of the blade and points anteriorly toward the glottis. This view makes it unnecessary to directly visualize the glottis and is useful when aligning the oral and pharyngeal axis via sniffing position and neck extension is difficult or impossible. Differing slightly from direct laryngoscopy, the video laryngoscope blade is inserted into the mouth in the midline under direct visualization and advanced into the hypopharynx to place the camera in appropriate proximity to the glottis. A stylet shaped with an anterior curvature to match the video laryngoscope blade is necessary to deliver the ETT to the glottic opening.

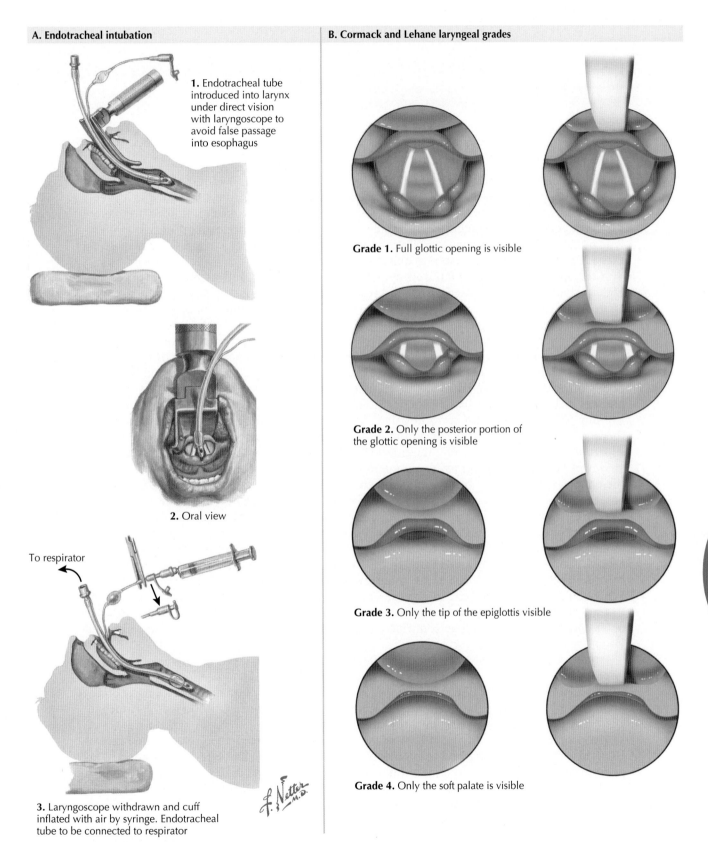

A. Endotracheal intubation

1. Endotracheal tube introduced into larynx under direct vision with laryngoscope to avoid false passage into esophagus

2. Oral view

To respirator

3. Laryngoscope withdrawn and cuff inflated with air by syringe. Endotracheal tube to be connected to respirator

B. Cormack and Lehane laryngeal grades

Grade 1. Full glottic opening is visible

Grade 2. Only the posterior portion of the glottic opening is visible

Grade 3. Only the tip of the epiglottis visible

Grade 4. Only the soft palate is visible

FIGURE 49.5 Laryngoscopy.

(B, Illustration courtesy of Mike Mustar, medical illustrator, MetroHealth Medical Center, Cleveland, OH.)

FIBEROPTIC BRONCHOSCOPY

Flexible fiberoptic bronchoscopy (FOB) is often the preferred intubation method in awake, spontaneously breathing patients. Awake airway placement should be considered in patients with a known or suspected difficult airway, patients with a full stomach not likely to tolerate the short period of apnea required for rapid sequence intubation, and patients in whom paralytic or ablation of spontaneous respiration may be detrimental (e.g., compressive mediastinal mass). However, awake intubation requires a cooperative patient.

After appropriate preparation and anesthesia, a fiberoptic bronchoscope with preloaded endotracheal tube can be used for airway placement via a nasopharyngeal or oropharyngeal approach. Application of a silicone spray or other lubricant to the bronchoscope ensures easy advancement of the ETT over the FOB.

The nasopharyngeal method may be preferred in patients undergoing maxillofacial or dental surgery, when mouth opening is severely limited or when orotracheal intubation is contraindicated. Understanding the anatomic structural relationships is paramount to avoid complications during an NTI. First, the scope is advanced through either nasal opening. The anatomic borders include the skull based superiorly, the nasal septum medially, the three turbinates laterally, and both the hard and soft palates inferiorly. Continuing with scope advancement, there are two channels; the safer and more transversable entry is the inferior pathway. The superior pathway is bordered by the inferior and middle turbinates and is seldomly used for airway placement. The lower pathway, and more preferred airway entry, runs along the floor of the nasal cavity. A slight tube rotation and gentle pressure advancement should guide the tube past the posterior element of the nasopharyngeal cavity. Once the ETT reaches the oropharynx, a jaw thrust may be necessary to anteriorly displace the tongue to provide a better view of the glottic opening. In some instances, combined fiberoptic and direct or video laryngoscopy may be necessary for adequate vocal cord visualization. Once the vocal cords are visualized, topical 4% lidocaine can be instilled through the bronchoscope to provide anesthesia to the vocal cords and below. This will ablate the cough reflex mediated by the vagus nerve (CN X). The FOB should then be advanced through the vocal cords at least to the level of the carina, and the ETT advanced along the scope for intubation. Once through the vocal cords, tracheal rings will be visible. Placement should be confirmed as described previously and can also be confirmed visually with bronchoscopy.

Pitfalls or challenges of NTI include challenging anatomy, poor laryngeal visualization, or improper tube selection. Typically, patients are able to accommodate the same-diameter ETT nasally as they can orally; however, selecting a one or one-half size smaller ETT for nasal placement may decrease nasal trauma during placement. Absolute contraindications to NTI include known skull base fractures, coagulopathy, and frank epistaxis.

The oropharyngeal method can be assisted by an oral airway designed to accommodate an ETT. This acts as a bite block and to anteriorly displace the tongue for better visualization. Oropharyngeal anesthesia with a form of inhaled or viscous lidocaine as described previously will block the gag reflex of the glossopharyngeal nerve (CN IV). The FOB is advanced through the oral airway past the base of the tongue and into the posterior oropharynx, where the epiglottis and glottic opening should become visible distally. Intubation is then achieved in a similar fashion to NTI by advancing the FOB through the glottic opening and advancing the ETT into place over the FOB.

FAILED INTUBATION

A difficult airway is defined by the American Society of Anesthesiologists (ASA) as a situation in which a conventionally trained anesthesiologist experiences difficulty with BMV, intubation, or both. Difficult direct laryngoscopy occurs when it is not possible to visualize any part of the vocal cords after multiple attempts at conventional laryngoscopy. Difficult tracheal intubation occurs when intubation requires multiple attempts, and failed intubation occurs when placement of ETT fails after multiple attempts.

The decision to intubate a patient in respiratory distress is often made in a life-threatening situation with only seconds to spare; thus it is critical to have contingency plans in the event that intubation is not successful on the first attempt. The ASA Task Force on the Difficult Airway first published an algorithm for clinician use in 1993. The most recent update was published in 2013 and is widely accepted as a model for the approach to the difficult airway for not just anesthesiologists, but any practitioner involved in airway placement.

When difficult intubation is encountered, rescue plans usually consist of BMV with adjuncts such as oral or nasopharyngeal airways or placement of a supraglottic device such as a laryngeal mask airway (LMA). In the event that ventilation via BMV or LMA is still inadequate, the sequence must rapidly and safely progress to a surgical airway such as the cricothyroidotomy or tracheostomy, reviewed in another chapter of this textbook, to prevent hypoxia and brain injury.

SUMMARY

Airway anatomy can be complex and challenging. Reliable knowledge of the airway structural relationships, various assessment tools, and detailed innervation can greatly assist in securing a definitive airway. Familiarity with normal airway anatomy can also help the airway specialist approach a difficult airway with more confidence even in the more emergent lifesaving situations.

SUGGESTED READINGS

Apfelbaum JL, et al. American Society of Anesthesiologists. Practice guidelines for management of the difficult airway: an updated report by the American Society of Anesthesiologists task force on management of the difficult airway. Anesthesiology 2013;118:251–70.

Kortbeek JB, Turki SA, Ali J, et al. Advanced trauma life support, 8th edition, the evidence of change. J Trauma 2008;64:1638–50.

Chest Tube Placement

Sofya H. Asfaw

INTRODUCTION

Chest tube placement may be a lifesaving maneuver. Chest tubes are generally inserted for pneumothorax, hemothorax, hemopneumothorax, empyema, chylothorax, bronchopleural fistula, and pleural effusion. Although there are no absolute contraindications to placement, caution is advised when considering placement in patients with coagulopathy or those who may be on antiplatelet agents or other anticoagulants. They are placed in emergent and non-emergent clinical situations, and depending on the indication and urgency, the technique may vary slightly. Understanding thoracic anatomy and key landmarks can aid in safe and efficient chest tube insertion.

THORACIC ANATOMY AND KEY LANDMARKS

The chest wall comprises multiple layers, which include the skin, subcutaneous tissue, intercostal muscles, and parietal pleura (Figs. 50.1 and 50.2). Placing a tube requires traversing these structures.

The key landmarks are the clavicular head; midclavicular line; the anterior, middle, and posterior axillary lines; and intercostal spaces with corresponding ribs. The anterior border of the latissimus dorsi, the lateral border of the pectoralis major, and a line superior to the horizontal level of the nipple has been described as the "triangle of safety" in chest tube placement. Ideal placement in most situations is the fourth/fifth intercostal space. Identifying this rib space is essential to proper insertion of a chest tube. In a male patient, the lower border of the pectoralis major muscle may be used as a landmark to identify the fourth/fifth rib space; however, in a female patient, the nipple should *not* be used as a landmark. Instead, the inframammary fold should be used to identify the fifth rib at the anterior axillary line. Failure to recognize these boundaries can result in complications such as placing a tube into or below the diaphragm, which can result in bleeding or injury to intra-abdominal or major vascular structures (see Fig. 50.1A).

The intercostal neurovascular bundle lies just below the inferior portion of the rib (see Fig. 50.2B). It is important to place the chest tube over the most superior portion of the rib to avoid injuring the intercostal neurovascular bundle. Recognizing the location of these important structures is a key concept in placement.

Misguided tube placement can also be avoided by understanding the differences between the left and right chest cavities (see Fig. 50.1B). The right lung is trilobar and the left is bilobar. The location of the horizontal fissure on the right and oblique fissure on the left is at approximately the fourth rib at the anterior axillary line. Staying below this rib can help avoid inadvertent placement of the tube within a fissure.

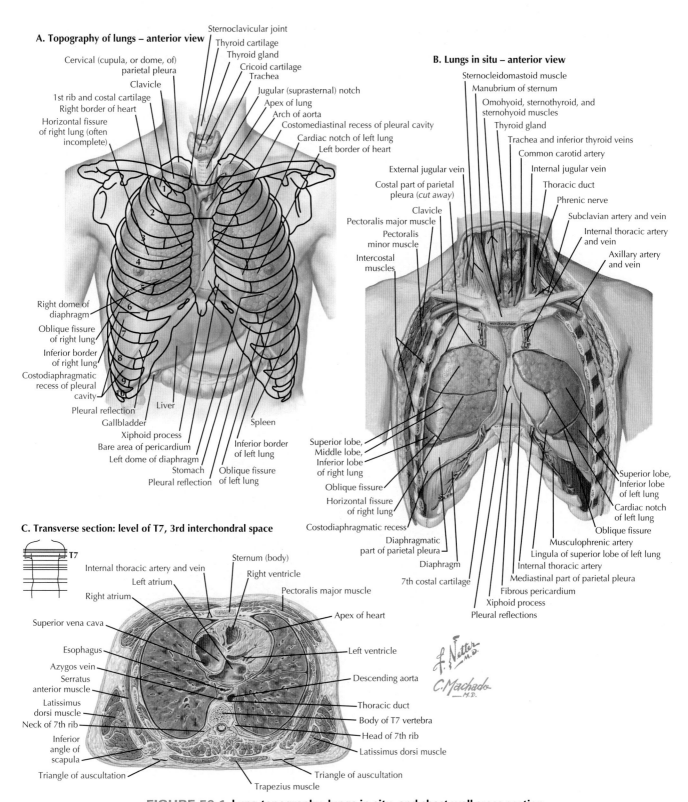

FIGURE 50.1 **Lung topography, lungs in situ, and chest wall cross section.**

A. Surface anatomy of the thorax

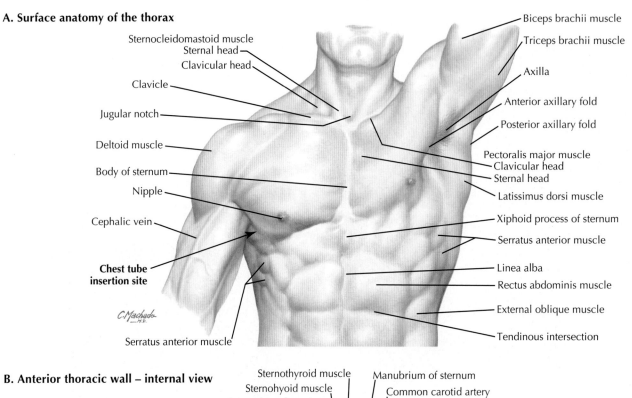

Sternocleidomastoid muscle
Sternal head
Clavicular head
Clavicle
Jugular notch
Deltoid muscle
Body of sternum
Nipple
Cephalic vein
Chest tube insertion site
Serratus anterior muscle

Biceps brachii muscle
Triceps brachii muscle
Axilla
Anterior axillary fold
Posterior axillary fold
Pectoralis major muscle
Clavicular head
Sternal head
Latissimus dorsi muscle
Xiphoid process of sternum
Serratus anterior muscle
Linea alba
Rectus abdominis muscle
External oblique muscle
Tendinous intersection

B. Anterior thoracic wall – internal view

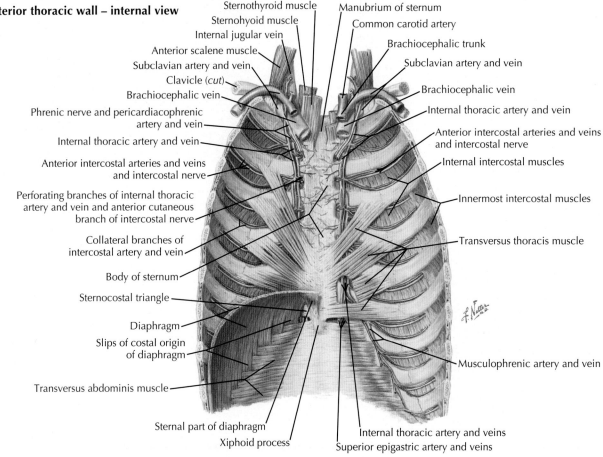

Sternothyroid muscle
Sternohyoid muscle
Internal jugular vein
Anterior scalene muscle
Subclavian artery and vein
Clavicle (cut)
Brachiocephalic vein
Phrenic nerve and pericardiacophrenic artery and vein
Internal thoracic artery and vein
Anterior intercostal arteries and veins and intercostal nerve
Perforating branches of internal thoracic artery and vein and anterior cutaneous branch of intercostal nerve
Collateral branches of intercostal artery and vein
Body of sternum
Sternocostal triangle
Diaphragm
Slips of costal origin of diaphragm
Transversus abdominis muscle

Manubrium of sternum
Common carotid artery
Brachiocephalic trunk
Subclavian artery and vein
Brachiocephalic vein
Internal thoracic artery and vein
Anterior intercostal arteries and veins and intercostal nerve
Internal intercostal muscles
Innermost intercostal muscles
Transversus thoracis muscle
Musculophrenic artery and vein

Sternal part of diaphragm
Xiphoid process
Internal thoracic artery and veins
Superior epigastric artery and veins

FIGURE 50.2 Anatomy of thorax.

TECHNIQUE AND STEPS

Experience and practice facilitate safe chest tube insertion, especially in an emergent situation. Proper patient position will also help to facilitate a safe placement.

Select an appropriate-size chest tube. For thicker, more viscous fluid, a larger tube is preferred, for example a 36-French or larger. For a simple pneumothorax, a smaller tube may be appropriate.

Begin by placing the patient in either a supine or semirecumbent position and abduct the patient's ipsilateral arm over or behind his or her head. Next, prepare the target area with an antiseptic solution such as chlorhexidine or povidone-iodine and place a sterile barrier to outline the field. Even in an emergent situation, this step is highly recommended. When the sterile field is marked, the nipple should be visible to help identify the appropriate landmarks.

As discussed in the last section, identifying landmarks is critical. Identify the anterior axillary line and the inframammary or subpectoral fold and palpate the rib at this location.

Infuse the intended location with local anesthetic. Start by anesthetizing the skin and soft tissue adjacent to the incision site. Then infuse deeper through the intercostal layers to the pleura. Slowly advance the needle while aspirating until the pleural space is encountered. Entry may be confirmed by aspiration of air (if the indication is for pneumothorax) or fluid. The pleura can then be anesthetized as well. In an emergent situation, administration of local anesthetic may not be possible.

Next, make an approximately 2-cm skin incision directly over the center of the rib, incising down to the periosteum of the rib. Using a Kelly clamp, tunnel through the incision, above the rib space, through the intercostal muscles and the parietal pleura. Apply gentle pressure using care to control the tip of the instrument and entry to the pleural space should be gained. Once the chest cavity is entered, insert one finger and gently sweep circumferentially to ensure that lung is away from the insertion site. The chest tube can then be placed through this tunnel with the assistance of the large Kelly clamp. To aid in insertion, the tube can be preloaded on the end of a Kelly clamp that can then be directed into the chest cavity (see Fig. 50.3). Once the tube has been inserted into the pleural cavity, it is important to ensure that the "sentinel hole" of the chest tube is within the pleural space as the tube will not work properly if it is not. After this has been accomplished, the tube is connected to a drainage system and secured to the skin with a large suture. Making sure the skin is securely closed around the tube is important to facilitate proper tube functioning. The tails of the suture are typically wrapped around the chest tube to anchor it into position. Additionally, placing a purse-string suture around the tube at the time of insertion facilitates an easy removal because this suture can be used to close the entry site at the time of tube removal. A nonocclusive petroleum based dressing is then applied around the insertion site of the chest tube, and the site is then appropriately dressed. After the tube is secured, a chest radiograph should be obtained to confirm placement.

An alternative to lateral tube positioning would be placement in the second/third interspace at the midclavicular line. This location is typically reserved for using a small-bore tube to evacuate a pneumothorax (see Fig. 50.3).

SPECIAL CONSIDERATIONS

Pregnancy

Pregnancy can present an uncommon circumstance for chest tube insertion. In the latter half of a pregnancy, the diaphragm can be displaced upward by an expanding uterus and other displaced intra-abdominal organs. As such, it is important to reconsider the usual anatomic placement of a chest tube. Instead of the typical fourth/fifth interspace placement, some authors advocate for insertion in as high as the third interspace to avoid a potential transdiaphragmatic placement. Additionally, attention to patient positioning is particularly important. As a pregnancy progresses, the gravid and enlarging uterus may place pressure on the inferior vena cava and impede venous return, especially when a patient is placed in a supine position for an extended period of time. In this particular population, if supine positioning is required for tube placement, safe and expeditious execution is recommended to avoid the physiologic disturbances associated with caval compression.

Ultrasound

Ultrasound is a modality that provides excellent visualization of not only fluid but also lung and thoracic structures (Fig. 50.3). When used, ultrasound can be diagnostic and therapeutic and aid in safer and more precise placement of pleural catheters than a conventional blind placement. Not only has it been shown to reduce hospital costs but also may reduce procedure-related risks. Although it may not be possible to use in an emergent situation, ultrasound guidance can be an ideal adjunct to placement in elective or nonurgent cases.

Hemostat technique

Preferred sites
1. For pneumothorax (2nd or 3rd interspace at midclavicular line)
2. For hemothorax (5th interspace at midaxillary line)

A. Skin incised and pleura entered by blunt dissection

B. Tube inserted into pleural cavity

C. Tube attached to underwater seal (with suction if indicated)

Note: For all techniques, local anesthesia is used; penetrate close to upper border of lower rib to avoid intercostal vessels. Aspirate first for free blood or free air (adherent lung)

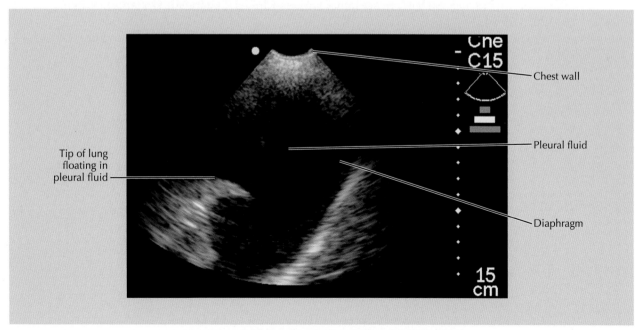

Chest wall

Pleural fluid

Tip of lung floating in pleural fluid

Diaphragm

FIGURE 50.3 Landmarks for chest tube placement.

SUGGESTED READINGS

Dev SP, Nascimiento B, Simone C, Chien V. Chest-tube insertion. N Engl J Med 2007;357:e15.

Hoth JJ, Kincaid EH, Meredith JW. Injuries to the chest. In: Ashley SW, editor. ACS Surgery: Principles and Practice. Hamilton, Ontario: Decker; 2012. www.acssurgery.com.

Ingelfinger J, Peris A, Tutino L, Cianchi G, Gensini G. Ultrasound guidance for pleural-catheter placement. N Engl J Med 2018;378:14 e19.

Varghese Jr TK. Chest trauma. In: Mulholland MH, et al., editors. Greenfield's Surgery: Scientific Principles and Practice. 5th ed. Philadelphia: Wolters Kluwer/Lippincott, Williams & Wilkins; 2011. p. 370–84.

Venuta F, Diso D, Anile M, Redina EA, Onorati I. Chest tubes: generalities. Thor Surg Clin 2017;27:1–5.

Emergency Thoracotomy for Trauma

Molly Flannagan

INTRODUCTION

Resuscitative emergency thoracotomy can be a lifesaving procedure for patients in traumatic cardiac arrest. As a salvage maneuver, the associated mortality is high, and the search to clarify indications has sparked controversy since its first description. Patients who are pulseless with signs of life after penetrating thoracic trauma have the highest chance of survival after emergency thoracotomy (Fig. 51.1A). Additional indications include penetrating extra-thoracic trauma and patients with signs of life after blunt injury. Knowledge of indications and anatomy is crucial to good patient outcomes.

SURGICAL PRINCIPLES

Five main maneuvers can be performed, depending on the findings:
1. Thoracotomy
2. Open pericardium
3. Cardiac massage
4. Damage control
5. Aortic cross-clamp

THORACOTOMY

Expeditious entry into the thoracic cavity is achieved through a left anterolateral thoracotomy incision in the fourth or fifth intercostal space (Fig. 51.1B). External landmarks for the fourth and fifth intercostal space are just below the nipple for men and in the inframammary fold for women (with the breast retracted). This incision is made with a scalpel and deepened through the musculature into the pleural space. Mayo scissors are used to extend the incision as shown (Fig. 51.1C).

For suspected or known injuries in the right chest, the incision can be extended medially across the sternum to make a clamshell thoracotomy (Fig. 51.1D). Care should be taken to ligate the internal thoracic arteries if extending to a clamshell incision to prevent iatrogenic blood loss.

Place a rib retractor for exposure with the handle positioned in the left axilla, which keeps the handle from interfering with extension to the right chest if it becomes necessary.

The endotracheal tube (ETT) can be advanced into the right mainstem bronchus, if necessary, to deflate the left lung and improve exposure to the thoracic structures.

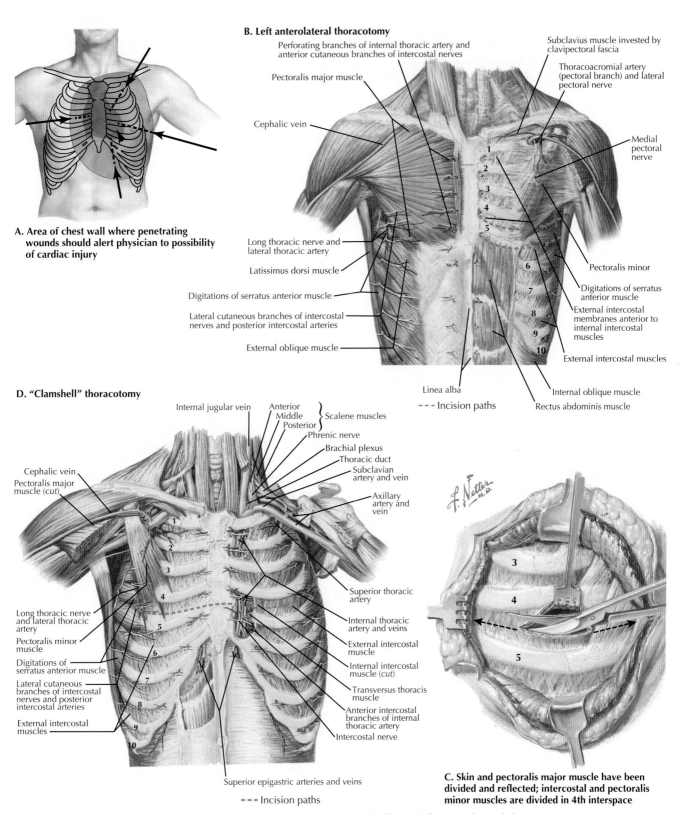

B. Left anterolateral thoracotomy

Perforating branches of internal thoracic artery and anterior cutaneous branches of intercostal nerves

Pectoralis major muscle

Cephalic vein

Long thoracic nerve and lateral thoracic artery

Latissimus dorsi muscle

Digitations of serratus anterior muscle

Lateral cutaneous branches of intercostal nerves and posterior intercostal arteries

External oblique muscle

Subclavius muscle invested by clavipectoral fascia

Thoracoacromial artery (pectoral branch) and lateral pectoral nerve

Medial pectoral nerve

Pectoralis minor

Digitations of serratus anterior muscle

External intercostal membranes anterior to internal intercostal muscles

External intercostal muscles

Internal oblique muscle

Rectus abdominis muscle

Linea alba

- - - Incision paths

A. Area of chest wall where penetrating wounds should alert physician to possibility of cardiac injury

D. "Clamshell" thoracotomy

Internal jugular vein

Anterior
Middle   Scalene muscles
Posterior

Phrenic nerve

Brachial plexus

Thoracic duct

Subclavian artery and vein

Axillary artery and vein

Cephalic vein

Pectoralis major muscle (cut)

Long thoracic nerve and lateral thoracic artery

Pectoralis minor muscle

Digitations of serratus anterior muscle

Lateral cutaneous branches of intercostal nerves and posterior intercostal arteries

External intercostal muscles

Superior thoracic artery

Internal thoracic artery and veins

External intercostal muscle

Internal intercostal muscle (cut)

Transversus thoracis muscle

Anterior intercostal branches of internal thoracic artery

Intercostal nerve

Superior epigastric arteries and veins

- - - Incision paths

C. Skin and pectoralis major muscle have been divided and reflected; intercostal and pectoralis minor muscles are divided in 4th interspace

FIGURE 51.1 Entry into thoracic cavity: "clamshell" and left anterolateral thoracotomy.

OPEN PERICARDIUM

Visualize the heart by pushing the left lung posteriorly. Bulging of the pericardium or visualization of pericardial blood is managed with immediate pericardiotomy. The pericardium is grasped with toothed forceps if possible, and an incision is made with a scalpel, anterior and parallel to the phrenic nerve (Fig. 51.2A). The incision is extended with Metzenbaum scissors (Fig. 51.2B), long enough to allow the delivery of the heart into the left chest. Temporary control of cardiac wounds is best managed with direct manual pressure until the patient can be transferred to the operating room (Fig. 51.2C).

Definitive management of cardiac injury is best managed in the operating room. Atrial and venous injuries are repaired with running 3-0 or 4-0 polypropylene suture (Fig. 51.2D). Ventricular injuries are repaired with pledgeted sutures. Wounds adjacent to the coronary arteries are repaired as shown (Fig. 51.2E).

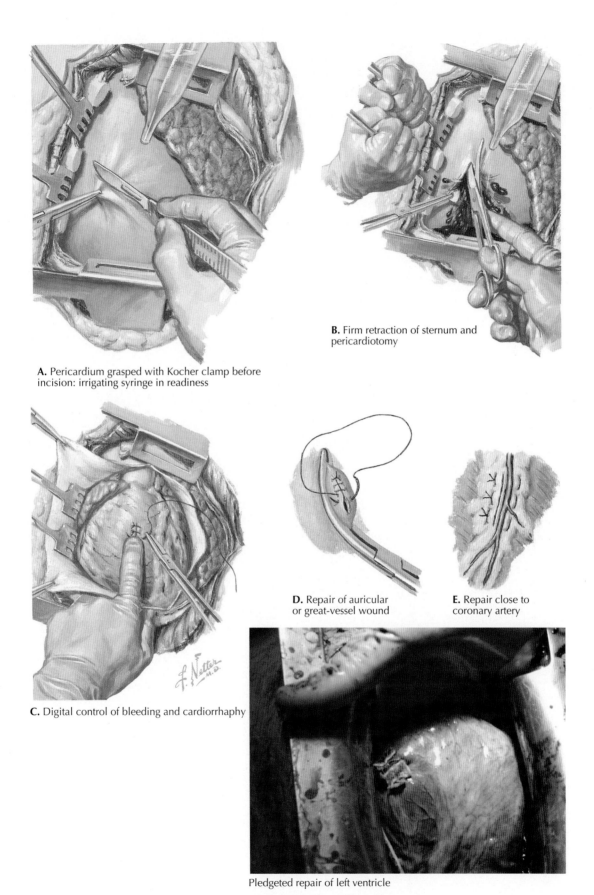

A. Pericardium grasped with Kocher clamp before incision: irrigating syringe in readiness

B. Firm retraction of sternum and pericardiotomy

C. Digital control of bleeding and cardiorrhaphy

D. Repair of auricular or great-vessel wound

E. Repair close to coronary artery

Pledgeted repair of left ventricle

FIGURE 51.2 **Pericardiotomy and cardiorrhaphy.**

CARDIAC MASSAGE

Open cardiac massage is performed by delivering the heart though the pericardial incision and using two flat palms with the wrists together to perform a hinged clapping motion. The thumbs should remain flat to prevent accidental perforation of the heart, and the heart is compressed from the apex to the base (Fig. 51.3).

A. Open cardiac massage

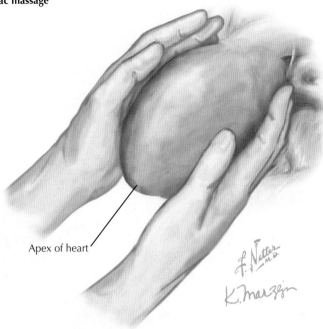

Apex of heart

B. Contents of the thorax: mediastinum

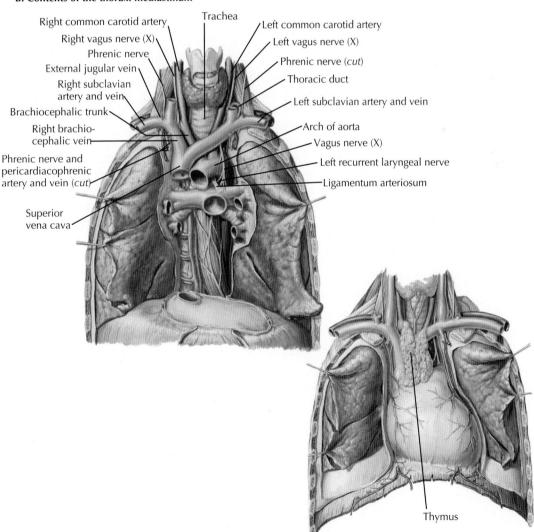

Right common carotid artery
Right vagus nerve (X)
Phrenic nerve
External jugular vein
Right subclavian artery and vein
Brachiocephalic trunk
Right brachiocephalic vein
Phrenic nerve and pericardiacophrenic artery and vein (cut)
Superior vena cava

Trachea

Left common carotid artery
Left vagus nerve (X)
Phrenic nerve (cut)
Thoracic duct
Left subclavian artery and vein
Arch of aorta
Vagus nerve (X)
Left recurrent laryngeal nerve
Ligamentum arteriosum

Thymus

FIGURE 51.3 Cardiac massage, left thoracotomy, and ligament incision.

DAMAGE CONTROL

Systematic assessment of the thoracic cavity is undertaken to identify and temporize life-threatening injuries. Cardiac injuries are stabilized as described above. Vascular and pulmonary injuries can be temporarily addressed with direct pressure, laparotomy pads, and sponge sticks. Once in the operating room, pulmonary injuries are best treated by nonanatomic resection, direct suture repair, or pulmonary tractotomy (Fig. 51.4A and B).

Major pulmonary hemorrhage can be controlled at the pulmonary hilum with a large vascular clamp (e.g., Satinsky) or with a hilar twist. To perform the hilar twist, first divide the inferior pulmonary ligament (Fig. 51.4C), taking care not to injure the inferior pulmonary vein. Then rotate the left lower lobe 180 degrees over the left upper lobe, compressing the main pulmonary vasculature. Pulmonary hilar occlusion is not well tolerated, risking irreversible injury to the lung, pneumonectomy, right heart failure, and arrhythmias, and should be used only as a last resort.

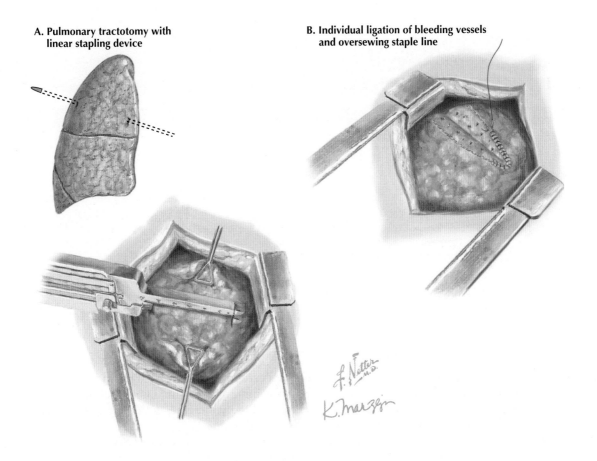

A. Pulmonary tractotomy with linear stapling device

B. Individual ligation of bleeding vessels and oversewing staple line

C. Incision of inferior pulmonary ligament

Heart in pericardium

Inferior pulmonary vein

Inferior pulmonary ligament

Diaphragm

Left lung

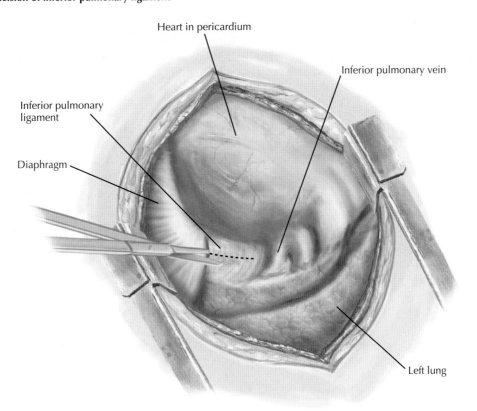

FIGURE 51.4 Pulmonary injuries.

AORTIC CROSS-CLAMP

The descending thoracic aorta is clamped to preserve cerebral and coronary blood flow and to stop subdiaphragmatic blood loss in patients with concomitant abdominal injuries (Fig. 51.5A). It should be undertaken with caution, because it can suddenly increase afterload and blood loss from proximal thoracic injuries, and it leads to visceral ischemia.

To accomplish this maneuver, retract the left lung anteriorly and divide the inferior pulmonary ligament. The aorta will be the first tubular longitudinal structure anterior to the thoracic vertebral bodies (Fig. 51.5B). Placement of a nasogastric or orogastric tube can help differentiate the esophagus from the floppy, empty aorta, which lies in a more anterior position.

The parietal pleura overlying the aorta is opened sharply, and blunt dissection is used to open a plane between the aorta and esophagus and in the prevertebral space. Care is taken to avoid injury to the intercostal vessels. The cross-clamp is then placed. It should be removed as soon as possible in the operating room to prevent visceral ischemia.

SUMMARY

Emergency thoracotomy can be a lifesaving procedure for patients in traumatic cardiac arrest. Patients with isolated penetrating cardiac injuries are the most likely to survive. Understanding the indications for emergency thoracotomy and thorough knowledge of thoracic anatomy are critical for safe performance of this procedure.

A. Thoracic and abdominal aorta

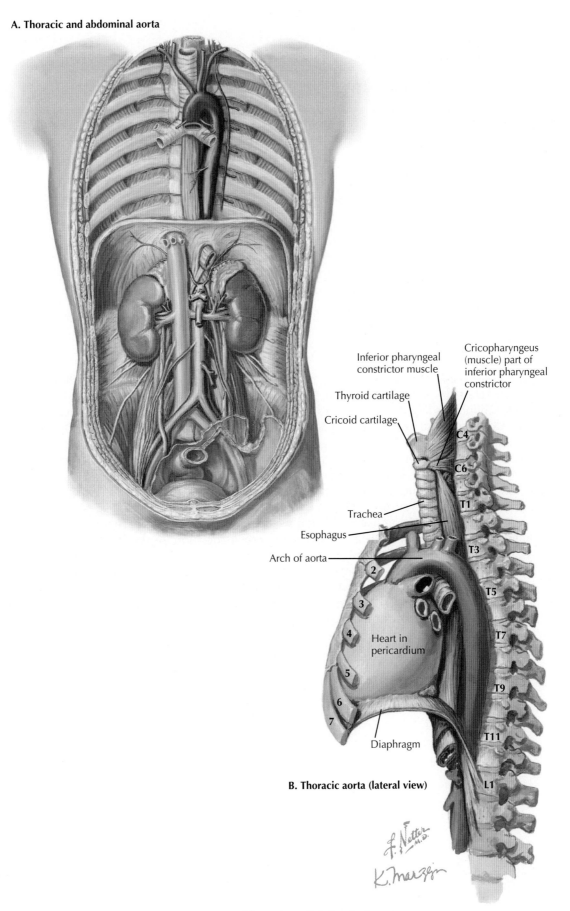

B. Thoracic aorta (lateral view)

FIGURE 51.5 **Thoracic and abdominal aorta.**

SUGGESTED READINGS

Hunt PA, Greaves I, Owens WA. Emergency thoracotomy in thoracic trauma-a review. Injury 2006;37(1):1–19. Epub 2005 Apr 20. Review.

Inaba K, Chouliaras K, Zakaluzny S, Swadron S, Mailhot T, Seif D, Teixeira P, Sivrikoz E, Ives et al. FAST ultrasound examination as a predictor of outcomes after resuscitative thoracotomy: a prospective evaluation. Ann Surg 2015;262(3):512–8; discussion 516–8.

Moore EE, Knudson MM, Burlew CC, Inaba K, Dicker RA, Biffl WL, Malhotra AK, Schreiber et al. Defining the limits of resuscitative emergency department thoracotomy: a contemporary Western Trauma Association perspective. J Trauma 2011;70(2):334–9.

Seamon MJ, Haut ER, Van Arendonk K, Barbosa RR, Chiu WC, Dente CJ, Fox N, Jawa RS, et al. An evidence-based approach to patient selection for emergency department thoracotomy: a practice management guideline from the Eastern Association for the Surgery of Trauma. J Trauma Acute Care Surg 2015;79(1):159–73.

Working Group, Ad Hoc Subcommittee on Outcomes, American College of Surgeons. Committee on Trauma. Practice management guidelines for emergency department thoracotomy. Working Group, Ad Hoc Subcommittee on Outcomes, American College of Surgeons-Committee on Trauma. J Am Coll Surg 2001;193(3):303–9.

Central Line Anatomy

Tony R. Capizzani

INTRODUCTION

Successful and safe insertion of a central venous catheter requires an understanding of the anatomic relationships associated with the larger veins of the body. These catheters can be used for fluid resuscitation, blood draws, hemodynamic monitoring, parental nutrition, and blood product administration. When bedside ultrasonography is used, these key anatomic relationships are even better observed during catheter placement. Ultrasound can be used to assist in assessing the patient, confirming safe catheter placement and reducing complications.

VENOUS CENTRAL ACCESS PREPARTION

There are numerous key factors for success in central venous access insertion. Any institution-recognized safety checklist and patient consent forms should always be completed. Refamiliarizing oneself with the anticipated anatomy provided by the figures in this chapter can assist with successful central line placement. There are key features for each specific central venous access approach. For the internal jugular and subclavian vein procedures, anatomy and identification of the central venous system is assisted by the Trendelenburg position. For all venous access procedures, proper sterile technique including chlorhexidine scrub and full body drape are necessary to reduce complications such as superficial, systemic, and line infections.

Procedural preparation should include a thorough review of preprocedural images such as plain chest radiography or prior venous ultrasounds. Additionally, bedside ultrasound can be used to access the vascular patency, anatomy, and surrounding deep tissue structural relationships. In the age of the electronic medical record, chart reviews of central access can also be completed with saved ultrasound anatomic images of successful venous access insertions.

Although numerous methods can be used for catheter insertion in the central venous system, this chapter focuses on the anatomy and details of the most commonly used techniques.

INTERNAL JUGULAR VENOUS CATHETERIZATION

The patient is placed in Trendelenburg position. An ultrasound can be used to confirm the anatomy of the internal jugular vein in between the sternal and clavicular heads of the sternocleidomastoid (SCM) muscle. The patient's head is often rotated 45 degrees to the contralateral side of the side desired for access. A shoulder roll can be used to extend the neck gently during this approach.

With use of ultrasound, the carotid artery is seen lateral to the internal jugular vein within the SCM triangle (Fig. 52.1). Within the cross-sectional ultrasonographic view, the needle may be inserted in perpendicular, oblique, and longitudinal approach to the probe. Most commonly, the needle is held in the perpendicular approach, which allows the needle shaft to be in parallel with the jugular vein. The skin puncture site should be 2 cm superior to the ipsilateral clavicle. As the needle tip punctures the vein, dark venous blood should be gently aspirated, confirming cannulation of the correct vessel.

At this point, the wire is guided through the needle and into the vein. The ultrasound probe can then be positioned in a longitudinal fashion to observe the wire in the correct trajectory and vessel. Using standard Seldinger technique, the needle is removed, and a sterile saline flushed catheter is manipulated over the guidewire. The wire can be safely removed, and the central line is secured in place and appropriately covered with a sterile dressing. In an adult, depending on which jugular vein is accessed, the catheter length inserted into the venous system is between 12 and 15 cm from the skin puncture site. A chest radiograph should be used to confirm this length and the tip of the catheter being located at the junction of the superior vena cava and right atrium.

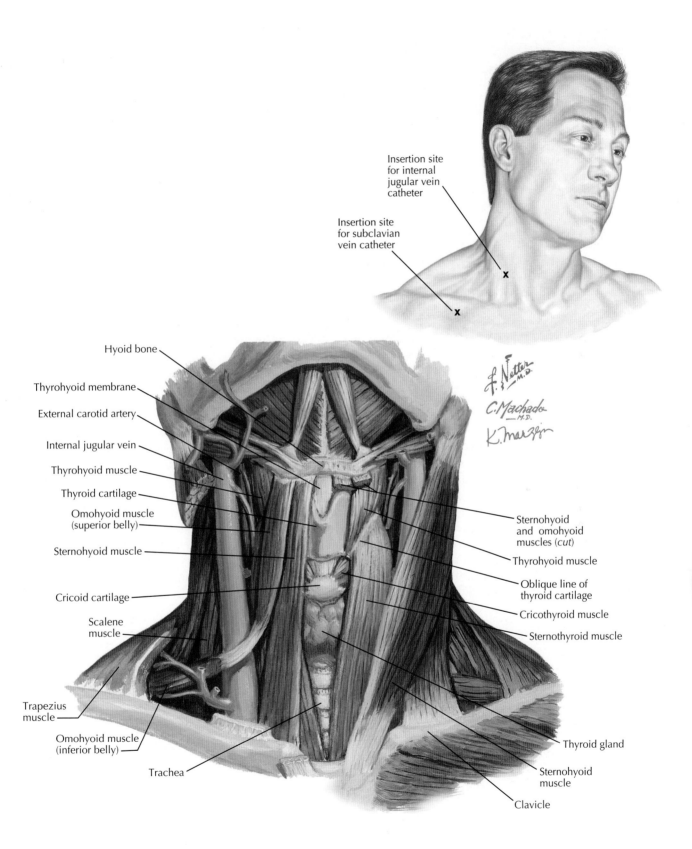

FIGURE 52.1 **Internal jugular vein anatomy and insertion sites for catheterization.**

INFRACLAVICULAR SUBCLAVIAN VENOUS CATHETERIZATION

Successful insertion again is assisted by the Trendelenburg position. In the adult there is often enough anatomic space lateral to the sternum to use ultrasound to distinguish between the subclavian artery and the subclavian vein. The subclavian vein is anterior and inferior to the subclavian artery at the palpable angle of the clavicle, at the medial third of the clavicle (Fig. 52.2).

The needle is inserted at the skin level 2 cm lateral to and 2 cm inferior to the angle of the clavicle in a trajectory toward the sternal notch. Care should be taken in staying anterior to the first rib and just inferior to the clavicle as the needle is advanced. The subclavian vein is punctured with the return of dark nonpulsatile blood. A sterile manometry technique can be used to visualize anticipated central venous pressure, and then the remaining CVL insertion is completed as previously described for the internal jugular vein.

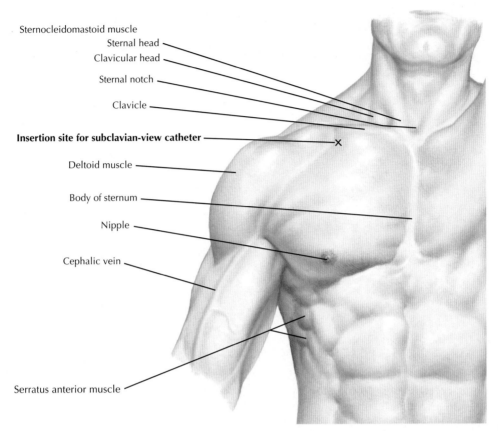

Sternocleidomastoid muscle

Sternal head

Clavicular head

Sternal notch

Clavicle

Insertion site for subclavian-view catheter

Deltoid muscle

Body of sternum

Nipple

Cephalic vein

Serratus anterior muscle

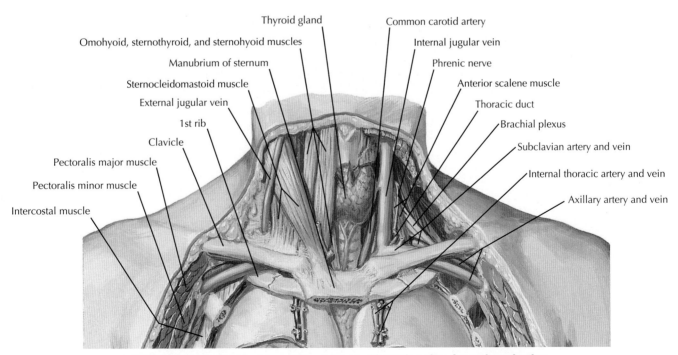

Thyroid gland

Omohyoid, sternothyroid, and sternohyoid muscles

Manubrium of sternum

Sternocleidomastoid muscle

External jugular vein

1st rib

Clavicle

Pectoralis major muscle

Pectoralis minor muscle

Intercostal muscle

Common carotid artery

Internal jugular vein

Phrenic nerve

Anterior scalene muscle

Thoracic duct

Brachial plexus

Subclavian artery and vein

Internal thoracic artery and vein

Axillary artery and vein

FIGURE 52.2 Subclavian vein anatomy and insertion sites for catheterization.

FEMORAL VENOUS CATHETERIZATION

Femoral venous access is often used in urgent or emergent clinical scenarios assisting observed cardiopulmonary arrest or trauma surgery patients requiring resuscitation. Anatomic structures such as the inguinal ligament and femoral pulse should be identified before the standard sterile drape and prep. The femoral vasculature lies within the femoral triangle. The triangle is bordered superiorly by the inguinal ligament, inframedially by the adductor longus muscle, and infralaterally by the sartorius muscle. The femoral arterial pulse can be palpated to help determine the more medial position of the femoral vein (Fig. 52.3). This medial-lateral relationship can also be visualized with bedside ultrasound. The needle trajectory should be at a slight angle, usually 30 to 45 degrees, to the patient's skin and at a minimum of 2 cm inferior to the inguinal ligament. Dark venous blood is aspirated, and the central line insertion is completed as previously described.

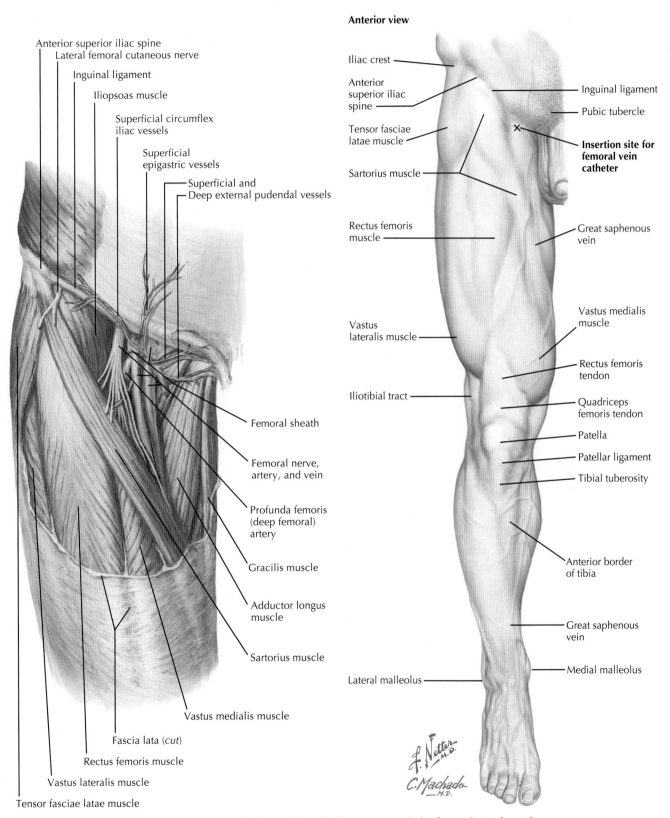

Anterior view

Anterior superior iliac spine
Lateral femoral cutaneous nerve
Inguinal ligament
Iliopsoas muscle
Superficial circumflex iliac vessels
Superficial epigastric vessels
Superficial and Deep external pudendal vessels
Femoral sheath
Femoral nerve, artery, and vein
Profunda femoris (deep femoral) artery
Gracilis muscle
Adductor longus muscle
Sartorius muscle
Vastus medialis muscle
Fascia lata (*cut*)
Rectus femoris muscle
Vastus lateralis muscle
Tensor fasciae latae muscle

Iliac crest
Anterior superior iliac spine
Tensor fasciae latae muscle
Sartorius muscle
Rectus femoris muscle
Vastus lateralis muscle
Iliotibial tract
Lateral malleolus

Inguinal ligament
Pubic tubercle
Insertion site for femoral vein catheter
Great saphenous vein
Vastus medialis muscle
Rectus femoris tendon
Quadriceps femoris tendon
Patella
Patellar ligament
Tibial tuberosity
Anterior border of tibia
Great saphenous vein
Medial malleolus

FIGURE 52.3 **Femoral vein and inguinal anatomy and site for catheter insertion.**

COMPLICATIONS

Complications can be largely avoided with proper preparation, anatomic knowledge often assisted by ultrasound, sterile technique, and a problem-solving skill set. Central line insertion can have associated immediate and late complications. For internal jugular and subclavian placed catheters, some immediate, more commonly observed complications include mispositioned central lines, arterial puncture, pneumothorax, hemothorax, and superficial hematomas. Immediate chest radiography and bedside confirming ultrasonography will help reduce or at least provide early diagnosis of these complications.

With all anatomic central line approaches, later complications can include catheter dislodgement, catheter site infections, central line–associated bacteremia, and even sepsis.

Unless other vessels are thrombosed or otherwise complicated, femoral lines are infrequently used in the ambulatory patient; they carry a higher infection risk because of the close proximity to the perineum.

SUGGESTED READINGS

Branner D, Lai S, Eman S, Tegtmeyer K. Central venous catheterization: subclavian vein. N Engl J Med 2007;357:e26.

Maurino P. Marino's the ICU Book. Hemodynamic Monitoring. 4th ed. Wolter's Kluwer Health; 2014. p. 123–71.

Oretga R, Song M, Hansen CJ, Barash P. Ultrasound-guided internal jugular vein cannulation. N Engl J Med 2010;362:e57.

Arterial Line Anatomy

Jeannine L. Marong

INTRODUCTION

Arterial lines are invasive procedures performed under sterile technique in the emergency, critical care, and operative settings to closely monitor blood pressure. They are most commonly placed in the radial artery but can also be placed in the axillary, brachial, femoral, and dorsalis pedis arteries. Arterial lines are also useful to have in place when frequent blood draws and blood gas analyses are needed.

RADIAL ARTERY

Because of its ease of accessibility, the radial artery is generally the vessel of choice when placing arterial lines. It can easily be palpated on the radial side of the wrist between the distal radius tendon and the flexor carpi radialis tendon (Fig. 53.1). If the blood pressure is low or vasculature is poor, the radial artery can be found via the aid of an ultrasound. If the radial artery cannot be cannulated successfully, alternative sites such as the axillary, brachial, femoral, and dorsalis pedis arteries can also be used, as described in more detail below.

A helpful, but not proven, examination that should be performed before radial artery cannulation is the Allen test. The Allen test is used to check for collateral circulation to the hand via the ulnar artery. This bedside test is performed by occluding the radial and ulnar arteries of one limb manually while the patient makes a fist. The hand will take on the characteristics of reduced blood flow until the ulnar artery is released while the radial remains occluded. If perfusion returns to the hand within seconds, then the collateral circulation provided by the ulnar artery is intact.

After assurance of the collateral circulation, the procedure can then be performed under sterile technique. For this procedure, an arterial line kit may be provided, or the use of a 20-gauge angiocatheter may be preferred, depending on the practitioner. The radial artery is cannulated via a catheter inserted at a 30- to 45-degree angle through the skin, subcutaneous tissue, and fascia of the ventral wrist. Once pulsatile blood flow has been encountered, the catheter can be secured into place and connected to intravenous tubing and a pressurized flush bag to start transducing or to obtain lab and gas samples.

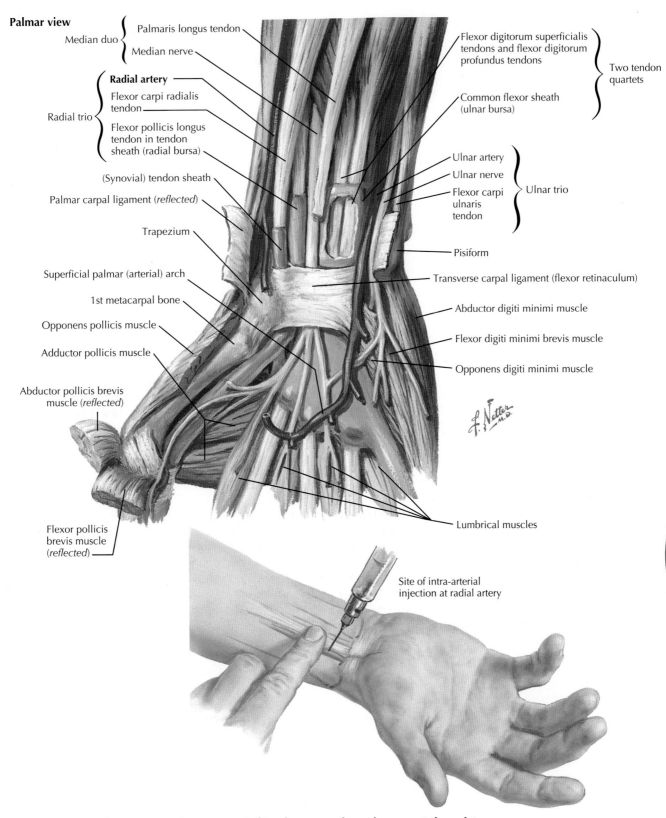

Palmar view

Median duo {
— Palmaris longus tendon
— Median nerve

Radial trio {
— **Radial artery**
— Flexor carpi radialis tendon
— Flexor pollicis longus tendon in tendon sheath (radial bursa)

(Synovial) tendon sheath
Palmar carpal ligament (*reflected*)
Trapezium
Superficial palmar (arterial) arch
1st metacarpal bone
Opponens pollicis muscle
Adductor pollicis muscle
Abductor pollicis brevis muscle (*reflected*)
Flexor pollicis brevis muscle (*reflected*)

Flexor digitorum superficialis tendons and flexor digitorum profundus tendons
Common flexor sheath (ulnar bursa)

} Two tendon quartets

Ulnar artery
Ulnar nerve
Flexor carpi ulnaris tendon
} Ulnar trio

Pisiform
Transverse carpal ligament (flexor retinaculum)
Abductor digiti minimi muscle
Flexor digiti minimi brevis muscle
Opponens digiti minimi muscle

Lumbrical muscles

Site of intra-arterial injection at radial artery

FIGURE 53.1 Arrangement of tendons, vessels, and nerves at the wrist.

AXILLARY ARTERY

Another access point for arterial line insertion in the upper extremity is the axillary artery. Caution must be taken when cannulating this artery because it lies in close proximity to the brachial plexus, and nerve injury may occur. On physical exam, patients are instructed to raise their arm over their head to most easily palpate the axillary artery. The artery can be found lateral to the axillary vein. Of its three sections, the part most available for arterial line insertion is the third and most distal segment located laterally to the pectoralis minor muscle in the chest (Fig. 53.2A). The remainder of the procedure follows that of the radial artery insertion.

BRACHIAL ARTERY

The brachial artery provides the majority of the blood flow to the humerus and the muscles in the upper arm and is an additional potential site for arterial line insertion in the upper extremity. Although limb ischemia is a potential concern, there is little evidence to support this feared complication. The brachial artery is formed from the axillary artery just below the teres major muscle. It then bifurcates into the radial and ulnar arteries after it traverses the flexor compartment of the arm (Fig. 53.2B). The brachial artery can be felt on physical exam between the biceps and triceps muscles that are proximal to the antecubital fossa. The artery is covered only by skin, subcutaneous tissue, and fascia and can be easily palpated on exam or with ultrasound guidance.

A. Axillary artery

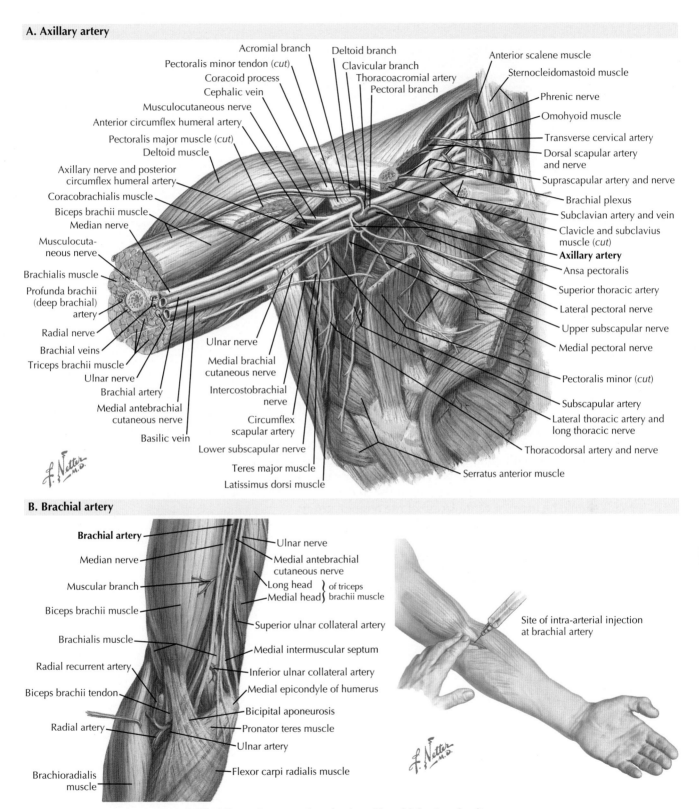

Acromial branch
Pectoralis minor tendon (cut)
Coracoid process
Cephalic vein
Musculocutaneous nerve
Anterior circumflex humeral artery
Pectoralis major muscle (cut)
Deltoid muscle
Axillary nerve and posterior circumflex humeral artery
Coracobrachialis muscle
Biceps brachii muscle
Median nerve
Musculocuta-neous nerve
Brachialis muscle
Profunda brachii (deep brachial) artery
Radial nerve
Brachial veins
Triceps brachii muscle
Ulnar nerve
Brachial artery
Medial antebrachial cutaneous nerve
Basilic vein

Deltoid branch
Clavicular branch
Thoracoacromial artery
Pectoral branch

Ulnar nerve
Medial brachial cutaneous nerve
Intercostobrachial nerve
Circumflex scapular artery
Lower subscapular nerve
Teres major muscle
Latissimus dorsi muscle

Anterior scalene muscle
Sternocleidomastoid muscle
Phrenic nerve
Omohyoid muscle
Transverse cervical artery
Dorsal scapular artery and nerve
Suprascapular artery and nerve
Brachial plexus
Subclavian artery and vein
Clavicle and subclavius muscle (cut)
Axillary artery
Ansa pectoralis
Superior thoracic artery
Lateral pectoral nerve
Upper subscapular nerve
Medial pectoral nerve
Pectoralis minor (cut)
Subscapular artery
Lateral thoracic artery and long thoracic nerve
Thoracodorsal artery and nerve
Serratus anterior muscle

B. Brachial artery

Brachial artery
Median nerve
Muscular branch
Biceps brachii muscle
Brachialis muscle
Radial recurrent artery
Biceps brachii tendon
Radial artery
Brachioradialis muscle

Ulnar nerve
Medial antebrachial cutaneous nerve
Long head } of triceps
Medial head } brachii muscle
Superior ulnar collateral artery
Medial intermuscular septum
Inferior ulnar collateral artery
Medial epicondyle of humerus
Bicipital aponeurosis
Pronator teres muscle
Ulnar artery
Flexor carpi radialis muscle

Site of intra-arterial injection at brachial artery

FIGURE 53.2 Axilla (dissection: anterior view) and brachial artery in situ.

FEMORAL AND DORSALIS PEDIS ARTERIES

Arterial insertion can also be performed in the lower extremity, using the femoral and dorsalis pedis arteries. The femoral artery lies medial to the femoral nerve and lateral to the femoral vein and is the continuation of the external iliac artery (Fig. 53.3). It can be palpated below the inguinal ligament, halfway between the anterior superior iliac spine and the pubic symphysis at the midinguinal point. In addition to the axillary and brachial artery, a longer catheter (12 cm) should be used for cannulation of the femoral artery.

Finally, the dorsalis pedis artery can be palpated between the first and second metatarsal bones over the dorsum of the foot. The artery is a continuation of the anterior tibialis artery that passes through the first intermetatarsal space to join with the plantar arch on the sole of the foot (Fig. 53.4).

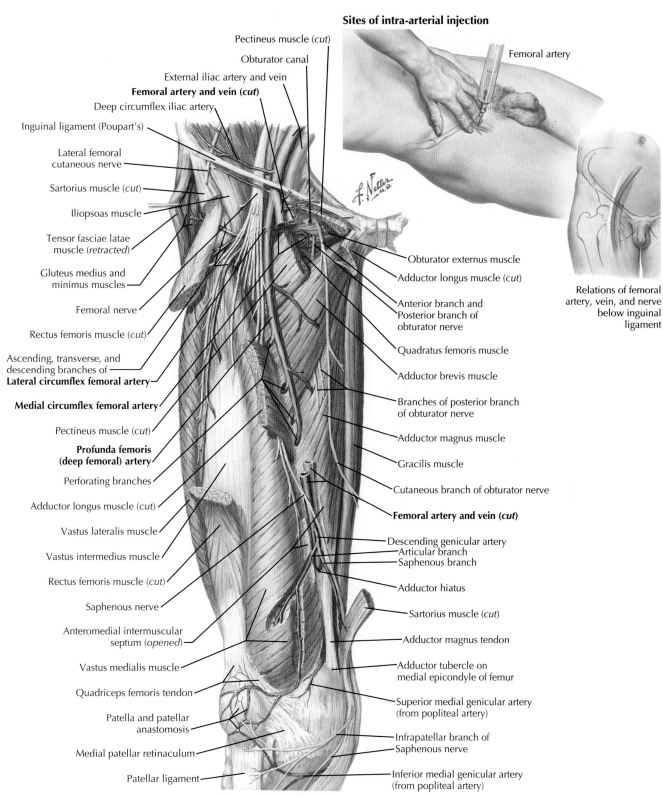

Sites of intra-arterial injection

Pectineus muscle (*cut*)

Obturator canal

External iliac artery and vein

Femoral artery and vein (cut)

Deep circumflex iliac artery

Inguinal ligament (Poupart's)

Lateral femoral cutaneous nerve

Sartorius muscle (*cut*)

Iliopsoas muscle

Tensor fasciae latae muscle (*retracted*)

Gluteus medius and minimus muscles

Femoral nerve

Rectus femoris muscle (*cut*)

Ascending, transverse, and descending branches of **Lateral circumflex femoral artery**

Medial circumflex femoral artery

Pectineus muscle (*cut*)

Profunda femoris (deep femoral) artery

Perforating branches

Adductor longus muscle (*cut*)

Vastus lateralis muscle

Vastus intermedius muscle

Rectus femoris muscle (*cut*)

Saphenous nerve

Anteromedial intermuscular septum (*opened*)

Vastus medialis muscle

Quadriceps femoris tendon

Patella and patellar anastomosis

Medial patellar retinaculum

Patellar ligament

Femoral artery

Relations of femoral artery, vein, and nerve below inguinal ligament

Obturator externus muscle

Adductor longus muscle (*cut*)

Anterior branch and Posterior branch of obturator nerve

Quadratus femoris muscle

Adductor brevis muscle

Branches of posterior branch of obturator nerve

Adductor magnus muscle

Gracilis muscle

Cutaneous branch of obturator nerve

Femoral artery and vein (cut)

Descending genicular artery
Articular branch
Saphenous branch

Adductor hiatus

Sartorius muscle (*cut*)

Adductor magnus tendon

Adductor tubercle on medial epicondyle of femur

Superior medial genicular artery (from popliteal artery)

Infrapatellar branch of Saphenous nerve

Inferior medial genicular artery (from popliteal artery)

FIGURE 53.3 Arteries and nerves of thigh: deep dissection (anterior view).

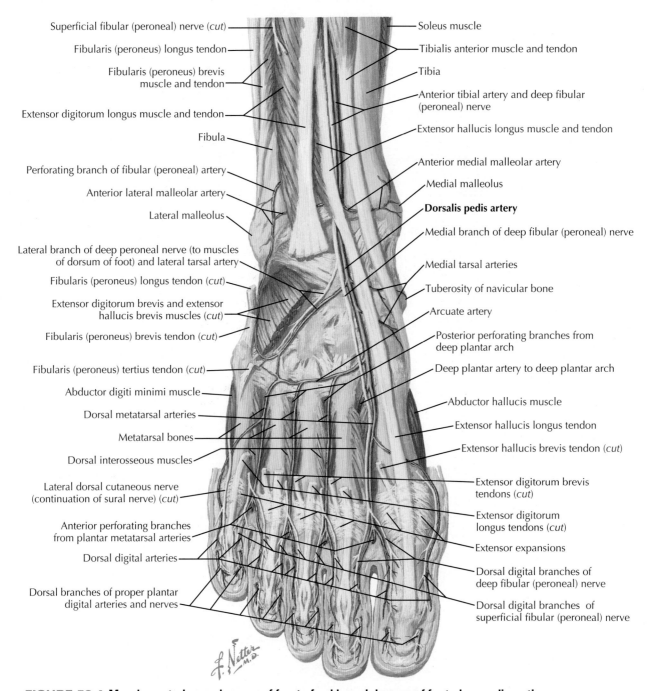

Superficial fibular (peroneal) nerve (*cut*)

Fibularis (peroneus) longus tendon

Fibularis (peroneus) brevis muscle and tendon

Extensor digitorum longus muscle and tendon

Fibula

Perforating branch of fibular (peroneal) artery

Anterior lateral malleolar artery

Lateral malleolus

Lateral branch of deep peroneal nerve (to muscles of dorsum of foot) and lateral tarsal artery

Fibularis (peroneus) longus tendon (*cut*)

Extensor digitorum brevis and extensor hallucis brevis muscles (*cut*)

Fibularis (peroneus) brevis tendon (*cut*)

Fibularis (peroneus) tertius tendon (*cut*)

Abductor digiti minimi muscle

Dorsal metatarsal arteries

Metatarsal bones

Dorsal interosseous muscles

Lateral dorsal cutaneous nerve (continuation of sural nerve) (*cut*)

Anterior perforating branches from plantar metatarsal arteries

Dorsal digital arteries

Dorsal branches of proper plantar digital arteries and nerves

Soleus muscle

Tibialis anterior muscle and tendon

Tibia

Anterior tibial artery and deep fibular (peroneal) nerve

Extensor hallucis longus muscle and tendon

Anterior medial malleolar artery

Medial malleolus

Dorsalis pedis artery

Medial branch of deep fibular (peroneal) nerve

Medial tarsal arteries

Tuberosity of navicular bone

Arcuate artery

Posterior perforating branches from deep plantar arch

Deep plantar artery to deep plantar arch

Abductor hallucis muscle

Extensor hallucis longus tendon

Extensor hallucis brevis tendon (*cut*)

Extensor digitorum brevis tendons (*cut*)

Extensor digitorum longus tendons (*cut*)

Extensor expansions

Dorsal digital branches of deep fibular (peroneal) nerve

Dorsal digital branches of superficial fibular (peroneal) nerve

FIGURE 53.4 Muscles, arteries, and nerves of front of ankle and dorsum of foot: deeper dissection.

SUGGESTED READINGS

Dibble C, Kohl B, Lankin P. Vascular access issues and procedures. The ICU Manual. 2nd ed. Elsevier Saunders; 2014. p. 105–8.

Hall-Craggs ECB. Anatomy as a Basis for Clinical Medicine. 2nd ed. New York: Urban & Schwarzenberg; 1990.

Slogoff S, Keats AS, Arlund C. On the safety of radial artery cannulation. Anesthesiology 1983;59:42–47.

Upper and Lower Extremity Fasciotomy

Rachael C. Sullivan

INTRODUCTION

Compartment syndrome of any extremity is a limb-threatening condition that must be recognized and treated in a timely fashion. Left untreated, compartment syndrome can lead to not only limb loss or functional impairment of the affected limb but also systemic consequences such as renal failure, worsening acidosis, and death.

Compartment syndrome is seen in both the upper and lower extremities, and the etiologies are similar. Blunt trauma leading to fractures and direct muscle injury, expanding hematomas, external compression, fluid extravasation, infection, reperfusion, and severe burns are some of the more common causes of compartment syndrome. Fasciotomy of the affected compartments is the definitive treatment of true compartment syndrome and must be performed in a timely fashion to prevent ongoing tissue injury.

ETIOLOGY OF COMPARTMENT SYNDROME

Compartment syndrome occurs when the pressure in the affected compartment rises above the pressure within the vessels of that compartment, leading to inadequate tissue perfusion. In the confines of a fixed space when the pressure is greater than 30 mm Hg, both capillary perfusion and venous outflow are impeded. Without timely intervention, this leads to tissue death.

Increased compartmental pressure can be due to constriction of the compartment, such as from fascial closure or contraction of the overlying skin because of scarring (Fig. 54.1), or external compression, such as from tight casts or dressings. Prolonged downtime with compression of a limb as seen in metabolic comas or traumatic falls can also lead to elevated compartmental pressure (see Fig. 54.1). Another common etiology of compartment syndrome is increased volume of fluid within the space. This can be due to a number of causes, including bleeding, infiltration of exogenous fluid such as intravenous (IV) extravasation (either from intravenous catheters in the upper extremity or intraosseous catheters in the lower extremity that have slipped from their intended positions), capillary leakage from reperfusion injury, severe burns, trauma (especially crush injuries), venous or lymphatic obstruction, or muscle swelling from overexertion (see Fig. 54.1). Reperfusion injury is commonly seen after revascularization procedures and trauma, and the concern is heightened if the limb was ischemic for greater than 4 to 6 hours. Prophylactic fasciotomy should be considered in these patients.

Constriction of compartment

Increased fluid content in compartment

External compression

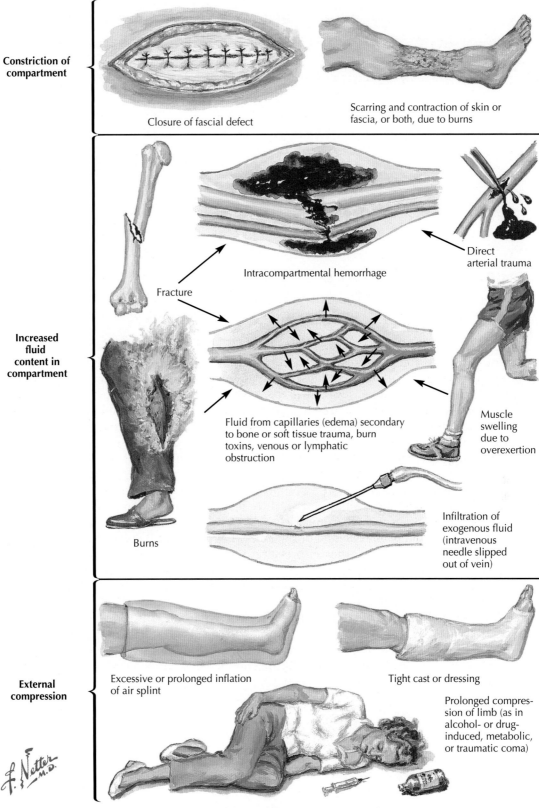

Closure of fascial defect

Scarring and contraction of skin or fascia, or both, due to burns

Fracture

Intracompartmental hemorrhage

Direct arterial trauma

Fluid from capillaries (edema) secondary to bone or soft tissue trauma, burn toxins, venous or lymphatic obstruction

Muscle swelling due to overexertion

Burns

Infiltration of exogenous fluid (intravenous needle slipped out of vein)

Excessive or prolonged inflation of air splint

Tight cast or dressing

Prolonged compression of limb (as in alcohol- or drug-induced, metabolic, or traumatic coma)

FIGURE 54.1 Etiology of compartment syndrome.

CLINICAL DIAGNOSIS AND DECISION MAKING

In cases of both upper and lower extremity compartment syndrome, a high index of suspicion must be maintained and, with suggestive clinical exam findings, will result in the diagnosis in most cases.

Pain, often out of proportion to exam, is the most common presenting symptom with compartment syndrome and is worsened with passive stretch (Fig. 54.2). Paresthesia and loss of light touch sensation resulting from the sensitivity of neurons to ischemia are other common early symptoms. These symptoms usually precede the development of diminished motor function and paralysis. In the upper extremity, forearm compartment syndrome most commonly affects the flexor (or volar) compartment. As such, pain with passive extension of finger and wrist extensors is most often seen. Paresthesia in the hand occurs because of the involvement of the median, ulnar, and radial nerves (Fig 54.3A). Less frequently, the dorsal compartments are involved.

Light touch sensation in the lower extremity can be assessed early on by testing the web space between the first and second toe, which is supplied by the deep peroneal nerve (Fig. 54.3B). Motor function of the major muscle groups of the lower extremity can be assessed by testing dorsiflexion and plantar flexion of the ankle and great toe. Pulselessness is a late sign; capillary flow may be restricted at lower pressures than the larger vessels. Thus, radial, ulnar, dorsalis pedis, and posterior tibialis pulses can often be palpated until later in the course of the disease. One must keep in mind that pulses may not be palpable at baseline in the presence of severe peripheral vascular disease.

For both upper and lower extremity compartment syndrome, the clinical situation must be taken into account. If a traumatic mechanism occurred, radiographs to identify fractures will help aid the diagnosis. In equivocal cases, compartmental pressure should be obtained (Fig. 54.4). Pressures greater than 30 mm Hg are considered abnormal, and urgent fasciotomy should be undertaken.

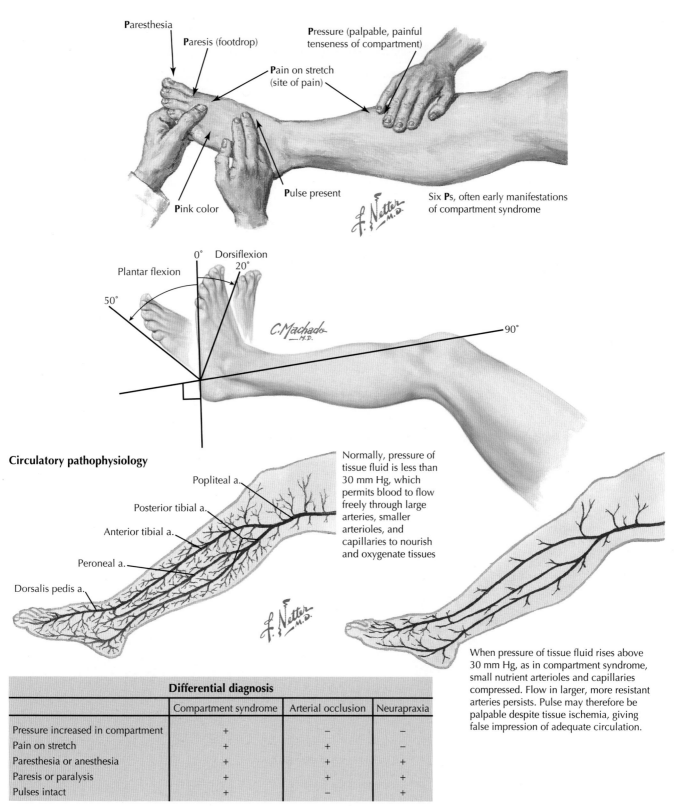

Paresthesia

Paresis (footdrop)

Pressure (palpable, painful tenseness of compartment)

Pain on stretch (site of pain)

Pulse present

Pink color

Six **P**s, often early manifestations of compartment syndrome

Plantar flexion

0° Dorsiflexion

20°

50°

90°

Circulatory pathophysiology

Popliteal a.

Posterior tibial a.

Anterior tibial a.

Peroneal a.

Dorsalis pedis a.

Normally, pressure of tissue fluid is less than 30 mm Hg, which permits blood to flow freely through large arteries, smaller arterioles, and capillaries to nourish and oxygenate tissues

When pressure of tissue fluid rises above 30 mm Hg, as in compartment syndrome, small nutrient arterioles and capillaries compressed. Flow in larger, more resistant arteries persists. Pulse may therefore be palpable despite tissue ischemia, giving false impression of adequate circulation.

Differential diagnosis			
	Compartment syndrome	Arterial occlusion	Neurapraxia
Pressure increased in compartment	+	−	−
Pain on stretch	+	+	−
Paresthesia or anesthesia	+	+	+
Paresis or paralysis	+	+	+
Pulses intact	+	−	+

FIGURE 54.2 Clinical diagnosis of compartment syndrome.

A. Nerves of upper limb

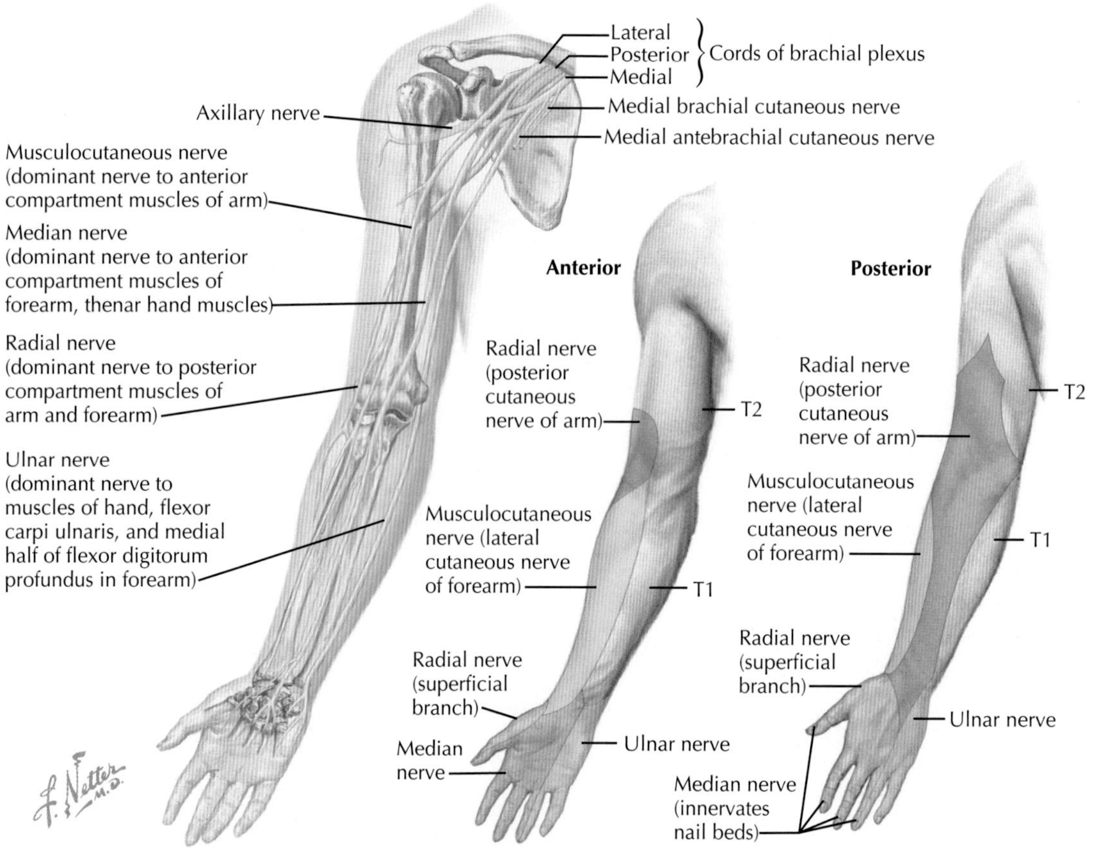

Lateral
Posterior } Cords of brachial plexus
Medial

Axillary nerve

Medial brachial cutaneous nerve
Medial antebrachial cutaneous nerve

Musculocutaneous nerve
(dominant nerve to anterior
compartment muscles of arm)

Median nerve
(dominant nerve to anterior
compartment muscles of
forearm, thenar hand muscles)

Radial nerve
(dominant nerve to posterior
compartment muscles of
arm and forearm)

Ulnar nerve
(dominant nerve to
muscles of hand, flexor
carpi ulnaris, and medial
half of flexor digitorum
profundus in forearm)

Anterior

Posterior

Radial nerve
(posterior
cutaneous
nerve of arm)

T2

Radial nerve
(posterior
cutaneous
nerve of arm)

T2

Musculocutaneous
nerve (lateral
cutaneous nerve
of forearm)

T1

Musculocutaneous
nerve (lateral
cutaneous nerve
of forearm)

T1

Radial nerve
(superficial
branch)

Radial nerve
(superficial
branch)

Ulnar nerve

Median
nerve

Ulnar nerve

Median nerve
(innervates
nail beds)

B. Common fibular (peroneal) nerve: mixed motor/sensory function

Common fibular
(peroneal) nerve
(*phantom*)

Lateral sural cutaneous
nerve (*phantom*)

Biceps femoris tendon

Articular branches

**Common fibular
(peroneal) nerve
(L4, 5, S1, 2)**

Recurrent articular nerve

Head of fibula

Extensor digitorum
longus muscle (*cut*)

Fibularis (peroneus)
longus muscle (*cut*)

**Deep fibular
(peroneal) nerve**

**Superficial fibular
(peroneal) nerve**

Tibialis anterior muscle

Branches of lateral
sural cutaneous nerve

Fibularis (peroneus)
longus muscle

Extensor digitorum
longus muscle

Fibularis (peroneus)
brevis muscle

Extensor hallucis
longus muscle

Medial dorsal
cutaneous nerve

Intermediate dorsal
cutaneous nerve

Lateral branch of deep fibular
(peroneal) nerve to

Inferior extensor
retinaculum (*partially cut*)

Extensor hallucis brevis
and
Extensor digitorum brevis
muscles

Lateral dorsal
cutaneous nerve
(branch of sural nerve)

Medial branch of deep
fibular (peroneal) nerve

Dorsal digital nerves

**Cutaneous
innervation**

Lateral sural
cutaneous nerve

Superficial fibular
(peroneal) nerve

Deep fibular
(peroneal) nerve

Sural nerve via
lateral dorsal
cutaneous branch

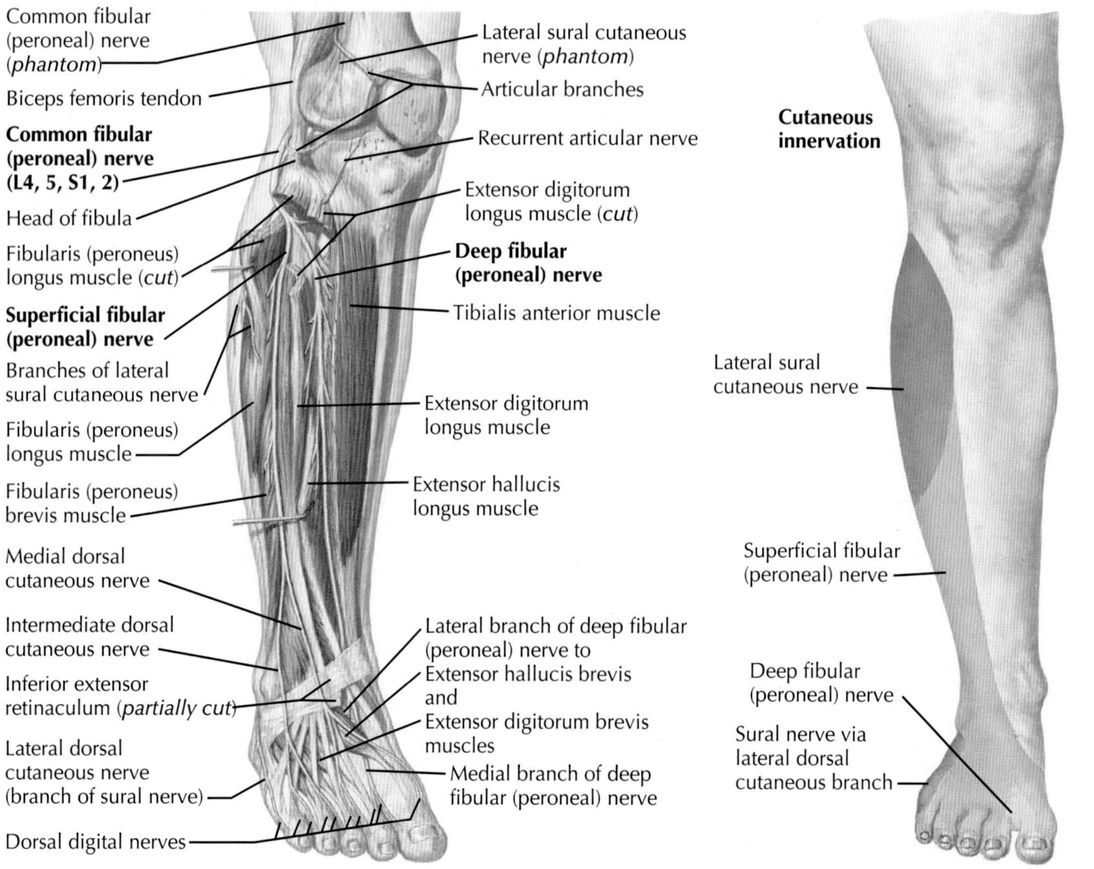

FIGURE 54.3 Upper and lower extremity innervation. (A) Nerves of upper limb. (B) Common fibular (peroneal) nerve: mixed motor/sensory function.

Wick catheter technique

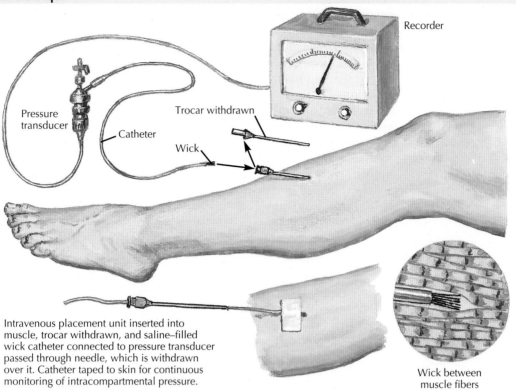

Intravenous placement unit inserted into muscle, trocar withdrawn, and saline–filled wick catheter connected to pressure transducer passed through needle, which is withdrawn over it. Catheter taped to skin for continuous monitoring of intracompartmental pressure.

Wick between muscle fibers

Slit catheter technique

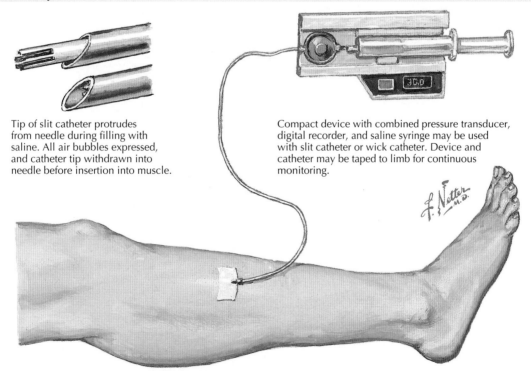

Tip of slit catheter protrudes from needle during filling with saline. All air bubbles expressed, and catheter tip withdrawn into needle before insertion into muscle.

Compact device with combined pressure transducer, digital recorder, and saline syringe may be used with slit catheter or wick catheter. Device and catheter may be taped to limb for continuous monitoring.

FIGURE 54.4 Measurement of intracompartmental pressure.

UPPER EXTREMITY COMPARTMENT SYNDROME

Upper extremity compartment syndrome occurs most often in the forearm, which houses one volar and two dorsal compartments. Of these, the volar compartment is the most commonly affected and has subcompartments divided by muscular septae (Fig. 54.5). The volar compartment contains the wrist and hand flexors and muscles of forearm pronation. This anatomic distinction creates a presenting sign of forearm compartment syndrome as exaggeration of the resting position: increased flexion of the wrist and digits, and exaggerated pronation of the forearm. The most superficial volar compartment houses the flexor carpi ulnaris, flexor palmaris longus, and the flexor carpi radialis, as well as the superficial portion of the pronator teres (Fig. 54.6). The most dorsal aspect of the volar compartment includes the flexor digitorum superficialis, flexor digitorum profundus, and the flexor pollicis longus.

There are two dorsal compartments, which contain the extensor muscles of the hand and wrist. The two dorsal compartments are divided into extrinsic digit extensors and the wrist extensors.

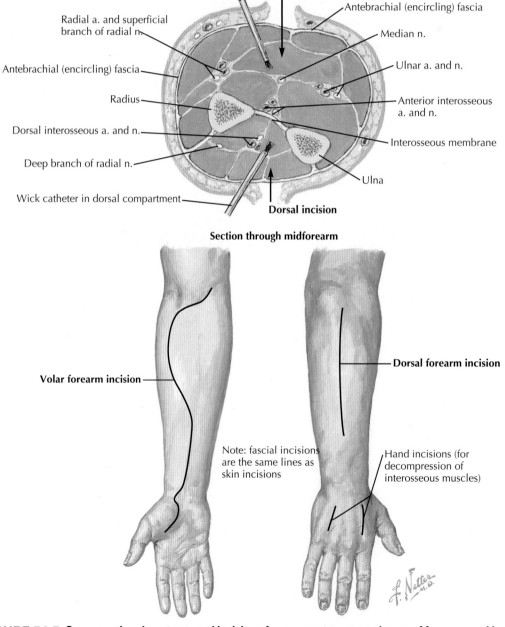

FIGURE 54.5 Cross-sectional anatomy and incisions for compartment syndrome of forearm and hand.

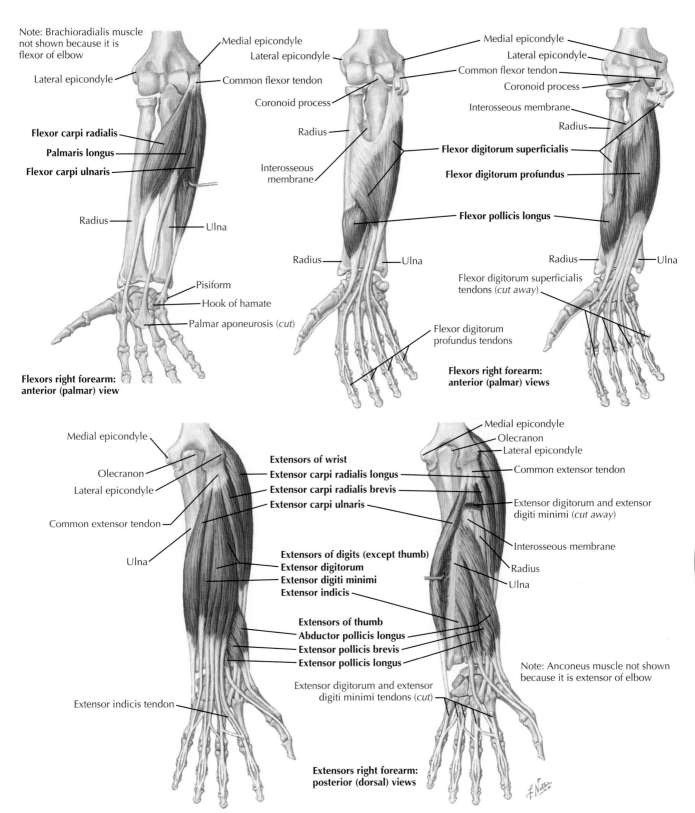

Note: Brachioradialis muscle not shown because it is flexor of elbow

Lateral epicondyle

Medial epicondyle

Lateral epicondyle

Common flexor tendon

Coronoid process

Flexor carpi radialis

Palmaris longus

Flexor carpi ulnaris

Radius

Ulna

Pisiform

Hook of hamate

Palmar aponeurosis (cut)

Radius

Interosseous membrane

Flexors right forearm: anterior (palmar) view

Medial epicondyle

Lateral epicondyle

Common flexor tendon

Coronoid process

Radius

Interosseous membrane

Radius

Ulna

Flexor digitorum profundus tendons

Flexors right forearm: anterior (palmar) views

Medial epicondyle

Lateral epicondyle

Common flexor tendon

Coronoid process

Interosseous membrane

Radius

Flexor digitorum superficialis

Flexor digitorum profundus

Flexor pollicis longus

Radius

Ulna

Flexor digitorum superficialis tendons (cut away)

Medial epicondyle

Olecranon

Lateral epicondyle

Common extensor tendon

Ulna

Medial epicondyle

Olecranon

Lateral epicondyle

Common extensor tendon

Extensors of wrist

Extensor carpi radialis longus

Extensor carpi radialis brevis

Extensor carpi ulnaris

Extensors of digits (except thumb)

Extensor digitorum

Extensor digiti minimi

Extensor indicis

Extensors of thumb

Abductor pollicis longus

Extensor pollicis brevis

Extensor pollicis longus

Extensor digitorum and extensor digiti minimi tendons (cut)

Extensor indicis tendon

Medial epicondyle

Olecranon

Lateral epicondyle

Common extensor tendon

Extensor digitorum and extensor digiti minimi (cut away)

Interosseous membrane

Radius

Ulna

Note: Anconeus muscle not shown because it is extensor of elbow

Extensors right forearm: posterior (dorsal) views

FIGURE 54.6 Individual muscles of forearm: flexors and extensors.

SURGICAL PRINCIPLES, ANATOMY, AND TECHNIQUE

Treatment of compartment syndrome involves complete decompressive fasciotomy. Because the volar aspect is the most commonly and severely affected, this compartment is initially incised. The volar forearm incision is made in a "lazy S" fashion proximally from above the elbow joint down through the wrist and extended distally through the wrist joint onto the palm (see Fig. 54.5). The carpal tunnel retinaculum should be released if there is distal involvement, which should be suspected if there is significant distal and/or hand edema.

The fascial incisions are made along the same line as the skin incision. The fascia overlying the compartments must be completely incised, and the septae within the volar compartment must also be fully opened for a complete decompression (see Figs. 54.5 and 54.7). The deeper subcompartment within the volar space, like the anterior compartment in the lower extremity, can be involved earlier, allowing for increased tissue destruction. Therefore dissecting deeply and incising the subcompartmental fascia encompassing this section is paramount in surgical therapy.

The ulnar nerve lies next to the flexor digitorum profundus muscle in the forearm, and the median nerve lies between the and the flexor digitorum profundus and flexor digitorum superficialis in the mid-forearm (see Figs. 54.3 and 54.7), and care must be taken to avoid inadvertent injury. The extent of involvement must be ascertained intraoperatively, and further surgical intervention of the dorsal forearm should be pursued if necessary.

If dorsal decompressive fasciotomy is indicated, one longitudinal incision 2 cm lateral and distal to the lateral epicondyle is used to access both compartments (see Fig. 54.5) and continued down to the junction of the extensor muscles in the mid-forearm. The fascia of both dorsal compartments can be incised through this incision. If the hand is involved, two dorsal hand incisions are used to access the interossei and adductor pollicis compartments (see Fig. 54.5).

The wounds are dressed with saline wet-to-dry dressings and changed daily. Once edema has abated, the fascia can be closed primarily if amenable. If fascial closure cannot be safely obtained, negative pressure–assisted therapy or healing by secondary intention with delayed skin grafting can be employed. The most common complications are bleeding, nerve injury, infection, and poor wound healing.

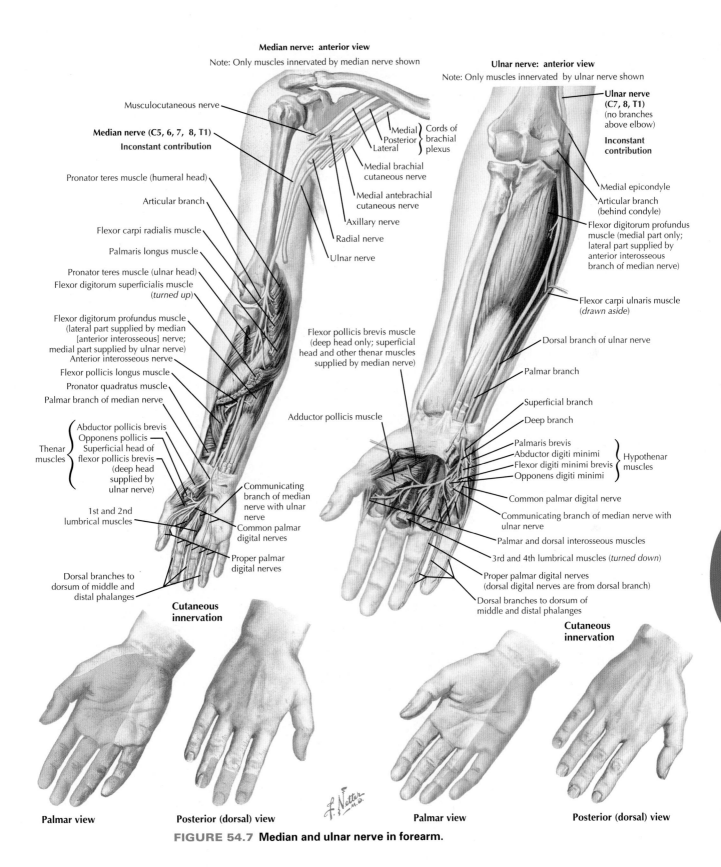

Median nerve: anterior view
Note: Only muscles innervated by median nerve shown

Ulnar nerve: anterior view
Note: Only muscles innervated by ulnar nerve shown

Musculocutaneous nerve

Median nerve (C5, 6, 7, 8, T1)
Inconstant contribution

Pronator teres muscle (humeral head)

Articular branch

Flexor carpi radialis muscle

Palmaris longus muscle

Pronator teres muscle (ulnar head)
Flexor digitorum superficialis muscle
(*turned up*)

Flexor digitorum profundus muscle
(lateral part supplied by median
[anterior interosseous] nerve;
medial part supplied by ulnar nerve)
Anterior interosseous nerve

Flexor pollicis longus muscle
Pronator quadratus muscle
Palmar branch of median nerve

Abductor pollicis brevis
Opponens pollicis
Thenar muscles { Superficial head of
flexor pollicis brevis
(deep head supplied by
ulnar nerve)

1st and 2nd
lumbrical muscles

Dorsal branches to
dorsum of middle and
distal phalanges

Medial
Posterior } Cords of
Lateral brachial
plexus

Medial brachial
cutaneous nerve

Medial antebrachial
cutaneous nerve

Axillary nerve

Radial nerve

Ulnar nerve

Flexor pollicis brevis muscle
(deep head only; superficial
head and other thenar muscles
supplied by median nerve)

Adductor pollicis muscle

Communicating
branch of median
nerve with ulnar
nerve
Common palmar
digital nerves

Proper palmar
digital nerves

Ulnar nerve
(C7, 8, T1)
(no branches
above elbow)

Inconstant
contribution

Medial epicondyle
Articular branch
(behind condyle)
Flexor digitorum profundus
muscle (medial part only;
lateral part supplied by
anterior interosseous
branch of median nerve)

Flexor carpi ulnaris muscle
(*drawn aside*)

Dorsal branch of ulnar nerve

Palmar branch

Superficial branch

Deep branch

Palmaris brevis
Abductor digiti minimi } Hypothenar
Flexor digiti minimi brevis muscles
Opponens digiti minimi

Common palmar digital nerve

Communicating branch of median nerve with
ulnar nerve

Palmar and dorsal interosseous muscles

3rd and 4th lumbrical muscles (*turned down*)

Proper palmar digital nerves
(dorsal digital nerves are from dorsal branch)

Dorsal branches to dorsum of
middle and distal phalanges

Cutaneous
innervation

Cutaneous
innervation

Palmar view **Posterior (dorsal) view**

Palmar view **Posterior (dorsal) view**

FIGURE 54.7 Median and ulnar nerve in forearm.

LOWER EXTREMITY COMPARTMENT SYNDROME

Compartment syndrome can occur within any compartment of the lower extremity, including the buttocks, thighs, lower leg, and foot but is most common in the lower leg. The lower leg is divided into four compartments: anterior, lateral, deep posterior, and superficial posterior (Fig. 54.8), and all of these compartments must be opened to ensure complete release. Of these compartments, the anterior compartment is more commonly and severely affected by increased compartmental pressures because of the scarcity of collateral arterial flow to this compartment. As with upper extremity compartment syndrome, treatment involves complete decompressive fasciotomy.

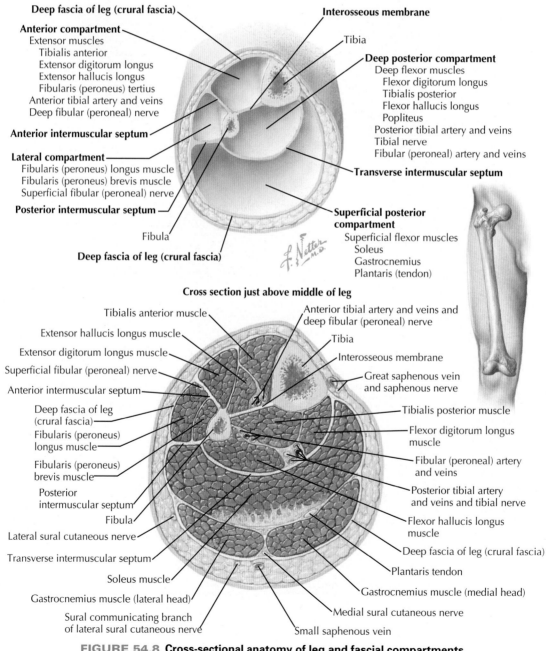

Cross section just above middle of leg

FIGURE 54.8 **Cross-sectional anatomy of leg and fascial compartments.**

SURGICAL PRINCIPLES, ANATOMY, AND TECHNIQUE

The objective in leg fasciotomy is to completely release all four compartments. The entire length of the fascia of the involved compartments must be opened to ensure adequate pressure release of the tissues. Inadequate lysis of fascia yields incomplete treatment, and further tissue damage can occur. The course of the arteries, veins, and nerves changes from proximal to distal within the compartments, and care must be taken while performing fasciotomies of the deep and superficial compartments (Figs. 54.9 and 54.10).

A four-compartment fasciotomy may be performed via one lateral incision, but the most common approach is via medial and lateral incisions (Fig. 54.11). The medial incision is used to decompress the deep and superficial posterior compartments and is made 2 cm posterior to the medial edge of the tibia for a length of approximately 10 cm. The fascia of the superficial posterior compartment is visualized and incised the entire length of the compartment from the proximal tibia to the medial malleolus. To access the deep posterior compartment, the gastrocnemius-soleus complex must be taken down from its tibial attachments proximally (Fig. 54.12). The long saphenous vein and its tributaries will be encountered during this dissection, and the tributaries can be ligated as necessary to facilitate complete fascial lysis (see Fig. 54.11). Additionally, the sensory saphenous nerve runs parallel to the long saphenous vein in the lower leg, and precautions should be taken to avoid this structure during the fasciotomy.

The lateral incision is used to decompress the anterior and lateral compartments and is made 1 cm anterior to the fibular head for approximately a length of 10 cm. The fascia of the anterior compartment is visualized and incised the length of the skin incision. This is then lengthened proximally and distally under the skin using scissors. The lateral compartment is similarly decompressed via the same incision. Care is taken to avoid the superficial peroneal nerve, which lies in the intramuscular septum between the anterior and lateral compartments.

The wounds are dressed with saline wet-to-dry dressings and changed daily. Once edema has abated, the fascia can usually be closed primarily. If fascial closure cannot be safely obtained, negative pressure-assisted therapy or healing by secondary intention with delayed skin grafting can be employed. The most common complications are bleeding, nerve injury, infection, and poor wound healing.

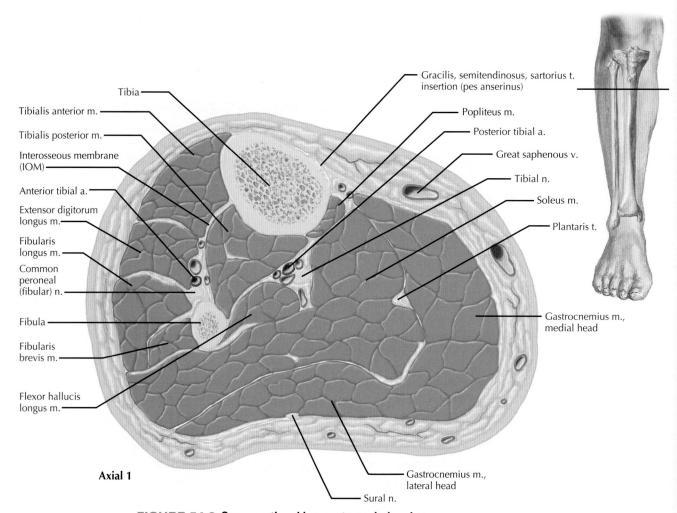

Tibia

Tibialis anterior m.

Tibialis posterior m.

Interosseous membrane (IOM)

Anterior tibial a.

Extensor digitorum longus m.

Fibularis longus m.

Common peroneal (fibular) n.

Fibula

Fibularis brevis m.

Flexor hallucis longus m.

Gracilis, semitendinosus, sartorius t. insertion (pes anserinus)

Popliteus m.

Posterior tibial a.

Great saphenous v.

Tibial n.

Soleus m.

Plantaris t.

Gastrocnemius m., medial head

Gastrocnemius m., lateral head

Sural n.

Axial 1

FIGURE 54.9 Cross-sectional leg anatomy, below knee.

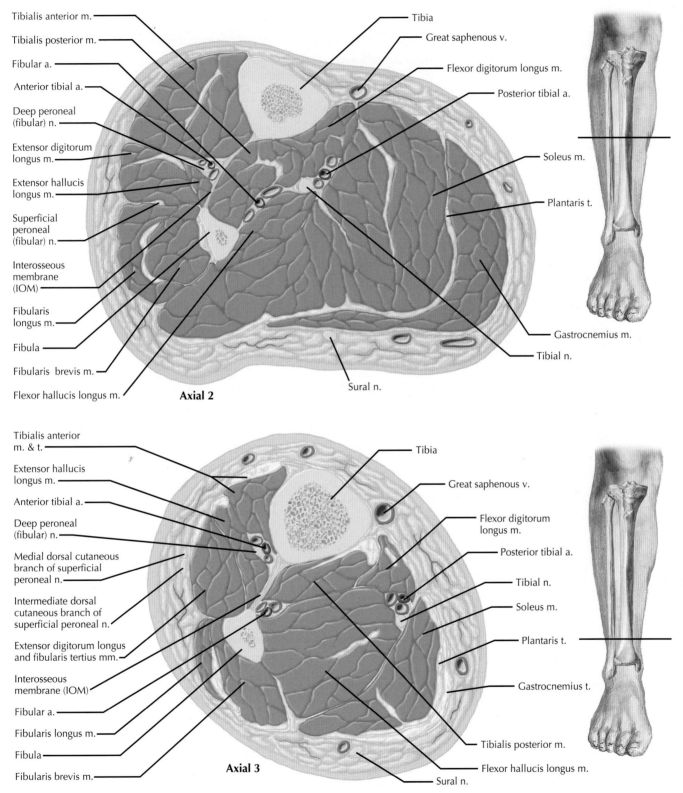

Tibialis anterior m.

Tibialis posterior m.

Fibular a.

Anterior tibial a.

Deep peroneal (fibular) n.

Extensor digitorum longus m.

Extensor hallucis longus m.

Superficial peroneal (fibular) n.

Interosseous membrane (IOM)

Fibularis longus m.

Fibula

Fibularis brevis m.

Flexor hallucis longus m.

Axial 2

Tibia

Great saphenous v.

Flexor digitorum longus m.

Posterior tibial a.

Soleus m.

Plantaris t.

Gastrocnemius m.

Tibial n.

Sural n.

Tibialis anterior m. & t.

Extensor hallucis longus m.

Anterior tibial a.

Deep peroneal (fibular) n.

Medial dorsal cutaneous branch of superficial peroneal n.

Intermediate dorsal cutaneous branch of superficial peroneal n.

Extensor digitorum longus and fibularis tertius mm.

Interosseous membrane (IOM)

Fibular a.

Fibularis longus m.

Fibula

Fibularis brevis m.

Axial 3

Tibia

Great saphenous v.

Flexor digitorum longus m.

Posterior tibial a.

Tibial n.

Soleus m.

Plantaris t.

Gastrocnemius t.

Tibialis posterior m.

Flexor hallucis longus m.

Sural n.

FIGURE 54.10 Cross-sectional leg anatomy, middle and lower tibia.

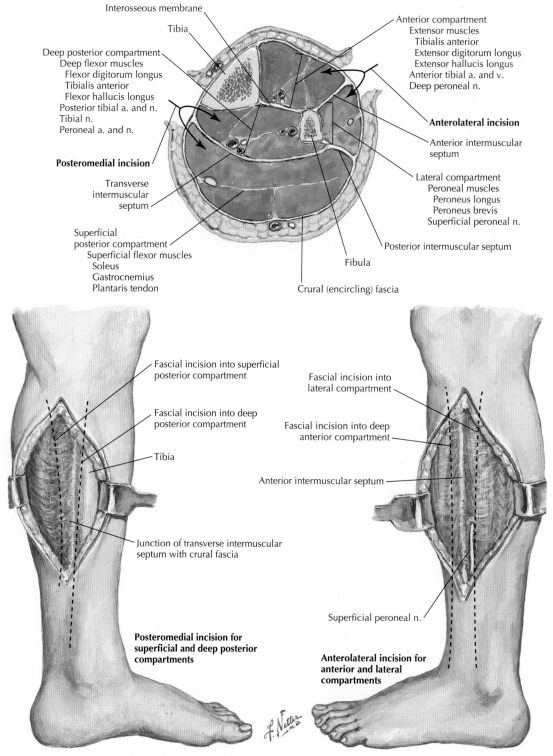

Interosseous membrane

Tibia

Deep posterior compartment
Deep flexor muscles
Flexor digitorum longus
Tibialis anterior
Flexor hallucis longus
Posterior tibial a. and n.
Tibial n.
Peroneal a. and n.

Posteromedial incision

Transverse
intermuscular
septum

Superficial
posterior compartment
Superficial flexor muscles
Soleus
Gastrocnemius
Plantaris tendon

Anterior compartment
Extensor muscles
Tibialis anterior
Extensor digitorum longus
Extensor hallucis longus
Anterior tibial a. and v.
Deep peroneal n.

Anterolateral incision

Anterior intermuscular
septum

Lateral compartment
Peroneal muscles
Peroneus longus
Peroneus brevis
Superficial peroneal n.

Posterior intermuscular septum

Fibula

Crural (encircling) fascia

Fascial incision into superficial
posterior compartment

Fascial incision into deep
posterior compartment

Tibia

Junction of transverse intermuscular
septum with crural fascia

**Posteromedial incision for
superficial and deep posterior
compartments**

Fascial incision into
lateral compartment

Fascial incision into deep
anterior compartment

Anterior intermuscular septum

Superficial peroneal n.

**Anterolateral incision for
anterior and lateral
compartments**

FIGURE 54.11 Incisions for compartment syndrome of leg.

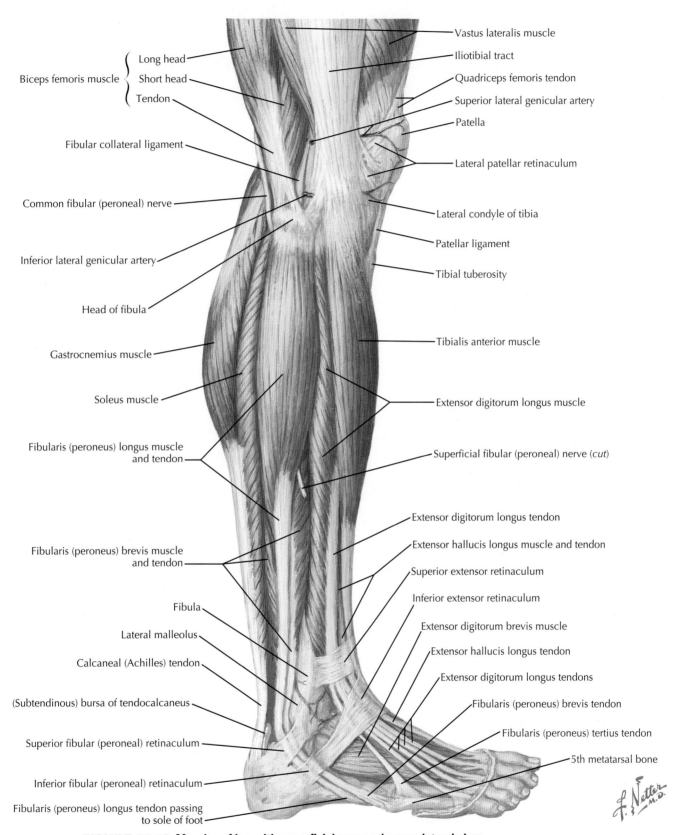

Vastus lateralis muscle

Iliotibial tract

Quadriceps femoris tendon

Superior lateral genicular artery

Patella

Lateral patellar retinaculum

Lateral condyle of tibia

Patellar ligament

Tibial tuberosity

Tibialis anterior muscle

Extensor digitorum longus muscle

Superficial fibular (peroneal) nerve (*cut*)

Extensor digitorum longus tendon

Extensor hallucis longus muscle and tendon

Superior extensor retinaculum

Inferior extensor retinaculum

Extensor digitorum brevis muscle

Extensor hallucis longus tendon

Extensor digitorum longus tendons

Fibularis (peroneus) brevis tendon

Fibularis (peroneus) tertius tendon

5th metatarsal bone

Biceps femoris muscle
Long head
Short head
Tendon

Fibular collateral ligament

Common fibular (peroneal) nerve

Inferior lateral genicular artery

Head of fibula

Gastrocnemius muscle

Soleus muscle

Fibularis (peroneus) longus muscle and tendon

Fibularis (peroneus) brevis muscle and tendon

Fibula

Lateral malleolus

Calcaneal (Achilles) tendon

(Subtendinous) bursa of tendocalcaneus

Superior fibular (peroneal) retinaculum

Inferior fibular (peroneal) retinaculum

Fibularis (peroneus) longus tendon passing to sole of foot

FIGURE 54.12 Muscles of leg with superficial peroneal nerve: lateral view.

SUGGESTED READINGS

Cha J, York B, Tawfik J. Forearm compartment syndrome. Eplasty 2014;14: ic10 Published online 2014 April 23.

Chandraprakasam T, Kumar RA. Acute compartment syndrome of forearm and hand. Indian J Plast Surg 2011;44(2):212–8.

Ellison E, Zollinger RM, Jr. Eds. Zollinger's Atlas of Surgical Operations. 10th ed. New York: McGraw-Hill.

Breast and Oncology

SECTION EDITOR: Stephen R. Grobmyer

Mastectomy: Partial and Total

Stephen R. Grobmyer

INTRODUCTION

Breast cancer is the most common cancer diagnosed and the second leading cause of cancer mortality in women. Major advances in recent years, including hormonal and monoclonal antibody therapy, have greatly improved outcomes in breast cancer patients. Historically, breast cancer has primarily been a surgically treated disease. In 1894, Halsted (per Dorland's) and Myers described the landmark radical mastectomy. This operation removes the breast tissue, nipple-areola complex, overlying skin, and pectoralis major and minor muscles, in addition to a complete axillary lymphadenectomy. Although the radical mastectomy is effective at improving survival, the procedure carries a high morbidity.

Since then, surgeons have developed techniques to minimize morbidity and maximize survival rates. These procedures include partial mastectomy, simple or total mastectomy, modified radical mastectomy, skin-sparing mastectomy, and nipple-sparing mastectomy. Together these procedures have maintained survival rates in properly selected patients while greatly reducing the morbidity of the Halsted radical mastectomy. The approach to surgical intervention is made on the basis of tumor size in relation to breast size, multifocal disease, bilateral disease, specific pathological considerations of the tumor, the patient's germline genetic status, and patient preference. This chapter addresses the most common surgical interventions: the partial mastectomy and total mastectomy.

PARTIAL MASTECTOMY

Breast-conserving surgery (i.e., partial mastectomy, lumpectomy, tylectomy, wide local excision, segmental mastectomy) can be considered for early stage disease (i.e., stages 0, I, and II). When combined with radiation therapy for properly selected patients, breast-conserving surgery has the same survival rate as modified radical mastectomy. Partial mastectomy is increasingly used because the oncologic outcomes are also the same, while improving aesthetics, quality of life, and psychological impact on the patient.

Partial mastectomy is often performed with axillary sentinel lymph node biopsy (SLNB) when the diagnosis of invasive cancer is made. Partial mastectomy can also be performed without SLNB for patients with noninvasive breast cancer, ductal carcinoma in situ (DCIS).

With breast conservation and aesthetics the focus of partial mastectomy, the choice of incision is of great importance (Fig. 55.1A). Circumareolar incisions provide good cosmesis. Curvilinear incisions that parallel Langer's lines of tension in the upper half of the breast also work well. In the inferior half of the breast, radial incisions provide good cosmesis. For palpable lesions, the incision should be made directly over the tumor. For nonpalpable tumors localized with a wire or other wireless localizing technologies (e.g., radioactive seed), care should be made to make the incision over the expected location of the tumor.

Small skin flaps are raised, and then dissection can be performed sharply or with electrocautery. Breast tissue can be grasped with an Adair clamp to facilitate dissection, but care should be used to avoid tearing or crushing the tissues (Fig. 55.1B).

Current guidelines recommend removal of invasive cancers with clear margins (i.e., no tumor on ink). Once removed, the specimen must be oriented so that if a margin is positive, an accurate margin re-excision can be performed (Fig. 55.1C).

Depending on the size of the breast and the size of the specimen being resected, oncoplastic techniques may be used. For large specimens that may cause dimpling of the skin or obvious deformity, rotation of a portion of breast tissue into the cavity may improve aesthetics. Also, for large breasts and a large specimen, breast reduction techniques in conjunction with partial mastectomy may be used to preserve symmetry and/or achieve desired cosmetic results.

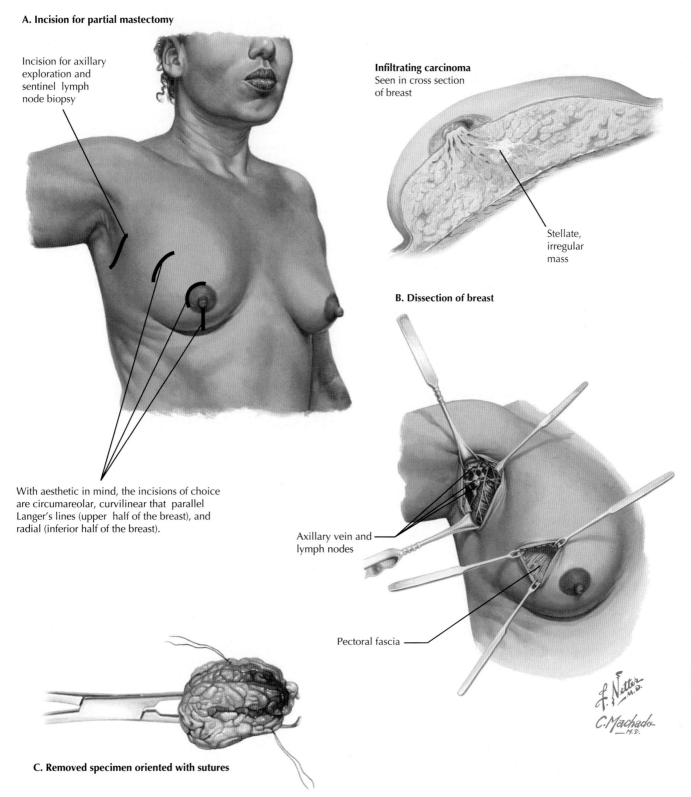

A. Incision for partial mastectomy

Incision for axillary
exploration and
sentinel lymph
node biopsy

Infiltrating carcinoma
Seen in cross section
of breast

Stellate,
irregular
mass

With aesthetic in mind, the incisions of choice
are circumareolar, curvilinear that parallel
Langer's lines (upper half of the breast), and
radial (inferior half of the breast).

B. Dissection of breast

Axillary vein and
lymph nodes

Pectoral fascia

C. Removed specimen oriented with sutures

FIGURE 55.1 **Partial mastectomy.**

TOTAL MASTECTOMY

When patients have large tumors in relation to breast size or multifocal disease without clinical node involvement, total mastectomy with sentinel node biopsy may be the treatment of choice. Another term for total mastectomy is simple mastectomy. Other factors, such as patient preference and genetic mutation status, also play an important role in determining surgical treatment options. There is increasing use of germline genetic testing to screen women at exceptionally high risk for developing breast cancer. Many of these genetically high-risk women with breast cancer chose bilateral mastectomy to treat the cancer and reduce their subsequent risk of developing breast cancer. In the case of risk-reducing mastectomy, a total mastectomy is performed.

MODIFIED RADICAL MASTECTOMY

For breast cancer patients with clinical nodal involvement having a mastectomy and in patients found to have metastatic disease in the sentinel node at the time of mastectomy, the procedure of choice is the modified radical mastectomy. This approach combines total mastectomy (discussed later) with axillary lymph node dissection (see Chapter 59, Axillary Lymphadenectomy and Lymphaticovenous Bypass).

For patients electing not to have immediate breast reconstruction, the incision for the procedure is typically an ellipse centered on the areola (Fig. 55.2A). This incision should encompass previous biopsy and excision scars.

Skin flaps are then raised, typically with the use of skin hooks or rakes to provide tension (Fig. 55.2B). The skin flaps should be approximately 7 to 10 mm and thick enough to avoid necrosis and buttonholes but thin enough to resect all breast tissue. The thickness of the flaps does vary with the body mass index (BMI) of the patient. Patients with higher BMI generally require thicker flaps. These flaps are carried superiorly to the level of the clavicle and inferiorly to the inframammary fold. The flaps should reach the lateral border of the sternum medially and the latissimus dorsi muscle laterally.

Fig. 55.2C shows a lateral view of the breast with the correct plane of dissection for mastectomy being deep to the pectoral fascia.

The breast is then dissected off the chest wall, starting superiorly at the clavicle (Fig. 55.2D and E). This dissection continues inferiorly deep to the retromammary fascia and investing fascia of the pectoralis major muscle. The breast tissue is retracted inferiorly as electrocautery is used to dissect the tissue and investing fascia of the pectoralis from the underlying muscle.

Care should be taken to identify perforating vessels from the pectoralis muscle to the breast tissue and divide them accordingly. These vessels can bleed briskly, and if divided too close to the pectoralis, they may retract into the muscle.

For a total mastectomy, once the dissection has reached the inframammary fold, the breast can be removed and the overlying skin closed with drains in place (Fig. 55.2F). If a modified radical mastectomy is performed, the lateral border of the breast that is attached to the axilla should be left in place, and the axillary lymph node dissection is completed. This approach will remove a single en-bloc specimen containing the breast and contents of the axilla.

BREAST REMOVAL AND RECONSTRUCTION

An important consideration of breast surgery is the reconstruction options. It is important to have a candid discussion with patients before any surgical intervention. Also, it is advisable to consult with a reconstructive plastic surgeon to devise an optimal treatment plan for each patient. Some patients may be candidates for mastectomy and reconstruction at the same surgery, whereas others require delayed reconstruction. Skin- and nipple-sparing mastectomy are options in selected patients to facilitate immediate reconstruction.

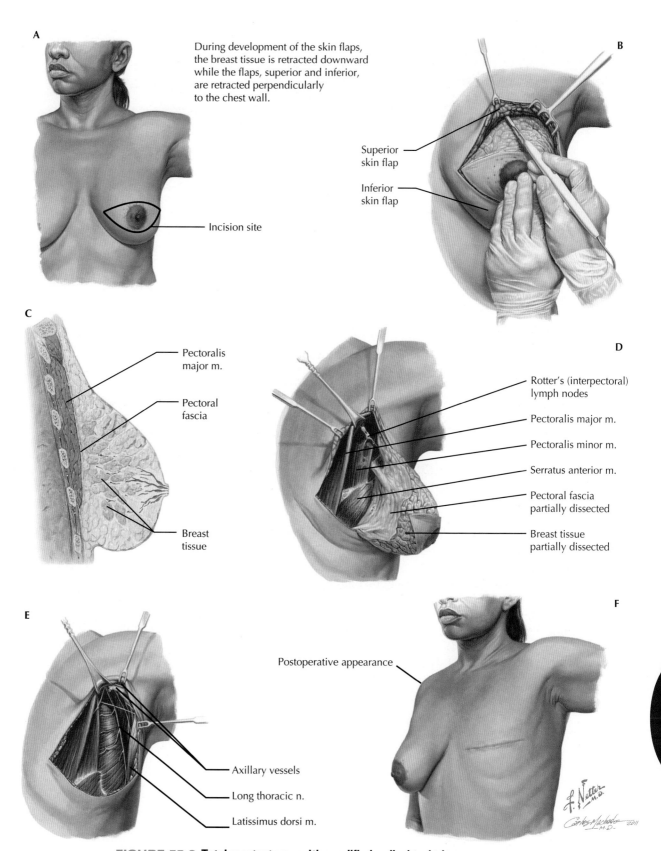

A

During development of the skin flaps, the breast tissue is retracted downward while the flaps, superior and inferior, are retracted perpendicularly to the chest wall.

Incision site

B

Superior skin flap

Inferior skin flap

C

Pectoralis major m.

Pectoral fascia

Breast tissue

D

Rotter's (interpectoral) lymph nodes

Pectoralis major m.

Pectoralis minor m.

Serratus anterior m.

Pectoral fascia partially dissected

Breast tissue partially dissected

E

Axillary vessels

Long thoracic n.

Latissimus dorsi m.

F

Postoperative appearance

FIGURE 55.2 **Total mastectomy with modified radical technique.**

SUMMARY

Discussion with the breast cancer patient and multidisciplinary team is essential to determine the most appropriate surgical approach. Skin-flap thickness is important; if too thin, there is risk of necrosis, and if too thick, risk of recurrence. When the surgeon is dissecting the investing fascia off the pectoralis major, the perforating vessels can be a source of postoperative bleeding, and care should be taken to ligate or cauterize them appropriately. Breast reconstruction options can affect aspects of the resection and should be planned in advance.

SUGGESTED READINGS

Clarke M, Collins R, Darby S, et al. Effects of radiotherapy and of differences in the extent of surgery for early breast cancer on local recurrence and 15-year survival: an overview of the randomised trials. Lancet 2005;366(9503):2087–106.

Crowe JP, Kim JA, Yetman R, et al. Nipple-sparing mastectomy: technique and results in 54 procedures. Arch Surg 2004;139(2):148–50.

Grobmyer SR, Pederson HJ, Valente S, et al. Evolving indications and long-term oncologic outcomes of risk-reducing bilateral nipple sparing mastectomy. BJS Open 2018: Nov;26:2018.

Lee GK, Sheckter CC. Breast reconstruction following breast cancer treatment-2018. JAMA 2018;320(12):1277–8.

Moo TA, Sanford R, Dang C, Morrow M. Overview of breast cancer therapy. PET Clin 2018;13(3):339–54.

Moran MS, Schnitt SJ, Giuliano AE, et al. Society of Surgical Oncology-American Society for Radiation Oncology consensus guideline on margins for breast-conserving surgery with whole-breast irradiation in stages I and II invasive breast cancer. J Clin Oncol 2014;32(14):1507–15.

Breast Reconstruction

Tripp Leavitt and Risal Djohan

INTRODUCTION

The modern treatment of breast cancer, in simplified terms, sets forth the goal to cure the patient of breast cancer without diminishing patient quality of life, which for many patients is heavily reliant on breast reconstruction. Although some patients may decline surgery to reconstruct the breast, all patients undergoing mastectomy should be offered a referral to a board-certified plastic surgeon for potential reconstructive surgery, per the standards set by the National Accreditation Program for Breast Centers (NAPBC). Today, breast cancer is more frequently diagnosed in its earlier stages as compared with prior decades, offering the potential to pursue oncologic resections that are less extensive, thereby opening up a wider range of reconstructive possibilities. Collaboration between plastic surgeons and breast surgeons is fundamental to achieving an optimal reconstructive outcome and depends on each understanding the pertinent anatomy and techniques relevant to the other's specialty.

Patients electing to undergo breast reconstruction after mastectomy are faced with two major decisions: whether to undergo autologous or implant-based reconstruction, and whether to stage their reconstruction. Certain practical limitations such as soft tissue availability, tumor stage and location, and need for radiation therapy may narrow the range of reconstructive options. However, through careful discussion with their multidisciplinary team, patients are left to make informed decisions that are most consistent with their personal goals and expectations.

ANATOMIC CONSIDERATIONS IN BREAST RECONSTRUCTION

First described by Phillip Blondeel, consideration of the breast in terms of its footprint, conus, and skin envelope are essential to achieving ideal breast aesthetics. The footprint is bordered by the clavicle, lateral sternum, anterior axillary line, and the inframammary fold (IMF). Obliteration of the IMF, whether the result of oncologic involvement or mastectomy overdissection, negatively affects the reconstruction because of loss of fascial attachments helping to support the volume of the breast or implant, which subsequently drop over time. The conus is representative of the three-dimensional shape, volume, projection, and contour of the breast. The large variety of modern implant sizes, shapes, and material compositions permits breast reconstruction that better emulates the patient's natural conus. Frequently the most important factor in breast reconstruction after mastectomy is the quality and quantity of the remaining skin envelope. Immediate reconstruction with a permanent implant cannot be performed if there is insufficient soft tissue remaining for coverage. In addition, much of the blood supply to the breast skin is derived from perforating branches of the intercostal, internal mammary, and thoracoacromial arteries, which are divided during mastectomy. Earlier cancer detection, coupled with an increasing prevalence of prophylactic mastectomies, and a greater concern for aesthetic outcomes have driven up the rate at which nipple-sparing and skin-sparing mastectomies are performed. Although these procedures offer the potential for a more aesthetic result, the skin envelope represents a larger area of tissue reliant on the subdermal plexus for perfusion, increasing the risk of tissue ischemia and subsequent wound-healing complications. As noted in the previous chapter, skin flap thickness is a critical variable in mastectomy surgery; a balance must be struck between minimizing the risks of disease recurrence versus soft tissue necrosis. Perfusion status of the mastectomy skin flap is very closely associated with flap thickness and should be carefully assessed in the operating room during the course of breast reconstruction (Fig. 56.1).

Tissue expanders are frequently relied upon to maintain or restore natural breast aesthetics. They may be required to achieve optimal results in larger reconstructions, allowing gradual filling of the breast skin envelope without compromising perfusion. They are also an option for patients who are likely to undergo radiation therapy, because they can be deflated while still maintaining the breast pocket, which would otherwise be heavily altered or ablated because of postradiation changes. Finally, in submuscular implant placement, as described below, tissue expansion may be required to fit an appropriately sized implant within the smaller submuscular pocket.

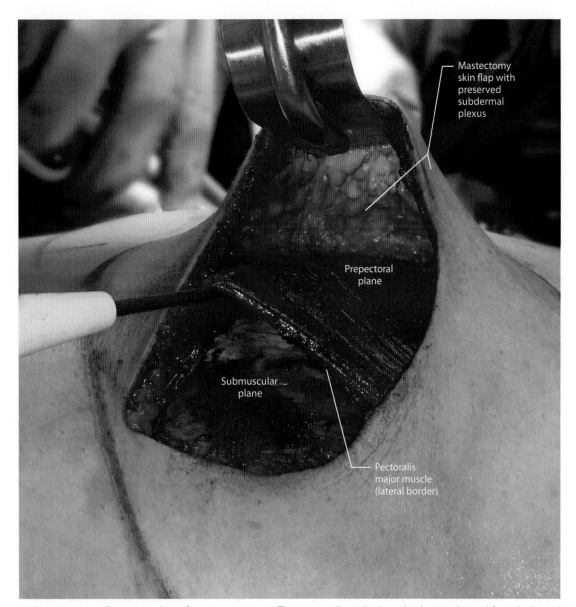

FIGURE 56.1 Breast pocket after mastectomy. The pectoralis major has also been released from its lateral and inferior attachments, demonstrating the available planes for implant insertion. Note the mastectomy skin flap demonstrating excellent thickness for reconstructive purposes, with no signs of tissue ischemia or translucency.

IMPLANT-BASED RECONSTRUCTION

Breast reconstruction with the use of a prosthetic implant remains the most common form of reconstruction after mastectomy. Implants can be placed at the time of mastectomy or during a separate procedure, referred to as immediate or delayed reconstruction, respectively. Alternatively, tissue expanders can be placed at the time of mastectomy and later replaced with permanent implants as part of "delayed-immediate" or staged reconstruction. These implants are placed in either the prepectoral or submuscular planes. The surgical approach is commonly via the pre-existing mastectomy incision (refer to Chapter 55).

In recent years, immediate reconstruction with prepectoral implants has become increasingly more common, primarily driven by greater demand for nipple-sparing mastectomies and the proliferation of acellular dermal matrices (ADM) in breast reconstruction. The ADM is placed over the implant and anchored to the chest wall at the boundaries of the breast, providing structural support and additional soft tissue coverage as it is gradually incorporated by the adjacent native tissue (Fig. 56.2A). The combination of ADM with the larger skin envelope preserved by nipple-sparing mastectomy facilitates a wider range of implant sizes, allowing more patients to forgo the time-consuming and often painful tissue expansion process to achieve the desired aesthetic result, without an increased risk for tissue necrosis.

Although relatively more involved from an anatomic perspective, the submuscular plane remains the most common site for implant placement in breast reconstruction. It is accessed by elevating the pectoralis major muscle from the anterior chest wall along its inferolateral border (occasionally with some inferomedial release), preserving its medial attachment along the sternum. This plane between the pectoralis major and the chest wall (and the pectoralis minor superiorly), is relatively avascular, with the exception of internal mammary perforators emerging just lateral to the sternal border, at the most medial extent of the dissection. Submuscular implant-based reconstruction can be further categorized as partial or complete submuscular implant placement. With partial submuscular placement, the inferior aspect of the implant protrudes from underneath the inferior border of the pectoralis major. Biologic mesh, generally composed of acellular dermal matrix, is frequently used in this type of reconstruction. By fixating it to the inferior border of the pectoralis major and the anterior chest wall at the internal mammary fold (IMF), a sling is created to augment the tissues supporting the implant, while supplementing the soft tissue coverage over the otherwise exposed lower segment of the implant (Fig. 56.2B). Alternatively, the serratus anterior muscle and/or fascia can be elevated from the lateral chest wall and advanced medially and sutured to the lateral border of the pectoralis major, to provide muscular coverage over the lower lateral implant surface, defining complete submuscular implant placement (Fig. 56.2C through G). Submuscular implant placement is generally preferred when there is evidence of ischemia of the mastectomy skin flaps, because the overlying muscle prevents implant extrusion in the event of full-thickness skin necrosis. Tissue expansion is frequently used in submuscular implant placement because of the limited implant volume that can be inserted at the time of mastectomy. The expansion process is frequently more painful with submuscular expanders, and the final result is compromised by animation deformity of the breasts during contraction of the pectoralis major, leading to patients frequently opting for prepectoral placement if they are a candidate.

Anatomic planes for implant-based breast reconstruction.

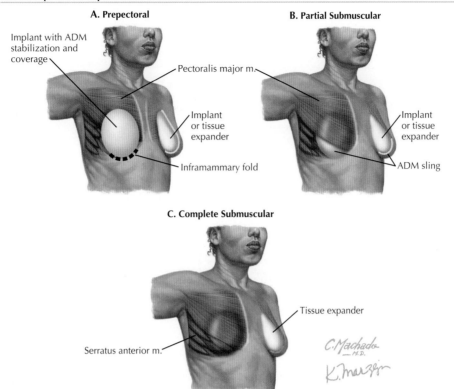

A. Prepectoral

Implant with ADM stabilization and coverage

Pectoralis major m.

Implant or tissue expander

Inframammary fold

B. Partial Submuscular

Implant or tissue expander

ADM sling

C. Complete Submuscular

Tissue expander

Serratus anterior m.

C. Machado M.D.
K. Marzsm

First stage of a delayed-immediate breast reconstruction performed at time of mastectomy, with complete submuscular tissue expander placement.

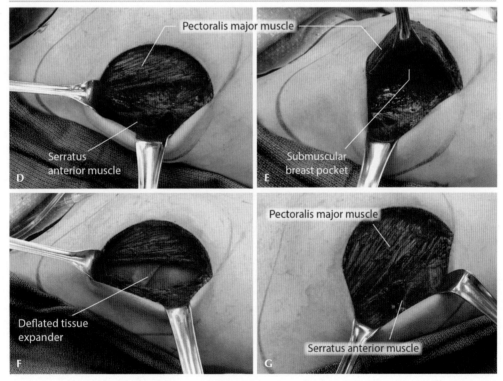

Pectoralis major muscle

Serratus anterior muscle

D

Submuscular breast pocket

E

Deflated tissue expander

F

Pectoralis major muscle

Serratus anterior muscle

G

FIGURE 56.2 Implant-based breast reconstruction. (A to C) Anatomic planes for implant-based breast reconstruction. *ADM,* Acellular dermal matrix. (D to G) First stage of a delayed-immediate breast reconstruction performed at time of mastectomy, with complete submuscular tissue expander placement. (D) The serratus anterior and pectoralis major muscles are observed within the mastectomy defect. (E) Elevation of the pectoralis muscle reveals the submuscular plane. (F) Elevation of the serratus anterior muscle along the lateral chest wall further enlarges the submuscular pocket within which the deflated tissue expander is inserted, providing additional soft tissue coverage. (G) The serratus anterior muscle is then approximated to the lateral border of the pectoralis major muscle, to provide complete coverage of the tissue expander, which can be slightly inflated if significant tension is not placed across the closure.

AUTOLOGOUS BREAST RECONSTRUCTION

A variety of reconstructive modalities exist that use the patient's own body tissues, often forgoing the need for breast implants, resulting in a more natural, longer-lasting result. Tissue can be transferred based on named blood vessels as a pedicled flap, or completely separated from its native blood supply and anastomosed at a distal site as free tissue transfer (free flap).

Abdominal Flaps in Breast Reconstruction

The abdomen is an ideal donor site for autologous reconstruction in that it provides a large volume of soft, malleable tissue of similar quality to the natural breast. Workhorse flaps from the abdomen used in breast reconstruction include deep inferior epigastric perforator (DIEP), free transverse rectus abdominis (TRAM), and pedicled TRAM flaps. Despite the variety of abdominally based flaps for breast reconstruction, the adipocutaneous portion of each is the same, generally incorporating a fusiform skin island from the suprapubic crease to just above the umbilicus, between the two anterior superior iliac spines. In the case of DIEP and TRAM flaps, the adipocutaneous tissue is perfused by vessels that pass from source vessel to skin surface, either through or between deep tissues, in this case muscle, defining them as myocutaneous perforators.

Deep Inferior Epigastric Perforator Flap

The DIEP flap preserves the full function of the rectus abdominis muscle, minimizing donor site morbidity while optimizing aesthetic result. The deep inferior epigastric artery branches from the external iliac artery just above the level of the inguinal ligament, traveling superiorly within the extraperitoneal fat before piercing the transversalis fascia (Fig. 56.3A). As it continues along its cephalad trajectory, it traverses superficially to the arcuate line, coursing along the posterior surface of the rectus abdominis. It is here that the artery assumes one of several types of branching pattern, until its terminal branches anastomose with branches derived from the superior epigastric artery. Commonly, the deep inferior epigastric artery divides into two branches with variable intramuscular courses, whose branches give rise to the medial and lateral row perforators supplying the overlying skin and adipose tissue (Fig. 56.3B). Less frequently, a single vessel may run centrally within the muscle, or there may be more than two major branches (Fig. 56.3C). At least one dominant perforator is identified for dissection, isolating its corresponding source vessel along its proximal, intramuscular course, eventually reaching the origin of the deep inferior epigastric artery, just superior to the inguinal ligament. The final stage of any free flap harvest is transection of the vascular pedicle near its origin as a longer pedicle increases the ease with which microsurgical anastomosis can be performed. Therefore it is at this level of the dissection that the deep inferior epigastric artery and vein are divided.

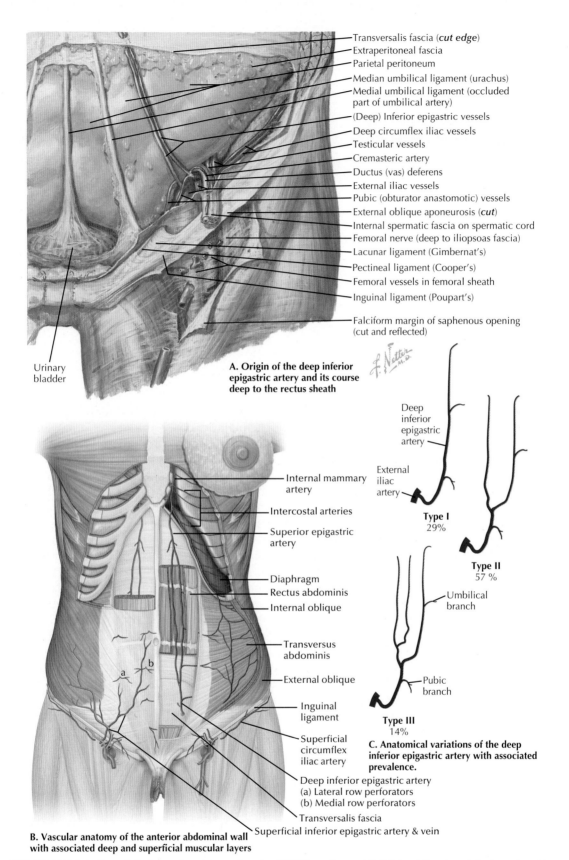

A. Origin of the deep inferior epigastric artery and its course deep to the rectus sheath

- Transversalis fascia (*cut edge*)
- Extraperitoneal fascia
- Parietal peritoneum
- Median umbilical ligament (urachus)
- Medial umbilical ligament (occluded part of umbilical artery)
- (Deep) Inferior epigastric vessels
- Deep circumflex iliac vessels
- Testicular vessels
- Cremasteric artery
- Ductus (vas) deferens
- External iliac vessels
- Pubic (obturator anastomotic) vessels
- External oblique aponeurosis (*cut*)
- Internal spermatic fascia on spermatic cord
- Femoral nerve (deep to iliopsoas fascia)
- Lacunar ligament (Gimbernat's)
- Pectineal ligament (Cooper's)
- Femoral vessels in femoral sheath
- Inguinal ligament (Poupart's)
- Falciform margin of saphenous opening (cut and reflected)

Urinary bladder

B. Vascular anatomy of the anterior abdominal wall with associated deep and superficial muscular layers

- Internal mammary artery
- Intercostal arteries
- Superior epigastric artery
- Diaphragm
- Rectus abdominis
- Internal oblique
- Transversus abdominis
- External oblique
- Inguinal ligament
- Superficial circumflex iliac artery
- Deep inferior epigastric artery
  (a) Lateral row perforators
  (b) Medial row perforators
- Transversalis fascia
- Superficial inferior epigastric artery & vein

C. Anatomical variations of the deep inferior epigastric artery with associated prevalence.

Deep inferior epigastric artery

External iliac artery

Type I 29%

Type II 57 %

Umbilical branch

Pubic branch

Type III 14%

FIGURE 56.3 Deep inferior epigastric perforator (DIEP) anatomy. (A) Origin of the deep inferior epigastric artery and its course deep to the rectus sheath. (B) Vascular anatomy of the anterior abdominal wall with associated deep and superficial muscular layers. (C) Anatomic variations of the deep inferior epigastric artery with associated prevalence. (*B, Reused with permission from Howard MA, Dickie SR. Comprehensive trunk anatomy. In: Song DH, Neligan PC, eds. Plastic Surgery: Lower Extremity, Trunk, and Burns. 4th ed. vol 4. Elsevier; 2018. Fig. 9-10, p 227. C, Phillips T J, Stella D L, Rozen W M, et al. Abdominal wall CT angiography: A detailed account of a newly established preoperative imaging technique. Radiology 2008; 249:32-44.*)

Deep Inferior Epigastric Perforator Flap (Continued)

Elevation of the DIEP or other abdominal free flap inherently severs the cutaneous sensory innervation supplying the skin paddle. Similarly, the majority of sensory nerves supplying the breast and nipple-areola complex are divided during mastectomy, resulting in breast hypoesthesia. Return of sensation is a slow and unreliable process but can be augmented in autologous reconstruction by coapting sensory nerves at the flap and recipient sites, often with the use of a nerve graft. Several nerves may also be encountered during intramuscular dissection of the perforators, segmental branches coursing from the lateral aspect of the rectus abdominis, traveling within or directly below the muscle. Within the muscle, these mixed segmental branches divide into their respective motor and sensory branches. Whereas the motor branch crosses over the deep inferior epigastric artery to innervate the medial aspect of the rectus abdominis, the sensory branch travels anteriorly to provide sensation to the overlying skin (Fig. 56.4A). These sensory branches should be carefully dissected for potential flap neurotization, optimizing the potential for sensory reinnervation of the breast flap. Ideally the motor branches encountered during flap elevation should be preserved to minimize weakness to the abdominal wall.

The superficial inferior epigastric vein (SIEV) is encountered early in flap dissection at the inferior abdominal incision. It is approximately midway between the anterior superior iliac spine and the pubic symphysis, above Scarpa's fascia (Fig. 56.3B). In a small subset of patients, the superficial system provides the dominant venous drainage to the adipocutaneous tissue harvested with the flap. Careful isolation and dissection of the SIEV allows its use as an additional venous conduit to supercharge venous outflow should the deep inferior epigastric vein provide inadequate outflow, determined by the presence of flap congestion after arterial and venous anastomosis.

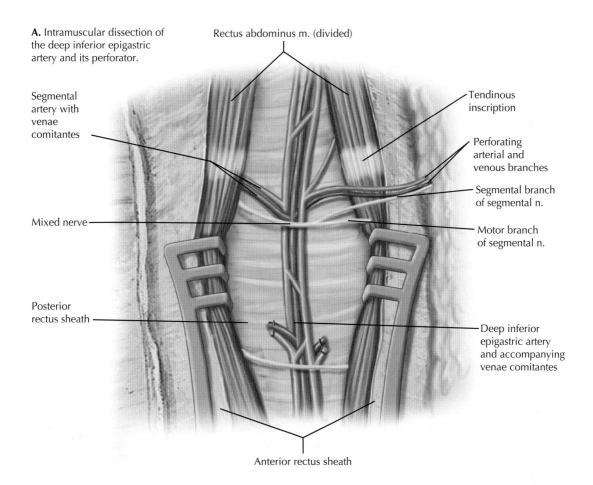

A. Intramuscular dissection of the deep inferior epigastric artery and its perforator.

Rectus abdominus m. (divided)

Tendinous inscription

Perforating arterial and venous branches

Segmental branch of segmental n.

Motor branch of segmental n.

Segmental artery with venae comitantes

Mixed nerve

Posterior rectus sheath

Deep inferior epigastric artery and accompanying venae comitantes

Anterior rectus sheath

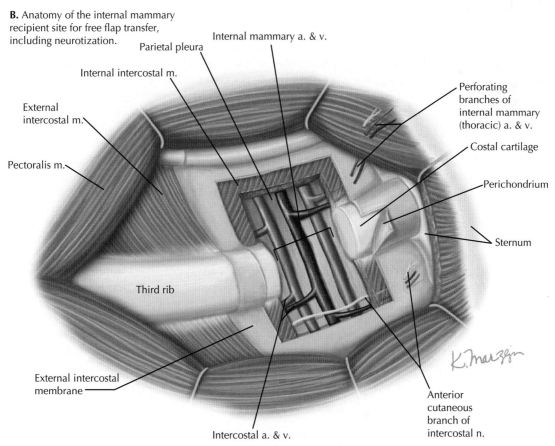

B. Anatomy of the internal mammary recipient site for free flap transfer, including neurotization.

Internal mammary a. & v.

Parietal pleura

Internal intercostal m.

External intercostal m.

Perforating branches of internal mammary (thoracic) a. & v.

Pectoralis m.

Costal cartilage

Perichondrium

Sternum

Third rib

External intercostal membrane

Intercostal a. & v.

Anterior cutaneous branch of intercostal n.

K. marzejn

FIGURE 56.4 DIEP flap vascular pedicle and recipient vessel dissection. (A) Intramuscular dissection of the deep inferior epigastric artery and its perforator. (B) Anatomy of the internal mammary recipient site for free flap transfer, including neurotization.

Free Transverse Rectus Abdominis Flap

The anatomy relevant to harvest of a free TRAM flap is similar to that of a DIEP flap, with each distinguished by the extent to with the rectus abdominis is preserved. Whereas perforator dissection in a DIEP flap preserves the entire rectus abdominis muscle, a free TRAM flap may sacrifice the entire width of the muscle across some of its length, or preserve the muscle to some degree, defined as a muscle-sparing (MS)-TRAM flap. Depending on the extent to which the rectus abdominis muscle is preserved, muscle-sparing free TRAM flaps are categorized as MS-0, where the full width is harvested; MS-1 with preservation of the lateral segment (or occasionally medial); MS-2 with preservation of lateral and medial segments; and MS-3 or DIEP flap, with preservation of the entire muscle (Fig. 56.5). Perforator size and arrangement, quantity of transferred abdominal tissue, and patient comorbidities factor into the decision to harvest a segment of muscle with the flap. The muscle is harvested as a conduit for myocutaneous perforators, rather than a source volume for the reconstructed breast. Before the advent of DIEP flaps, TRAM flaps were the workhorse flap in free-autologous tissue transfer for breast reconstruction. However, because of the risk for abdominal wall weakness and contour abnormalities, they are progressively falling out of favor.

Recipient Vessels for Free Autologous Tissue Transfer

Free tissue transfer in breast reconstruction relies on vascular anastomosis to the internal mammary (thoracic) artery and its branches or to the thoracodorsal artery. The internal mammary vessels are commonly accessed at the level of the third costal cartilage, as distal to the fourth rib, the internal mammary veins become much smaller and bifurcate, complicating vascular anastomosis. The internal mammary artery (IMA) and vein (IMV) run below the costal cartilage, which is removed in a subperichondrial plane after division of the pectoralis major muscle along the length of its fibers. The posterior perichondrium is then removed to reveal the underlying IMA, usually accompanied by paired IMVs (Fig. 56.4B). Adjacent intercostal musculature can also be removed to improve exposure and allow greater vessel mobility for anastomosis. The anterior cutaneous branch of the intercostal nerve assumes a more superficial course as it travels medially in this region, initially traveling deep to the internal intercostal muscle at the inferior costal margin. This sensory nerve can be isolated for neurotization of any identified segmental sensory nerve to the abdominal flap, usually from the T11 or T12 levels. Access to the internal mammary vessels can also be achieved via a rib-sparing technique, excising only the intercostal musculature. The internal mammary vessels also give off perforating branches, which emerge near the sternal border and can be used as recipient vessels, without need for complete isolation of the IMA and IMV. However, these vessels are relatively smaller and thus inconsistently an option for microvascular anastomosis. If immediate autologous reconstruction is pursued in the setting of mastectomy with axillary lymphadenectomy, the thoracodorsal vessels are usually exposed and require little additional dissection to prepare them as recipient vessels.

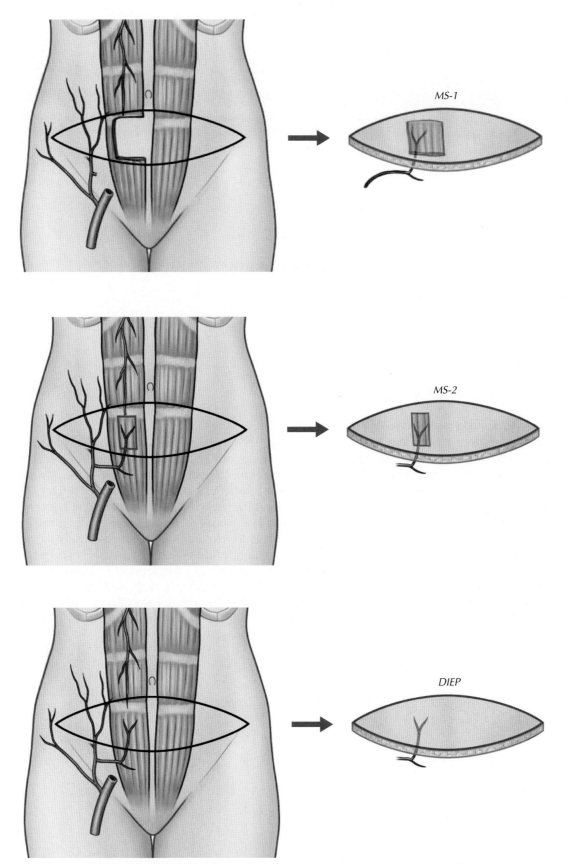

FIGURE 56.5 Classification of muscle-sparing transverse rectus abdominis muscle flaps.
DIEP, Deep inferior epigastric perforator; *MS,* muscle-sparing. (*Reused with permission from Nahabedian MY. The free TRAM flap. In: Song DH, Neligan PC, eds. Plastic Surgery: The Breast. 4th ed, vol 5. Elsevier; 2018. Fig. 20-4, p 352.*)

Pedicled Transverse Rectus Abdominis Flaps

Similar to a free TRAM flap, a pedicled TRAM relies on the rectus abdominis muscle to act as a conduit for the vessels supplying the adipocutaneous portion of the flap. However, the flap is perfused by vessels originating from the superior epigastric artery. Because the vascular pedicle is not divided, it must be tunneled in a subcutaneous plane into the breast pocket, differentiating it from a free flap (Fig. 56.6). Although the pedicled TRAM can also be harvested in a muscle-sparing fashion, almost the entire length is sacrificed with division of the muscle at approximately the level of the arcuate line. At this level, the inferior epigastric vessels are also divided. Superiorly, careful dissection of the subcutaneous tunnel to the breast pocket is needed to prevent distortion of the IMF, without it being so small as to risk tension or kinking of the vascular pedicle. The eighth intercostal nerve should be identified and divided during flap dissection as it enters the muscle near the costal margin, usually at its deep surface. Division of this nerve facilitates necessary muscle atrophy, reducing pedicle bulk within the epigastric region, which is an inherent disadvantage relative to free tissue transfer.

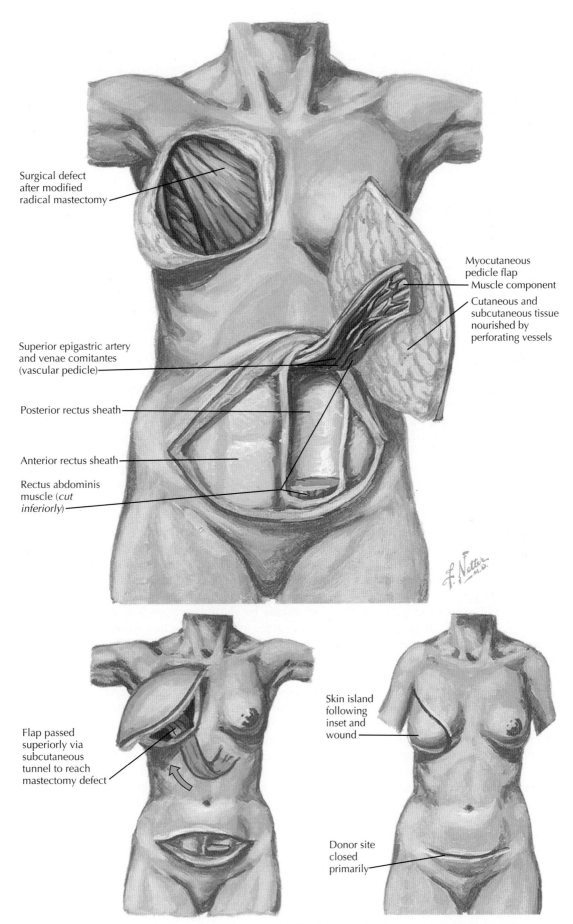

Surgical defect after modified radical mastectomy

Myocutaneous pedicle flap
Muscle component

Cutaneous and subcutaneous tissue nourished by perforating vessels

Superior epigastric artery and venae comitantes (vascular pedicle)

Posterior rectus sheath

Anterior rectus sheath

Rectus abdominis muscle (*cut inferiorly*)

Flap passed superiorly via subcutaneous tunnel to reach mastectomy defect

Skin island following inset and wound

Donor site closed primarily

FIGURE 56.6 Pedicled transverse rectus abdominis muscle flap in breast reconstruction.

Alternatives to Abdominally Based Flaps

Latissimus Dorsi Myocutaneous Flap

The latissimus dorsi muscle is another source of autologous tissue frequently used in breast reconstruction, harvested as a pedicled myocutaneous flap. Therefore, unlike abdominal free tissue transfer, the procedure does not require microsurgical techniques, and patients are able to recovery more quickly. It is an excellent salvage option in cases in which prior reconstructive modalities have failed, for managing complications associated with radiation therapy, or for those with morbid obesity, prior abdominal surgery, or current tobacco use, as its robust axial blood supply is more resistant to the associated postoperative complications.

The latissimus dorsi is a large superficial posterior trunk muscle, originating from the lower thoracic spine, the posterior iliac crest, and the thoracolumbar fascia (Fig. 56.7A). It inserts at the intertubercular groove of the humerus, acting to adduct the arm and internally rotate the shoulder. Although harvest of this muscle may result in shoulder weakness or stiffness, functional deficits are frequently negligible and respond well to postoperative physical therapy.

The tip of the scapula, posterior iliac crest, and dorsal midline are useful surface markers identifying the superior, inferior, and medial borders of the muscle, respectively. Medially, several large lumbar and intercostal artery perforators course through the muscle and will be ligated as the muscle is released from its midline attachments. The inferior muscle fibers of the trapezius also overlie the superomedial aspect of the latissimus dorsi and should be protected during dissection. At its lateral border, care must be taken to separate the latissimus from the underlying serratus anterior muscle, which may be accidentally incorporated into the flap harvest if an incorrect plane is followed. Inferiorly, the muscle is divided near its caudal origin, taking care not to violate the underlying paraspinous or external oblique fascia to reduce the risk of developing a lumbar hernia. Finally, at its superolateral border, the latissimus dorsi must be distinguished from the teres minor, to which it may be closely associated, as both course toward their respective humeral insertions.

The latissimus dorsi muscle is perfused primarily by the thoracodorsal artery, which arises as a branch from the subscapular artery. As it courses inferiorly, the thoracodorsal artery gives off a branch to the serratus anterior muscle just before it enters the deep surface latissimus dorsi, dividing into transverse and descending branches within the substance of the muscle. A robust network of myocutaneous perforators supply the overlying skin, allowing for harvest of a variety of skin island sizes and orientations depending on reconstructive needs (Fig. 56.7B).

During dissection of the vascular pedicle for flap harvest, or alternatively during axillary dissection, the thoracodorsal artery can be differentiated from nearby structures as it travels as a neurovascular bundle, accompanied by the thoracodorsal nerve and vein. Once the muscle is freed along its superficial and deep surfaces, its tendinous insertion is divided with care taken to avoid injury to the neurovascular pedicle, as well as the teres minor insertion. Ideally, the thoracodorsal nerve is cut to prevent postoperative animation deformity. However, this complication is rarely significant to the patient, even if the nerve is left intact, so long as the muscular insertion is completely divided. The myocutaneous flap is then transposed through a subcutaneous tunnel high in the axilla, into the breast pocket for inset. Additional breast volume can be achieved with a tissue expander or permanent implant, which will be inserted between the native pectoralis major muscle and the overlying latissimus dorsi flap.

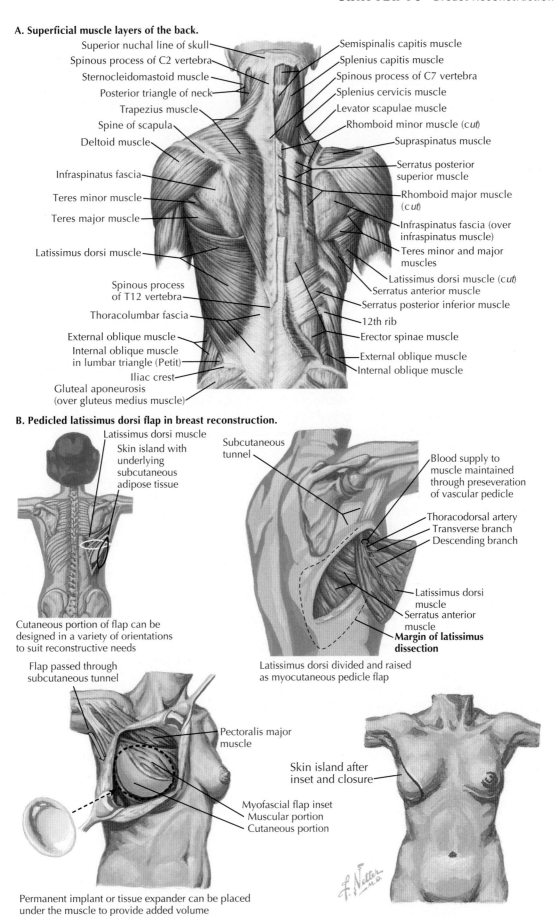

A. Superficial muscle layers of the back.

Superior nuchal line of skull
Spinous process of C2 vertebra
Sternocleidomastoid muscle
Posterior triangle of neck
Trapezius muscle
Spine of scapula
Deltoid muscle
Infraspinatus fascia
Teres minor muscle
Teres major muscle
Latissimus dorsi muscle
Spinous process of T12 vertebra
Thoracolumbar fascia
External oblique muscle
Internal oblique muscle in lumbar triangle (Petit)
Iliac crest
Gluteal aponeurosis (over gluteus medius muscle)

Semispinalis capitis muscle
Splenius capitis muscle
Spinous process of C7 vertebra
Splenius cervicis muscle
Levator scapulae muscle
Rhomboid minor muscle (cut)
Supraspinatus muscle
Serratus posterior superior muscle
Rhomboid major muscle (cut)
Infraspinatus fascia (over infraspinatus muscle)
Teres minor and major muscles
Latissimus dorsi muscle (cut)
Serratus anterior muscle
Serratus posterior inferior muscle
12th rib
Erector spinae muscle
External oblique muscle
Internal oblique muscle

B. Pedicled latissimus dorsi flap in breast reconstruction.

Latissimus dorsi muscle
Skin island with underlying subcutaneous adipose tissue

Cutaneous portion of flap can be designed in a variety of orientations to suit reconstructive needs

Subcutaneous tunnel

Blood supply to muscle maintained through preseveration of vascular pedicle
Thoracodorsal artery
Transverse branch
Descending branch
Latissimus dorsi muscle
Serratus anterior muscle
Margin of latissimus dissection

Latissimus dorsi divided and raised as myocutaneous pedicle flap

Flap passed through subcutaneous tunnel

Pectoralis major muscle

Myofascial flap inset
Muscular portion
Cutaneous portion

Skin island after inset and closure

Permanent implant or tissue expander can be placed under the muscle to provide added volume

FIGURE 56.7 Breast reconstruction with latissimus dorsi pedicled myocutaneous flap. (A) Superficial muscle layers of the back. (B) Pedicled latissimus dorsi flap in breast reconstruction.

Alternative Free Flaps for Breast Reconstruction

The medial thigh has become a popular alternative donor site in breast reconstruction, from which the transverse upper gracilis (TUG) flap can be harvested. This myocutaneous flap is designed with a transverse elliptical skin island adjacent to the groin crease and is harvested with a segment of the underlying gracilis muscle. This flap is perfused by the medial circumflex femoral vessels, which course through the intermuscular septum between the adductor longus and gracilis muscles. The vascular pedicle is dissected proximally and divided at its origin from the profunda femoris artery. Transfer and inset of this free flap is performed in a manner similar to that previously described for abdominally based free flaps.

The gluteal region provides further alternatives for autologous tissue transfer in breast reconstruction, commonly as superior (SGAP) and inferior (IGAP) gluteal artery perforator flaps. Harvested as fasciocutaneous free flaps, perforators from the superior or inferior gluteal arteries are identified with Doppler ultrasonography. Deep to the crural fascia, these vessels are traced along their intramuscular course until adequate pedicle length is achieved for tension-free anastomosis to either the internal mammary or the thoracodorsal vessels. Careful dissection is required because of the large number of side branches encountered. Many variations of these flaps exist which are beyond the scope of this chapter.

SUGGESTED READINGS

Blondeel PN, Hijjawi J, Depypere H, Roche N, Van Landuyt K. Shaping the breast in aesthetic and reconstructive breast surgery: an easy three-step principle. Part II—Breast reconstruction after total mastectomy. Plast Reconstr Surg 2009;123(3):794–805.

Haddock NT, Teotia SS. Five steps to internal mammary vessel preparation in less than 15 minutes. Plast Reconstr Surg 2017;140(5):884–6.

Neligan P. Plastic Surgery. 4th ed. London: Elsevier; 2018.

Sigalove S, Maxwell GP, Sigalove NM, et al. Prepectoral implant-based breast reconstruction: rationale, indications, and preliminary results. Plast Reconstr Surg 2017;139(2):287–94.

Wei F-C, Mardini S. Flaps and Reconstructive Surgery. 2nd ed. Elsevier; 2017.

Zenn MR, Jones GE. Reconstructive Surgery: anatomy, technique, and clinical applications. St. Louis, MO: Quality Medical Pub.; 2012.

Central Duct Excision and Nipple Discharge

Debra Pratt

INTRODUCTION

Nipple discharge is the third most common breast complaint for which women will see a physician. The majority of nipple discharge is benign. Nipple discharge can be characterized as physiologic or pathological. Physiologic nipple discharge is often bilateral, expressed from multiple ducts, and color can range from green to creamy. Pathological nipple discharge is spontaneous, unilateral, single duct, and bloody or serous (Fig. 57.1). The causes of pathological nipple discharge include benign papilloma, ductal ectasia, and malignancy (reported in 5% to 15% of cases). The goal of the nipple discharge evaluation is to determine which patients need surgery to rule out malignancy.

PREOPERATIVE WORKUP

The evaluation of the patient with nipple discharge starts with a history and physical exam. The history reviews risk factors for breast cancer, rules out infection or trauma, and helps determine if the nipple discharge is physiologic or pathological. The physical exam will determine if there is a breast mass present and help confirm the character of the nipple discharge (expressed/spontaneous, unilateral/bilateral, single duct/multiple ducts, and color).

The pathological nipple discharge is further evaluated with a diagnostic mammogram and retroareolar ultrasound. The mammogram rules out additional nonpalpable abnormalities in the breast. The retroareolar ultrasound helps identify masses within the duct that are not detected on mammography.

Galactography, magnetic resonance imaging (MRI), MRI galactography, and ductoscopy (Fig. 57.1A) are other studies available to further evaluate the potential lesion that may be the cause of the nipple discharge. Their sensitivities range from 52% to 67%, whereas the specificities range from 92% to 25% (MRI). None of these modalities are able to replace histopathological diagnosis. Removal of the duct that is the source of the nipple discharge is needed for pathological examination (Fig. 57.1C).

A. Ductoscopy

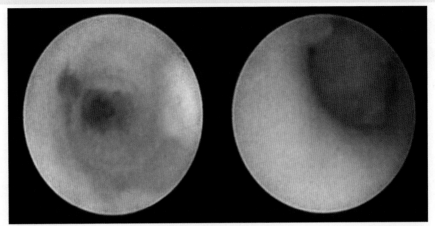

Ductoscopy can differentiate normal ducts (*left*) from intraductal papilloma (*right*) and provide therapeutic options.

B. Clinical considerations with nipple discharge

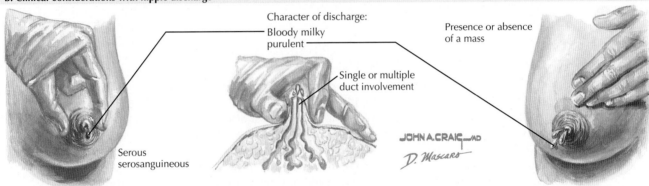

Character of discharge:
Bloody milky
purulent

Presence or absence
of a mass

Single or multiple
duct involvement

Serous
serosanguineous

JOHN A. CRAIG—MD
D. Mascaro

C. Management algorithm for nipple discharge

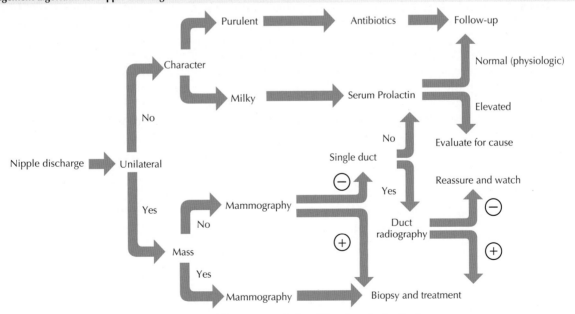

FIGURE 57.1 Management algorithm for nipple discharge.

SURGICAL PRINCIPLES AND TECHNIQUE

The nipple discharge must be present the day of the procedure to help identify the correct duct. Advising the patient to not express the nipple for discharge during the week before surgery can be helpful. The procedure can be done with a local anesthesia (nipple block) with sedation.

The duct is identified by expressing the discharge and then cannulated. Cannulation has been described with a lacrimal probe, injection with methylene blue, nonabsorbable stitch, or a ductoscope (Fig. 57.2). An incision is made at the nipple areolar border near the cannulated duct. The skin of the areola is made into a flap (taking care to preserve the blood supply to the skin by avoiding making it too thin). The cannulated duct is identified and divided close to the nipple. This duct is then removed with a length extending from the nipple level to the proximal breast tissue for a distance of at least 5 cm. (If using ductoscopy, one can see the exact location and precisely design the surgical extent around it.) The majority of pathological lesions are identified within 5 cm of the nipple. The defect is closed by approximating the breast tissue. If there is concern for nipple inversion, a star stitch with absorbable suture can be placed on the underside of the nipple to maintain eversion. The incision is then closed in two layers with absorbable suture.

Women need to be counseled on the effect of the surgery on sensation, potential to nurse, and cosmesis.

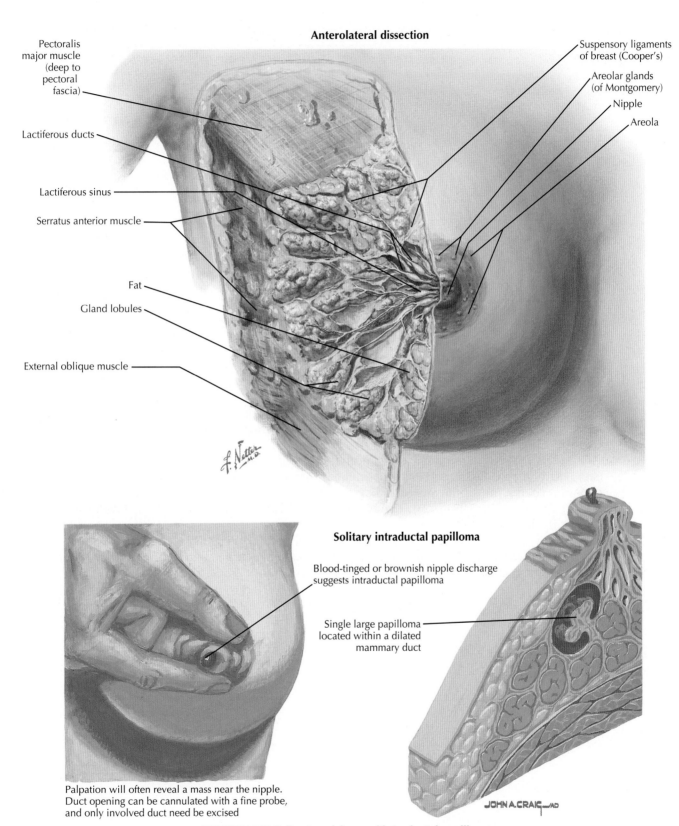

Anterolateral dissection

Pectoralis major muscle (deep to pectoral fascia)

Lactiferous ducts

Lactiferous sinus

Serratus anterior muscle

Fat

Gland lobules

External oblique muscle

Suspensory ligaments of breast (Cooper's)

Areolar glands (of Montgomery)

Nipple

Areola

Solitary intraductal papilloma

Blood-tinged or brownish nipple discharge suggests intraductal papilloma

Single large papilloma located within a dilated mammary duct

Palpation will often reveal a mass near the nipple. Duct opening can be cannulated with a fine probe, and only involved duct need be excised

JOHN A. CRAIG—AD

FIGURE 57.2 Duct excision and intraductal papilloma.

SUGGESTED READINGS

Grunwald S, et al. Diagnostic value of ductoscopy and the diagnosis of nipple discharge and intraductal proliferations in comparison to standard. Methods Onkologie 2007;30:243–8. https://doi.org/10.1159/000100848.

Gui C, et al. INTEND II randomized clinical trial of intraoperative duct endoscopy and pathological nipple discharge. Published online 21 September 2018 in Wiley Online Library (www.bjs.co.uk). https://doi.org/10.1002/bjs.10990.

Harris JR, Lippman ME, Morrow M, Kent Osborne C. Diseases of the Breast. 5th ed. Wolters Kluwer Health Adis (ESP); 2014.

Waaijer, L. et al Systematic review and meta-analysis of the diagnostic accuracy of the ductoscopy in patients with pathological nipple discharge. Published online 23 March 2016 in Wiley Online Library (www.bjs.co.uk). https://doi.org/0.1002/bjs.10125.

Sentinel Lymph Node Biopsy

Kelsey E. Larson

INTRODUCTION

Several cancers, particularly breast cancer and melanoma, are similar in that regional lymph node metastasis greatly affects treatment, prognosis, recurrence rates, adjuvant therapy recommendations, and survival. Therefore accurate assessment and management of regional lymph node disease are of great interest in these patients. Historically, complete lymph node dissection was the standard of care for everyone with invasive breast cancer and melanoma. Although associated with high morbidity, including rates of lymphedema up to 40%, the operation was required to treat regional lymph node disease, to correctly stage the patient, and to allow for appropriate adjuvant radiation and systemic therapy recommendations.

Sentinel lymph node biopsy (SLNB) has dramatically changed the management of breast cancer and melanoma patients. Although first described in 1977, years of research were required to prove the technique accurate and applicable. After the Z11 study in the early 2000s, SLNB was adopted as the standard of care for breast cancer patients with T1-T3 disease who are clinically node negative. During a similar timeframe, the Multicenter Selective Lymphadenectomy Trial (MSLT-1) helped to establish SLNB as the standard of care in clinically node-negative melanoma patients as well.

SELECTION OF DYE/RADIOTRACER AND INJECTION SITES

For breast cancer, the choice of single-agent (blue dye or radiocolloid alone) versus dual-agent (both blue dye and radiocolloid) mapping has been the subject of multiple studies. Although some studies show equivalence between these techniques, the dual tracer technique has been associated with improved sensitivity and specificity and thus is often preferred. However, there are no current national guidelines regarding dye use for SLNB, so the final choice of blue dye or radiolabeled colloid is dictated by surgeon preference and patient characteristics. Blue dye should never be used in pregnancy. In addition, it is important to remember the potential side effects of methylene blue (skin necrosis) and isosulfan blue (anaphylaxis) when selecting an agent for lymphatic mapping.

For breast cancer, the injection site for the blue dye or the radiotracer can be either peritumoral or periareola (Fig. 58.1). Intradermal injection is contraindicated because of skin discoloration, so most injections are done into the breast parenchyma or subdermal levels. The injection may be performed in nuclear medicine preoperatively but may also be performed intraoperatively by the breast surgeon at the start of the case.

For melanoma, intradermal injection of the dye is recommended and is usually performed around the site of the tumor (or around the biopsy site if the primary tumor was previously removed). Any discoloration of the skin is irrelevant because the skin is removed as part of wide local excision. Most often dual tracer technique is used for melanoma. Whereas breast cancers drain to the axillary lymph nodes preferentially, variable lymphatic drainage is common with melanoma depending on location. Thus the radionucleotide injection for melanoma is often performed preoperatively in nuclear medicine so that lymphoscintigraphy can be used to identify the draining nodal basin. If injected in the operating room, it can be more difficult to identify the appropriate nodal basin using the gamma probe alone.

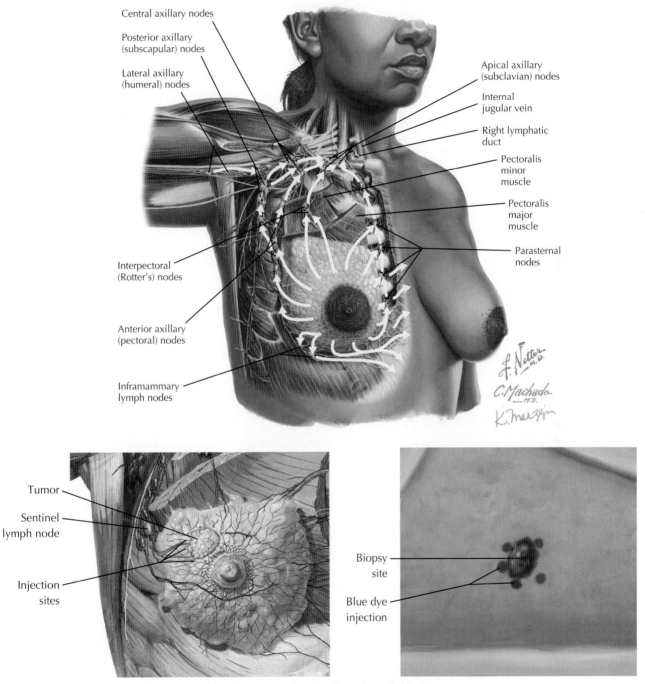

Central axillary nodes

Posterior axillary (subscapular) nodes

Lateral axillary (humeral) nodes

Apical axillary (subclavian) nodes

Internal jugular vein

Right lymphatic duct

Pectoralis minor muscle

Pectoralis major muscle

Parasternal nodes

Interpectoral (Rotter's) nodes

Anterior axillary (pectoral) nodes

Inframammary lymph nodes

Tumor

Sentinel lymph node

Injection sites

Biopsy site

Blue dye injection

FIGURE 58.1 Sentinel lymph node biopsy.

LYMPHATIC DRAINAGE PATTERNS

The lymphatic drainage of the breast and overlying skin are the same: the axillary lymph nodes. Because both peritumoral and periareolar injections work equally well for SLNB mapping in breast cancer, some surgeons use the same injection site for every case, whereas others vary the location. For example, a large upper outer quadrant tumor may not map as well from a periareolar injection, or dye injected behind the nipple areolar complex in nipple-sparing mastectomy may make for more difficult visualization and dissection in this area.

Unlike breast cancer, the variable locations of cutaneous melanoma lead to SLNB being performed in differing anatomic regions. Often, upper-extremity melanomas will drain to the axillary lymph nodes, although epitrochlear lymph nodes may also contain the sentinel node in distal tumors (Fig. 58.2A). Lesions of the scalp typically drain to the posterior cervical lymph nodes, whereas lesions of the face and oral cavity usually drain to the anterior cervical lymph nodes (Fig. 58.2B). Lower-extremity tumors can drain into the popliteal or inguinal node basins (Fig. 58.2C and D). Thus lymphoscintigraphy is important to correctly identify SLNB location in melanoma.

SURGICAL APPROACH

Incisions for the sentinel lymph node biopsies are guided by the expected location of sentinel nodes.

For breast cancer or melanoma mapping to the axilla, a curvilinear incision 1 to 2 fingerwidths below the axillary hairline is almost uniformly used. This approach allows excellent access to the axilla for SLNB, as well as ability to extend the incision if subsequent axillary dissection is required. Dissection for SLNB first proceeds through subcutaneous fatty tissue and then through the clavipectoral fascia into the axilla. The nodes that are targets for SLNB (and axillary dissection, if required) lie deep to the clavipectoral fascia and may be either level 1 or level 2.

Preoperative lymphoscintigraphy for patients with melanoma will indicate if there is an epitrochlear or popliteal sentinel node in tumors of the distal extremity. If a node is found in these beds, a small axial incision over the bed will suffice. If the sentinel node is in the inguinal region, a 2- to 3-cm axial incision below the inguinal ligament should provide the necessary exposure. However, these incisions can be tailored to the location of the sentinel nodes seen on lymphoscintigraphy and identified by the gamma probe in the operating room.

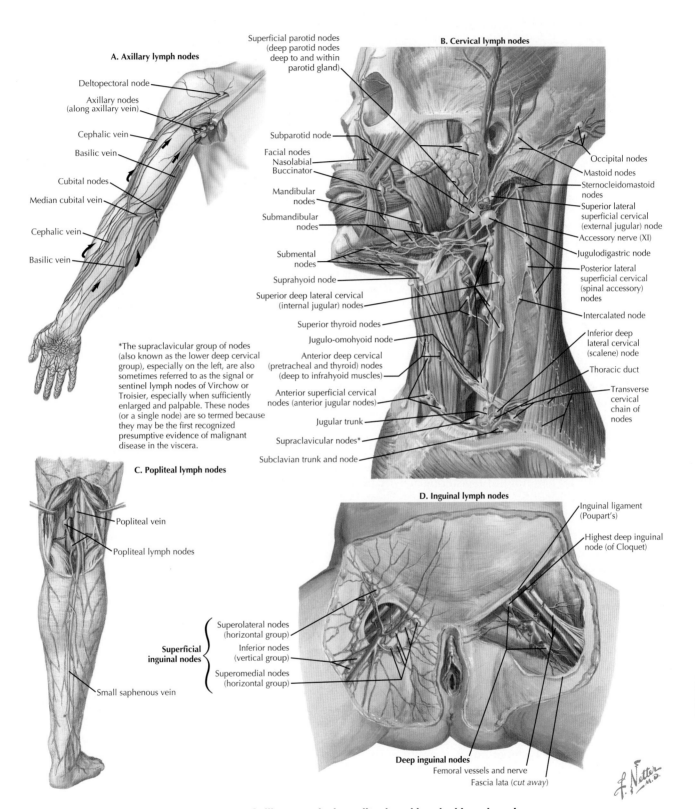

A. Axillary lymph nodes

Deltopectoral node

Axillary nodes (along axillary vein)

Cephalic vein

Basilic vein

Cubital nodes

Median cubital vein

Cephalic vein

Basilic vein

*The supraclavicular group of nodes (also known as the lower deep cervical group), especially on the left, are also sometimes referred to as the signal or sentinel lymph nodes of Virchow or Troisier, especially when sufficiently enlarged and palpable. These nodes (or a single node) are so termed because they may be the first recognized presumptive evidence of malignant disease in the viscera.

Superficial parotid nodes (deep parotid nodes deep to and within parotid gland)

B. Cervical lymph nodes

Subparotid node

Facial nodes
Nasolabial
Buccinator

Mandibular nodes

Submandibular nodes

Submental nodes

Suprahyoid node

Superior deep lateral cervical (internal jugular) nodes

Superior thyroid nodes

Jugulo-omohyoid node

Anterior deep cervical (pretracheal and thyroid) nodes (deep to infrahyoid muscles)

Anterior superficial cervical nodes (anterior jugular nodes)

Jugular trunk

Supraclavicular nodes*

Subclavian trunk and node

Occipital nodes

Mastoid nodes

Sternocleidomastoid nodes

Superior lateral superficial cervical (external jugular) node

Accessory nerve (XI)

Jugulodigastric node

Posterior lateral superficial cervical (spinal accessory) nodes

Intercalated node

Inferior deep lateral cervical (scalene) node

Thoracic duct

Transverse cervical chain of nodes

C. Popliteal lymph nodes

Popliteal vein

Popliteal lymph nodes

Small saphenous vein

D. Inguinal lymph nodes

Inguinal ligament (Poupart's)

Highest deep inguinal node (of Cloquet)

Superolateral nodes (horizontal group)

Superficial inguinal nodes

Inferior nodes (vertical group)

Superomedial nodes (horizontal group)

Deep inguinal nodes
Femoral vessels and nerve
Fascia lata (*cut away*)

FIGURE 58.2 Axillary, cervical, popliteal, and inguinal lymph nodes.

OPERATIVE IDENTIFICATION OF THE SENTINEL LYMPH NODE

After entering the anatomic area of the sentinel node, the surgeon begins localized dissection. If blue dye is used, careful dissection is performed until a blue node is discovered. All nodes that are dyed blue should be removed. If radiolabeled colloid is used, a gamma probe will guide the dissection (Fig. 58.3A). It is important to search for the node with the highest level of radioactivity. This node, as well as all nodes with more than 10% of the highest count, should be removed for pathological evaluation. Thus an appropriate SLNB operation removes all nodes that are "hot" (positive with the gamma probe and within 10% of the highest number) and blue.

It is important to understand the relationship between the injection site and the direction the probe is pointing. In a phenomenon referred to as "shine through," pointing the gamma probe in the direction of the injection site could cause falsely elevated counts and mislead the approach of the dissection. For example, if the dye were injected into the breast in the upper outer quadrant, angling the gamma probe toward this area may pick up gamma signal from the breast injection site (breast parenchyma) rather than a true sentinel node. It is also important to understand this principle as it applies to the lymph nodes. After identifying a "hot" lymph node (Fig. 58.3B), the surgeon should examine the tissue directly behind it to ensure that the node is truly hot and not just registering activity from another deeper node (Fig. 58.3C).

WIRE OR SEED LOCALIZATION OF SENTINEL LYMPH NODE AFTER NEOADJUVANT CHEMOTHERAPY IN BREAST CANCER

For patients who are known to have N1 or N2 lymph node–positive disease, who receive neoadjuvant chemotherapy, and who have a good response to systemic treatment such that they become clinically node negative, SLNB may be appropriate. The surgeon or radiologist performing the initial image-guided lymph node biopsy should place a clip to mark the positive node. After chemotherapy, this clip is then localized using a wire or seed in a similar fashion to how localization is performed for lumpectomy. The localized, clipped node is removed in addition to the nodes identified in the standard sentinel lymph node fashion.

LYMPHEDEMA RISK

One benefit of SLNB is a lower risk of lymphedema compared with a complete axillary dissection and/or complete lymphadenectomy. The rate of lymphedema with SLNB is around 5% to 7%. Removal of excessive number of lymph nodes increases the risk of lymphedema after SLNB; thus it is important that only the true sentinel lymph nodes (those that are hot and/or blue) are removed. Removing additional adjacent nonsentinel nodes does not improve the accuracy of SLNB staging and should not be done.

A. Gamma counter unit

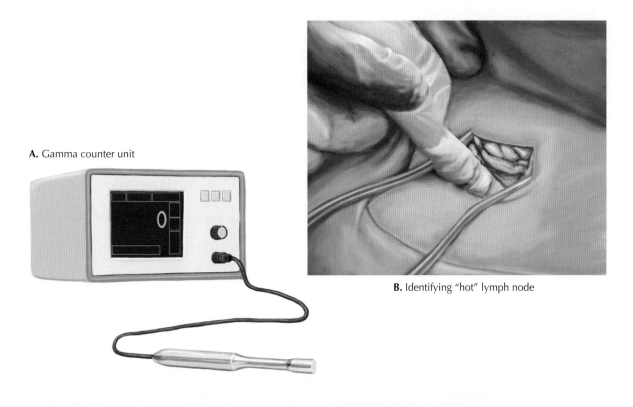

B. Identifying "hot" lymph node

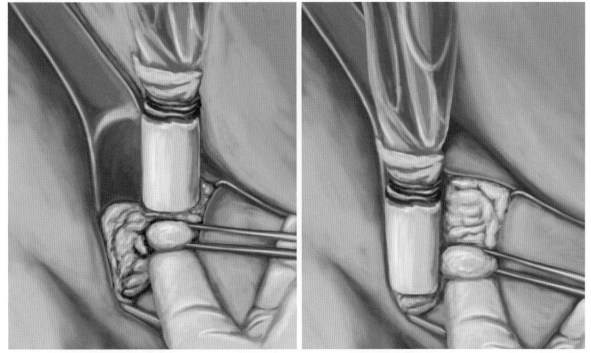

C. After identifying a "hot" lymph node (*left*), the tissue directly behind it should be examined to ensure that the node is truly "hot" and not just registering background from another node (*right*).

FIGURE 58.3 Identification of "hot" lymph node.

SUGGESTED READINGS

Bagaria SP, Faries MB, Morton DL. Sentinel node biopsy in melanoma: technical considerations of the procedure as performed at the John Wayne Cancer Institute. J Surg Oncol 2010;101(8):669–76.

Giuliano AE, Ballman KV, McCall L, et al. Effect of axillary dissection vs no axillary dissection on 10-year overall survival among women with invasive breast cancer and sentinel node metastasis: the ACOSOG Z0011 (Alliance) randomized clinical trial. JAMA 2017;318(10):918–26.

Lynch MA, Jackson J, Kim JA, Leeming RA. Optimal number of radioactive sentinel lymph nodes to remove for accurate axillary staging of breast cancer. Surgery 2008;144(4):525–31; discussion 531–2.

Menes TS, Schachter J, Steinmetz AP, Hardoff R, Gutman H. Lymphatic drainage to the popliteal basin in distal lower extremity malignant melanoma. Arch Surg 2004;139(9):1002–6.

Morton DL, Chocran AJ, Thompson FJ, et al. Sentinel node biopsy for early-stage melanoma: accuracy and morbidity in MSLT-1, an international multicenter trial. Ann Surg 2005;242(3):302–11.

Sloan P. Head and neck sentinel lymph node biopsy: current state of the art. Head Neck Pathol 2009;3(3):231–7.

Axillary Lymphadenectomy and Lymphaticovenous Bypass

Stephanie A. Valente and Graham Schwarz

INTRODUCTION

British surgeon Sir Berkeley Moynihan stated, "Surgery of cancer is not the surgery of the organs; it is the surgery of the lymphatic system." This statement is especially true of breast cancer and melanoma, in which specific operations are carried out to remove regional lymph node metastases. Axillary lymph node dissection (ALND) was traditionally the standard of care for staging as well as treating these patients. However, in the 1990s sentinel lymph node biopsy (SLNB) changed the way surgeons stage and treat both breast cancer and melanoma (see Chapter 58, Sentinel Lymph Node Biopsy).

Patients who undergo ALND have either had an SLNB performed, which has shown metastatic disease in lymph nodes, or have locally advanced disease with cancer in their lymph node(s) (LN) at the time of their presentation. Cancer that has spread to LN is at a more advanced stage with possibility of distant metastatic spread and higher risk of local/regional recurrence.

AXILLARY LYMPH NODE DISSECTION

A thorough ALND involves extensive dissection around important neurovascular structures.

The boundaries of the axilla are the axillary vein superiorly, serratus anterior muscle and chest wall medially, subscapularis and teres minor posteriorly, latissimus dorsi posteriorly and laterally, and pectoralis minor and major muscles anteriorly (Fig. 59.1A). These structures create a pyramid, with the apex positioned superiorly.

The lymph nodes of the axilla are divided into levels I, II, and III, on the basis of their anatomic location in relation to the pectoralis minor (Fig. 59.1B). Level I nodes are lateral to the lateral edge of the pectoralis minor muscle, level II nodes are posterior to the pectoralis minor, and level III nodes are medial to the medial edge. Lymph nodes are also located between the pectoralis minor and major muscles (Rotter's interpectoral nodes). The lymph nodes are enveloped into a fatty axillary tissue, which also contains important neurovascular structures that must be preserved during dissection, as described later.

For surgical excision the patient should be positioned with the arm abducted 90 degrees. If the patient is undergoing a modified radical mastectomy, access to the axilla is gained through lateral extension of the mastectomy incision (see Chapter 55). Otherwise, an oblique incision at the inferior margin of the axillary hairline extending from the lateral edge of the pectoralis muscle to the medial edge of the latissimus muscle is typically used (Fig. 59.2A). If present, a scar from previous SLNB should be used.

The initial step in ALND is creating skin flaps. The flaps should be raised superiorly to the level of the axillary vein and inferiorly to the fourth or fifth rib. Laterally, the flaps should extend to the latissimus dorsi and medially to the pectoralis major. If the ALND is part of a modified radical mastectomy, these flaps may be already raised as part of the mastectomy.

A. Axillary vessels and muscles

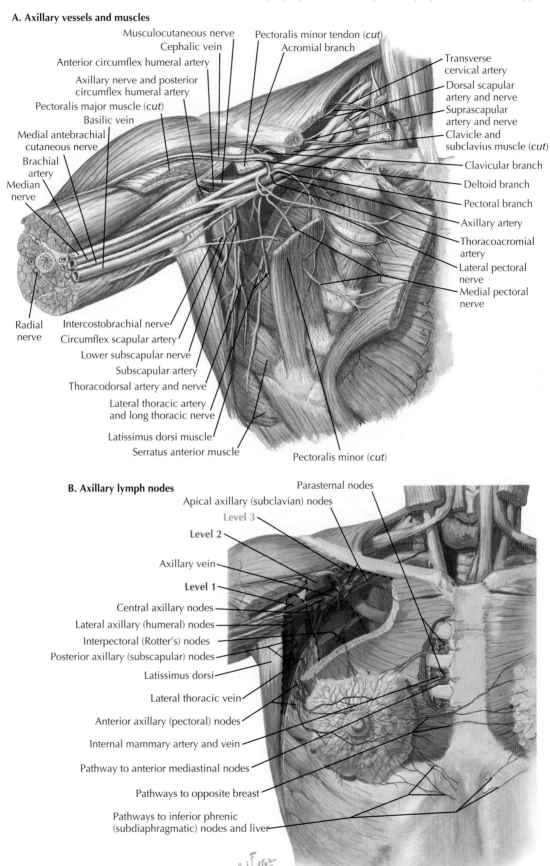

Musculocutaneous nerve
Cephalic vein
Anterior circumflex humeral artery
Axillary nerve and posterior circumflex humeral artery
Pectoralis major muscle (cut)
Basilic vein
Medial antebrachial cutaneous nerve
Brachial artery
Median nerve
Radial nerve
Intercostobrachial nerve
Circumflex scapular artery
Lower subscapular nerve
Subscapular artery
Thoracodorsal artery and nerve
Lateral thoracic artery and long thoracic nerve
Latissimus dorsi muscle
Serratus anterior muscle

Pectoralis minor tendon (cut)
Acromial branch
Pectoralis minor (cut)

Transverse cervical artery
Dorsal scapular artery and nerve
Suprascapular artery and nerve
Clavicle and subclavius muscle (cut)
Clavicular branch
Deltoid branch
Pectoral branch
Axillary artery
Thoracoacromial artery
Lateral pectoral nerve
Medial pectoral nerve

B. Axillary lymph nodes

Apical axillary (subclavian) nodes
Level 3
Level 2
Axillary vein
Level 1
Central axillary nodes
Lateral axillary (humeral) nodes
Interpectoral (Rotter's) nodes
Posterior axillary (subscapular) nodes
Latissimus dorsi
Lateral thoracic vein
Anterior axillary (pectoral) nodes
Internal mammary artery and vein
Pathway to anterior mediastinal nodes
Pathways to opposite breast
Pathways to inferior phrenic (subdiaphragmatic) nodes and liver

Parasternal nodes

FIGURE 59.1 Axilla (dissection) and lymph vessels/nodes of mammary gland.

AXILLARY LYMPH NODE DISSECTION (Continued)

After raising the skin flaps, the surgeon should open the clavipectoral fascia and bluntly dissect through the axillary fat pad to carefully identify the axillary vein superiorly. The axillary vein can be identified coursing horizontally in the superior portion of the dissection field, inferior and anterior to the axillary artery (Fig. 59.2B). Once it is identified, starting at the lateral edge of the pectoralis muscle and moving laterally toward the arm, dissection will identify the lateral thoracic vein (LTV) approximately 2 to 3 cm from the lateral chest wall, draining into the inferior-medial portion of the axillary vein. The LTV drains the lateral portion of the breast and can be ligated and divided if needed to gain exposure into the axillary area, but only after the thoracodorsal bundle (TDB) has been identified. Consistently located deep and slightly lateral to the LTV is the TDB, which includes the nerve, artery, and vein running to the latissimus dorsi muscle. The bundle consists of the nerve located lateral, the vein medial, and the artery positioned in middle. The TDB should be identified and preserved along its entire course to its insertion into the medial edge of the latissimus muscle. The thoracodorsal nerve provides motor function to the latissimus dorsi muscle, and transection results in loss in ability of muscle abduction. The long thoracic nerve runs parallel to the TBD along the lateral deep surface of the serratus anterior muscle and provides motor function to the muscle. Transection results in inability to keep the scapula flat against the posterior chest wall, giving the "winged scapula" phenomenon. The nerve should be identified and preserved along its course.

Approximately 2 cm inferior to the axillary vein is the intercostobrachial sensory nerve. This nerve runs from the second intercostal rib space and transverses across the axilla to provide sensory innervation to the medial portion of the upper inner arm. It courses behind the LTV but anterior to the TDB. Although it can be sacrificed if involved with prominent adenopathy, an attempt should be made to preserve the intercostobrachial nerve.

Coursing along on the undersurface of the pectoralis muscles are important neurovascular structures, which should also be identified and preserved. The medial pectoral nerve innervates the pectoralis major muscle, and the lateral pectoral nerve innervates the pectoralis minor muscle. These nerves course with artery and vein branches from the thoracoacromial trunk off the axillary vessels, enter laterally, and then run on the underside of these muscles. Medial retraction of the pectoralis major and minor muscles will expose level II lymph nodes for dissection.

Once all the axillary anatomic structures have been identified, resection of level I and II lymph nodes can safely be performed. Currently, there is little indication to remove level III nodes, which therefore are typically not dissected, unless there is gross nodal involvement.

Superior dissection begins under the pectoralis minor muscle to remove level II lymphatics. Lymphatic channels and blood vessels should be clipped before ligation. After the superior dissection is completed, the specimen can be retracted inferiorly and the remainder of the lymphatic tissue (level I nodes) removed. Dissection should be performed medial to the serratus anterior muscle, posteriorly to the subscapularis muscle, laterally to the anterior edge of the latissimus dorsi muscle, and inferiorly to the level of the fourth rib, with care to remove all of the lymph nodes in this area, while preserving the neurovascular structures previously discussed (see Fig. 59.2B).

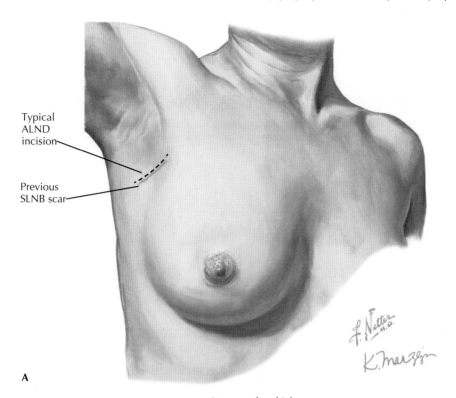

Typical
ALND
incision

Previous
SLNB scar

A

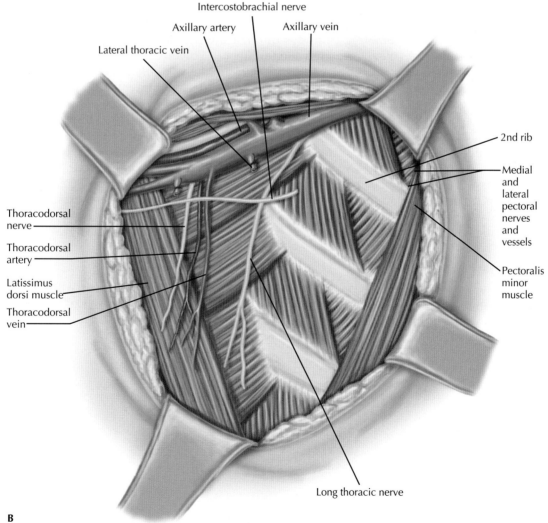

Intercostobrachial nerve

Axillary artery

Axillary vein

Lateral thoracic vein

2nd rib

Medial
and
lateral
pectoral
nerves
and
vessels

Thoracodorsal
nerve

Thoracodorsal
artery

Pectoralis
minor
muscle

Latissimus
dorsi muscle

Thoracodorsal
vein

Long thoracic nerve

B

FIGURE 59.2 Axillary lymph node dissection.

AXILLARY REVERSE MAPPING AND LYMPHATICOVENOUS BYPASS

The axilla is a crossroads for lymphatic drainage from the breast, trunk, back, and upper extremity. Axillary lymphadenectomy may result in lymphatic obstruction and subsequent development of lymphedema, a condition marked by accumulation of protein-rich lymphatic fluid in the extremity accompanied by progressive limb enlargement. Identification and differentiation of lymphatic drainage pathways through the use of tracer-based mapping during ALND or SLNB may allow for preservation of upper-extremity lymphatic vessels as they course through the axilla (Fig. 59.3A). This may mitigate the risk of lymphedema. Combinations of blue dye (isosulfan, methylene blue), radiotracer (technetium 99), and fluorophores (indocyanine green, fluorescein) injected into the upper extremity have been used for axillary lymphatic mapping to allow upper extremity lymphatic vessel visualization and preservation when indicated. When level I and II lymph nodes are removed during ALND, multiple upper arm efferent lymphatics coursing toward the thoracic duct will be inevitably transected. When axillary reverse mapping is employed, transected lymphatics can be identified. Lymphaticovenous bypass (LVB) may then be performed to immediately reconstruct the newly created lymphatic gap. This microsurgical procedure involves creating one or more anastomoses between transected lymphatic channels and competent recipient venous tributaries, thereby restoring anterograde flow and physiologic drainage of lymph into the venous system (Fig. 59.3B).

SUMMARY

Careful attention to neurovascular structures coursing through lymphatic beds will prevent injury during axillary lymphadenectomy. Importantly, only tissue inferior to the axillary vein is removed. Lymphatic mapping and lymphaticovenous bypass may be used as adjunctive procedures during lymphadenectomy to preserve and restore lymphatic continuity.

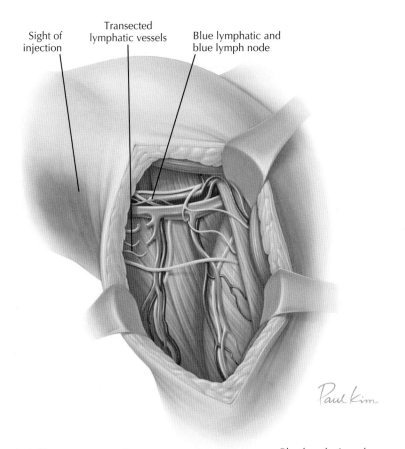

Sight of injection

Transected lymphatic vessels

Blue lymphatic and blue lymph node

Paul Kim

A. Axillary reverse mapping

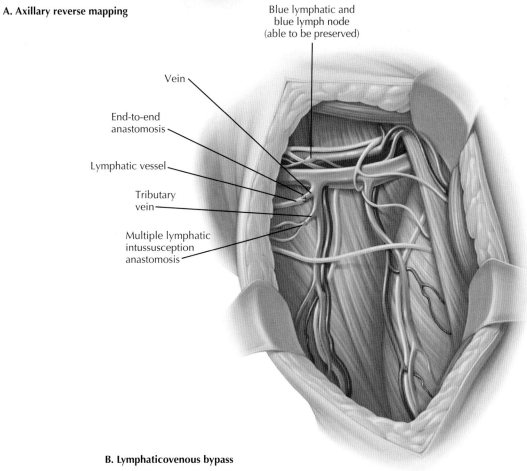

Blue lymphatic and blue lymph node (able to be preserved)

Vein

End-to-end anastomosis

Lymphatic vessel

Tributary vein

Multiple lymphatic intussusception anastomosis

B. Lymphaticovenous bypass

FIGURE 59.3 Axillary reverse mapping and lymphaticovenous bypass.

SUGGESTED READINGS

Anthony DJ, Basnayake BMOD, Ganga NMG, Mathangasinghe Y, Malalasekera AP. An improved technical trick for identification of the thoracodorsal nerve during axillary clearance surgery: a cadaveric dissection study. Patient Saf Surg 2018;12:18.

Boccardo F, Casabona F, De Cian F, et al. Lymphedema microsurgical preventive healing approach: a new technique for primary prevention of arm lymphedema after mastectomy. Ann Surg Oncol 2009;16(3):703–8. https://doi.org/10.1245/s10434-008-0270-y.

Petrek JA, Blackwood MM. Axillary dissection: current practice and technique. Curr Probl Surg 1995;32(4):257–323.

Schwarz G, Grobmyer SR, Djohan RD, Bernard S, Cakmakoglu C, Knackstedt R, Valente SA. Reverse axillary mapping and lymphaticovenous bypass: lymphedema prevention through enhanced lymphatic visualization and restoration of flow. J Surg Oncol 2019;120(2):160–7.

Shilad S, Cakmakoglu C, Schwarz G, Valente S, Djohan R, Grobmyer S. Triple mapping to optimize axillary management in breast cancer patients after neoadjuvant therapy. Ann Surg Oncol 2018;25(10):3106. https://doi.org/10.1245/s10434-018-6645-9.

Inguinal and Pelvic Lymphadenectomy

Eileen A. O'Halloran and Jeffrey M. Farma

INTRODUCTION

Inguinal lymph node dissection (ILND) is performed for therapeutic and staging purposes in neoplasms such as melanoma, penile cancer, and Merkel cell carcinoma and less commonly for sarcomas, squamous cell carcinoma, and vulvar, anal, and rectal cancers. Elective ILND is performed in T1b or greater penile cancers. In most diseases, the presence of clinically positive inguinal lymph nodes is an indication for ILND. In the absence of clinically positive nodes, sentinel lymphadenectomy is often offered to stage the lymph node basin. Historically, ILND was offered to patients with melanoma who have a positive sentinel node. More recently, prospective randomized data have demonstrated no improvement in melanoma-specific or overall survival in patients undergoing ILND for a positive sentinel node versus those undergoing ultrasound surveillance. Currently, ILND is often more selective and reserved for patients with significant sentinel node tumor burden and high-risk primary tumors.

Inguinal lymph node dissection is not without risks, with current rates of complications exceeding 50% in some series. Complications can include, but are not limited to, superficial and deep wound infections, wound dehiscence, seroma, lymphocele, hematoma, and lymphedema. A thorough understanding of the anatomy of the inguinal region is vital to minimize complications of this procedure. In the inguinal region, superficial nodes are those found superficial to the fascia lata proximally, whereas the deep nodes are defined as being deep to the fascia and adjacent to the femoral vessels (Fig. 60.1A). Inguinal lymph node dissection for oncologic indications involves removal of both levels of nodes.

In the operating room, the patient is placed in the supine position with the operative leg gently flexed, abducted, and externally rotated. Perioperative antibiotics should be administered. Pre- and postoperative evaluations by physical therapists specializing in lymphedema treatment and prevention are advocated, because the rate of lymphedema approaches 20%.

INGUINAL LYMPHADENECTOMY

The borders of an inguinal lymph node dissection are defined by the sartorius muscle laterally, the adductor longus muscle medially, and the inguinal ligament superiorly. The sartorius courses medially across the thigh, creating a triangle containing lymphatic tissue (Fig. 60.1B). The lymph tissue surrounds the greater saphenous vein medially and extends laterally and superiorly toward the anterior superior iliac spine (ASIS). These are the primary nodes removed during an ILND.

Inguinal lymphadenectomy begins with an incision made along the long axis of the limb, starting at the inguinal ligament overlying the femoral vessels in the central portion of the triangle and extending below the groin crease (Fig. 60.1C). Dissection is carried down to the superficial fascia, or Camper's fascia, as no lymphatics travel superficial to this fascial layer. Flaps are developed just deep to Camper's fascia. The superficial lymphatic tissue 2 to 3 cm superior to the inguinal ligament is cleared by carrying the subcutaneous flaps laterally to an area just medial to the anterior superior iliac crest. Dissection is carried medially to expose the aponeurosis of the external oblique, the superficial inguinal ring, and the femoral sheath, containing the femoral artery, the femoral vein, and the femoral nerve. Care should be taken to identify the greater saphenous vein, which will be found superficial to the fascia of the medial thigh. The caudal dissection is begun at the adductor longus muscle, just below the inguinal ligament. The fascia of the adductor muscle and sartorius are incised. Dissection is continued inferiorly, along the medial border of the sartorius muscle and the lateral aspect of the adductor longus, to approach the apex of the femoral triangle (Fig. 60.1D). The femoral artery is then exposed and skeletonized superiorly, thus revealing the femoral vein. Distally the femoral vein lies posterior to the artery and then becomes more superficial and medial to the artery as one moves proximally in the femoral triangle (Fig. 60.1E). The areolar and fatty node-bearing tissue is reflected from the femoral vessels in the cephalad direction, and the vessels should be skeletonized. The femoral nerve and its branches should be identified and carefully protected. At the saphenofemoral junction, the saphenous vein can be ligated and divided or skeletonized and spared depending on involvement. Commonly there may be smaller separate venous branches going to the lymph node packet that must be ligated separately. The remaining attachments to the nodal packet are then divided and the specimen is removed. Coverage of the exposed femoral vessels is often needed after inguinal lymphadenectomy, which can be achieved using a sartorius muscle transposition. This maneuver involves detaching the sartorius from its tendinous insertion on the ASIS and rotating it medially over the femoral vessels. This flap is then sutured into place along the inguinal ligament. Care should be taken to ensure that its medial blood supply remains intact. Placement of a drain in the surgical bed, which should exit the skin lateral to the incision, helps in the prevention and management of postoperative lymphocele and seroma. Early ambulation and appropriate pharmacologic prophylaxis are essential to decrease the incidence of postoperative deep vein thrombosis.

A. Superficial nodes of the inguinal region

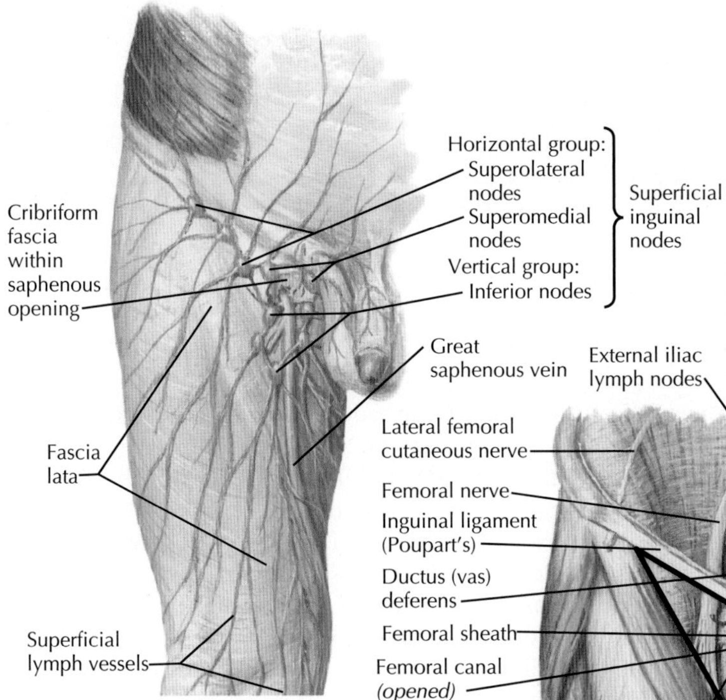

Cribriform fascia within saphenous opening

Horizontal group:
Superolateral nodes
Superomedial nodes
Vertical group:
Inferior nodes

Superficial inguinal nodes

Fascia lata

Great saphenous vein

Superficial lymph vessels

B. The black triangle depicts the borders of an inguinal lymph node dissection: the sartorius muscle laterally, the adductor longus muscle medially, and the inguinal ligament superiorly.

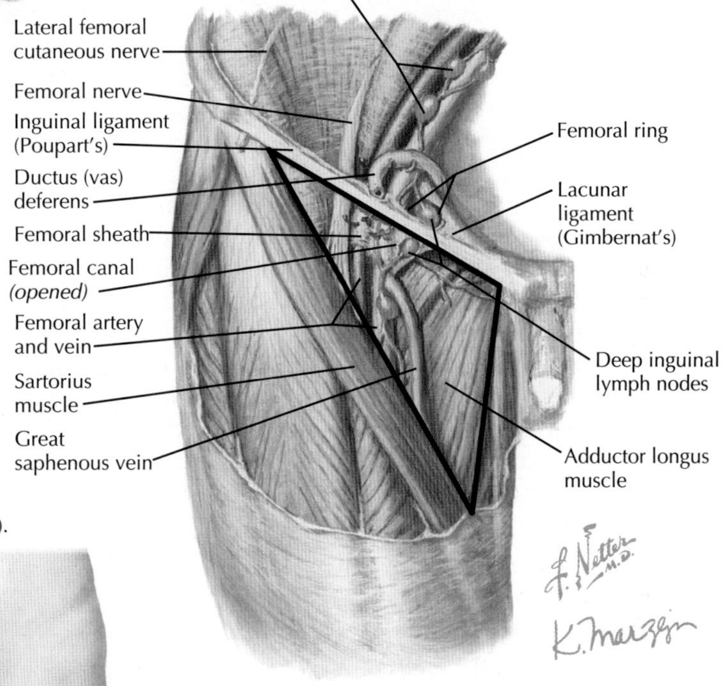

External iliac lymph nodes

Lateral femoral cutaneous nerve

Femoral nerve

Inguinal ligament (Poupart's)

Ductus (vas) deferens

Femoral sheath

Femoral canal *(opened)*

Femoral artery and vein

Sartorius muscle

Great saphenous vein

Femoral ring

Lacunar ligament (Gimbernat's)

Deep inguinal lymph nodes

Adductor longus muscle

C. The blue line depicts the incision made for an open inguinal lymph node dissection. If a pelvic node dissection is to be included in the procedure, an oblique extension approaching the anterior superior iliac spine is made (red).

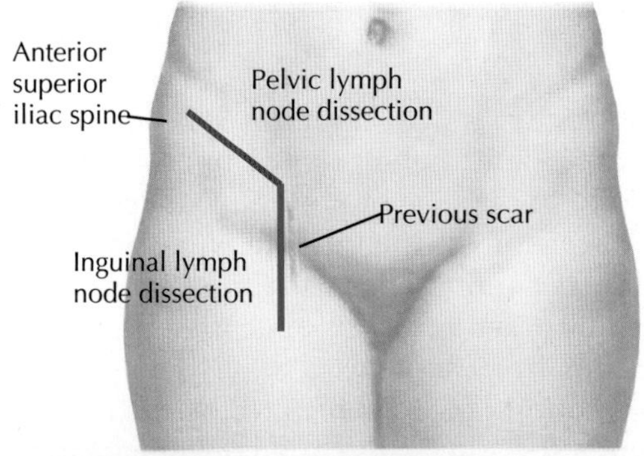

Anterior superior iliac spine

Pelvic lymph node dissection

Previous scar

Inguinal lymph node dissection

D. Inguinal dissection after the fascia of the adductor longus and sartorius are incised, revealing the contents of the femoral sheath.

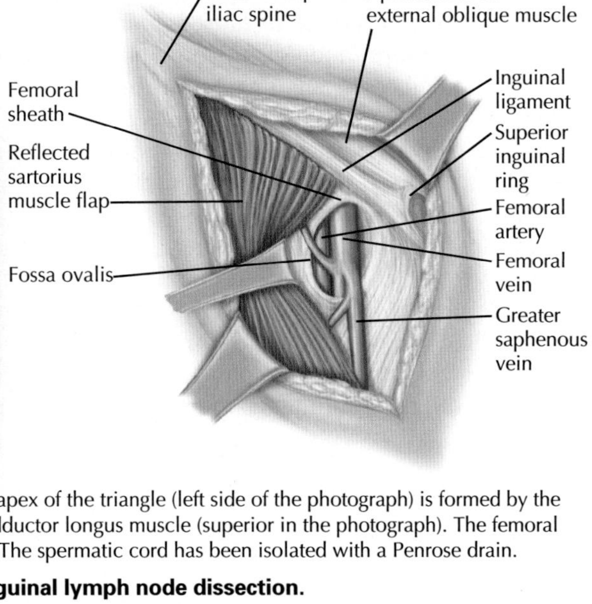

Anterior superior iliac spine

Aponeurosis of external oblique muscle

Femoral sheath

Reflected sartorius muscle flap

Fossa ovalis

Inguinal ligament

Superior inguinal ring

Femoral artery

Femoral vein

Greater saphenous vein

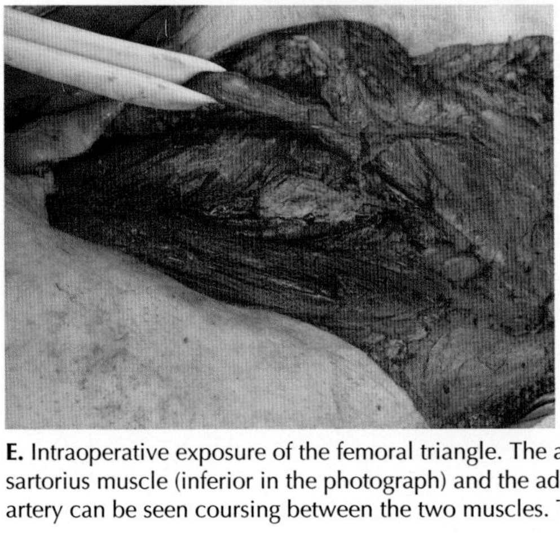

E. Intraoperative exposure of the femoral triangle. The apex of the triangle (left side of the photograph) is formed by the sartorius muscle (inferior in the photograph) and the adductor longus muscle (superior in the photograph). The femoral artery can be seen coursing between the two muscles. The spermatic cord has been isolated with a Penrose drain.

FIGURE 60.1 Inguinal lymph node dissection.

MINIMALLY INVASIVE APPROACHES TO INGUINAL LYMPH NODE DISSECTION

Laparoendoscopic and robotic approaches to inguinal lymphadenectomy are becoming more common. In these procedures, a subcutaneous space is created at the distal apex of the femoral triangle described earlier using blunt and sharp dissection just under the dermis to allow for port placement. Three ports are placed approximately 3 cm medial, distal, and lateral to the apex of the triangle, where the adductor longus and sartorius muscles meet (Fig. 60.2). Insufflation is initiated to elevate the cutaneous flap off of Camper's fascia; dissection is then carried proximally to create space between the subcutaneous tissue and the underlying nodal tissue, superficial to Scarpa's fascia up to the external oblique aponeurosis. The separation is carried laterally to identify and incise the sartorius muscle fascia. The dissection then proceeds medially to identify the adductor longus; care should be taken to identify the crossing saphenous vein. The specimen is then grasped and reflected superficially and cephalad, and the apex of the triangle is dissected. This reflection and dissection is continued cephalad, exposing and skeletonizing the femoral vessels to up to the saphenofemoral junction. The proximal ligation of the saphenous vein occurs at the fossa ovalis over the saphenofemoral junction so that a segment of the saphenous vein is excised with the specimen. The nodal packet is dissected free from its remaining attachments and removed from the patient in a sterile specimen pouch or with a wound protector. A drain is introduced into the lateral trocar, and insufflation is released.

PELVIC LYMPH NODE DISSECTION

The decision to perform a lateral pelvic node dissection is dependent upon the location of the clinically positive node and is often supported by cross-sectional imaging. Pelvic node dissection is pursued if radiographic lymphadenopathy is identified in the iliac or obturator nodes. Some surgeons base the decision to perform a pelvic node dissection on the intraoperative positivity of Cloquet's node, which is the lowest of the external iliac lymph nodes and found deep to the inguinal ligament, but many are moving away from this practice. Pelvic node dissection may also be considered if three or more inguinofemoral nodes are positive.

If a pelvic lymph node dissection is performed as a continuation of an ILND, the skin incision is extended cephalad and laterally to approach the ASIS. Alternatively, an oblique incision medial to the ASIS directed inferomedially is used (Fig. 60.1C). Access to the lateral pelvic nodes begins with detachment of the inguinal ligament from the anterior superior iliac spine. Medial reflection of this ligament, or division of the aponeurosis of the external oblique, the internal oblique, and the transversus, will expose the lymphatic tissue of the deep inguinal region. Frequently, a retroperitoneal approach is used in this location, sweeping the peritoneum to expose the vessels and lymph nodes. This tissue can be carefully cleared off the iliac vessels and removed. During the dissection, the lymph nodes from the common, external, and internal iliac vessels and obturator space should be removed. Special care must be taken to identify and protect the ureter and obturator nerve during this dissection. At the completion of the dissection, the inguinal ligament must be reapproximated or the incised fascial layers must be closed.

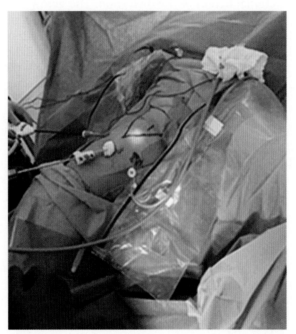

FIGURE 60.2 **External view of a laparoscopic inguinal lymph node dissection.**

MINIMALLY INVASIVE APPROACHES TO PELVIC NODE DISSECTION

Laparoscopic and robotic pelvic lymph node dissections are performed via an intra-abdominal approach. Ports are placed periumbilically and in bilateral lower quadrants to perform this operation. The procedure is begun by opening the peritoneum to access the paravesical space, lateral to the umbilical ligament and medial to the external iliac vein. The ureter is identified crossing superficial to the internal iliac vessels and is lifted off the vessels. The ureter is retracted medially with the peritoneal reflection as the vessels are followed cephalad to the common iliac artery, which is the cranial extent of the dissection. The genitofemoral nerve can be seen lateral to the common iliac artery and should be preserved. The genitofemoral nerve is the lateral extent of the dissection, while the distal aspect of the dissection is the deep circumflex iliac vein. At the distal extent of the dissection, the pubic ramus will be visible. The dissection can proceed cephalad to caudal or caudal to cephalad, skeletonizing the vessels and removing all the fibrofatty tissue from the vessels in one specimen. The psoas major muscle is identified medial to the external iliac artery, and the lymphatic tissue overlying the psoas is dissected free, laterally to medially. Liberating the fibrofatty tissue from the medial aspect of the psoas major muscle permits access to the obturator fossa and reveals the pelvic sidewall. Continuing to dissect the nodal packet from the medial aspect of the external iliac vessels will reveal the obturator nerve, which should be preserved. Carefully separating the nodal packet from the obturator nerve completes the dissection. The nodal packet can be removed with a sterile specimen pouch or wound protector.

SUMMARY

The indications for inguinal and pelvic lymphadenectomy are evolving and vary depending on the primary tumor. Detailed knowledge of inguinal and pelvic anatomy and careful attention to neurovascular structures coursing through lymphatic beds help prevent injury and postoperative complications after inguinal and pelvic lymphadenectomy.

SUGGESTED READINGS

Cesmebasi A, Baker A, Du Plessis M, et al. The surgical anatomy of the inguinal lymphatics. Am Surg 2015;81(4):365–9.

Dzwierzynski WW. Complete lymph node dissection for regional nodal metastasis. Clin Plast Surg 2010;37(1):113–25.

Elsamra SE, Poch MA. Robotic inguinal lymphadenectomy for penile cancer: the why, how, and what. Transl Adrol Urol 2017;6(5):826–32.

Faries MB, Thompson JF, Cochran A, et al. The impact on morbidity and length of stay of early versus delayed complete lymphadenectomy in melanoma: results of the multicenter selective lymphadenectomy trial (I). Ann Surg Oncol 2010;17(12):3324–9.

Faries MB, Thompson JF, Cochran AJ, et al. Completion dissection or observation for sentinel-node metastasis in melanoma. N Engl J Med 2017;376:2211–22.

Jakub JW, Terando AM, Sarnaik A, et al. Safety and feasibility of minimally invasive inguinal lymph node dissection in patients with melanoma (SAFE-MILND): report of a prospective multi-institutional trial. Ann Surg 2017;265(1):192–6.

Leiter U, Stadler R, Mauch C, et al. Complete lymph node dissection versus no dissection in patients with sentinel lymph node biopsy positive melanoma (DeCOG-SLT): a multicentre, randomised, phase 3 trial. Lancet Oncol 2016;17:757–67.

Retroperitoneal Sarcoma

Daniel J. Kagedan and Gary N. Mann

VIDEO

 61.1 Retroperitoneal Sarcoma

INTRODUCTION

Retroperitoneal sarcomas (RPS) are a heterogeneous group of rare mesenchymal neoplasms, accounting for 0.15% of all malignancies and approximately 15% of adult soft tissue sarcomas. Recurrence is common, approximately 50% at 5 years (all grades and subtypes combined). Approaches to management of primary and recurrent RPS are diverse, which necessitates highly individualized treatment decisions for patients.

Adequate surgical resection remains the cornerstone of curative treatment for RPS. An accurate pathological diagnosis is important, ideally obtained preoperatively through image-guided core biopsy of the mass. Lymphoma, testicular metastases, and primary adrenal tumors should be ruled out in patients with retroperitoneal masses. Optimal therapy is dictated by patient factors (performance status, goals of treatment), tumor biology (grade, histologic subtype, size, relationship to key anatomic structures), and tumor location. Multidisciplinary input can determine the role for neoadjuvant and adjuvant treatment and optimally sequence chemotherapy, radiation therapy, and surgery. A particular tumor's sensitivity to certain treatments, and its propensity to recur locally (e.g., liposarcoma) versus distantly (e.g., leiomyosarcoma), may prioritize radiation over chemotherapy or vice versa.

Contrast-enhanced computed tomography (CT) scans of the chest, abdomen, and pelvis should be performed to delineate the extent of the tumor, elucidate its relationship to surrounding structures, and identify possible distant metastases. Anticipating which structures may be involved preoperatively enables effective surgeon and patient preparation for resection.

Complete margin-negative resection is the standard of care for RPS. These tumors can create intense reactions in surrounding tissues, rendering it difficult to assess whether the tumors are invading, rather than just compressing, surrounding structures. Where the technology and expertise are available, intraoperative radiation therapy may be used if there is involvement of, or close proximity to, important structures or viscera, reducing the toxicity to these structure(s) while treating the cancer.

UNDERSTANDING OF ANATOMY AND PREPARATION FOR SURGERY

RPS can involve any intra-abdominal and/or retroperitoneal structure (Fig. 61.1). Their frequently massive size distorts normal anatomy and obscures key structures, landmarks, and planes, both on preoperative imaging and intraoperative assessment (Fig. 61.2). Cross-sectional imaging obtained preoperatively should be carefully scrutinized and used to plan the operation and anticipate intraoperative challenges and determinants of resectability. Assembling a multidisciplinary surgical team may be required if one appreciates the potential for vascular resection/reconstruction, plastic surgery reconstruction, and urologic or neurologic resection/reconstruction. Other potential preoperative interventions include assessment of split-kidney function and the need for ureteral stenting, nerve monitoring, bowel preparation, or stoma marking, as dictated by the preoperative evaluation of the tumor.

Incisions for this operation are varied. A standard midline laparotomy incision works well for most cases. Groin sarcomas may benefit from an abdominoinguinal incision. In other situations, placement of the patient in the lateral decubitus position and performing a curvilinear flank or thoracoabdominal incision may allow the best exposure.

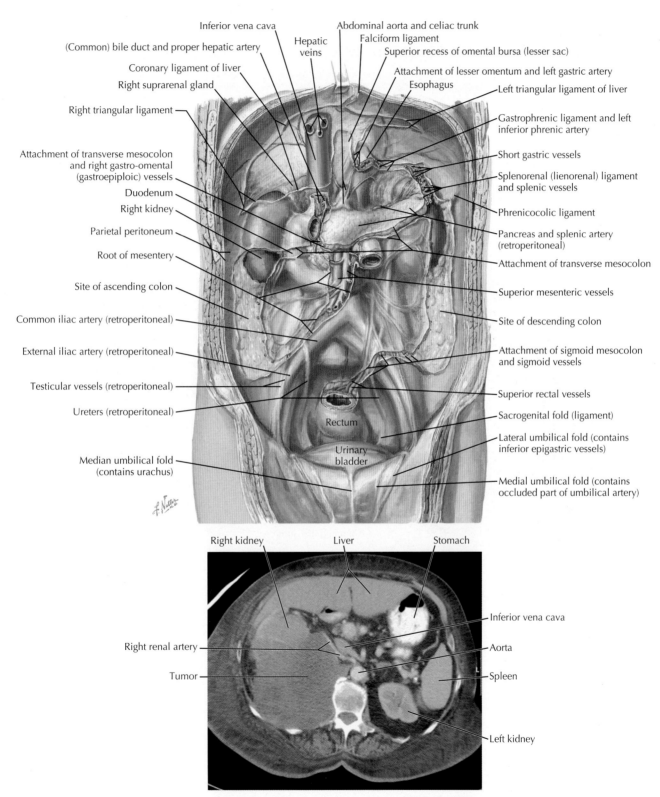

FIGURE 61.1 Retroperitoneal anatomy and computed tomography (CT) scan of large tumor.

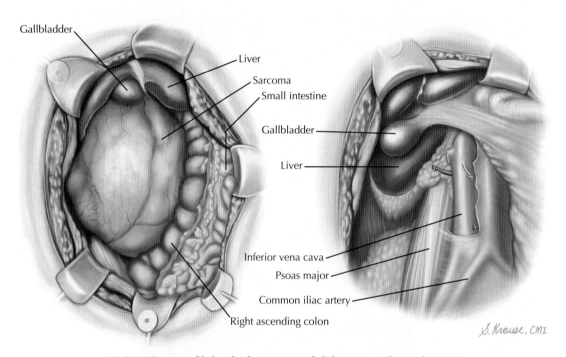

Gallbladder

Liver

Sarcoma

Small intestine

Gallbladder

Liver

Inferior vena cava

Psoas major

Common iliac artery

Right ascending colon

S. Krause, CMI

FIGURE 61.2 Abdominal exposure of right retroperitoneal tumor.

CONDUCT OF THE OPERATION (BOX 61.1)

Once the incision has been made, the first step should be a thorough exploration of the abdomen, evaluating for unanticipated metastases or other findings, such as involvement of viscera that may not have been apparent from preoperative imaging. Adequate exposure with one of the aforementioned incisions and a multiquadrant abdominal wall retractor (such as the Omni or Thompson retractor) is performed (Fig. 61.3). All vital (unresectable) structures potentially involved by the tumor should be identified; once these have been accounted for, all the remaining structures are resectable. Some of these structures cannot be assessed initially and may require significant dissection and mobilization before a determination regarding resectability can be made. Mobilization should proceed circumferentially, approaching a tumor from multiple angles, to avoid working in a hole. Helpful initial maneuvers include right or left colon mobilization along the lateral peritoneal reflection (white line of Toldt), and the Kocher maneuver. An early decision to perform colectomy, and bowel mobilization with medial mesenteric control and division, greatly facilitates the operation, particularly centrally near the great vessels. Key to mobilization are the principles of traction and countertraction, which are paramount for exposure as the surgeon proceeds with the operation.

Once full exposure of the tumor is obtained, a more detailed assessment can be made regarding which surrounding structures are involved. Margin status has a major impact on survival rate, so every attempt should be made for an en bloc, margin-negative resection. This often means that the kidney, portions of the colon, vascular structures, and/or distal pancreas and spleen are resected (see Fig. 61.3). Rarely a pancreaticoduodenectomy or liver resection may be required for right-sided tumors, greatly increasing the complexity of the operation. Various approaches to the extent of RPS resection have been described, including limited margin resection (tumor only or enucleation), wide margin resection (tumor plus involved organs en bloc), and compartmental resection (systematic resection of uninvolved contiguous organs/structures).

Box 61.1 Key Operative Steps in RPS Resection

---

1. Appropriate incision
2. Exploration with assessment for unexpected findings/metastases
3. Exposure with multiquadrant retraction
4. Circumferential mobilization with traction and counter-traction
5. Identification of key structures (all remaining are expendable)
6. Resection of tumor (marginal vs. compartmental)
7. Reconstruction

SUMMARY

Complete surgical resection affords the only opportunity for curative treatment of RPS. Accurate preoperative tissue diagnosis enables appropriate selection and sequencing of pre- and postoperative therapies, taking into account patient factors and disease biology. Preoperative imaging and intraoperative exposure are key to understanding the altered anatomy encountered, and resection should follow established surgical principles. Involving experienced surgeons and those with relevant expertise specific to the structures involved by the tumor enables successful resection.

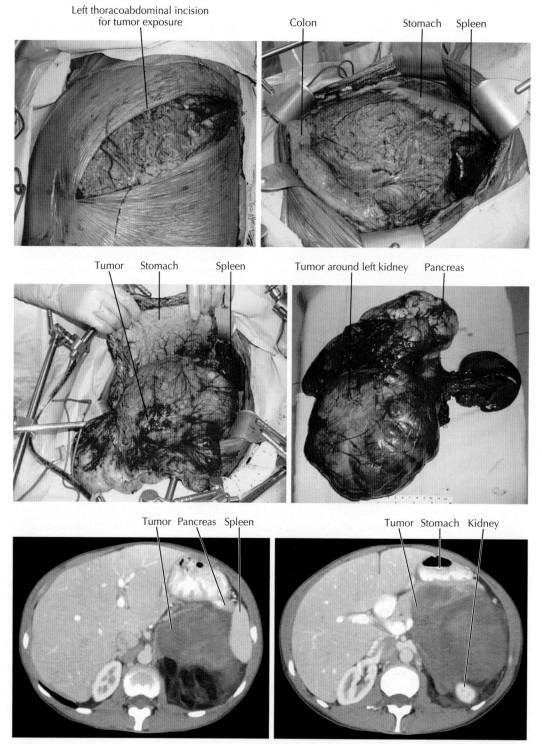

FIGURE 61.3 Computed tomography (CT) scan and resection of retroperitoneal sarcoma involving left kidney, distal pancreas, and spleen.

SUGGESTED READINGS

Gronchi A, Strauss DC, Miceli R, et al. Variability in patterns of recurrence after resection of primary retroperitoneal sarcoma (RPS): a report on 1007 patients from the multi-institutional collaborative RPS working group. Ann Surg 2016;263(5):1002–9.

Kelly KJ, Yoon SS, Kuk D, et al. Comparison of perioperative radiation therapy and surgery versus surgery alone in 204 patients with primary retroperitoneal sarcoma: a retrospective 2-institution study. Ann Surg 2015;262(1):156–62.

Lewis JJ, Leung D, Woodruff JM, Brennan MF. Retroperitoneal soft-tissue sarcoma: analysis of 500 patients treated and followed at a single institution. Ann Surg 1998;228(3):355–65.

Trans-Atlantic RPS Working Group. Management of primary retroperitoneal sarcoma (RPS) in the adult: a consensus approach from the Trans-Atlantic RPS Working Group. Ann Surg Oncol 2015;22(1):256–63.

Hysterectomy for Benign and Malignant Conditions

Chad M. Michener

INTRODUCTION

Hysterectomy remains one of the most common surgical procedures in women and is performed for benign and malignant conditions. The surgical approach varies by pathology, anatomic variations in disease and patients, and the skill set of the surgeon. In the United States, hysterectomy rates have been declining over the last two decades. Abdominal hysterectomy remains the most common approach. However, laparoscopic and robotic-assisted approaches are slowly reducing the proportion of abdominal hysterectomy. This chapter focuses on anatomy pertinent to completion of extrafascial abdominal and laparoscopic or robotic hysterectomy (minimally invasive hysterectomy, or MIH); the basic anatomy and steps are similar among procedures.

SURGICAL ANATOMY

An excellent understanding of the anatomic relationships between the ligamentous attachments and vascular supply to the uterus and the proximity to surrounding structures is a prerequisite to performing a safe and efficient hysterectomy. Although pathology can alter the anatomy of the pelvis, an understanding of normal anatomic relationships allows for easy transition between abdominal hysterectomy and MIH, because the sequence of events is very much the same in these varying surgical approaches. An excellent knowledge of the retroperitoneal anatomy will pay significant dividends when the surgeon is faced with a difficult case involving intraperitoneal adhesions from prior inflammation, endometriosis, or tumor implants, or when the anatomy is distorted by large uterine leiomyoma.

ROUND AND BROAD LIGAMENTS

These ligaments are typically the entry point to performing hysterectomy, as transection of the round ligament allows access into the retroperitoneal space to begin freeing the ligamentous attachments to the uterus and cervix. The round ligaments arise from the lateral aspect of the fundus on either side of the uterus and extend laterally and anteriorly to exit the pelvis through the deep inguinal canal (Fig. 62.1 and see 62.4A) and end by attaching to the subcutaneous tissue of the labia majora.

The broad ligament is formed by an anteroposterior layer of peritoneum that is draped over the uterus, round ligaments, and utero-ovarian ligaments, ending as it blends with the parietal peritoneum of the anterior and posterior cul-de-sacs, pelvic sidewalls, and superolaterally covers the suspensory ligament of the ovary (Figs. 62.1 and 62.2), also known as the infundibulopelvic ligament. Low in the pelvis the two layers form an envelope on either side of the uterus that cover retroperitoneal structures and connective tissue traveling to and from the uterus within the parametrium.

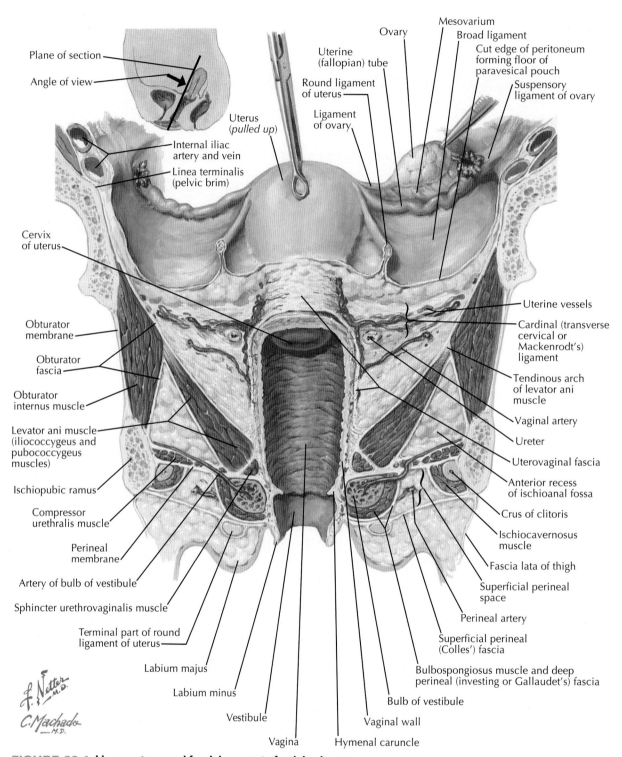

FIGURE 62.1 Ligamentous and fascial support of pelvic viscera.
Note the round ligaments inserting anterior to the fallopian tubes at the corneal regions of the uterus and portion of the broad ligament.

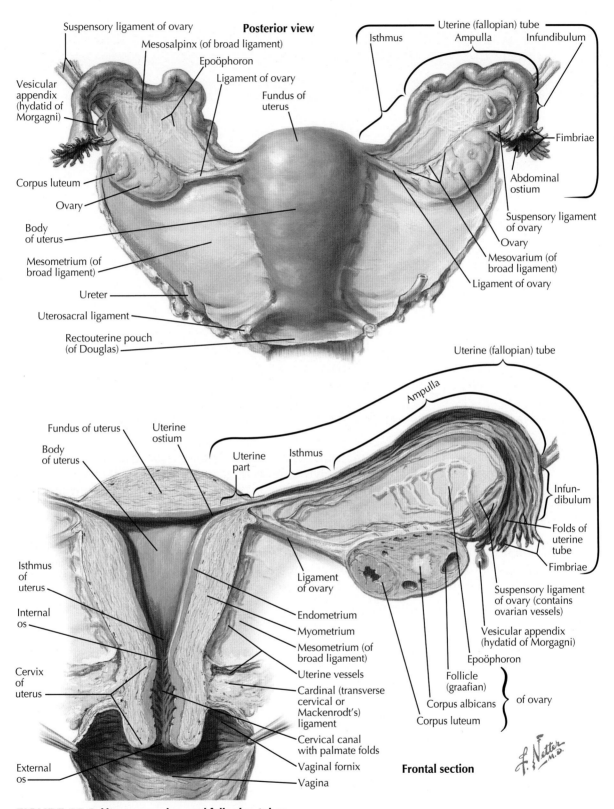

Posterior view

Suspensory ligament of ovary

Mesosalpinx (of broad ligament)

Epoöphoron

Ligament of ovary

Fundus of uterus

Vesicular appendix (hydatid of Morgagni)

Corpus luteum

Ovary

Body of uterus

Mesometrium (of broad ligament)

Ureter

Uterosacral ligament

Rectouterine pouch (of Douglas)

Isthmus

Uterine (fallopian) tube

Ampulla

Infundibulum

Fimbriae

Abdominal ostium

Suspensory ligament of ovary

Ovary

Mesovarium (of broad ligament)

Ligament of ovary

Uterine (fallopian) tube

Ampulla

Fundus of uterus

Body of uterus

Uterine ostium

Uterine part

Isthmus

Infundibulum

Folds of uterine tube

Fimbriae

Suspensory ligament of ovary (contains ovarian vessels)

Vesicular appendix (hydatid of Morgagni)

Epoöphoron

Follicle (graafian)

Corpus albicans

Corpus luteum

of ovary

Isthmus of uterus

Internal os

Cervix of uterus

External os

Endometrium

Myometrium

Mesometrium (of broad ligament)

Uterine vessels

Cardinal (transverse cervical or Mackenrodt's) ligament

Cervical canal with palmate folds

Vaginal fornix

Vagina

Ligament of ovary

Frontal section

FIGURE 62.2 Uterus, ovaries, and fallopian tubes.
Note that the broad ligament forms the mesosalpinx and continues below the ovary to envelop the cardinal ligament and uterine blood supply and laterally to cover the suspensory ligament of the ovary.

CARDINAL AND UTEROSACRAL LIGAMENTS AND POTENTIAL SPACES

The cardinal ligament, also known as the transverse cervical or Mackenrodt's ligament, extends laterally from the cervix and divides the pelvis into two potential spaces on either side (Fig. 62.3). Anterior to the cardinal ligament is the paravesical space bound anteriorly by the bladder and laterally by the levator ani and obturator internus muscles. Posterior to the cardinal ligament is the pararectal space bound posteriorly by the sacrum and laterally by the internal iliac vessels. These spaces should be understood because they play an important role in radical hysterectomy and can help get around significant intraperitoneal pathology. The uterosacral ligaments arise on a broad base from the midportion of the sacrum and extend in a curvilinear fashion anteromedially to insert onto the lower lateral aspect of the cervix.

Female: superior view (peritoneum and loose areolar tissue removed)

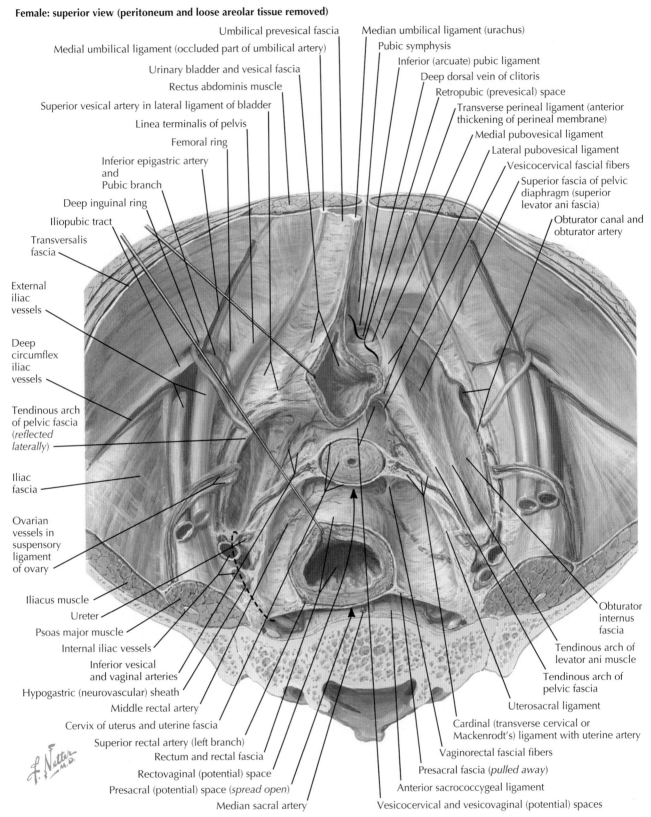

FIGURE 62.3 Pelvic cross section with peritoneum removed.
Note the cardinal ligament containing the uterine vessels and dividing the pelvis into anterior and posterior compartments. The paravesical and pararectal spaces are potential spaces just anterior and posterior to the cardinal ligament on each side.

PELVIC VASCULATURE AND RELATIONSHIP OF THE URETER

The uterine blood supply is derived from both ovarian arteries that originate directly from the aorta and the uterine artery, which is a branch of anterior division of the internal iliac artery. Additional branches important in pelvic surgical anatomy are the obturator, umbilical, vaginal, and inferior vesical arteries (Fig. 62.4). The uterine artery branches medially and travels within the cardinal ligament just anterior to the ureter to enter the uterus at the cervicouterine junction. Note that the ureter is typically 1.5 to 2.5 cm from the cervix in this region and is the most common place for iatrogenic ureteral injury during hysterectomy (see Fig. 62.4B). Detailed knowledge of the relationships among the uterus, cervix, pelvic vasculature, and ureter is critical to avoiding injury of the ureter or pelvic vessels.

Additional sites of ureteral injury during hysterectomy are near the pelvic brim during ligation and transection of the suspensory ligament of the ovary, where the ureter crosses over the common iliac vessels and runs just posterior to the ovarian vessels (see Fig. 62.4A). Identification of the ureter on the medial leaf of the broad ligament in this location will minimize the risk of this injury. The ureter then continues down into the pelvis on the medial leaf of the broad ligament, passes beneath the uterine artery, and turns anterior and medial to enter the base of the bladder near the cervicovaginal junction. The ureter can be injured here during transection of the vagina or during closure of the vaginal cuff.

Identification of the ureter is often easier if you dissect proximally in the retroperitoneal space until near the bifurcation of the common iliac artery. In open cases, two fingers can be "walked" along the iliac vessels toward the aorta, and a gentle lifting motion will expose the ureter on the medial leaf of the broad ligament.

HYSTERECTOMY

Hysterectomy may be performed with or without removal of the fallopian tubes and ovaries, depending on indications for surgery as well as patient age and wishes. Benign indications for hysterectomy include abnormal uterine bleeding, uterine leiomyoma, endometriosis, and as part of treatment for pelvic organ prolapse. Malignant indications include endometrial hyperplasia and carcinoma, uterine sarcoma, carcinoma of the ovary or fallopian tube, early stage cervical carcinoma, and occasionally in women with gestational trophoblastic disease. Approaches vary by indication; modified radical and radical hysterectomy are more common for cervical carcinoma as well as advanced cases of endometrial and ovarian carcinoma. The remainder of this section focuses on simple hysterectomy.

A. Arteries and veins of pelvic organs: anterior view

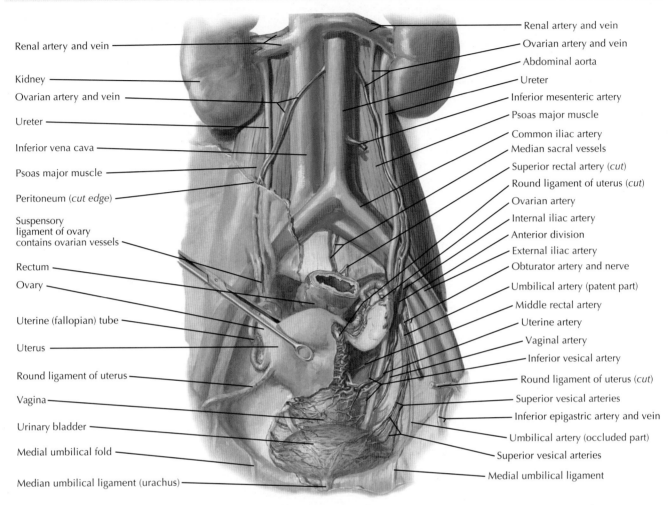

Renal artery and vein

Kidney

Ovarian artery and vein

Ureter

Inferior vena cava

Psoas major muscle

Peritoneum (*cut edge*)

Suspensory ligament of ovary contains ovarian vessels

Rectum

Ovary

Uterine (fallopian) tube

Uterus

Round ligament of uterus

Vagina

Urinary bladder

Medial umbilical fold

Median umbilical ligament (urachus)

Renal artery and vein

Ovarian artery and vein

Abdominal aorta

Ureter

Inferior mesenteric artery

Psoas major muscle

Common iliac artery

Median sacral vessels

Superior rectal artery (*cut*)

Round ligament of uterus (*cut*)

Ovarian artery

Internal iliac artery

Anterior division

External iliac artery

Obturator artery and nerve

Umbilical artery (patent part)

Middle rectal artery

Uterine artery

Vaginal artery

Inferior vesical artery

Round ligament of uterus (*cut*)

Superior vesical arteries

Inferior epigastric artery and vein

Umbilical artery (occluded part)

Superior vesical arteries

Medial umbilical ligament

B. Injuries to the ureter

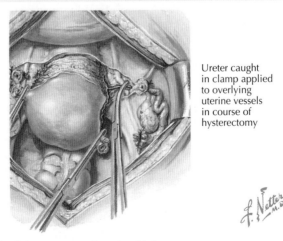

Ureter caught in clamp applied to overlying uterine vessels in course of hysterectomy

FIGURE 62.4 Arteries and veins of pelvic organs and ureteral injury.
Note the anatomic relationships between the ureter and the uterine and ovarian vasculature, especially at the most common sites of injury: the pelvic brim, the junction of the uterine artery, and at the lateral vesicovaginal junction.

SURGICAL APPROACH

The route chosen for completion of hysterectomy depends on several factors: pathology being treated, anatomic considerations, prior abdominal and pelvic surgery, as well as patient and physician preference. Vaginal hysterectomy is commonly used for pelvic organ prolapse and removal of small to moderate-size uteri but remains an underused route. The use of MIH (laparoscopic or robotic) continues to increase and is now replacing abdominal hysterectomy as the most common route for hysterectomy in many centers. MIH may be used for benign and malignant pathology and can be used for simple extrafascial, modified radical, and radical hysterectomy. An abdominal approach is required when there is a very large uterus, extensive peritoneal pathology (metastatic ovarian carcinoma), or when patient factors, such as an extensive history of abdominal surgery or adhesions, dictate.

The choice of incision for an open abdominal hysterectomy will depend on surgical indications, patient factors, and uterine size or anatomy. A midline vertical incision is more common for patients with very large uteri and extensive peritoneal disease necessitating upper abdominal access. A low transverse abdominal incision is often used for benign disease with a uterine size below the level of the umbilicus. Regardless of incision type, once the peritoneal cavity is entered, exploration of the pelvic and abdominal compartments by visualization (open and laparoscopic cases) and palpation (open cases) should be carried out and pelvic washings obtained if indicated. For open cases a self-retaining wound retractor should be placed and the bowel packed into the upper abdomen with moistened sponges or towels. For laparoscopic cases, the patient should be placed into steep Trendelenburg position and the bowels excluded from the pelvis using gravity and an atraumatic bowel grasper.

ACCESSING THE RETROPERITONEUM

Once abdominopelvic access and appropriate exposure have been obtained, the pertinent pelvic surface anatomy should be identified (Fig. 62.5A) and restored to normal where possible. For open hysterectomy, place a large Kelly clamp on both cornual regions of the uterus. For laparoscopic cases, placement of a uterine manipulator with a colpotomy ring will aid in maintaining upward traction on the uterus during dissection and facilitate colpotomy. From here, the steps of the operation are similar regardless of surgical approach, and steps are outlined for comparison in Table 62.1. The round ligaments should be cauterized and divided with either monopolar cautery or a vessel-sealing device. Alternatively they may be clamped, transected, and ligated with a heavy absorbable tie (Fig. 62.5B and C). The retroperitoneal spaces can then be opened with cautery or serial bites with the vessel-sealing device by extending the peritoneal incision inferiorly and medially to begin creation of the bladder flap along the vesicouterine peritoneum or cephalad to mobilize the suspensory ligament of the ovary. A similar dissection on the contralateral side of the pelvis will allow for dissection of the bladder flap. Once the vesicouterine peritoneum has been incised all of the way across, ensure that there is upward traction on the uterus, then carry the dissection inferiorly down the cervix and onto the upper vagina. Gentle traction and monopolar cautery can be used to facilitate dissection, while constant upward traction on the uterus helps to lateralize the ureters at the cervicovaginal junction. If there has been a prior cesarean section and there is a thick scar between the bladder and lower uterine segment, dissecting from lateral to medial will help gain access to the appropriate avascular plane just below the scar and allow for mobility of the bladder. Now that the bladder flap has been made and the sidewalls have been opened bilaterally, blunt dissection in the retroperitoneal space should be used to identify the ureters and retroperitoneal vessels (Fig. 62.5D). Constant upward traction on the uterus will aid in dissection of the bladder flap and allow the ureters to roll inferiorly and laterally to maximize distance between the ureter and clamps and/or cautery.

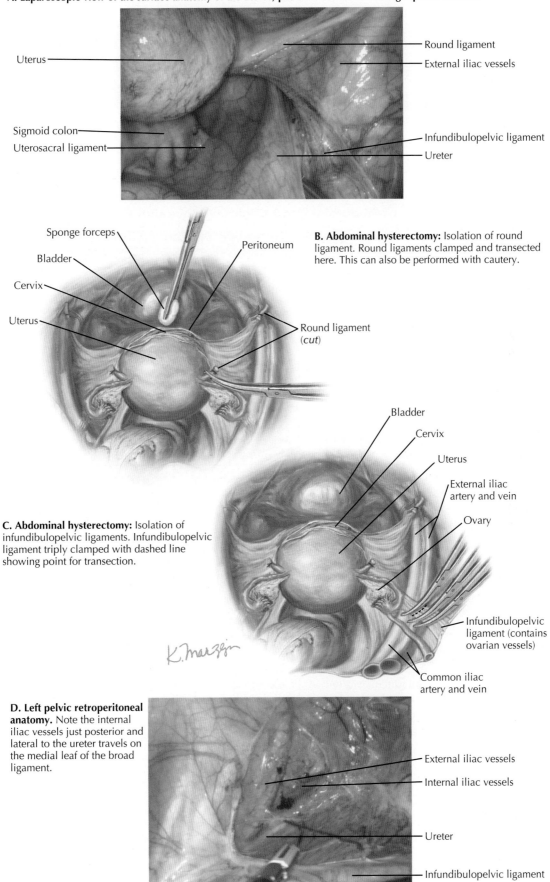

A. Laparoscopic view of the surface anatomy of the uterus, posterior cul de sac and right pelvic sidewall

Uterus

Round ligament

External iliac vessels

Sigmoid colon

Uterosacral ligament

Infundibulopelvic ligament

Ureter

Sponge forceps

Peritoneum

Bladder

Cervix

Uterus

Round ligament (*cut*)

B. Abdominal hysterectomy: Isolation of round ligament. Round ligaments clamped and transected here. This can also be performed with cautery.

Bladder

Cervix

Uterus

External iliac artery and vein

Ovary

C. Abdominal hysterectomy: Isolation of infundibulopelvic ligaments. Infundibulopelvic ligament triply clamped with dashed line showing point for transection.

Infundibulopelvic ligament (contains ovarian vessels)

Common iliac artery and vein

D. Left pelvic retroperitoneal anatomy. Note the internal iliac vessels just posterior and lateral to the ureter travels on the medial leaf of the broad ligament.

External iliac vessels

Internal iliac vessels

Ureter

Infundibulopelvic ligament

FIGURE 62.5 Accessing the retroperitoneum.

Table 62.1 Steps of Abdominal and Minimally Invasive Hysterectomy

Abdominal	Minimally Invasive
Clamp uterine cornu with Kelly clamps	Place uterine manipulator
Transect round ligaments with cautery	Cauterize and transect round ligaments with VS
Open pelvic sidewall with cautery	Open pelvic sidewall with cautery
Create bladder flap with cautery	Create bladder flap with cautery or VS
Identify ureters retroperitoneally	Identify ureters retroperitoneally
Create window in broad ligament	Create window in broad ligament
Clamp, transect, and ligate IP or utero-ovarian ligament with Heaney clamps	Use VS to cauterize and transect IP or utero-ovarian ligament
Skeletonize uterine vessels with cautery and ensure upward traction on uterus	Skeletonize uterine vessels with VS or cautery and ensure upward traction on uterus
Clamp, transect, and suture uterine vessels with Heaney clamps at cervicouterine junction	Cauterize and transect uterine vessels with VS at the cervico-uterine junction
Clamp, transect, and suture small bite just medial to previous pedicle to move ureter laterally	Cauterize and transect a small pedicle just medial to previous pedicle to move ureter laterally
Continue to clamp, transect, and suture pedicles medial to previous serially with straight Ballentine clamps until the cervicovaginal junction is reached	Continue to cauterize and transect pedicles medial to previous serially until the vessels are outside of the colpotomy ring (the upper vaginal fornix)
Ensure that bladder flap is 1.5–2 cm below planned colpotomy site (palpate cervix)	Ensure that bladder flap is 1.5–2 cm below planned colpotomy site
Clamp across the upper vagina and uterosacral ligaments with strongly curved Zeppelin clamp and place transfixation suture	Perform circumferential colpotomy with a monopolar hook or spatula
Close remaining vagina cuff with running (0-PGA or barbed absorbable) or figure-of-eight 0-PGA suture	Close vaginal cuff incorporating uterosacral ligaments with running barbed absorbable suture or running or figure-of-eight 0-PGA suture
Copiously irrigate pelvic and check all site for hemostasis	Copiously irrigate pelvic and check all site for hemostasis
Abdominal closure	Port site closure

MANAGEMENT OF THE OVARIES

If removing the ovaries, the surgeon should create a window through the peritoneum parallel to the suspensory ligament of the ovary between the ureter and ovarian vessels. The vessels should then be doubly clamped with Kelly or Heaney clamps, divided and ligated with a heavy absorbable suture for open cases (Fig. 62.5B and C), or cauterized and divided with a vessel-sealing device. (For additional information on oophorectomy, see Chapter 63.) If the ovaries are to remain in situ, identify the ureter and create a window in the peritoneum between the ureter and the utero-ovarian ligament just inferior to the ovary. Either doubly clamp, transect, and ligate or cauterize and transect the utero-ovarian ligament.

UTERINE BLOOD SUPPLY AND MOBILIZATION

The uterine vessels should be skeletonized using monopolar cautery to incise the broad ligament down toward the uterine vessels. Here the path of the ureter should be considered before placing curved Heaney clamps on the uterine vessels at the cervicouterine junction. The clamp should be placed so that the curve is inward with the tip just bouncing off of the uterus rather than curving outward toward the ureter (Fig. 62.4B) to avoid ureteral injury. Similarly, during laparoscopic hysterectomy, the vessel-sealing device should approach from a slight angle and bounce off of the uterus as it is closed (Fig. 62.6) to avoid ureteral injury.

For abdominal hysterectomy, an absorbable 0 suture should be placed just below and just off of the lateral aspect of the tip of the clamp for open procedures to avoid ligating the ureter at this location. Serial bites are then taken along the cardinal ligaments on either side of the cervix until the cervicovaginal junction is reached. For abdominal hysterectomy, this is done using serial clamping with straight Heaney clamps, transection with a scalpel, and ligation. Each bite should be taken medial to the last, and the sutures passed just under the lateral aspect of the tip of the clamp. Palpation of the tip of the cervix can be done through the vaginal wall between the thumb and forefinger to ensure that the appropriate level of dissection has been reached. For laparoscopic cases the cardinal ligaments are cauterized and transected with the vessel-sealing device until the vascular packet created is outside of the colpotomy ring (if used) or below the cervicovaginal junction.

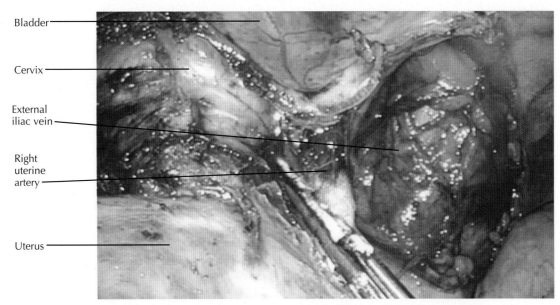

FIGURE 62.6 Laparoscopic transection of the right uterine artery and vein.
Note the location at the cervico-uterine junction and slight oblique angle of approach.

COLPOTOMY AND VAGINAL CLOSURE

Before separating the cervix and vagina, ensure that there is upward traction on the uterus and that the bladder flap has been mobilized approximately 2 cm below the cervix to facilitate vaginal closure without incorporation of the bladder and/or ureters. For abdominal hysterectomy, place a strongly curved clamp (Heaney or Zeppelin) across the upper vagina and uterosacral ligaments just below the level of the cervix. Transect the vagina with heavy curved scissors and remove the specimen from the pelvis. The angles of the vagina are sutured along with the distal uterosacral ligament using an absorbable 0 transfixation suture. The remainder of the vaginal cuff can be closed with running or figure-of-eight sutures. For laparoscopic cases, the vagina is transected over the colpotomy ring using a monopolar spatula or hook. Once the cervix has been detached, the specimen can be removed vaginally or can be placed into a laparoscopic specimen retrieval bag and then morcellated and/or removed by enlarging one of the laparoscopic incisions. The vaginal cuff can be closed with an absorbable 0 suture or a synthetic barbed absorbable suture in a running fashion. Care should be taken to include bites through the uterosacral ligaments on each side to help with suspension of the vaginal cuff as these fall away from the cut edge of the vagina during laparoscopic colpotomy.

After closure of the vaginal cuff, the pelvis should be irrigated and each site of dissection carefully inspected for hemostasis and integrity of the remaining structures. Cystoscopy can be used to evaluate ureteral patency if desired, whereas some surgeons are now exploring intravenous fluorescein to assess ureteral jets. Once hemostasis and ureteral integrity are confirmed all instruments, retractors and packing should be removed. The bowel should be placed back into anatomic position and the abdomen closed in standard fashion.

MODIFIED RADICAL AND RADICAL HYSTERECTOMY

Modified radical and radical hysterectomy are classically used for the surgical treatment of cervical cancer. However, endometrial carcinoma with cervical involvement, ovarian cancers, and occasionally benign pathology may necessitate a more extended hysterectomy. The initial steps for these procedures remain the same up through transection of the ovarian vessels or uterine ligament. Typically, radical hysterectomy includes pelvic lymphadenectomy (Fig. 62.7). The pelvic lymph nodes include those of the distal half of the common iliac artery down to the circumflex iliac vein. The lateral extent of the dissection is bound by the genitofemoral nerve and the medial extent to the superior vesical artery. The lymph nodes posterior to the external iliac vein in the obturator space should be removed down to the obturator nerve. Care should be taken to identify the obturator nerve before clamping or cauterizing and structures in this space to avoid injury to the nerve.

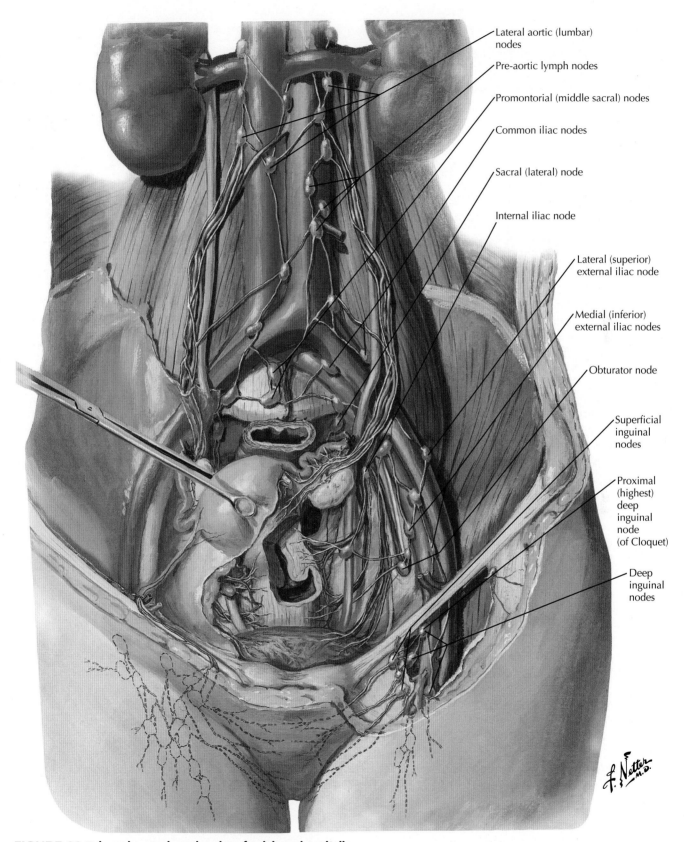

Lateral aortic (lumbar) nodes

Pre-aortic lymph nodes

Promontorial (middle sacral) nodes

Common iliac nodes

Sacral (lateral) node

Internal iliac node

Lateral (superior) external iliac node

Medial (inferior) external iliac nodes

Obturator node

Superficial inguinal nodes

Proximal (highest) deep inguinal node (of Cloquet)

Deep inguinal nodes

FIGURE 62.7 Lymph vessels and nodes of pelvis and genitalia.
Note the anatomic relationship of aortic and pelvic lymph nodes that drain the uterus, cervix, and adnexa.

MODIFIED RADICAL AND RADICAL HYSTERECTOMY (Continued)

Once lymphadenectomy has been completed, follow the internal iliac artery inferiorly until the uterine artery can be seen branching off of the medial aspect (see Fig. 62.4). This should be isolated by blunt dissection with either a right-angle clamp or a laparoscopic vessel sealer. The uterine artery should be clamped and transected or cauterized and transected just lateral to the ureter for modified radical or at its origin from the internal iliac for radical hysterectomy. The artery is then mobilized over the ureter, and the uterine veins are identified and transected. For open cases, place a vessel loop around the ureter for traction. Using a right-angle clamp or a laparoscopic vessel sealer dissect just anterior to the ureter within the tunnel until the anterior vesicouterine ligament is reached. The veins just off the corner of the bladder (bladder pillars) can bleed significantly. Carefully clamp, transect, and ligate or cauterize and transect the ligament. The uterus should be retracted anteriorly to expose the posterior cul de sac. The peritoneum overlying the pouch of Douglas should be incised with cautery to open the rectovaginal space (see Fig. 62.2). The space is carefully dissected with sharp and blunt dissection to expose the uterosacral ligaments. These should be cauterized or clamped and transected. In open cases this pedicle should be suture ligated with an absorbable 0 suture, taking care to avoid injury to the anterior rectum. With the uterus mobilized, the ureter can be retracted laterally and the parametrium on each side serially transected with curved Heaney clamps or a vessel-sealing device. The dissection should begin laterally from the internal iliac artery inferiorly and in toward the upper vagina. This frees the remaining attachments of the ureter. The cervicovaginal junction is identified, and dissection of the bladder down the upper half of the vagina is confirmed. The vagina is then clamped below the tumor using Wertheim clamp, and then the curved Heaney clamp is placed on either side approximately 3 to 4 cm below this clamp. The vagina is transected with curved scissors, and the specimen removed from the field. The vagina is closed in a manner similar to that for simple hysterectomy followed by irrigation, inspection, and closure of the abdomen.

SUGGESTED READINGS

Jones HW, Rock JA, editors. Telinde's Operative Gynecology. 11th ed. Philadelphia: Wolters Kluwer; 2015.

Michener CM, Falcone T. Laparoscopic hysterectomy. In: Baggish M, Karram M, editors. Atlas of Pelvic Anatomy and Gynecologic Surgery. 4th ed. Philadelphia: Elsevier; 2016.

Schellhas H, Baggish M. Radical hysterectomy. In: Baggish M, Karram M, editors. Atlas of Pelvic Anatomy and Gynecologic Surgery. 4th ed. Philadelphia: Elsevier; 2016.

Wright JD, et al. Nationwide trends in the performance of inpatient hysterectomy in the united states. Obstet Gynecol 2013;122(2 Pt 1):233–41. PMID: 23969789.

Oophorectomy for Benign and Malignant Conditions

Morgan Gruner and Robert DeBernardo

INTRODUCTION

The ovary is a complex organ from both a histologic and a functional standpoint. As a result, numerous tumors, benign and malignant, can arise in the adnexa. The surgical approach is often determined by the pathology as well as the desire to preserve gonadal function and fertility.

Although the majority of tumors arising in the ovary are benign, especially in younger women, proper surgical management of ovarian or tubal malignancy is much more complex. Epithelial ovarian and tubal malignancies tend to metastasize early and spread along peritoneal surfaces throughout the abdomen. These surgeries are designed to render the patient with minimal residual disease and often require pelvic peritonectomy with en bloc rectosigmoid resection to clear the pelvis. Complete cytoreductive surgery often includes equally radical upper abdominal resection. Multiple studies have shown that complete cytoreduction of metastatic disease affects overall survival rates and progression-free survival rates in women with epithelial ovarian malignancy. Overall survival rates of 66 to 120 months is achievable, even in women with advanced disease.

PREOPERATIVE IMAGING

Preoperative imaging of an adnexal mass helps not only to characterize the tumor but also to assess for ascites, hydronephrosis, lymphadenopathy, and omental implants that may affect the preoperative counseling and surgical approach. Ultrasonography is the most frequently used modality to assess a pelvic mass. It is readily accessible, noninvasive, and provides excellent delineation of ovarian tumors. The ultrasonographer should comment on lesion size, cystic/solid components, complexity, and Doppler flow along with evidence of hydronephrosis and ascites. Although magnetic resonance imaging (MRI) can provide significantly more information about an ovarian tumor, in reality MRI is rarely helpful in triaging an adnexal mass. Advanced imaging may help determine the extent of the lesion and provide useful information in planning complex surgical resections. Most lesions believed to be complex should be removed in all age groups. Computed tomography (CT) scans are essential to evaluate the retroperitoneum and upper abdomen in women with an ovarian mass that may be malignant.

SURGICAL APPROACH

The most prudent approach to a patient with an adnexal mass is made on the basis of the patient's age, desire for future fertility, desire for hormonal preservation, and imaging characteristics. Almost all pelvic masses in children, premenopausal girls, and postmenopausal women should be evaluated. Triage is made on the basis of imaging characteristics, symptoms, and concern for malignancy. Low-risk lesions, especially in premenopausal women, can often be followed for spontaneous resolution, especially if these are primarily cystic in nature. Solid masses or complex masses in any age group are more likely to be malignant and usually require surgical evaluation. Tumor markers (e.g., CA125) should be obtained preoperatively, although these may be informative in only 90% of cases. The surgical approach, whether laparoscopic, robotic, or conventional laparotomy, depends on the nature of the lesion and the likelihood of identifying a malignancy.

ANATOMY AND DISSECTION OF THE ADNEXA

The adnexa refers to the ovary, fallopian tube, the gonadal vessels, and its vascular attachment to the uterus, all of which is covered by peritoneum. An intimate understanding of the vascular supply to the adnexa and the relationship to the underlying ureter and uterus is required before commencing surgery (Fig. 63.1). The ovarian artery originates from the aorta beneath the renal vessels. It courses in the retroperitoneum and attaches to the ovary. The artery supplies the ovary and fallopian tube and then anastomoses with branches of the uterine vessels, forming the utero-ovarian pedicle. The general principles are similar regardless of surgical approach (open, laparoscopic, or robotic).

Anterior view

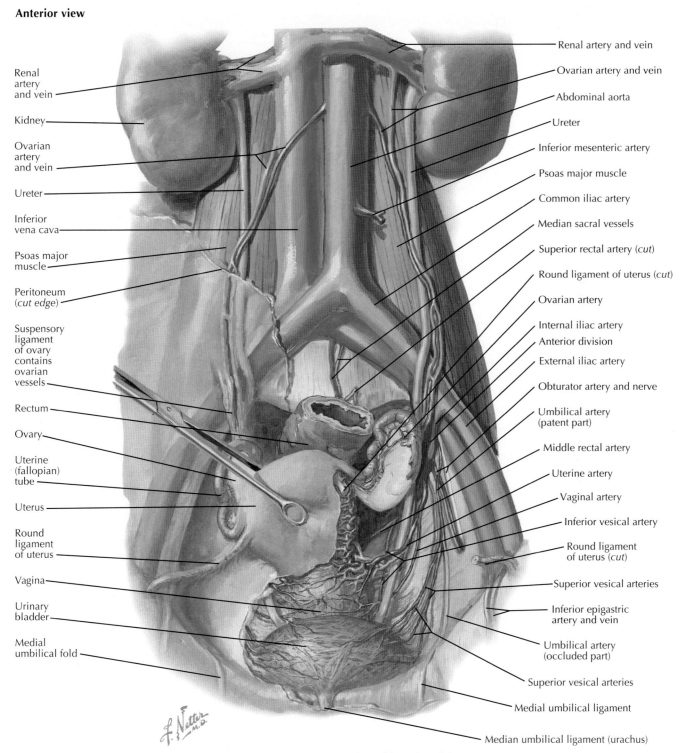

Renal artery and vein

Kidney

Ovarian artery and vein

Ureter

Inferior vena cava

Psoas major muscle

Peritoneum (*cut edge*)

Suspensory ligament of ovary contains ovarian vessels

Rectum

Ovary

Uterine (fallopian) tube

Uterus

Round ligament of uterus

Vagina

Urinary bladder

Medial umbilical fold

Renal artery and vein

Ovarian artery and vein

Abdominal aorta

Ureter

Inferior mesenteric artery

Psoas major muscle

Common iliac artery

Median sacral vessels

Superior rectal artery (*cut*)

Round ligament of uterus (*cut*)

Ovarian artery

Internal iliac artery

Anterior division

External iliac artery

Obturator artery and nerve

Umbilical artery (patent part)

Middle rectal artery

Uterine artery

Vaginal artery

Inferior vesical artery

Round ligament of uterus (*cut*)

Superior vesical arteries

Inferior epigastric artery and vein

Umbilical artery (occluded part)

Superior vesical arteries

Medial umbilical ligament

Median umbilical ligament (urachus)

FIGURE 63.1 Arteries and veins of female pelvic organs.

Gonadal Vessels and Infundibulopelvic Ligament

The initial step when removing a pelvic mass is to open the retroperitoneum and identify the gonadal vessels and ureter. The gonadal blood supply, or infundibulopelvic (IP) ligament, originates from the aorta and runs parallel to the ureter. The ureter and IP cross into the pelvis over the bifurcation of the common iliac vessels (Fig. 63.2A). The ureter is deep to the gonadal vessels. Although the ureter and IP may sometimes be identified through the peritoneum, some pathology my obscure adequate visualization, increasing the likelihood of unintended ureteral injury.

To identify the gonadal vessel and ureter, the peritoneum is incised lateral to the IP along the psoas muscle and external iliac artery and can be extended to the white line of Toldt. Gentle dissection with a large Kelly clamp along the sacrum parallel to the rectosigmoid will develop this space. When the peritoneum is open in this fashion, the gonadal vessels will be at the top of the medial reflection of the peritoneum, the ureter on the medial leaf as well but beneath the IP, and the iliac vessels will be identified laterally.

The IP can then be isolated, clamped, and cut, with the ureter under direct visualization. The adnexa can be elevated out of the pelvis and its peritoneal attachments mobilized until reaching its attachment to the uterus, the utero-ovarian pedicle (Fig. 63.2B).

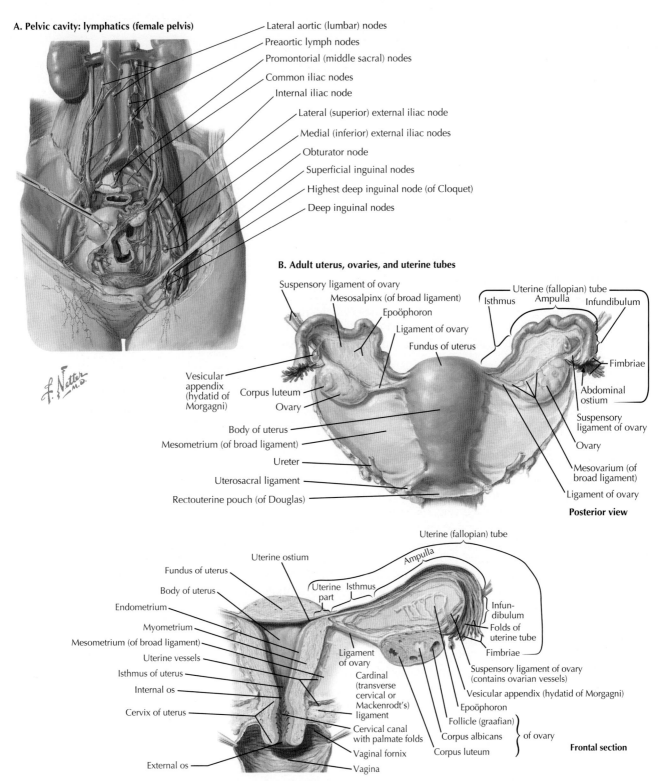

A. Pelvic cavity: lymphatics (female pelvis)

Lateral aortic (lumbar) nodes
Preaortic lymph nodes
Promontorial (middle sacral) nodes
Common iliac nodes
Internal iliac node
Lateral (superior) external iliac node
Medial (inferior) external iliac nodes
Obturator node
Superficial inguinal nodes
Highest deep inguinal node (of Cloquet)
Deep inguinal nodes

B. Adult uterus, ovaries, and uterine tubes

Suspensory ligament of ovary
Mesosalpinx (of broad ligament)
Epoöphoron
Ligament of ovary
Fundus of uterus

Uterine (fallopian) tube
Isthmus   Ampulla   Infundibulum

Vesicular appendix (hydatid of Morgagni)
Corpus luteum
Ovary
Body of uterus
Mesometrium (of broad ligament)
Ureter
Uterosacral ligament
Rectouterine pouch (of Douglas)

Fimbriae
Abdominal ostium
Suspensory ligament of ovary
Ovary
Mesovarium (of broad ligament)
Ligament of ovary

Posterior view

Uterine (fallopian) tube
Ampulla

Uterine ostium
Fundus of uterus
Body of uterus
Endometrium
Myometrium
Mesometrium (of broad ligament)
Uterine vessels
Isthmus of uterus
Internal os
Cervix of uterus

Uterine part   Isthmus

Infundibulum
Folds of uterine tube
Fimbriae
Suspensory ligament of ovary (contains ovarian vessels)
Vesicular appendix (hydatid of Morgagni)
Epoöphoron
Follicle (graafian)
Corpus albicans   } of ovary
Corpus luteum

Ligament of ovary
Cardinal (transverse cervical or Mackenrodt's) ligament
Cervical canal with palmate folds
Vaginal fornix
External os
Vagina

Frontal section

FIGURE 63.2 Pelvic cavity lymphatics and adult uterus, ovaries, and tubes.

Utero-ovarian Vessels

The utero-ovarian vessels are supplied by the gonadal vessels cephalad and the uterine vessels caudad. This pedicle must be secured when removing the ovary, unless the uterus is concurrently being removed. Unlike the gonadal vessels, the utero-ovarian pedicle is poorly defined in many patients, and securing it can be challenging; a large clamp (e.g., Heaney) with a suture ligature works best. A vascular stapling device or energy device is frequently used in laparoscopic cases.

It is important to recognize that the ureter is deep and lateral to the utero-ovarian pedicle, except when the tumor is encasing the pelvic side wall, as can be seen in endometriosis or, more often, ovarian malignancy. In those cases, it is wise to identify the ureter at the pelvic brim and follow it into the pelvic pathology to avoid injury.

LARGE MASSES AND MODIFIED APPROACHES

Some ovarian tumors can grow to be greater than 20 or 30 cm before they are identified. In these cases, it may not be possible to isolate the blood supply and identify the ureter before removing the mass itself (Fig. 63.3A).

It is preferable to remove an ovarian mass intact, without rupture, to avoid seeding the peritoneum should malignancy exist. In cases of malignancy, the surgical approach should be modified in one of two ways. If the utero-ovarian pedicle can be identified, the safest approach is to sacrifice this pedicle first and proceed with the operation described earlier, but in reverse. This approach allows for the mobilization of the adnexa cephalad by incising the peritoneum along the pelvic side wall, thus allowing for the ureter to drop away from the gonadal blood supply. Once the dissection is carried to the pelvic brim, the IP is generally easily isolated and secured.

In some cases, neither the IP nor the utero-ovarian pedicle can be identified, and the mass can often be delivered through the incision and the adnexa itself clamped. In our experience, there is little chance of inadvertently injuring the ureter because it runs deep to the IP pedicle (Fig. 63.3B).

Nonetheless, it is prudent to dissect the retroperitoneum once the mass has been removed and identify the ureter to ensure it has not been injured.

A. Clear cell carcinoma of ovary

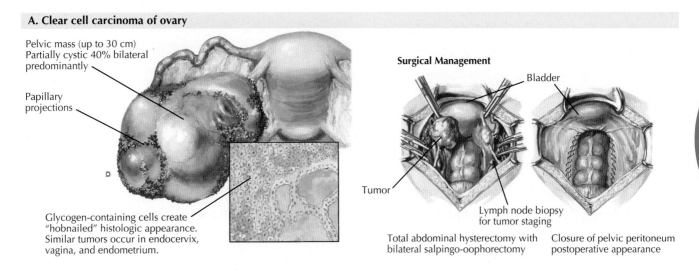

Pelvic mass (up to 30 cm)
Partially cystic 40% bilateral
predominantly

Papillary
projections

Glycogen-containing cells create
"hobnailed" histologic appearance.
Similar tumors occur in endocervix,
vagina, and endometrium.

Surgical Management

Bladder

Tumor

Lymph node biopsy
for tumor staging

Total abdominal hysterectomy with
bilateral salpingo-oophorectomy

Closure of pelvic peritoneum
postoperative appearance

B. Diagnosis of ovarian neoplasms

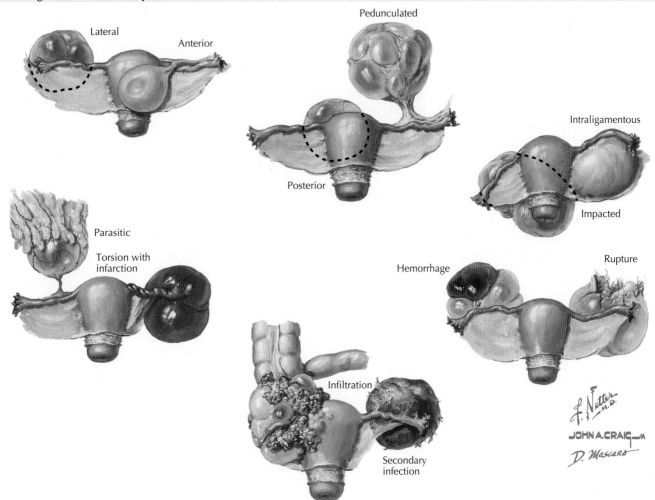

Lateral

Anterior

Pedunculated

Posterior

Intraligamentous

Impacted

Parasitic

Torsion with
infarction

Hemorrhage

Rupture

Infiltration

Secondary
infection

FIGURE 63.3 Ovarian carcinomas: diagnosis and management.

RADICAL OOPHORECTOMY

In rare cases in which the previous techniques fail, or more often in the setting of an advanced pelvic malignancy, a more radical surgical approach becomes necessary. This is often the case when there is extensive pelvic pathology, such as stage IV endometriosis or advanced ovarian malignancy. Not only are the normal anatomic landmarks obscured, but the pelvic peritoneum is extensively involved in the disease process.

The resection of the adnexa in these patients starts in the upper abdomen at or near the origin of the gonadal blood supply. Generally, the white line of Toldt is developed bilaterally and the abdominal ureter and gonadal blood supply identified. It may be helpful to isolate the ureters at this point on vessel loops to keep them under continuous surveillance. Gentle tension facilitates the dissection. The gonadal vessels can be sacrificed at their origin or anywhere along their abdominal path. In the setting of an ovarian malignancy, the peritoneum overlying the gutters is incorporated along with this pedicle and taken en bloc into the pelvis, incorporating any extra-pelvic disease (Fig. 63.4A).

The dissection is then carried into the pelvis proper. Staying in the retroperitoneum, any involved peritoneal surfaces are included circumferentially to encompass the tumor. Anteriorly, the lateral pelvic side wall peritoneum is mobilized off the external iliac vessels and psoas muscle with gentle traction and monopolar cautery. The round ligaments are sacrificed at this point, and the bladder peritoneum can be resected when necessary, often without need for partial cystectomy.

This peritoneum is contiguous with the peritoneum overlying the uterus. Advanced ovarian malignant disease almost always involves the posterior pelvic peritoneum and sigmoid mesentery, requiring rectosigmoid resection to eradicate the disease completely (see Chapter 30, Low Anterior Resection With Total Mesorectal Excision and Anastomosis). Once the sigmoid is transected, the retroperitoneal dissection is carried laterally to encompass the anterior dissection and posteriorly along the sacrum. Similar to a colorectal malignancy, the dissection continues behind the rectum in the plane between the pre-sacral fascia and mesorectum (Fig. 63.4B).

Unlike a situation involving colorectal cancer, the objective here is not to obtain gross margins, but to debulk gross tumor to microscopic, residual disease. In the majority of cases, the tumor respects the peritoneum, and the dissection down to the level of the levator muscles is unnecessary. Once beyond the rectal reflection, the rectum can be skeletonized.

At this point, the adnexal structures are completely incorporated in the surgical specimen. The procedure is completed by isolating the uterine arteries, either at their origins or just medial to where they cross the ureters. Dissection is carried down along the cervix until the cervico-vaginal refection is identified. A colpotomy is performed and the rectovaginal septum developed. The rectum can then be transected with a stapling device and the specimen removed (Fig. 63.4C).

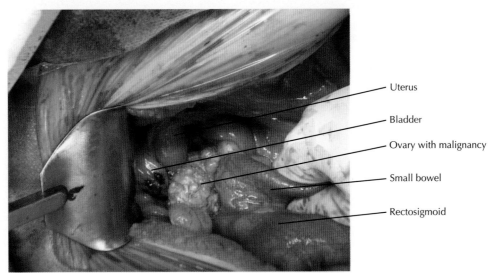

Uterus

Bladder

Ovary with malignancy

Small bowel

Rectosigmoid

A. Ovarian malignancy invading rectosigmoid, uterus, and pelvic peritoneum

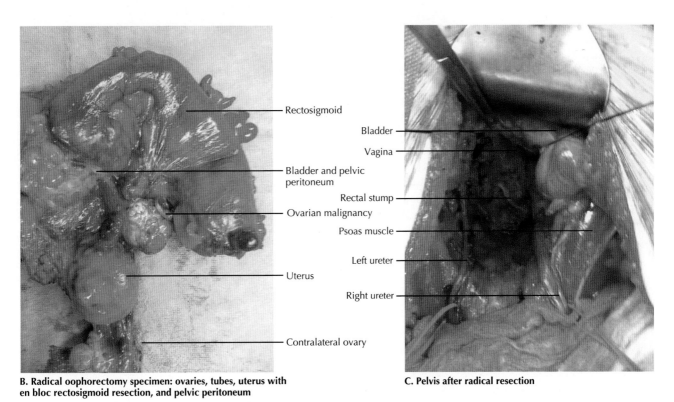

Rectosigmoid

Bladder and pelvic peritoneum

Ovarian malignancy

Uterus

Contralateral ovary

B. Radical oophorectomy specimen: ovaries, tubes, uterus with en bloc rectosigmoid resection, and pelvic peritoneum

Bladder

Vagina

Rectal stump

Psoas muscle

Left ureter

Right ureter

C. Pelvis after radical resection

FIGURE 63.4 Ovarian malignancy and radical oophorectomy.

SUGGESTED READINGS

Alcázar JL, Royo P, Jurado M, et al. Triage for surgical management of ovarian tumors in asymptomatic women: assessment of an ultrasound-based scoring system. Ultrasound Obstet Gynecol 2008;32(2):220–5.

Chang SJ, Bristow RE. Evolution of surgical treatment paradigms for advanced-stage ovarian cancer: redefining "optimal" residual disease. Gynecol Oncol 2012;125(2):483–92.

Esselen KM, Rodriguez N, Growdon W, et al. Patterns of recurrence in advanced epithelial ovarian, fallopian tube and peritoneal cancers treated with intraperitoneal chemotherapy. Gynecol Oncol 2012;127(1):51–4.

Giuntoli 2nd RL, Vang RS, Bristow RE. Evaluation and management of adnexal masses during pregnancy. Clin Obstet Gynecol 2006;49(3):492–505.

Moore RG, Miller MC, Disilvestro P, et al. Evaluation of the diagnostic accuracy of the risk of ovarian malignancy algorithm in women with a pelvic mass. Obstet Gynecol 2011;118(2 Pt 1):280–8.

Reconstructive Surgery for Pelvic Floor Disorders

Beri M. Ridgeway

INTRODUCTION

Pelvic floor disorders are a group of conditions that affect pelvic floor function. The pelvic floor includes the ligaments, muscles, nerves, and connective tissue that support the pelvic organs, specifically the bladder, vagina, uterus, bowel, and rectum. Pelvic floor disorders, including pelvic organ prolapse, urinary incontinence, and fecal incontinence, greatly affect quality of life. Risk factors for pelvic floor disorders include pregnancy and birth (especially vaginal birth), aging, chronic heavy lifting and straining, hysterectomy, and genetic factors. Pelvic floor disorders are extremely common in women. In a population-based survey, 24% of all women suffered from pelvic floor disorders, with 16% of women experiencing urinary incontinence, 3% of women experiencing prolapse symptoms, and 9% of women experiencing fecal incontinence. The results also demonstrated that the prevalence of pelvic floor disorders increases significantly with age and that many women suffer from more than one pelvic floor disorder.

Pelvic floor disorders highlight an interesting relationship between anatomy and function. Many women who suffer from pelvic floor disorders have anatomic changes visible on physical examination, and with surgical correction of the anatomic abnormality, the pelvic floor disorder functionally improves. However, some women who have pelvic floor disorders have normal-appearing anatomy, and many women who have abnormal-appearing anatomy have normal function and do not have pelvic floor symptoms.

RECONSTRUCTIVE SURGERY FOR PELVIC FLOOR DISORDERS

Reconstructive surgery for pelvic floor disorders encompasses a variety of procedures, including urethral support via sutures (Burch urethropexy) or a fascial or polypropylene sling to treat stress urinary incontinence; anal sphincter reconstruction to treat fecal incontinence; and diverse procedures to treat pelvic organ prolapse. This chapter focuses on reconstructive surgery for pelvic organ prolapse. Pelvic organ prolapse occurs when the connective tissue attaching the muscles, bones, and organs is compromised, leading to inappropriate support of the pelvic organs. The result is the organs dropping toward or through the vaginal opening. Patients often can see or feel this tissue protruding at or beyond the vaginal opening (Fig. 64.1). Besides feeling the sensation of bulge and pressure, patients may note pain or discomfort and have trouble emptying their bladder and bowels. Reconstructive surgery aims to restore anatomy and relieve these troubling symptoms.

Female: midsagittal section

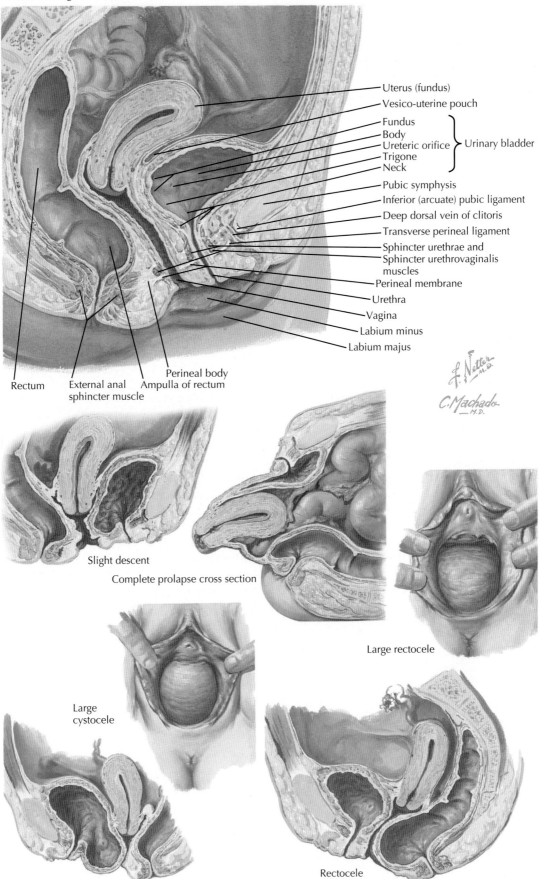

Uterus (fundus)
Vesico-uterine pouch
Fundus ⎫
Body ⎪
Ureteric orifice ⎬ Urinary bladder
Trigone ⎪
Neck ⎭
Pubic symphysis
Inferior (arcuate) pubic ligament
Deep dorsal vein of clitoris
Transverse perineal ligament
Sphincter urethrae and
Sphincter urethrovaginalis muscles
Perineal membrane
Urethra
Vagina
Labium minus
Labium majus

Rectum   External anal sphincter muscle   Ampulla of rectum   Perineal body

Slight descent

Complete prolapse cross section

Large rectocele

Large cystocele

Rectocele

FIGURE 64.1 Pelvic organ prolapse.

PELVIC FLOOR ANATOMY

A description of these procedures relies on an understanding of normal anatomy of the pelvic floor and how the pelvic organs are supported. The pelvic floor consists of the coccygeus muscle (also known as the pelvic diaphragm) and a set of muscles called the levator ani. The levator ani spans the pelvic floor, connecting to the bony pelvis, and consists of three muscles: the puborectalis, pubococcygeus, and ileococcygeus (Fig. 64.2A). There are three anatomic levels of pelvic support, as described by John DeLancey (Fig. 64.2B). Level 1 support is the most cephalad and is defined as the cardinal-uterosacral ligament complex. This provides apical attachment of the uterus and vaginal vault to the bony sacrum. Level 2 support is defined by the arcus tendineus fascia pelvis and the fascia overlying the levator ani muscles, which provide support to the middle part of the vagina. Level 3 support is provided by the urogenital diaphragm and the perineal body, which provide support to the lower part of the vagina.

Pelvic reconstructive surgery attempts to restore the anatomic deficits with the goal of restoring function and quality of life. Of the three levels of support, level 1 support, or apical support, is the most critical. Multiple studies demonstrate that a significant proportion of vaginal support is attributed to apical support. Real-world experience confirms this: if the vaginal apex or uterus is not supported well, the chance of long-term successful outcomes after prolapse repair is low.

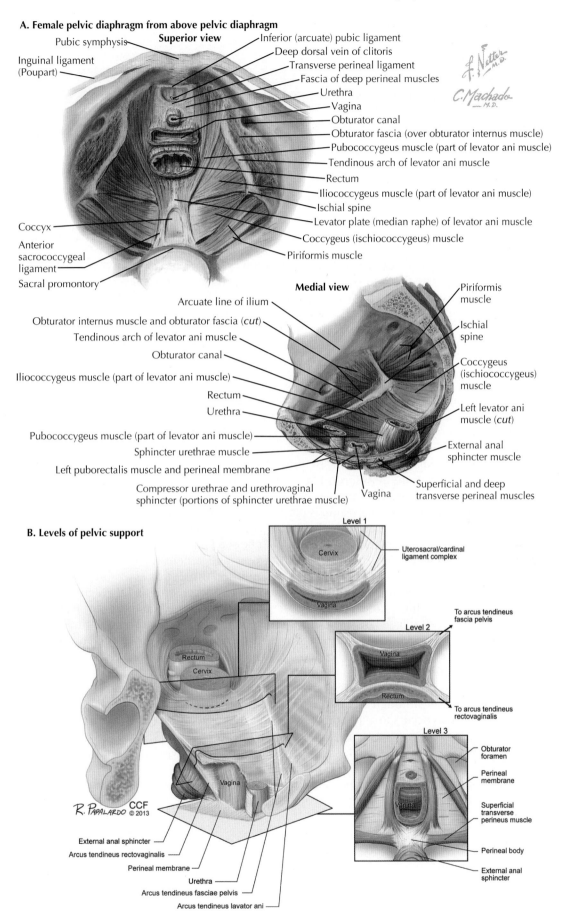

FIGURE 64.2 Pelvic floor anatomy. (B, Reprinted with permission, Cleveland Clinic Center for Medical Art & Photography © 2012-2019. All Rights Reserved.)

SURGICAL APPROACHES TO SUSPEND VAGINAL APEX

Colpopexy comes from the Greek words *colpo,* meaning "vagina," and *pexy,* meaning "fixing (in place) or fastening." The three most common and well-studied approaches to restoring apical (level 1) support in pelvic organ prolapse are uterosacral ligament colpopexy, sacrospinous ligament colpopexy, and sacral colpopexy. As colpopexy's meaning indicates, all three procedures involve resuspending the top of the vagina to a stronger and higher area in the pelvis, leaving the vagina in an anatomic position to restore function.

UTEROSACRAL LIGAMENT COLPOPEXY

The uterosacral ligament colpopexy attaches the top of the vagina to the mid-portion of the uterosacral ligament. The uterosacral ligament is a band of connective tissue that connects the posterior vagina, cervix, and lower uterus to the sacrum. There are two uterosacral ligaments, one on each side. The uterosacral ligament measures approximately 12 × 2 cm and travels along the sidewall medial to the ureter. Before uterosacral ligament colpopexy, the patient is placed in the high lithotomy position using stirrups. A transvaginal hysterectomy is typically performed, allowing access to the intraperitoneal cavity. The bowel is packed away with moistened laparotomy sponges. An Allis clamp is placed on the uterosacral ligament insertion at the vaginal cuff and traction is applied. This allows the uterosacral ligament to be seen through the peritoneum and fat. The uterosacral ligament should be seen moving cephalad and medial as it approaches the sacrum. The mid-portion of the uterosacral ligament is located at or above the ischial spine. This area is grasped with a long Allis clamp, and three sutures of absorbable suture are placed lateral to medial through the uterosacral ligament, each one slightly higher than the last (Fig. 64.3A). Once this is done bilaterally, the packs are removed, and the sutures are run through the vaginal cuff (Fig. 64.3B). The distal suture is run through the anterior and posterior cuff at each corner, the middle uterosacral stitch is run through the anterior and posterior cuff halfway between the corner and midline, and the proximal uterosacral stitch is run through the anterior and posterior mid-portion of the cuff. The vagina is elevated using retractors and the stitches are tied down, attaching the vagina to six points of the uterosacral ligament. Significant complications are rare, although one of the most common intraoperative complications is ureteral obstruction. This occurs in approximately 5% of cases and has to do with the proximity of the ureter to the uterosacral ligament (see Fig. 64.3). Sutures placed through the ligament and tied to the vagina can move the pelvic sidewall peritoneum medially. This can pull and kink the ureter. For this reason, cystoscopy to evaluate ureteral efflux is required after this procedure. If ureteral kinking occurs, the uterosacral ligament sutures can be removed, and the ureter immediately returns to normal function in almost all cases.

A. The uterosacral ligament and related anatomy

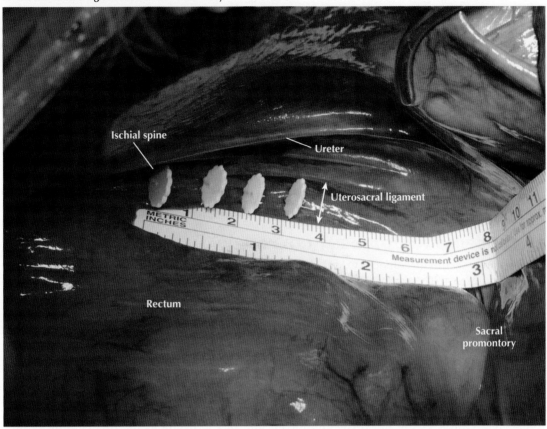

B. The uterosacral ligament colpopexy

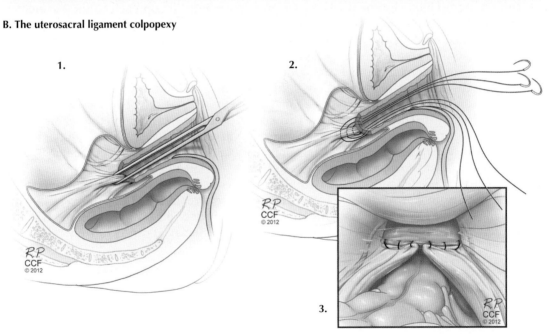

FIGURE 64.3 Uterosacral ligament colpopexy. *(Reprinted with permission, Cleveland Clinic Center for Medical Art & Photography © 2019. All Rights Reserved.)*

SACROSPINOUS LIGAMENT COLPOPEXY

Sacrospinous ligament colpopexy uses an anchor point in the pelvis not originally involved in level 1 support. The sacrospinous ligament is a thin, triangular ligament that extends from the ischial spine to the sacrum and lies superior to the sacrotuberous ligament (Fig. 64.4A). It measures approximately 5 cm. The sacrospinous ligament functions to prevent the ilium from rotating past the sacrum. Anatomically, it divides the sciatic foramen into the greater and lesser sciatic foramen. The sacrospinous ligament provides a strong attachment point for the vagina, but great care must be taken given the surrounding anatomy. The pudendal nerve and vessels pass behind the sacrospinous ligament close to the ischial spine. The inferior gluteal artery, branching from the internal iliac artery, passes behind the sacrospinous ligament and is vulnerable above the top portion of the sacrospinous ligament. To prevent nerve or vascular injury, it is critical to use the medioinferior portion of the ligament for vaginal attachment. To perform sacrospinous ligament colpopexy, an extraperitoneal approach to the ligament is performed, which can be approached from the vaginal apex or posterior vagina. Sharp dissection is performed until an avascular plane is encountered. Blunt dissection is performed until the sacrospinous ligament is reached. The sacrospinous ligament is cleared of overlying fat and connective tissue. A combination of two to four permanent and delayed absorbable sutures are placed through the medioinferior portion of the ligament. These sutures are then run through the vagina, similar to the uterosacral ligament colpopexy (Fig. 64.4B). The vagina is elevated and the sutures are tied down, placing the vaginal cuff in direct opposition to the ligament. The sacrospinous ligament colpopexy can be performed unilateral or bilateral, although the majority of data available describe the unilateral approach. Because of its location in the pelvis, after sacrospinous ligament colpopexy, the vagina lies subtly deviated to one side (if unilateral) and at a flatter angle (deviated toward the rectum). Unlike with the uterosacral ligament colpopexy, ureteral injury is unlikely, and cystoscopy is not absolutely required. Postoperatively, buttock pain on the side the colpopexy was performed is commonly described. Unless the pain is severe or neurologic symptoms are present, this complaint can be managed conservatively, with most pain resolving by 6 weeks.

A. Bones and ligaments of the pelvis

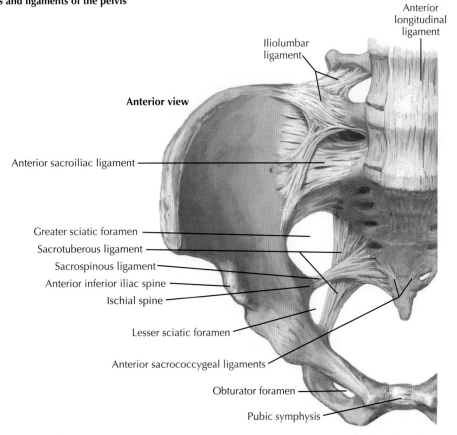

Anterior longitudinal ligament

Iliolumbar ligament

Anterior view

Anterior sacroiliac ligament

Greater sciatic foramen

Sacrotuberous ligament

Sacrospinous ligament

Anterior inferior iliac spine

Ischial spine

Lesser sciatic foramen

Anterior sacrococcygeal ligaments

Obturator foramen

Pubic symphysis

B. Sacrospinous ligament colpopexy

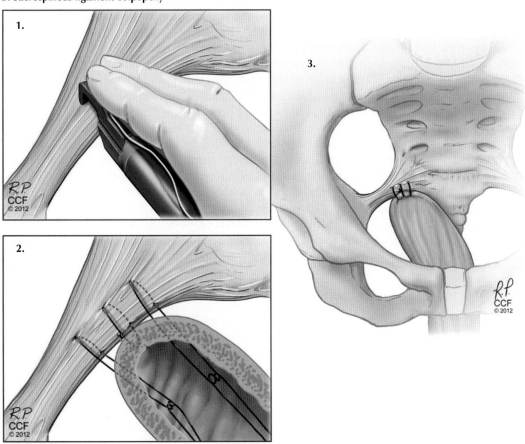

1.

2.

3.

FIGURE 64.4 Sacrospinous ligament colpopexy. *(B, Reprinted with permission, Cleveland Clinic Center for Medical Art & Photography © 2012-2019. All Rights Reserved.)*

SACRAL COLPOPEXY

Sacral colpopexy can be performed laparoscopically, robotically, or via an open abdominal approach. After gaining intra-abdominal access, the peritoneum overlying the sacral promontory is elevated and opened. Great care must be taken because the aortic bifurcation and vena cava is superior; the ureter is to the right side; and the sigmoid colon and left common iliac vein are located to the left side (Fig. 64.5). Once the peritoneum is opened, additional dissection is performed until the sacrum can be seen. The anterior longitudinal ligament of the sacral level of the spine is identified and cleared of overlying connective tissue. Attention to avoid the middle sacral artery, branching from the aorta and running in the middle of the anterior longitudinal ligament, is critical because injuring this vessel can lead to life-threatening bleeding that is difficult to control. The peritoneal incision is carried caudad toward the vagina with the ureter and sigmoid in view. Peritoneal flaps are created on each side. The bladder and vagina are separated sharply until the trigone is reached, and the rectum and vagina are separated sharply for 5 to 8 cm. A graft, most often polypropylene mesh, is sewn to the anterior and posterior vagina using delayed absorbable suture and permanent suture. The tail of the graft is attached to the sacral portion of the anterior longitudinal ligament using permanent suture. This graft creates a bridge between the sacrum and the vagina, elevating the vagina and anchoring it to a strong fixation point. The graft is then covered with the peritoneal flaps. Cystoscopy should be performed to evaluate the bladder integrity and ureteral patency.

All three approaches to apical prolapse provide level 1 support to the vagina. They are associated with good anatomic and functional outcomes but confer different risk profiles.

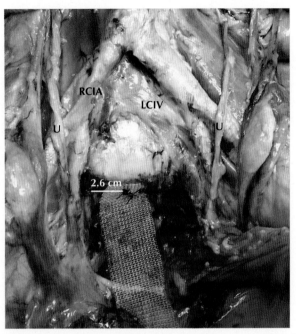

FIGURE 64.5 The sacral promontory and related anatomy. *LCIV,* Left common iliac vein; *RCIA,* right common iliac artery; *U,* ureter. *(Courtesy of Dr. Karl Jallad, Cleveland Clinic.)*

SUGGESTED READINGS

DeLancey JO. Anatomic aspects of vaginal eversion after hysterectomy. Am J Obstet Gynecol 1992;1666:1717–24.

DeLancey JO. What's new in the functional anatomy of pelvic organ prolapse? Curr Opin Obstet Gynecol 2016;28(5):420–9.

Maher C, Feiner B, Baessler K, Christmann-Schmid C, Haya N, Brown J. Surgery for women with apical vaginal prolapse. Cochrane Database Syst Rev 2016;10:CD012376.

Maldonado PA, Wai CY. Pelvic organ prolapse: new concepts in pelvic floor anatomy. Obstet Gynecol Clin North Am 2016;43(1):15–26.

Nygaard I, Barber MD, Burgio KL, Kenton K, Meikle S, Schaffer J, et al. Prevalence of symptomatic pelvic floor disorders in US women. JAMA 2008;300(11):1311–6.

Walters MD, Ridgeway BM. Surgical treatment of vaginal apex prolapse. Obstet Gynecol 2013;121(2 Pt 1):354–74.

Laparoscopic Transperitoneal Radical Nephrectomy

Riccardo Bertolo and Lee Ponsky

INTRODUCTION

Renal cell carcinoma (RCC) represents the most frequent cause of renal neoplasm and is the third most common malignancy in men and women. The widespread use of abdominal imaging has significantly increased the diagnosis of renal masses. Current guidelines recommend elective partial nephrectomy as the standard surgical treatment for renal tumors smaller than 4 cm in maximum diameter and favor partial nephrectomy over radical nephrectomy for tumors 4 to 7 cm when technically feasible. For larger renal tumors (>7 cm), radical nephrectomy is still regarded as the reference standard.

Since the introduction of laparoscopic radical nephrectomy by Clayman and colleagues in 1990, the minimally invasive approach to the removal of the kidney has become the "gold standard." Laparoscopic radical nephrectomy has demonstrated comparable oncologic outcomes to those seen with the open approach, but less morbidity, shorter hospital stay, less pain, quicker recovery, and improved cosmesis.

In more recent years, the advent of the robotic approach has prompted the adoption of robot-assisted laparoscopy for radical nephrectomy. Nevertheless, the higher costs of robotic surgery have limited the widespread use of robotic radical nephrectomy because of the equivalent results obtained with the standard laparoscopic approach.

PREOPERATIVE IMAGING

In the majority of the cases, the first diagnosis is incidental and performed by ultrasonography. Typically, a contrast-enhanced computed tomography (CT) scan or a magnetic resonance imaging (MRI) is obtained before surgery for a more precise mapping of the kidney anatomy and vasculature, the perirenal fat, and relation to adjacent organs. Also, CT and MRI allow for the identification of potential tumor thrombus and provide preoperative clinical staging. It is also prudent to visualize the contralateral kidney parenchyma to evaluate the renal function. Cross-sectional images are usually sufficient, but coronal images can be extremely helpful (Fig. 65.1A). More recently, the use of more advanced software allows for three-dimensional reconstruction of the CT scan and the MRI, improving the understanding of the anatomy and the preoperative planning (Fig. 65.1B).

SURGICAL APPROACH

Laparoscopic radical nephrectomy can be performed by using either a transperitoneal or a retroperitoneal approach. Both techniques have been demonstrated to be safe and effective. The transperitoneal approach is more common, but it is helpful for surgeons to be able to perform the retroperitoneal approach, particularly for patients with previous abdominal surgeries or other contraindications to the transperitoneal approach. The retroperitoneal approach also offers the ability to control the renal hilum almost immediately. However, with limited recognizable landmarks for orientation using the retroperitoneal approach, the majority of laparoscopic radical nephrectomies are performed by a transperitoneal approach.

PATIENT POSITIONING AND TROCAR PLACEMENT

For left radical nephrectomy, the patient is placed in the right lateral decubitus with the left flank up. The patient is centered over the break in the bed. The lower leg is bent and the top leg straight, and the dependent hip, knee, and ankle padded appropriately. Pillows can be placed between the legs. An axillary roll should be placed under the axilla to protect from nerve damage. The patient's lower arm is placed straight out on an arm board, and the upper arm should be secured to an upper arm board. The upper arm must be safely positioned away from the working field to ensure full access for the laparoscopic instruments.

It is important to secure the patient to the table with heavy tape wrapped around the patient (preferably directly to skin) and table several times to prevent the patient from moving or sliding during surgery. For the transperitoneal approach, the patient can be rotated posteriorly just before being secured to the table. It is also helpful to plan for the extraction site, possibly marking it before positioning and including it in the prepped and draped area. Ports placement has been described in several ways and depends on surgeon preference.

The Veress needle is typically used for access, although the Hasson cut-down technique is also appropriate. Correct placement of the right-handed port is typically marked half the distance between the anterior superior iliac spine and the umbilicus, then moved superiorly up to the level of the umbilicus. This would typically be a 10-mm port. The middle camera port is typically placed just lateral to the rectus abdominis muscle, approximately in line with the tip of the 12th rib. The left-handed, typically 5-mm port is approximately at the junction of the lateral aspect of the rectus muscle and the subcostal border.

A. Computed tomography (CT) scans of kidney cancers

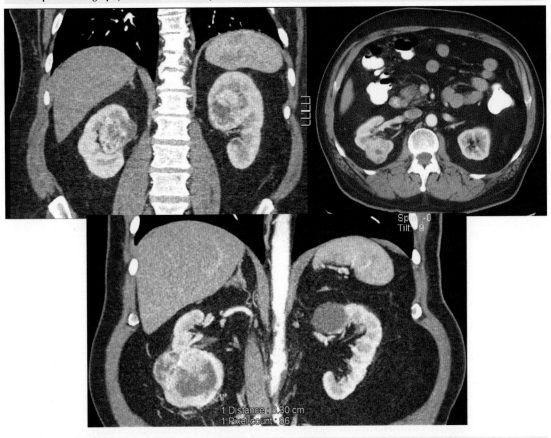

B. 3D reconstructions of kidney cancers performed by different software

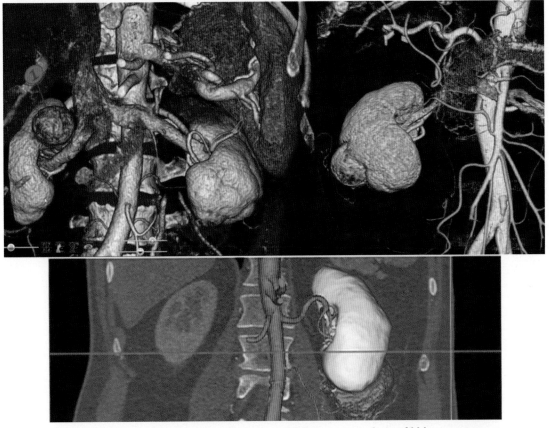

FIGURE 65.1 Computed tomography and 3D reconstructions of kidney cancers.

MOBILIZATION OF THE COLON

Once getting the access to the abdominal cavity, the first step is to reflect the colon. Although the standard description of mobilizing the colon describes incising along the white line of Toldt, it is not necessary to incise that laterally; in fact, it could be more challenging to incise that laterally, because the peritoneum must be dissected off Gerota's fascia posteriorly and reflected medially to expose the retroperitoneum and kidney (Fig. 65.2).

It is important to incise the peritoneum lateral to the colon. If the white line of Toldt is incised, the surgeon must be certain not to continue to follow that plane posteriorly, to prevent dissecting the kidney's lateral attachments, complicating the dissection. It is useful to leave the kidney's lateral attachments until after the hilum is controlled; the lateral attachments help "retract" the kidney up, avoiding the need of using one of the instruments for kidney retraction. This peritoneal layer is very thin; the surgeon must stay outside Gerota's fascia but avoid entering the posterior mesentery. There is a clear difference in the appearance of the fat layers of Gerota's fascia (paler yellow) and posterior mesentery (brighter yellow).

It is often helpful to free up the upper-pole attachments between the spleen and kidney to avoid capsular tear of the spleen from a retraction injury. It is important to reflect the colon far enough superiorly to ensure sufficient access to the upper pole of the kidney, and low enough to ensure access to the ureter below the lower pole.

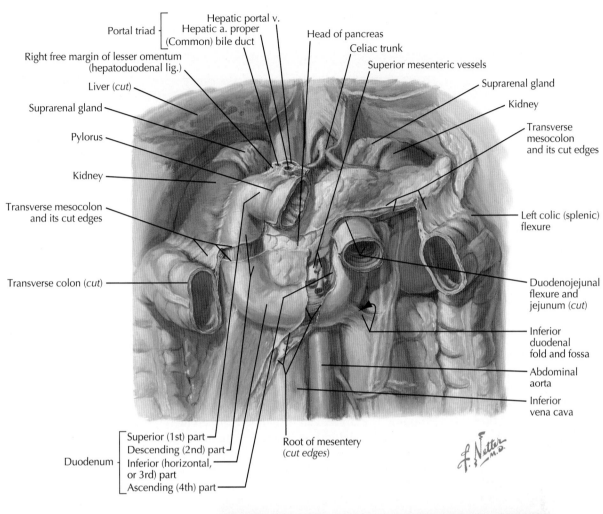

Portal triad
— Hepatic portal v.
— Hepatic a. proper
— (Common) bile duct
Head of pancreas
Celiac trunk
Superior mesenteric vessels
Suprarenal gland
Kidney
Transverse mesocolon and its cut edges
Right free margin of lesser omentum (hepatoduodenal lig.)
Liver (cut)
Suprarenal gland
Pylorus
Kidney
Transverse mesocolon and its cut edges
Transverse colon (cut)
Left colic (splenic) flexure
Duodenojejunal flexure and jejunum (cut)
Inferior duodenal fold and fossa
Abdominal aorta
Inferior vena cava
Duodenum
— Superior (1st) part
— Descending (2nd) part
— Inferior (horizontal, or 3rd) part
— Ascending (4th) part
Root of mesentery (cut edges)

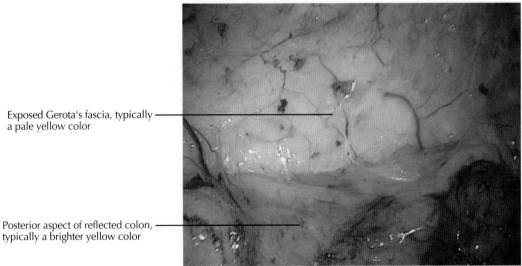

Exposed Gerota's fascia, typically a pale yellow color

Posterior aspect of reflected colon, typically a brighter yellow color

Posterior aspect of the mesentery reflected medially off the Gerota's fascia. The Gerota's fascia is more pale than the posterior mesenteric fat.

FIGURE 65.2 Reflected colon and mesentery medially; kidney and Gerota's fascia laterally.

DISSECTION

Ureter

Once the colon is reflected, the next step is to dissect the ureter. Starting below the lower pole of the kidney, the surgeon should dissect lateral to the aorta, identifying the ureter and gonadal vein (Fig. 65.3). Once identified, the ureter should be retracted laterally, exposing the psoas muscle posteriorly. At that point, the ureter can be clipped and divided with the lateral attachments to the ureter all the way to the abdominal side wall. The proximal end of the divided ureter can then be used for gentle retraction to help follow the psoas muscle, ureter, and gonadal vein (on the left) as landmarks up to the renal hilum.

Renal Hilum

With the transperitoneal approach, the renal vein is typically anterior to the renal artery. Once the attachments overlying the hilum are divided, the renal artery should be identified posterior to the renal vein. Some variation may be seen, because the renal artery can be directly posterior, inferior, or slightly superior to the renal vein, but typically is directly posterior (Fig. 65.4A).

The renal artery should be controlled and divided before dividing the renal vein. The surgeon should be cautious because accessory arteries or veins and lumbar vessels may require control. As discussed, the preoperative imaging, particularly with software-based reconstruction, is typically helpful, but these accessory vessels are not always identified, and the renal hilum should be dissected with great care.

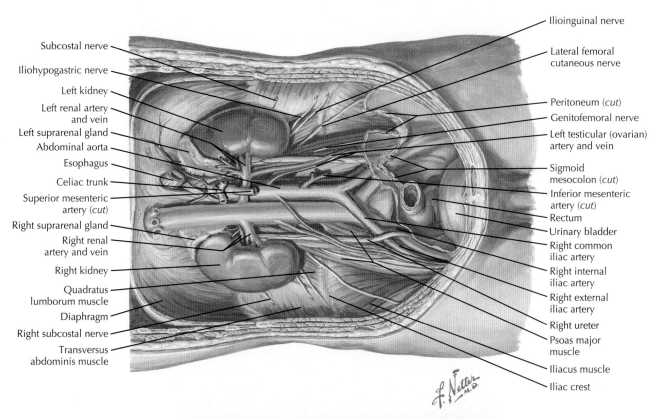

Subcostal nerve

Iliohypogastric nerve

Left kidney

Left renal artery and vein

Left suprarenal gland

Abdominal aorta

Esophagus

Celiac trunk

Superior mesenteric artery (cut)

Right suprarenal gland

Right renal artery and vein

Right kidney

Quadratus lumborum muscle

Diaphragm

Right subcostal nerve

Transversus abdominis muscle

Ilioinguinal nerve

Lateral femoral cutaneous nerve

Peritoneum (cut)

Genitofemoral nerve

Left testicular (ovarian) artery and vein

Sigmoid mesocolon (cut)

Inferior mesenteric artery (cut)

Rectum

Urinary bladder

Right common iliac artery

Right internal iliac artery

Right external iliac artery

Right ureter

Psoas major muscle

Iliacus muscle

Iliac crest

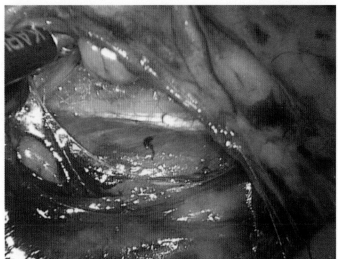

The left ureter and gonadal vein are retracted up, exposing the psoas muscle posteriorly.

FIGURE 65.3 **Anatomic relations of kidney and psoas exposure.**

Adrenal Gland

The original description of radical nephrectomy involved removal of the adrenal gland, but more recent evidence showed that the removal of the adrenal gland may not be necessary for all radical nephrectomies. This is why the adrenal gland is often preserved in many contemporary radical nephrectomy series.

To preserve the adrenal gland, the dissection should start immediately superior to the renal vein (Fig. 65.4B). On the left, the renal vein should be divided distal to the adrenal vein insertion into the renal vein. The adrenal gland should be dissected from the upper pole of the kidney. On the right side, special caution is taken because the right adrenal vein is short, with its insertion directly into the vena cava.

Lateral Attachments Divided

Once the ureter, the hilum, and the upper pole attachments are divided, the kidney's lateral attachments can be divided, freeing up the kidney completely. Care should be taken to stay outside Gerota's fascia but avoiding the abdominal side wall.

EXTRACTION

Once free from all attachments, the kidney should be placed into an EndoCatch bag for removal. For specimen retrieval, a Pfannenstiel or a Gibson incision is often used. Once the kidney is removed, the extraction incision and the ports incisions are closed.

A. Demonstrates the renal vein typically anterior to the renal artery

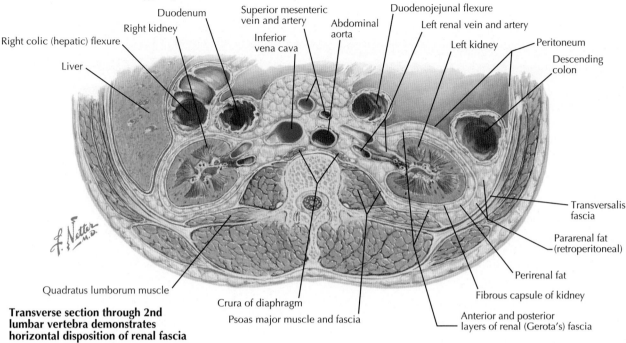

Transverse section through 2nd lumbar vertebra demonstrates horizontal disposition of renal fascia

B. Demonstrates the relationship between the adrenal and upper pole of the kidney

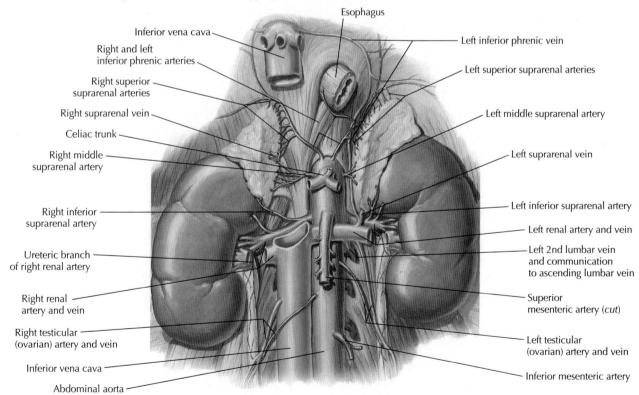

FIGURE 65.4 Relationships of renal vessels and adrenal gland.

SUGGESTED READINGS

Allan JD, Tolley DA, Kaouk JH, et al. Laparoscopic radical nephrectomy. Eur Urol 2001;40(1):17–23. Review.

Choi JE, You JH, Kim DK, et al. Comparison of perioperative outcomes between robotic and laparoscopic partial nephrectomy: a systematic review and meta-analysis. Eur Urol 2015;67(5):891–901. https://doi.org/10.1016/j.eururo.2014.12.028. Epub 2015 Jan 6.

Desai MM, Strzempkowski B, Matin SF, et al. Prospective randomized comparison of transperitoneal versus retroperitoneal laparoscopic radical nephrectomy. J Urol 2005;173(1):38–41.

Jeong IG, Khandwala YS, Kim JH, et al. Association of robotic-assisted vs laparoscopic radical nephrectomy with perioperative outcomes and health care costs, 2003 to 2015. JAMA 2017;318(16):1561–8. https://doi.org/10.1001/jama.2017.14586.

Ponsky L, Cherullo E, Moinzadeh A, et al. The Hem-o-lok clip is safe for laparoscopic nephrectomy: a multi-institutional review. Urology 2008;71(4):593–6.

Radical Prostatectomy

Riccardo Bertolo, Jihad Kaouk, and Robert Abouassaly

 VIDEO

66.1 Robotic Prostatectomy

INTRODUCTION

Radical prostatectomy is the "gold standard" in the surgical treatment of localized prostate cancer. Current evidence confirms a survival advantage over the absence of treatment in men with prostate cancer. Traditionally, radical prostatectomy was performed in the open retropubic or transperineal approach. The advent of minimally invasive techniques (pure and robot-assisted laparoscopy) allowing for improved visualization, has increased the understanding of prostate anatomy and surrounding structures and reduced the morbidity associated with radical prostatectomy.

In addition, over the last decade, the use of minimally invasive approaches has dramatically increased, particularly robot-assisted laparoscopic radical prostatectomy (Fig. 66.1A), which facilitates laparoscopic suturing.

Prostatectomy can result in urinary incontinence and erectile dysfunction because of the damage to the urethral-sphincter complex and the periprostatic neurovascular bundles. Current 1-year data report that urinary continence is achieved in approximately 90% of patients, and erectile function is recovered in most men with good preoperative function.

PROSTATE CANCER: THERAPEUTIC PRINCIPLES

Once the diagnosis of prostate cancer is made on biopsy, staging is obtained depending on the patient's Gleason score, prostate-specific antigen (PSA), clinical stage, and life expectancy.

Staging can include pelvic computed tomography (CT) or, more recently, magnetic resonance imaging (MRI). A bone scan can be performed to exclude bone metastases. If the malignancy has a high probability of being localized to the prostate, treatment options are discussed with the patient, including active surveillance, radiation therapy, or surgery, depending on disease factors, life expectancy, and patient preference.

Radical prostatectomy is generally considered in men with life expectancy greater than 10 years who have prostate cancer at significant risk of progression. The variation in prostate size and shape, as well as its location deep in the pelvis between the bladder and the urethra and adjacent to the rectum, make surgical extirpation challenging (Fig. 66.1B). Additionally, the prostate is surrounded by a venous plexus and the neurovascular bundles responsible for erection. Therefore the surgical dissection required during radical prostatectomy should be performed meticulously by a surgeon with detailed knowledge of the anatomic relationships of the prostate.

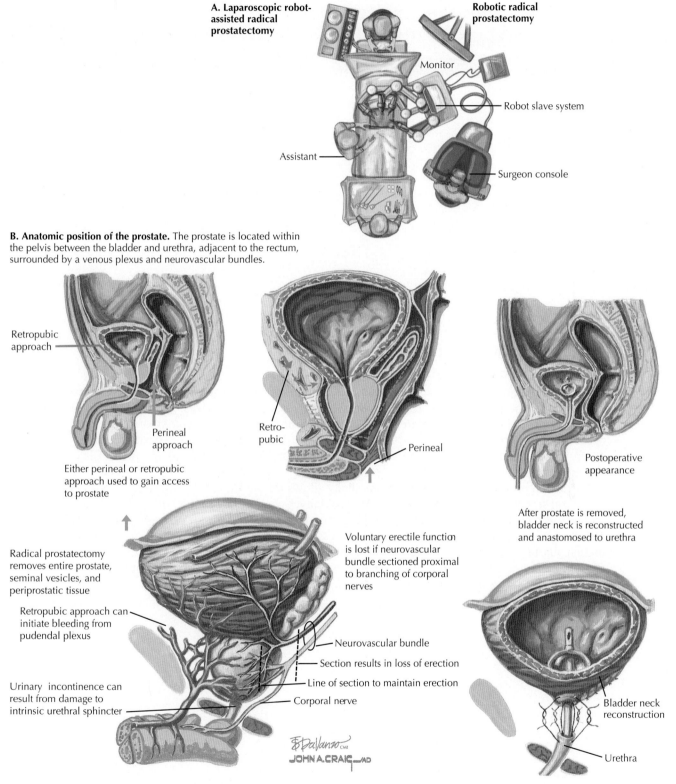

A. Laparoscopic robot-assisted radical prostatectomy

Robotic radical prostatectomy

Monitor

Robot slave system

Assistant

Surgeon console

B. Anatomic position of the prostate. The prostate is located within the pelvis between the bladder and urethra, adjacent to the rectum, surrounded by a venous plexus and neurovascular bundles.

Retropubic approach

Perineal approach

Either perineal or retropubic approach used to gain access to prostate

Retro-pubic

Perineal

Postoperative appearance

After prostate is removed, bladder neck is reconstructed and anastomosed to urethra

Radical prostatectomy removes entire prostate, seminal vesicles, and periprostatic tissue

Retropubic approach can initiate bleeding from pudendal plexus

Urinary incontinence can result from damage to intrinsic urethral sphincter

Voluntary erectile function is lost if neurovascular bundle sectioned proximal to branching of corporal nerves

Neurovascular bundle

Section results in loss of erection

Line of section to maintain erection

Corporal nerve

Bladder neck reconstruction

Urethra

FIGURE 66.1 Robot-assisted prostatectomy and surgical approaches to prostate.

SURGICAL APPROACH

Posterior Prostatic Dissection

After the induction of pneumoperitoneum and gaining access to the peritoneal cavity, initial inspection of the pelvis is performed to identify the relevant landmarks: the medial umbilical ligaments and the vasa deferentia. The rectovesical cul-de-sac (pouch of Douglas) is approached, and the courses of the vasa deferentia are identified through the peritoneum (Fig. 66.2A through D). The peritoneum is incised, and the ampulla of the vas deferens is isolated and transected.

Retraction on the vas deferens ventromedially allows for identification and dissection of the ipsilateral seminal vesicle. The artery to the seminal vesicle is either clipped or controlled with bipolar electrocautery. The procedure is repeated on the contralateral side. The seminal vesicles and vasa are retracted ventrally, exposing Denonvilliers' fascia (Fig. 66.2E and F). This fascia is incised sharply just dorsal to the base of the prostate. This approach allows entry into a plane containing perirectal fat so that the surgeon can carefully dissect the prostate off of the rectum in an antegrade direction toward the prostatic apex.

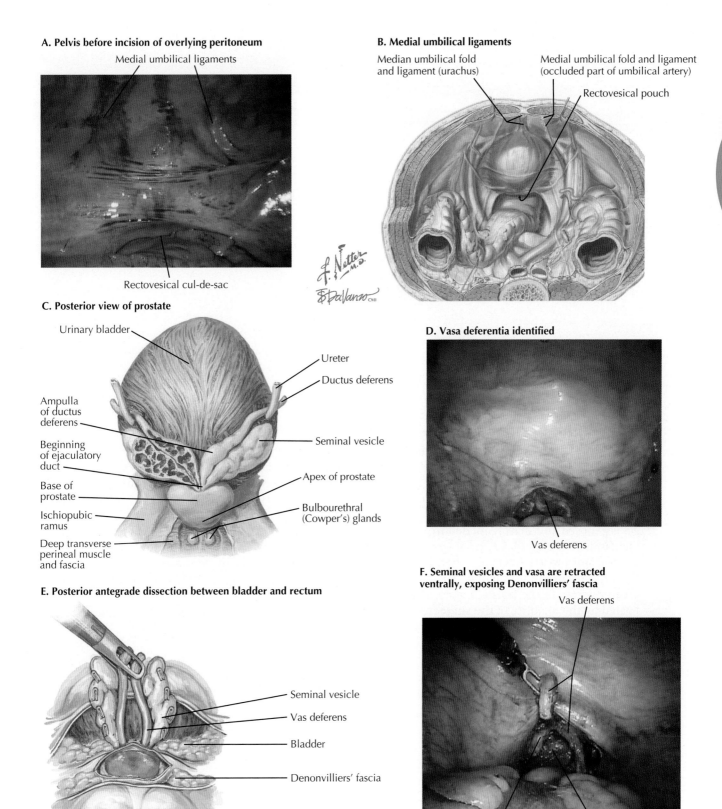

A. Pelvis before incision of overlying peritoneum

Medial umbilical ligaments

Rectovesical cul-de-sac

B. Medial umbilical ligaments

Median umbilical fold and ligament (urachus)

Medial umbilical fold and ligament (occluded part of umbilical artery)

Rectovesical pouch

C. Posterior view of prostate

Urinary bladder

Ureter

Ductus deferens

Ampulla of ductus deferens

Beginning of ejaculatory duct

Seminal vesicle

Apex of prostate

Base of prostate

Bulbourethral (Cowper's) glands

Ischiopubic ramus

Deep transverse perineal muscle and fascia

D. Vasa deferentia identified

Vas deferens

E. Posterior antegrade dissection between bladder and rectum

Seminal vesicle

Vas deferens

Bladder

Denonvilliers' fascia

Rectum

F. Seminal vesicles and vasa are retracted ventrally, exposing Denonvilliers' fascia

Vas deferens

Seminal vesicle

Denonvilliers' fascia

FIGURE 66.2 Posterior prostatic dissection.

Development of the Space of Retzius

The urachus and medial umbilical ligaments are then transected with electrocautery just inferior to the umbilicus (Fig. 66.3). The bladder is carefully dissected off of the anterior abdominal wall just deep to the posterior rectus sheath and transversalis fascia. The lateral limits of the dissection are the lateral borders of the medial umbilical ligaments.

The bladder is then swept off of the iliac vessels and obturator muscles. The endopelvic fascia is exposed and sharply incised from the base of the prostate to the puboprostatic ligaments bilaterally. The superficial dorsal vein is coagulated with bipolar electrocautery and transected. Levator ani muscle fibers are then swept off of the lateral aspects of the prostate, exposing the prostate-urethral junction. The puboprostatic ligaments are sharply transected, allowing greater access to the prostatic apex. The deep dorsal venous complex (DVC) is then suture-ligated by the majority of the surgeons, even though suture ligation is not mandatory.

A. The urachus and medial umbilical ligaments are transected inferior to the umbilicus

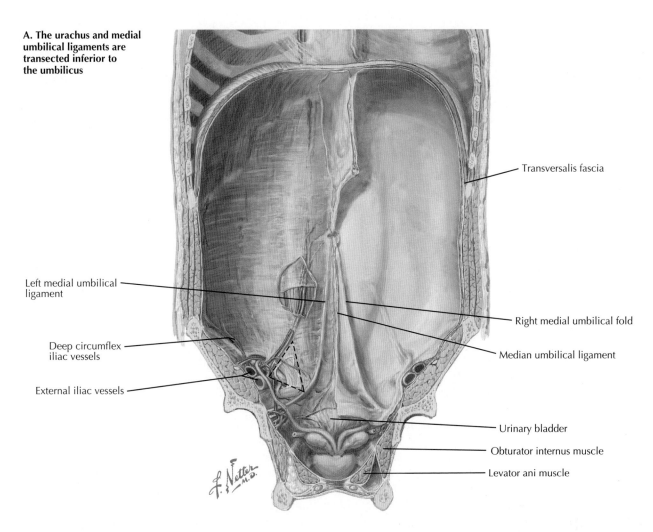

Transversalis fascia

Left medial umbilical ligament

Deep circumflex iliac vessels

External iliac vessels

Right medial umbilical fold

Median umbilical ligament

Urinary bladder

Obturator internus muscle

Levator ani muscle

B. The bladder is dissected off of the anterior abdominal wall and swept off of the iliac vessels and obturator muscles. The endopelvic fascia is then sharply incised.

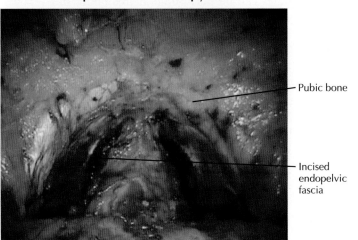

Pubic bone

Incised endopelvic fascia

C. The dorsal venous complex is suture ligated.

Ligated DVC

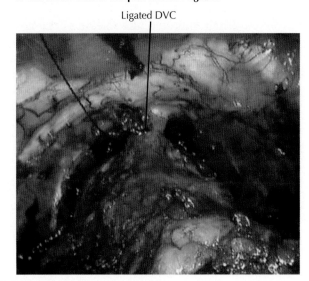

FIGURE 66.3 Development of space of Retzius. *DVC,* Dorsal venous complex.

Bladder Neck Dissection

The contour of the prostate, the pliability of the tissues, and the balloon from the urethral catheter are used to identify the bladder neck just proximal to the base of the prostate. Electrocautery is then used to dissect the anterior, lateral, and posterior bladder neck off of the base of the prostate (Fig. 66.4A).

If present, an enlarged median lobe of the prostate is identified during this step. The dissection will be modified accordingly to ensure complete excision with the prostate specimen.

Care is taken by the surgeon during the posterior bladder neck dissection to avoid ureteral injury. It is ideal when the surgeon is able to identify the ureteral orifices. Once through the posterior bladder neck, the surgeon can enter the posterior plane developed earlier in the procedure, and the transected vasa deferentia and seminal vesicles can be visualized and grasped for retraction.

Neurovascular Bundle Preservation

When indicated, the release of the neurovascular bundles can be performed at this point, or after control of the vascular pedicles to the prostate (Fig. 66.4B). The levator ani fascia is sharply incised over the anterolateral prostate, preserving the underlying prostatic fascia. This incision is carried distal beyond the prostatic apex and proximal to the vascular pedicles.

The dissection is then carried dorsally along the surface of the prostate until the posterior plane is entered, and the neurovascular bundles are completely released off of the prostatic surface. In many patients, during this step, venous or small arterial tributaries coursing between the neurovascular bundles and the prostate are encountered.

A. Bladder neck dissection

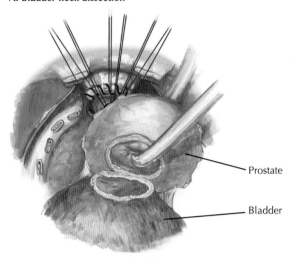

Prostate

Bladder

Division of bladder neck

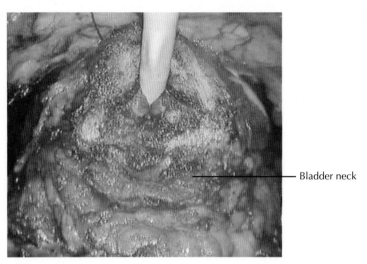

Bladder neck

B. Neurovascular bundle preservation. The neurovascular bundles are completely released off of the prostatic surface.

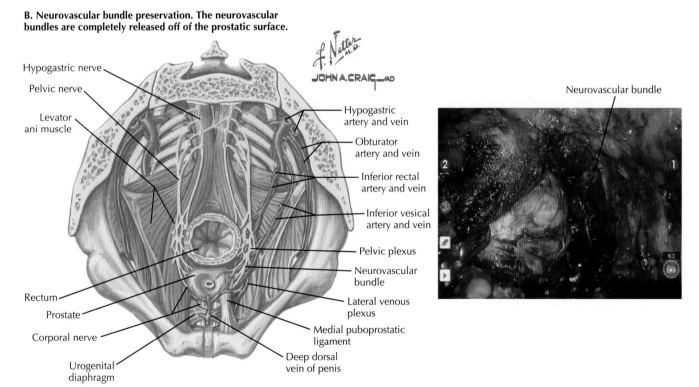

Hypogastric nerve

Pelvic nerve

Levator ani muscle

Hypogastric artery and vein

Obturator artery and vein

Inferior rectal artery and vein

Inferior vesical artery and vein

Pelvic plexus

Neurovascular bundle

Lateral venous plexus

Rectum

Prostate

Corporal nerve

Medial puboprostatic ligament

Deep dorsal vein of penis

Urogenital diaphragm

Neurovascular bundle

FIGURE 66.4 Bladder neck dissection and neurovascular bundle.

Prostatic Pedicle Ligation and Division of the Deep Dorsal Venous Plexus

The base of the prostate is left attached by the vascular pedicles (Fig. 66.5). The seminal vesicles and vasa are retracted anteriorly and contralaterally, defining the prostatic pedicles at the 5 and 7 o'clock positions. The pedicles are then clipped or suture-ligated and transected sharply.

The DVC is transected immediately proximal to the previously placed suture. If bleeding from the DVC occurs, repeated suture ligation can be required to achieve adequate hemostasis. Once the DVC is completely divided, the prostate can be retracted farther out of the pelvis, to stretch the urethra, so that the junction between the prostatic apex and the urethra is better visualized.

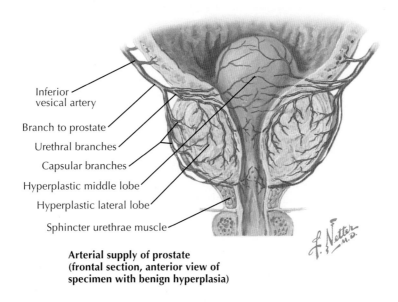

Inferior
vesical artery

Branch to prostate

Urethral branches

Capsular branches

Hyperplastic middle lobe

Hyperplastic lateral lobe

Sphincter urethrae muscle

**Arterial supply of prostate
(frontal section, anterior view of
specimen with benign hyperplasia)**

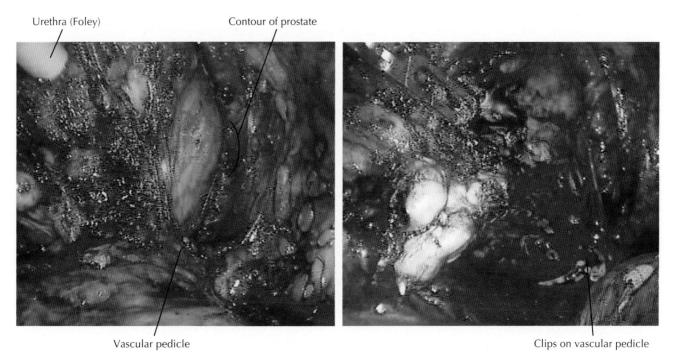

Urethra (Foley)

Contour of prostate

Vascular pedicle

Clips on vascular pedicle

FIGURE 66.5 Prostatic pedicle ligation and division of deep dorsal venous plexus.

Division of Urethra

The apex of the prostate is further defined with careful dissection around the urethra (Fig. 66.6A). Inspection is performed to confirm the neurovascular bundles are dissected off the prostatic apex to ensure that the bundles will not be inadvertently transected during the division of the urethra. The anterior urethra is then divided sharply just distal to the prostatic apex.

Care is taken to inspect the contour of the posterior prostatic apex before dividing the posterior urethra. Indeed, different apical shapes can be encountered. In some cases, the posterior prostatic apex can protrude beyond the anterior apex, requiring a more distal dissection in this area. Once the urethra is divided, the prostate is free to be moved out of the pelvic fossa into the peritoneal cavity and placed in a specimen bag for later retrieval.

Vesicourethral Anastomosis

A sutured vesicourethral anastomosis is then fashioned. Generally, two running sutures are performed in opposite directions from the mid-posterior to the mid-anterior bladder neck (Fig. 66.6B). Adequate apposition of the posterior bladder neck is needed to avoid postoperative urine leaks, because this is the area of greatest tension. To perform a high-quality tension-free anastomosis, several authors have described pairing the anastomosis with either posterior or anterior reconstruction, with the aim of restoring the original anatomy as much as possible.

A urethral catheter guides the completion of the anastomosis. After completing the anastomosis, most surgeons leave a closed suction drain in the prevesical space. Ideally, the drain should not be directly at the anastomosis to avoid suction causing leakage.

Specimen Extraction

Traditionally, the largest periumbilical camera port incision (10–12 mm) is chosen for the specimen retrieval. Incisions in the fascia and skin are extended accordingly to allow safe extraction of the prostate specimen entrapped in an EndoCatch bag. Fascial and skin incisions are then closed and dressings applied.

ALTERNATIVE APPROACHES

The standard approach with dissection in the space of Retzius has been described; however, some authors have described a complete posterior approach to prostatectomy (the so-called "Retzius sparing" approach). Additionally, with the aim of expediting the postoperative recovery and improving cosmesis, the idea of performing a robotic procedure through a single abdominal incision is being considered with the advent of single-port–dedicated robotic platforms. Such techniques could spur the discovery of different access routes to the prostate, including the Retzius-sparing and the transperineal approach originally described in open surgery literature, with a goal of leaving as much anatomy untouched as possible, to maximize the functional outcomes of the patient. Ideally, with all of these approaches in the armamentarium of the surgeon, each approach could be individually tailored based on patient's and disease's characteristics.

A. Division of the urethra

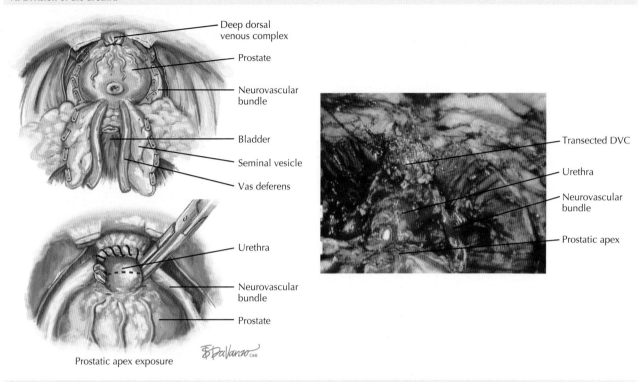

Deep dorsal venous complex

Prostate

Neurovascular bundle

Bladder

Seminal vesicle

Vas deferens

Urethra

Neurovascular bundle

Prostate

Prostatic apex exposure

Transected DVC

Urethra

Neurovascular bundle

Prostatic apex

B. Vesicourethral anastomosis. The anastomosis is created by running two sutures in opposite directions from the midposterior neck to the midanterior bladder neck.

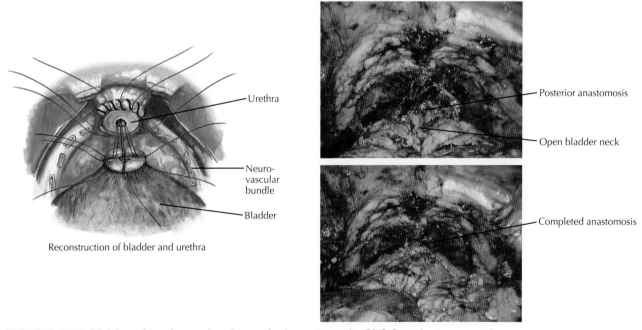

Urethra

Neurovascular bundle

Bladder

Reconstruction of bladder and urethra

Posterior anastomosis

Open bladder neck

Completed anastomosis

FIGURE 66.6 Division of urethra and vesicourethral anastomosis. *DVC,* Dorsal venous complex.

SUGGESTED READINGS

Bill-Axelson A, Holmberg L, Ruutu M, et al. Radical prostatectomy versus watchful waiting in early prostate cancer. N Engl J Med 2011;364:1708.

Ficarra V, Novara G, Artibani W, et al. Retropubic, laparoscopic, and robot-assisted radical prostatectomy: a systematic review and cumulative analysis of comparative studies. Eur Urol 2009;55:1037.

Kaouk J, Garisto J, Bertolo R. Different approaches to the prostate: the upcoming role of a purpose-built single-port robotic system. Arab J Urol 2018;16:302–6.

Walz J, Epstein JI, Ganzer R, et al. A critical analysis of the current knowledge of surgical anatomy of the prostate related to optimisation of cancer control and preservation of continence and erection in candidates for radical prostatectomy: an update. Eur Urol 2016;70(2):301–11. https://doi.org/10.1016/j.eururo.2016.01.026. Epub 2016 Feb 2.

Radical Cystectomy

Riccardo Bertolo, Juan Garisto, and Jihad Kaouk

INTRODUCTION

In the United States, bladder cancer is the fourth most common type in men and the ninth most common type of cancer in women. When not muscle invasive, bladder cancer can often be treated with transurethral resections and possible intravesical immunotherapy or chemotherapy with cystoscopic surveillance. For muscle-invasive bladder cancer or for tumors with high-grade features and invasion into the lamina propria (T1) without metastatic disease, radical cystectomy with urinary diversion remains the gold standard treatment. Other indications for cystectomy include refractory disease to intravesical immunotherapy or chemotherapy, and as a palliative procedure for patients with severely symptomatic metastatic or locally advanced bladder cancer necessitating acute hospital care and readmissions.

Pelvic lymphadenectomy is performed regardless of gender. Radical cystectomy in men typically involves the removal of the bladder, distal ureters, prostate, and seminal vesicles. For radical cystoprostatectomy, advances in surgical technique have included nerve-sparing procedures aimed to preserve potency in men and, in selected cases, prostate-sparing procedures. Moreover, techniques for orthotopic bladder substitution have been developed.

In women not seeking a "sexual-sparing" procedure and who have extensive disease, anterior pelvic exenteration is traditionally performed, including cystectomy, salpingo-oophorectomy, hysterectomy, urethrectomy, and resection of the anterior third of the vaginal wall. More recent data have challenged the anterior pelvic exenteration in females and supported a more limited resection in patients without extensive disease, preserving the anterior vaginal wall, uterus, ovaries, and pelvic supporting ligaments, with undoubted benefit on functional outcomes.

SURGICAL APPROACH

Radical cystectomy has traditionally been performed through a low abdominal midline incision, although minimally invasive approaches may now be offered. Although some surgeons are choosing the robot-assisted approach for performing the extirpative phase of the procedure, the open approach still remains the gold standard. For the reconstructive phase, there are reports of successfully completed minimally invasive intracorporeal urinary diversions. Nevertheless, the post-cystectomy method of urinary diversion is still generally completed with an extracorporeal approach. Whatever approach used, standardized surgical steps are used.

Bladder Mobilization

After incision of the skin and anterior and posterior layers of the anterior abdominal wall fascia, the extraperitoneal space is entered. The space of Retzius is developed to mobilize the bladder away from the symphysis pubis anteriorly and to expose the external iliac artery and vein on each side.

The peritoneum is opened and extended laterally from the medial umbilical ligament to the internal inguinal rings. The urachus is divided high near the level of the umbilicus and subsequently used for retraction. Anatomically, an avascular plane of fibroareolar connective tissue can be followed, between the posterior rectus sheath and the peritoneum and along the medial umbilical ligaments. Care should be taken to avoid injury to the inferior epigastric arteries, which course in this plane and serve as the primary blood supply to the rectus abdominis muscle.

The sigmoid colon is often adherent laterally to the side wall and occasionally to the bladder. It is mobilized medially at this point by opening the peritoneum at the white line of Toldt. The peritoneal wings previously left in place by developing the space of Retzius and opening the peritoneum from the umbilicus to the inguinal ring are easily seen and divided with electrocautery to the level of the vas deferens in the male patient. The vas deferens is divided with the understanding that vascular structures are associated with both vasa. The use of ties is generally preferred to allow later identification of the seminal vesicles (Fig. 67.1A and B).

Dissection of Ureters

After bilateral ligation of the vas deferens, the immediate posterior peritoneum along the bladder and above the sigmoid is opened. This approach allows identification of the ureters as they cross over the iliac vessels and anterior mobilization of the bladder off the proximal rectum to the level of the prostate and seminal vesicles. This maneuver can be done with a gentle blunt movement, however great care must be taken because this loose plane of connective tissue becomes dense at the level of the prostate and cannot always be easily bluntly dissected. There is the potential risk of rectal injury. The left ureter is identified posterior to the sigmoid colon, in a position often more medial than expected. The retroperitoneal space behind the sigmoid colon at the level of the sacral promontory is opened to allow the ureter to be passed to the other side after its division. The right ureter is found by dividing the visible peritoneal fold overlying it (Fig. 67.1C).

The ureters are mobilized cephalad approximately 5 cm and then caudad down to the ureterovesical junction. Care must be taken to preserve soft tissue around the ureter. The periureteral blood supply is enveloped in this layer, and excellent vascularity will aid in a successful, patent anastomosis for the urinary diversion. The distal 5 mm of each ureter can then be divided and sent as a frozen section to ensure adequacy of the margin. In some cases of in-situ carcinoma, several frozen sections may have to be sent before an adequate margin is achieved. However, this practice has come under debate in recent years, with contradictory conclusions regarding the value of a negative margin in reducing risk of upper tract cancer recurrence. This dissection allows for clear visualization of the common, external, and internal iliac arteries and prepares the surgeon to commence with pelvic lymphadenectomy.

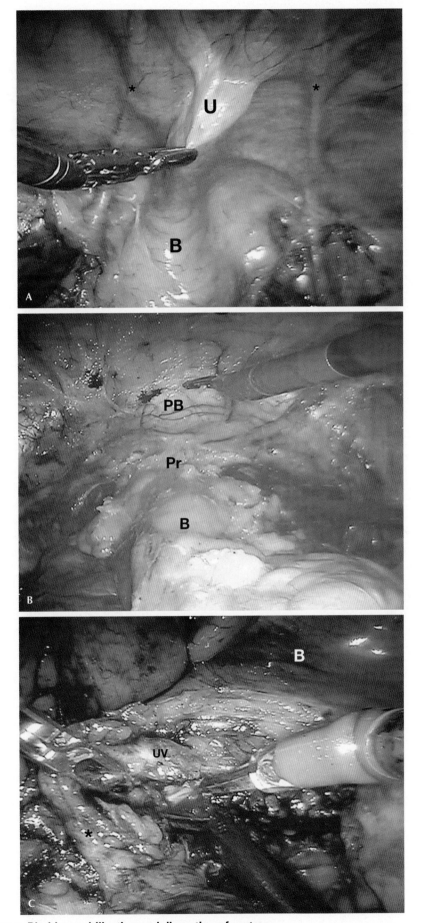

FIGURE 67.1 Bladder mobilization and dissection of ureters.
* (in A), Umbilical arteries; * (in C), ureter; *B,* bladder; *PB,* pubic bone; *Pr,* prostate; *U,* urachus; *UV,* uretero-vescical junction.

Pelvic Lymph Nodes Dissection

Limits of the lymph nodes dissection can vary depending on the extent of disease. It has been demonstrated that 25 to 30 lymph nodes should be resected to determine nodal status and that this can be curative in some cases of micrometastatic nodal disease. The most limited dissection should at least include all fibroadipose and lymphatic tissue between the external iliac artery laterally, the internal iliac artery medially, the crossing of the ureter at the common iliac artery cranially, the circumflex iliac vein or inguinal ligament of Cooper caudally, and the obturator nerve inferiorly. More extensive dissection can extend to the genitofemoral nerve laterally and the bifurcation of the aorta cranially or even to the inferior mesenteric artery (Fig. 67.2).

Two important anatomic notes during the lymph node dissection are the frequent presence of an accessory obturator vein draining into the external iliac vein and the proximity of the obturator nerve during dissection. Injury to the obturator nerve will result in difficulty adducting the ipsilateral lower extremity. Conversely, the obturator artery and vein can be sacrificed with no adverse sequelae.

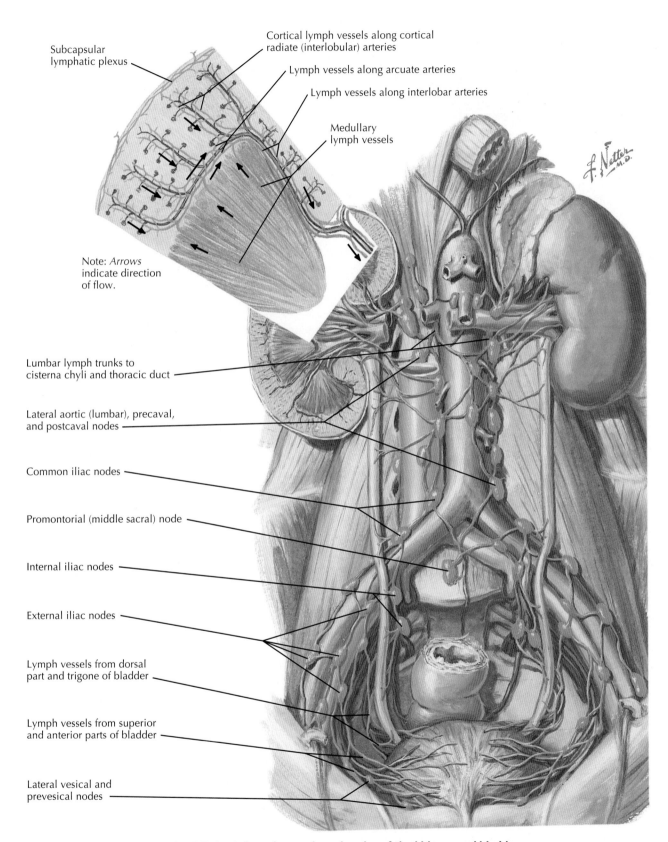

Subcapsular lymphatic plexus

Cortical lymph vessels along cortical radiate (interlobular) arteries

Lymph vessels along arcuate arteries

Lymph vessels along interlobar arteries

Medullary lymph vessels

Note: *Arrows* indicate direction of flow.

Lumbar lymph trunks to cisterna chyli and thoracic duct

Lateral aortic (lumbar), precaval, and postcaval nodes

Common iliac nodes

Promontorial (middle sacral) node

Internal iliac nodes

External iliac nodes

Lymph vessels from dorsal part and trigone of bladder

Lymph vessels from superior and anterior parts of bladder

Lateral vesical and prevesical nodes

FIGURE 67.2 Lymph vessels and nodes of the kidneys and bladder.

Pedicle Dissection

Knowledge of the vascular anatomy is the key to successful dissection of the lateral and posterior pedicles of the bladder. With the internal iliac artery already exposed and the vas deferens divided, the superior vesical artery, the first anterior branch of the internal iliac artery, can be safely ligated near its origin from the internal iliac artery (Fig. 67.3A).

The remainder of the vascular supply to the bladder and prostate is carried in vessels of small enough caliber that collective division between stapling devices, clips, thermal dissectors, or ligation can be accomplished without individual identification. It is extremely important to remember that the use of stapling devices or thermal dissectors will divide tissues irrespective of tissue planes, and precise knowledge of the patient's anatomy is critical to avoid injury to adjacent structures.

After ligating the superior vesicle artery, the surgeon can divide the remaining lateral and posterior pedicles of the bladder as previously described, to the level of the endopelvic fascia. Anterior retraction of the bladder exposes the pedicles, facilitating their division. Using a combination of sharp and blunt dissection, the surgeon brings the bladder with the seminal vesicles forward off the rectum. The posterior pedicles can now be visualized, posteromedial to the divided ureteral stump. This pedicle is divided to the level of the seminal vesicles with a thermal dissector or surgical stapler. Continuing distally, a plane may be developed between the rectum posteriorly and the posterior lamina of Denonvilliers' fascia anteriorly, taking care to stay anterior to the prerectal fat.

The space posterior to the prostate is developed caudally as close to the prostatic apex as possible. Here the surgeon may choose to continue with either nerve-sparing or non–nerve-sparing technique. Care should be taken to avoid damaging any of the autonomic nerves from the pelvic plexuses, because these nerves innervate the urinary sphincters and will play an important role in postoperative continence if an orthotopic urinary diversion is constructed (Fig. 67.3B). To preserve the autonomic plexus, an incision should be made between the lateral pelvic fascia and Denonvilliers' fascia to find the neurovascular bundles that lie posterolaterally along the prostate (Fig. 67.3C and D).

Urethral Ligation

After dissection of the pedicles, urethral ligation is completed in a manner similar to a prostatectomy.

Continuing caudally from the previously developed space of Retzius, the space anterior to the prostate is first opened, and the prostate is separated from its anterior attachments to the pubis. The endopelvic fascia and puboprostatic ligaments are exposed anteriorly, and the endopelvic fascia is opened, revealing the muscular attachments of the levator ani muscles to the prostate. With the endopelvic fascia open bilaterally, the anterior prostatic fascia, the extension of the endopelvic fascia over the prostate, can be suture ligated. The dorsal venous complex (Santorini's plexus) is located within this fascia (Fig. 67.3E).

The lateral edges of the prostate are dissected from the remaining muscular attachments of the levator ani muscle. The urethra is then freed with blunt dissection, isolated, and divided. This approach exposes the triangular extension of Denonvilliers' fascia. When incised, this exposes the rectum. Any remaining pedicle attachments of the bladder or prostate are then divided. The specimen, including the bladder, terminal ureters, seminal vesicles, and prostate, can then be removed en bloc. Anastomotic sutures can be placed in the remaining proximal urethra if orthotopic urinary diversion is planned.

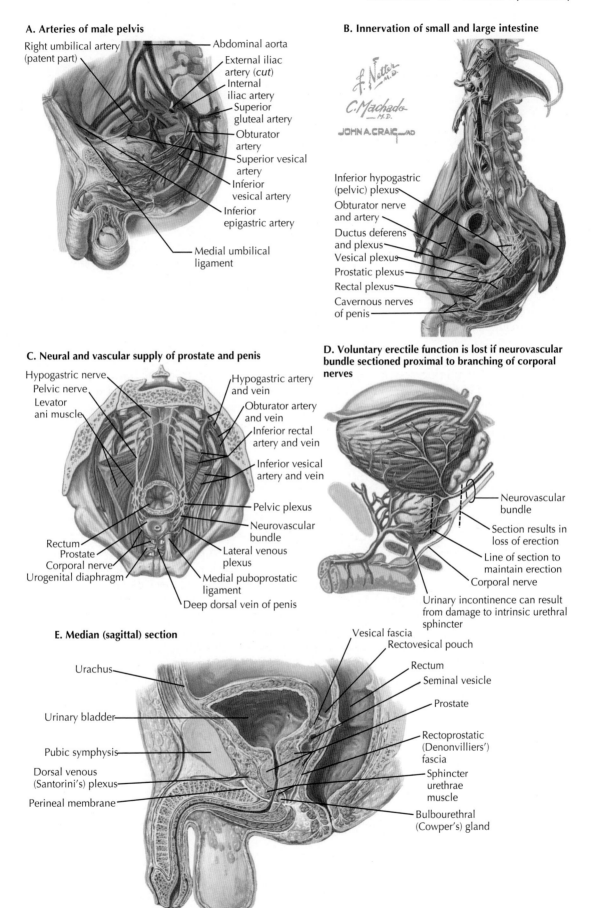

A. Arteries of male pelvis

Right umbilical artery (patent part)
Abdominal aorta
External iliac artery (*cut*)
Internal iliac artery
Superior gluteal artery
Obturator artery
Superior vesical artery
Inferior vesical artery
Inferior epigastric artery
Medial umbilical ligament

B. Innervation of small and large intestine

Inferior hypogastric (pelvic) plexus
Obturator nerve and artery
Ductus deferens and plexus
Vesical plexus
Prostatic plexus
Rectal plexus
Cavernous nerves of penis

C. Neural and vascular supply of prostate and penis

Hypogastric nerve
Pelvic nerve
Levator ani muscle
Hypogastric artery and vein
Obturator artery and vein
Inferior rectal artery and vein
Inferior vesical artery and vein
Pelvic plexus
Neurovascular bundle
Lateral venous plexus
Medial puboprostatic ligament
Deep dorsal vein of penis
Rectum
Prostate
Corporal nerve
Urogenital diaphragm

D. Voluntary erectile function is lost if neurovascular bundle sectioned proximal to branching of corporal nerves

Neurovascular bundle
Section results in loss of erection
Line of section to maintain erection
Corporal nerve
Urinary incontinence can result from damage to intrinsic urethral sphincter

E. Median (sagittal) section

Urachus
Urinary bladder
Pubic symphysis
Dorsal venous (Santorini's) plexus
Perineal membrane
Vesical fascia
Rectovesical pouch
Rectum
Seminal vesicle
Prostate
Rectoprostatic (Denonvilliers') fascia
Sphincter urethrae muscle
Bulbourethral (Cowper's) gland

FIGURE 67.3 Male: vascular supply of pelvic organs and erectile function.

ANTERIOR PELVIC EXENTERATION

As mentioned earlier, anterior pelvic exenteration is traditionally performed in female patients who have extensive disease. It includes cystectomy, salpingo-oophorectomy, hysterectomy, urethrectomy, and resection of the anterior one-third of the vaginal wall.

After a lower abdominal midline incision, the peritoneum is incised laterally toward the round ligaments, which are then ligated. An anterior retraction stitch on the fundus of the uterus facilitates exposure of the uterine vessels. First, the ovarian vessels and infundibulopelvic ligaments are ligated, which allows for better exposure because the intestines can be packed upward into the abdomen away from the pelvis. The ureters are traced to the vascular supply of the uterus. The uterine vessels are suture ligated at their origin from the internal iliac vessels to mobilize and expose the ureters to the ureterovesical junction, where they are ligated (Fig. 67.4A). The uterus is then mobilized laterally from its attachments at the cervix and inferior ligaments. The uterus can be left attached anteriorly to the posterior aspect of the bladder to be removed en bloc with the specimen.

Bladder Mobilization

The technique for division of the lateral pedicles varies depending on whether a vagina-sparing procedure is being performed. The lateral blood supply is isolated as it branches from the internal iliac artery, and the inferior uterine arteries must be ligated. The bladder is mobilized medially away from the lateral walls of the pelvis to expose the endopelvic fascia, the perirectal fat pad, and the lateral pedicles. A povidone-iodine swab stick in the vagina is elevated cranially and ventrally to aid exposure of the apex of the vagina, which is opened immediately distal to the cervix into the posterior vagina by cautery. The incision at the apex of the vagina can be continued down bilaterally on the anterolateral sides of the vagina to the bladder neck.

The anterior vaginal wall is usually spared when the disease appears confined to the bladder or when cystectomy is being performed for benign disease. If vaginal sparing is not possible, on entering the vagina anteriorly, the surgeon can divide the lateral bladder pedicles en bloc with the anterior wall of the vagina, using thermal dissectors or suture ligation (Fig. 67.4B). Staples and clips should be avoided in this situation because these objects may migrate into the vagina postoperatively. The lateral pedicles with the remaining small, unnamed vessels can be ligated to the level of the endopelvic fascia.

Vagina-Sparing Technique

Alternatively, if the vagina is to be spared fully, or in cases of limited disease and previous hysterectomy, the space between the anterior vagina and the posterior bladder wall is developed, taking care to dissect close to the anterior vaginal wall. If hysterectomy is required, a circumferential incision of the vagina close to the vaginal apex allows for removal of the cervix and uterus. Closure of the vagina depends on the method of urethrectomy described below (see Fig. 67.4B).

A.

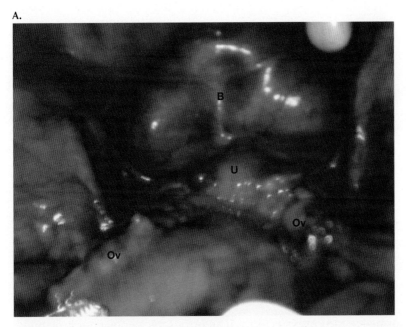

B. Female bladder and urethra

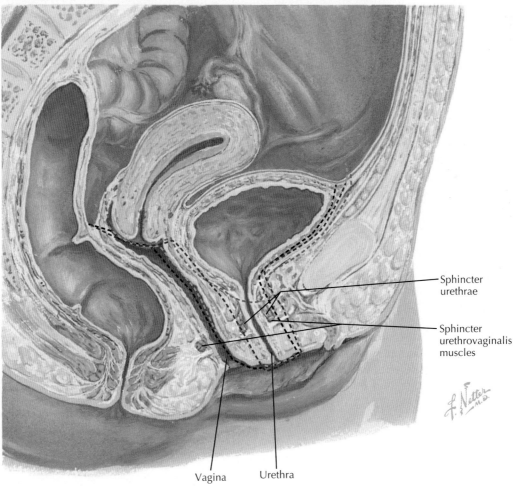

Sphincter urethrae

Sphincter urethrovaginalis muscles

Vagina   Urethra

\- - - En bloc resection of bladder, uterus, anterior 1/3 of vagina, and urethra

\- - - Resection of bladder and uterus, with preservation of vagina and urethra to allow for more successful reconstruction

\- - - Resection of bladder, uterus, anterior 1/3 of vagina, and urethra, with preservation of small portion of distal anterior vagina

\- - - Resection of bladder, uterus, and urethra with preservation of vagina

FIGURE 67.4 Female: vascular supply of pelvic organs and anterior exenteration resections. *B,* Bladder; *Ov,* ovary; *U,* uterus.

Urethrectomy

A urethrectomy can be performed in radical cystectomy. If an orthotopic neobladder is planned, a frozen section of the urethra can be sent to confirm a negative margin, in which case the urethra can be left intact to aid in maintenance of continence with the neobladder. Otherwise, to perform a complete urethrectomy, the patient must be positioned to allow for access to the introitus.

The labia are retracted laterally to expose the urethra. If vagina-sparing techniques are not used, a U-shaped incision can be made from the top of the introitus surrounding the anterior vaginal wall and carried around the urethra (Fig. 67.5A). Within the pelvis, the pubourethral suspensory ligaments, corresponding to the puboprostatic ligaments in men, are ligated to release the bladder and urethra. The dorsal vein complex superior to the urethra is isolated and ligated. Any other periurethral attachments are released circumferentially and passed in continuity through the vaginal incision into the pelvis.

Alternatively, a circular incision can be made around the urethra. The portion of the anterior vagina below the bladder neck is left in the pelvis to support the reconstruction of the vagina. The urethra is sharply dissected off the anterior vaginal wall and, after ligation of all other periurethral attachments, passed into the pelvis (see Fig. 67.4B).

Vaginal Reconstruction

When the anterior wall of the vagina is removed, vaginal reconstruction is necessary. Classically, the posterior wall of the vagina can be folded forward toward the apex as a flap for coverage of the introital defect (Fig. 67.5B). The reconstruction is completed with an absorbable suture, typically 2-0 polyglycolic acid or its equivalent. This maneuver will shorten the vagina. Alternatively, the lateral edges of the vagina can be approximated. Often this leads to a very narrow, nonfunctional vagina, and the suture line may be under tension. Preservation of the anterior vagina is recommended when considering construction of an orthotopic neobladder. Overlapping suture lines between the vagina and neobladder may predispose to fistula formation.

A

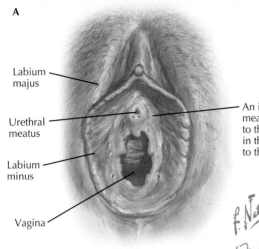

Labium majus

Urethral meatus

Labium minus

Vagina

An inverted U-shaped incision can be made around the urethral meatus, and the urethra is mobilized. The venous plexus anterior to the urethra is ligated within the pelvis, and the incisions made in the anterolateral vaginal wall within the pelvis are connected to the dissection at the perineum.

B

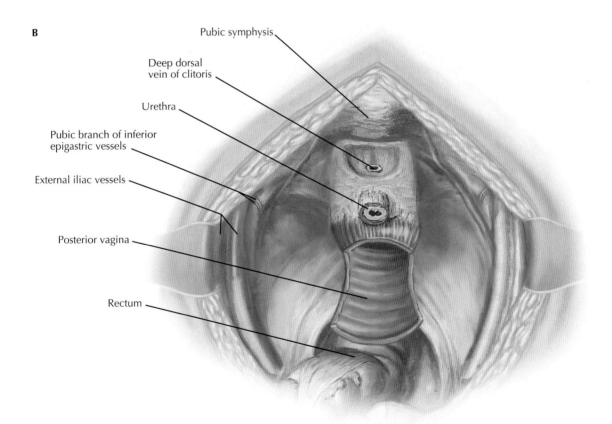

Pubic symphysis

Deep dorsal vein of clitoris

Urethra

Pubic branch of inferior epigastric vessels

External iliac vessels

Posterior vagina

Rectum

FIGURE 67.5 Urethral incision and resection.

SUGGESTED READINGS

Chang SS. Radical cystectomy. In: Smith J, Howards SS, Preminger GM, Hinman F, editors. Hinman's Atlas of Urologic Surgery. Philadelphia: Saunders-Elsevier; 2012.

Gakis G, Efstathiou J, Lerner SP, et al. ICUD-EAU International Consultation on Bladder Cancer 2012: Radical cystectomy and bladder preservation for muscle-invasive urothelial carcinoma of the bladder. Eur Urol 2013;63:45–57.

Ghonheim MA. Radical cystectomy in men. In: Graham SD, Keane TE, editors. Glenn's Urologic Surgery. Philadelphia: Lippincott, Williams & Wilkins; 2009.

Parekh DJ, Reis IM, Castle EP, et al. Robot-assisted radical cystectomy versus open radical cystectomy in patients with bladder cancer (RAZOR): an open-label, randomised, phase 3, non-inferiority trial. Lancet 2018;391:2525–36.

Weizer AZ, Lee CT. Radical cystectomy in women. In: Graham SD, Keane TE, editors. Glenn's Urologic Surgery. Philadelphia: Lippincott, Williams & Wilkins; 2009.

Retroperitoneal Lymph Node Dissection

Eric A. Klein, Georges-Pascal Haber, and Lewis J. Thomas IV

BILATERAL RETROPERITONEAL LYMPH NODE DISSECTION (RPLND)

Classically, a midline incision is made running from the xiphoid to just below the umbilicus. The peritoneum is entered, and the bowel retracted cephalad. The posterior peritoneum from the right lower quadrant (just inferior to the cecum/appendix) is then incised up to the ligament of Treitz, exposing the retroperitoneum. Care must be taken during this step to avoid injury to the right ureter, which courses across this plane of dissection just below the posterior peritoneum. Further mobilization of the right colon can be done by incising the white line of Toldt and rotating the ascending colon and cecum medially and cephalad. With the bowel mobilized and retroperitoneum exposed, the duodenum/pancreas are carefully dissected off the great vessels and retracted cephalad. A self-retaining retractor is then placed (such as a Bookwalter), and the bowel is packed out of the operative field; this is best achieved by keeping the bowel in the abdomen retracted under the abdominal wall, which limits the venous and lymphatic congestion that comes with placing the bowel on the patient's chest in a "bowel bag" and may contribute to earlier return of bowel function postoperatively. The primary blood supply to the bowel is from the superior mesenteric artery (SMA), which should be palpable at the superior margin of the retroperitoneal exposure. Retractors should be placed carefully to avoid compression of this critical vessel.

BILATERAL RETROPERITONEAL LYMPH NODE DISSECTION (RPLND) (Continued)

Exposure is critical for safe and oncologically sound RPLND. Ideal exposure should allow for visualization of the great vessels from the superior aspect of the renal vessels down to the bifurcation of the common iliac vessels. Identification of the critical retroperitoneal structures is paramount. Both ureters should be identified because they serve as the lateral boundaries of the full-template dissection. The aorta and vena cava as well as the left renal vein should be readily identifiable. In addition, the root of the inferior mesenteric artery (IMA) should be identified. This is a critical landmark as postganglionic sympathetic nerve fibers, which subserve ejaculation, coalesce around the origin of the IMA on the anterior surface of the aorta, forming the hypogastric plexus. Damage to this plexus can result in loss of ejaculation. Anatomy of the sympathetic nerve fibers through the operative field is shown in Fig. 68.1A. Left-sided retroperitoneal anatomy is shown in Fig. 68.1B. Right-sided retroperitoneal anatomy along with a common anatomic variant (accessory lower pole renal artery) is demonstrated in Fig. 68.1C. Assessment for anatomic variants on imaging is critical prior to surgery.

The lymph node dissection is then initiated using a "split and roll" technique. The nodal and fatty tissue overlying the anterior surface of the left renal vein is split and rolled caudally. This dissection is carried back to the inferior vena cava (IVC), and then caudally along the IVC, rolling the tissue into the paracaval and interaortocaval regions, respectively. The dissection should be in the plane that preserves the adventitia of the major vessels. During the dissection of the anterior surface of the vena cava, the right gonadal vein is ligated and divided. Dissection is carried down to the confluence of the common iliac veins. Dissection is avoided in the presacral space between the iliac vessels, because this is the site of nerve confluence and the hypogastric plexus. Once the vena cava and left renal vein have been exposed, attention is then turned to either exposure of the aorta or the precaval nodal dissection. The aorta is generally exposed first by performing a "split and roll" of the nodal and fatty tissue overlying the anterior surface of the aorta from the crossing of the left renal vein down to the IMA. Dissection caudal to the IMA is not performed at this time because this is where the postganglionic sympathetic fibers cross anterior to the aorta. With the aorta exposed, the bilateral renal arteries can then be identified as well as any lower-pole accessory renal arteries.

At this point, the critical vascular structures should all be identifiable, including the aorta, IVC, IMA, right renal arteries, right and left renal veins, and bilateral gonadal veins (with the right gonadal vein divided).

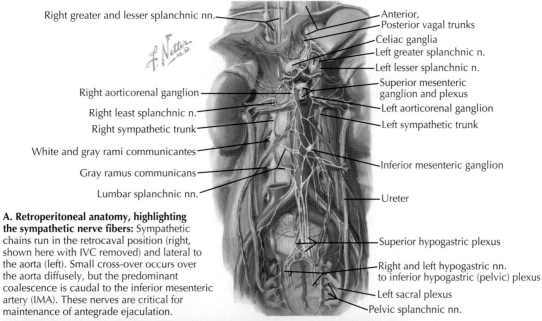

Right greater and lesser splanchnic nn.
Anterior,
Posterior vagal trunks
Celiac ganglia
Left greater splanchnic n.
Left lesser splanchnic n.
Right aorticorenal ganglion
Superior mesenteric ganglion and plexus
Right least splanchnic n.
Left aorticorenal ganglion
Right sympathetic trunk
Left sympathetic trunk
White and gray rami communicantes
Gray ramus communicans
Inferior mesenteric ganglion
Lumbar splanchnic nn.
Ureter
Superior hypogastric plexus
Right and left hypogastric nn. to inferior hypogastric (pelvic) plexus
Left sacral plexus
Pelvic splanchnic nn.

A. Retroperitoneal anatomy, highlighting the sympathetic nerve fibers: Sympathetic chains run in the retrocaval position (right, shown here with IVC removed) and lateral to the aorta (left). Small cross-over occurs over the aorta diffusely, but the predominant coalescence is caudal to the inferior mesenteric artery (IMA). These nerves are critical for maintenance of antegrade ejaculation.

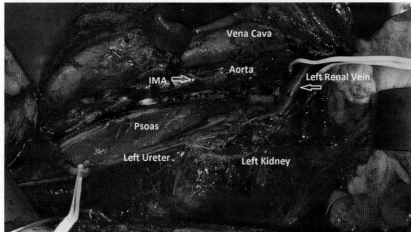

Vena Cava
Aorta
Left Renal Vein
IMA
Psoas
Left Ureter
Left Kidney

B. Common left sided anatomy including the left ureter (lateral border of paraaortic dissection), the left renal vein (superior border), and the aorta (medial border). Particular care should be taken with the cephalad portion of the dissection where the left gonadal vein, left renal lumbar veins, and the left sympathetic trunk are all present. This is a common site of "in-field" recurrence after RPLND.

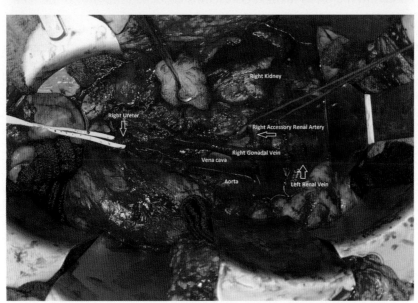

Right Kidney
Right Ureter
Right Accessory Renal Artery
Right Gonadal Vein
Vena cava
Aorta
Left Renal Vein

C. Aberrant anatomy can often complicate retroperitoneal lymph node dissection. Preoperative attention to imaging can help avoid inadvertent injury to aberrant anatomic structures. Here, right lower pole accessory renal artery is shown coursing just caudal and posterior to the right gonadal vein (anterior to the vena cava).

FIGURE 68.1 Retroperitoneal anatomy.

BILATERAL RETROPERITONEAL LYMPH NODE DISSECTION (RPLND) (Continued)

Attention is then turned to IVC mobilization. With the anterior surface of the IVC exposed, the "split and roll" technique is then used to expose the lumbar veins. The IVC is retracted to the patient's left and anterior, and the nodal/fatty tissue is rolled lateral. This should expose the right-sided lumbar veins, which are ligated and divided. It is critical to understand that lumbar vein anatomy can vary significantly, so meticulous and careful dissection is required to prevent hemorrhage. However, typically two to three right-sided lumbar veins are encountered. The largest right-sided vein is often at or just superior to the level of the right gonadal vein confluence. Significant care must be taken when dissecting out this vein because the right renal artery and the most superior lumbar splanchnic nerve (LSN) run near this large lumbar vein. Two additional right-sided lumbar veins are often encountered, with one in the middle of the IVC and another at the caudal aspect near the iliac confluence. This is illustrated in Fig. 68.2A. Once the right-sided lumbar veins have been controlled, the paracaval packet can be excised. With excision of any packet, control of the cephalad and caudad aspects with clips or liberal cautery is advised to try and prevent lymphatic leak. This is particularly important during the interaortocaval and paraaortic dissection, in which large lymphatics draining into the cisterna chyli can be encountered at the cephalad aspect. For the paracaval dissection, the boundaries are the cephalad aspect of the right renal vein, the IVC, the right ureter, the right common iliac vein, and the psoas muscle posteriorly. Careful lateral dissection of the tissue off Gerota's fascia is also important, because this is a possible site of right ureteral injury. In addition, care should be taken to avoid dissection into the psoas fascia, because this can lead to injury to the ilioinguinal or iliohypogastric nerves.

Attention is then turned to the interaortocaval lymph node dissection. If the tissue overlying the anterior aspect of the aorta has not been split, then that should be performed at this time. The interaortocaval tissue is then inspected, and the right aortic nerve plexus can often be identified, dissected free of the tissue (sharply to prevent cautery injury), and looped with vessel loops. These nerves can then be traced proximally to help identify the lumbar sympathetic nerve roots. The left-sided lumbar veins must then be controlled. The IVC is retracted to the patient's right and anterior, while the nodal/fatty tissue is rolled into the interaortocaval region; this should allow exposure of the left-sided lumbar veins, which are then ligated and divided as shown in Fig. 68.2B. The most prominent left-sided lumbar vein typically arises from a confluence of smaller veins and is approximately at the level of the IMA. However, the truncal nature of this large vein can lead to significant variation, with small lumbar veins draining directly into the IVC rather than this common lumbar trunk (meaning more lumbar veins flowing into the IVC). On average, two left-sided veins are typically encountered: the large truncal vein at the level of the IMA and another vein more caudal near the iliac confluence.

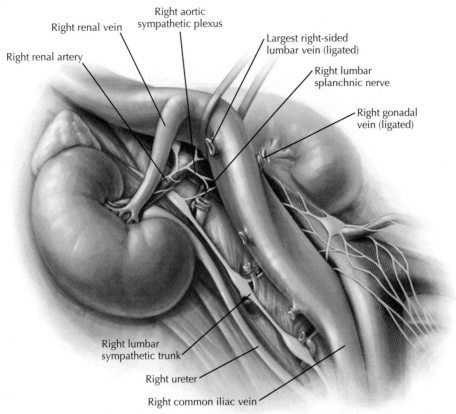

Right renal vein

Right aortic sympathetic plexus

Right renal artery

Largest right-sided lumbar vein (ligated)

Right lumbar splanchnic nerve

Right gonadal vein (ligated)

Right lumbar sympathetic trunk

Right ureter

Right common iliac vein

A. Once the right-sided lumbar veins have been ligated and divided, the IVC can be retracted medially and the roots of the right-sided lumbar splanchnic nerves identified. Identification of the nerves prior to paracaval packet excision is critical to successful nerve sparing.

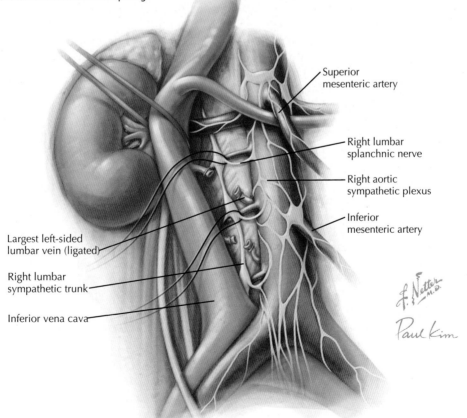

Superior mesenteric artery

Right lumbar splanchnic nerve

Right aortic sympathetic plexus

Inferior mesenteric artery

Largest left-sided lumbar vein (ligated)

Right lumbar sympathetic trunk

Inferior vena cava

B. Once the left-sided lumbar veins have been ligated and divided, the IVC can be retracted laterally. The previously identified lumbar splanchnic nerves can then be traced into the interaortocaval space and dissected free from the interaortocaval packet.

FIGURE 68.2 Paracaval and interaortocaval nodal dissection.

BILATERAL RETROPERITONEAL LYMPH NODE DISSECTION (RPLND) (Continued)

Once the left and right lumbar veins have been identified, ligated, and divided, the IVC can be fully mobilized, allowing access to the retrocaval space and identification of the origins of the right LSNs. A minimum of two LSNs can often be identified, although variants with additional nerves do exist. The superior LSN is usually just medial and superior to the right superior lumbar vein, whereas the inferior LSN is typically just superomedial to the left common truncal lumbar vein. Once the LSNs have been identified at their retrocaval origins and ideally dissected free to the right-sided aortic plexus, attention can be turned to mobilization of the aorta. The right sympathetic trunk, right-sided LSNs, and their relationship to the great vessels are demonstrated in Fig. 68.3.

With the right-sided aortic plexus identified, the preaortic tissue inferior to the IMA can then be carefully dissected, taking care to preserve the plexi that typically sit in close proximity to the IMA. Often the IMA can be spared (particularly in chemo-naive cases), although it can be ligated/divided to improve exposure, with blood supply to the left colon continuing through the marginal artery of Drummond. Once the preaortic tissue has been split, a "split and roll" technique is used to dissect in the aortic adventitial layer and identify the lumbar arteries. Care should be taken to preserve the testicular artery contralateral to the original testicular tumor. Unlike the veins, the lumbar arteries are defined paired structures, located at approximately the same distance from one another. The middle pair of arteries is commonly located at the same level as the IMA. The aorta is retracted to the patient's left with the interaortocaval tissue retracted to the right to identify the right-sided lumbar arteries. These are ligated and then divided. The right-sided arteries can then be used to identify the location of the left-sided arteries. Before full mobilization of the aorta, an effort should be made to identify the left-sided aortic nerve plexus. Similar to the right, identification and isolation of the nerve plexus can then allow for proximal dissection and identification of the left LSNs. Once the left aortic plexus has been identified, the left lumbar arteries can be exposed (with retraction of the aorta to the right and the paraaortic tissue to the left) and then ligated and divided. This should then permit complete mobilization of the aorta.

A. Common right sided anatomy including the right ureter (lateral border of paracaval dissection), the right renal vein (superior border), and the vena cava (medial border). Right-sided lumbar splanchnic nerves are looped (red vessel-loops)

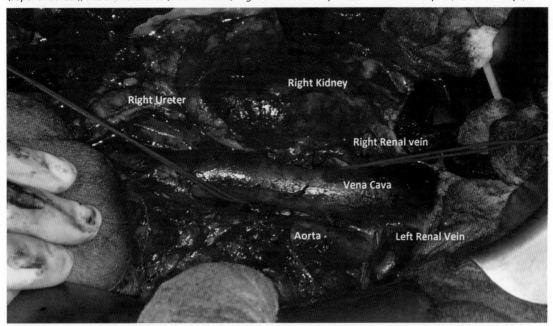

B. The right-sided sympathetic trunk and origins of the right-sided lumbar splanchnic nerves can now be visualized with the cava retracted laterally. Prospective identification of the sympathetic trunk laterally to the cava, and the nerves medially allows for nerve preservation.

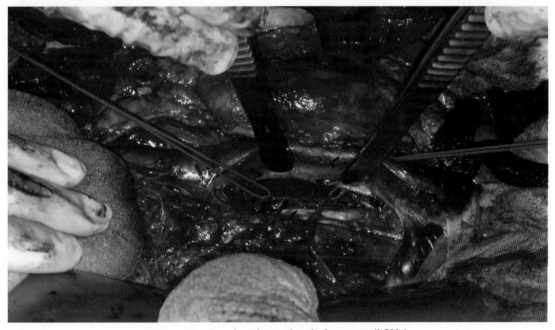

FIGURE 68.3 Lumbar splanchnic nerves (LSNs).

BILATERAL RETROPERITONEAL LYMPH NODE DISSECTION (RPLND) (Continued)

Once the great vessels are fully mobilized and the right-sided LSNs and right-sided aortic plexus identified and skeletonized, then the interaortocaval tissue can be dissected out. The boundaries of dissection are the superior edge of the left renal vein superiorly (should be mobilized caudal by the initial split and roll), the anterior spinous ligament posteriorly, and the common iliac confluence distally. Care must be taken during the interaortocaval dissection to avoid injury to the right-sided nerves, particularly as they cross over the aorta inferior to the IMA.

Attention is then turned to the para-aortic dissection. The boundaries of dissection are the cephalad edge of the left renal vein, the aorta, left ureter, psoas muscle posteriorly, and left common iliac artery bifurcation distally. Identification of the left ureter before dissection is advised, because the packet often lies in close proximity to the ureter. In addition, care should be taken during the para-aortic dissection, because this is one of the most common sites of in-field recurrence theorized to be from inadequate exposure of the renal vessels (due to the need to mobilize and reflect the pancreas superiorly) as well as difficulty controlling lumbar veins, which may drain into the left renal vein just left lateral to the aorta. The presence of such a lumbar vein can also complicate the dissection of left-sided LSNs, particularly the most superior left-sided nerves, which may run near the lumbar vein (either superior or inferior). Often medial visceral rotation of the descending colon will be needed to complete the caudal portion of the para-aortic dissection. This is done by incising along the white line of Toldt, similar to the ascending colon/cecal mobilization. Alternatively, in thin patients, the cut edge of the mesentery can often be lifted slightly, and dissection of the paraaortic packet can be performed under the mesentery and inferior mesenteric vein (IMV).

Once the major lymph node packets have been dissected out, the ipsilateral gonadal vein and cord are identified, having been previously tagged during the radical orchiectomy, and dissected out.

If identifiable, the posterior peritoneum can then be reapproximated. The viscera are then repositioned in the anatomic position. The midline wound is closed in multiple layers. Drain placement is typically not advocated, particularly if there is no apparent chylous leak at the time of the dissection.

VARIATIONS

Robotic

Robotic-assisted laparoscopy is becoming a more common method for performing RPLND. Laparoscopic techniques avoid the large midline incision, and the pneumoperitoneum can reduce small venous bleeding, leading to less intraoperative blood loss. However, vascular injury and significant hemorrhage are still a feared complication, and these procedures should be done only by those with advanced minimally invasive skills.

The robotic approach is typically done with the patient in Trendelenburg position. Ports are placed caudal to the umbilicus, and the robot is brought in either over the patient's shoulder (S or Si) or from the patient's side (Xi). The assistant stands opposite the robot, and an assistant port is placed on this side.

With the patient in Trendelenburg position, the bowel falls cephalad, revealing the posterior peritoneum. An incision similar to the open technique (from cecum up to the ligament of Treitz) is performed. The cephalad edge of the incised posterior peritoneum can then be tacked up to the anterior abdominal wall to provide retraction of the viscera.

Once the retroperitoneum has been adequately exposed, the procedure can proceed similar to the open procedure, although often the dissection proceeds distal to proximal (along the IVC and then the renal vein) rather than starting at the cephalad extent and working distally. Polymer clips are often used to secure the lumbar vasculature.

Extraperitoneal

An extraperitoneal approach to RPLND has been advocated as a possible method for reducing bowel handling and improving perioperative return of bowel function. In addition, this approach may limit the development of small bowel obstruction later in life, which can be one of the long-standing sequelae of the procedure.

The extraperitoneal approach is similar to the transperitoneal approach, with a long midline incision made from the subxiphoid to the subumbilical location. Starting at the caudal aspect of the incision, the surgeon incises the fascial layers, taking care not to enter the peritoneum. The peritoneum is then bluntly dissected off the abdominal wall (starting anterior and moving lateral and then posterior) and then dissected off the vasculature and psoas musculature, revealing the retroperitoneal structures. Peritonotomies are common but can be closed primarily if small, preserving the extraperitoneal approach. The superior portion of the peritoneal sac dissection is often somewhat fibrosed and is a common site of peritonotomies.

Postchemotherapy/Salvage

Although anatomy and technique of postchemotherapy RPLND are similar to chemotherapy-naive dissection, the procedure is notoriously harder because of potential residual bulky tissue as well as obliteration of tissue planes from tumor necrosis and inflammation induced by chemotherapy. Clinicians should inform patients of the high potential for not being able to preserve nerves adequate for antegrade ejaculation, as well as the possibility for significant additional procedures, such as nephrectomy or vascular reconstruction in rare cases. As in chemotherapy-naive RPLND, complete oncologic resection and skeletonization of the great vessels are critical to RPLND success and favorable long-term outcomes. Nerve preservation should always be secondary to complete oncologic resection.

Template

Templated RPLNDs were previously considered the standard of care, particularly for clinical stage I disease, because they allowed the preservation of the LSN, aortic plexi, and hypogastric plexus (preserving antegrade ejaculation). However, with the development of nerve-sparing procedures, template dissections have fallen out of favor. This is especially true as the bulk of the time and morbidity of the procedure are unchanged by using a template dissection (exposure of the whole retroperitoneum, mobilization and control of the lumbar vasculature). The classic bilateral template dissection as described above is illustrated in Fig. 68.4.

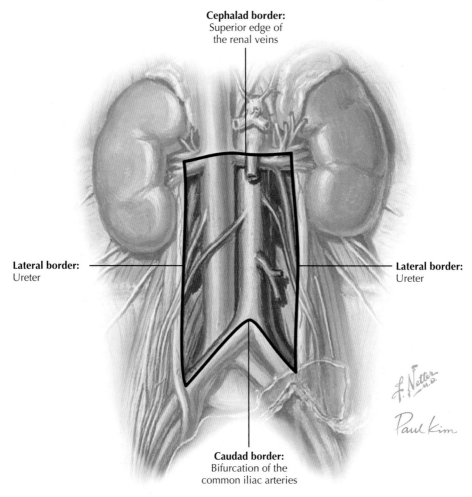

FIGURE 68.4 Standard bilateral template dissection.

SUGGESTED READINGS

Beveridge TS, et al. Anatomy of the infrarenal aortic plexus: implications for nerve-sparing retroperitoneal lymph node dissection. Western Graduate and Postdoctoral Studies; April 2018.

Beveridge TS, et al. Retroperitoneal lymph node dissection: anatomical and technical considerations from a cadaveric study. J Urol 2016;196:1764–71.

Jewett MA, et al. Nerve-sparing retroperitoneal lymphadenectomy. Urol Clin North Am 2007;34(2):149–58.

Large, et al. Retroperitoneal lymph node dissection: reassessment of modified templates. BJU Int 2009;104:1369–75.

Stepanian S, et al. Robot-assisted laparoscopic retroperitoneal lymph node dissection for testicular cancer: evolution of the technique. Eur Urol 2016;70(4):661–7.

Syan-Bhanvadia S, et al. Midline extraperitoneal approach to retroperitoneal lymph node dissection in testicular cancer: minimizing surgical morbidity. Eur Urol 2017;72:814–20.

Index

Page numbers followed by "f" indicate figures; "t," tables; "b," boxes.